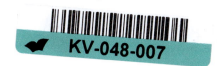
Breast Cancer Research Protocols

METHODS IN MOLECULAR MEDICINE™

John M. Walker, Series Editor

125. **Myeloid Leukemia:** *Methods and Protocols,* edited by *Harry Iland, Mark Hertzberg, and Paula Marlton, 2006*

124. **Magnetic Resonance Imaging:** *Methods and Biological Applications,* edited by *Pottumarthi V. Prasadi, 2006*

123. **Marijuana and Cannabinoid Research:** *Methods and Protocols,* edited by *Emmanuel S. Onaivi, 2006*

122. **Placenta Research Methods and Protocols:** *Volume 2,* edited by *Michael J. Soares and Joan S. Hunt, 2006*

121. **Placenta Research Methods and Protocols:** *Volume 1,* edited by *Michael J. Soares and Joan S. Hunt, 2006*

120. **Breast Cancer Research Protocols,** edited by *Susan A. Brooks and Adrian Harris, 2006*

119. **Human Papillomaviruses:** *Methods and Protocols,* edited by *Clare Davy and John Doorbar, 2005*

118. **Antifungal Agents:** *Methods and Protocols,* edited by *Erika J. Ernst and P. David Rogers, 2005*

117. **Fibrosis Research:** *Methods and Protocols,* edited by *John Varga, David A. Brenner, and Sem H. Phan, 2005*

116. **Inteferon Methods and Protocols,** edited by *Daniel J. J. Carr, 2005*

115. **Lymphoma:** *Methods and Protocols,* edited by *Timothy Illidge and Peter W. M. Johnson, 2005*

114. **Microarrays in Clinical Diagnostics,** edited by *Thomas O. Joos and Paolo Fortina, 2005*

113. **Multiple Myeloma:** *Methods and Protocols,* edited by *Ross D. Brown and P. Joy Ho, 2005*

112. **Molecular Cardiology:** *Methods and Protocols,* edited by *Zhongjie Sun, 2005*

111. **Chemosensitivity:** *Volume 2, In Vivo Models, Imaging, and Molecular Regulators,* edited by *Rosalyn D. Blumethal, 2005*

110. **Chemosensitivity:** *Volume 1, In Vitro Assays,* edited by *Rosalyn D. Blumethal, 2005*

109. **Adoptive Immunotherapy:** *Methods and Protocols,* edited by *Burkhard Ludewig and Matthias W. Hoffman, 2005*

108. **Hypertension:** *Methods and Protocols,* edited by *Jérôme P. Fennell and Andrew H. Baker, 2005*

107. **Human Cell Culture Protocols,** *Second Edition,* edited by *Joanna Picot, 2005*

106. **Antisense Therapeutics,** *Second Edition,* edited by *M. Ian Phillips, 2005*

105. **Developmental Hematopoiesis:** *Methods and Protocols,* edited by *Margaret H. Baron, 2005*

104. **Stroke Genomics:** *Methods and Reviews,* edited by *Simon J. Read and David Virley, 2004*

103. **Pancreatic Cancer:** *Methods and Protocols,* edited by *Gloria H. Su, 2004*

102. **Autoimmunity:** *Methods and Protocols,* edited by *Andras Perl, 2004*

101. **Cartilage and Osteoarthritis:** *Volume 2, Structure and In Vivo Analysis,* edited by *Frédéric De Ceuninck, Massimo Sabatini, and Philippe Pastoureau, 2004*

100. **Cartilage and Osteoarthritis:** *Volume 1, Cellular and Molecular Tools,* edited by *Massimo Sabatini, Philippe Pastoureau, and Frédéric De Ceuninck, 2004*

99. **Pain Research:** *Methods and Protocols,* edited by *David Z. Luo, 2004*

98. **Tumor Necrosis Factor:** *Methods and Protocols,* edited by *Angelo Corti and Pietro Ghezzi, 2004*

97. **Molecular Diagnosis of Cancer:** *Methods and Protocols, Second Edition,* edited by *Joseph E. Roulston and John M. S. Bartlett, 2004*

96. **Hepatitis B and D Protocols:** *Volume 2, Immunology, Model Systems, and Clinical Studies,* edited by *Robert K. Hamatake and Johnson Y. N. Lau, 2004*

95. **Hepatitis B and D Protocols:** *Volume 1, Detection, Genotypes, and Characterization,* edited by *Robert K. Hamatake and Johnson Y. N. Lau, 2004*

94. **Molecular Diagnosis of Infectious Diseases,** *Second Edition,* edited by *Jochen Decker and Udo Reischl, 2004*

93. **Anticoagulants, Antiplatelets, and Thrombolytics,** edited by *Shaker A. Mousa, 2004*

92. **Molecular Diagnosis of Genetic Diseases,** *Second Edition,* edited by *Rob Elles and Roger Mountford, 2004*

91. **Pediatric Hematology:** *Methods and Protocols,* edited by *Nicholas J. Goulden and Colin G. Steward, 2003*

90. **Suicide Gene Therapy:** *Methods and Reviews,* edited by *Caroline J. Springer, 2004*

89. **The Blood–Brain Barrier:** *Biology and Research Protocols,* edited by *Sukriti Nag, 2003*

88. **Cancer Cell Culture:** *Methods and Protocols,* edited by *Simon P. Langdon, 2003*

87. **Vaccine Protocols,** *Second Edition,* edited by *Andrew Robinson, Michael J. Hudson, and Martin P. Cranage, 2003*

86. **Renal Disease:** *Techniques and Protocols,* edited by *Michael S. Goligorsky, 2003*

METHODS IN MOLECULAR MEDICINE™

Breast Cancer Research Protocols

Edited by

Susan A. Brooks

School of Biological and Molecular Sciences
Oxford Brookes University
Headington, Oxford, UK

Adrian Harris

Medical Oncology Unit
The Churchill Hospital
Headington, Oxford, UK

HUMANA PRESS ✳ TOTOWA, NEW JERSEY

www.humanapress.com

Production Editor: Amy Thau

Cover design by Patricia F. Cleary

Cover Illustration:Figure 1B from Chapter 21, "Fluorescence *In Situ* Hybridization Assessment of c-*myc* Gene Amplification in Breast Tumor Tissues," by Patricia Gorman and Rebecca Roylance.

Printed in the United States of America 10 9 8 7 6 5 4 3 2 1
eISBN: 159259-969-9
ISSN: 1543-1894
Library of Congress Cataloging-in-Publication Data

Breast cancer research protocols / edited by Susan A. Brooks and Adrian
Harris.
    p. ; cm. -- (Methods in molecular medicine, ISSN 1543-1894 ; 120)
  Includes bibliographical references and index.
  ISBN 1-58829-191-X (alk. paper)
  1. Breast--Cancer--Laboratory manuals.
  [DNLM: 1. Breast Neoplasms--genetics. 2. Breast Neoplasms--pathology. 3.
Biopsy--methods. 4. Clinical Protocols--methods. 5. Genetic Techniques.
WP 870 B82398 2005] I. Brooks, Susan A. II. Harris, Adrian, 1950- III.
Series.
  RC280.B8B68788 2005
  616.99'449'0072--dc22
                                    2005010939

Preface

Throughout the world, breast cancer has increased in incidence in the last decade. Conversely, there has been a decrease in mortality as a result of an emerging combined therapy approach that includes systemic application of treatment modalities, such as chemotherapy and hormone therapy, combined with early detection. Based on the molecular understanding of the disease, many new treatments have been introduced into the clinic in the last five years, including antibody therapy to *HER2*, pure antiestrogens, and aromatase inhibitors. It is vital for breast cancer research to be able to link studies on cell lines and in preclinical models to studies of human tumor material. There are also many new technologies involving large-scale analysis for the expression of genes, such as proteomics and gene array analysis. Unprecedented opportunities have arisen for clinical application. Ultimately, these each need to be tested in randomized prospective studies modulating the target of interest.

Breast Cancer Research Protocols aims to cover the majority of the techniques that would be necessary for a research scientist or clinician intending to enter into this field and initiate research, as well as to communicate with others on methodologies and approaches. Because of the dramatic increase in the diagnosis and therapy of breast cancer, it is particularly important that these approaches be integrated for patient benefit in the long run.

Thus, this book of protocols initially covers how to collect and handle human breast tumor samples appropriately, and how to extract them for their constituent DNA, RNA, or proteins. Because samples are often quite small, the technology of handling biopsies appropriately is important. The new methods of analyzing gene expression are also described, as breast cancer has actually been one of the areas where this has been successfully applied.

One of the most important areas in breast cancer treatment is understanding prognosis and being able to select patients that are at highest risk. This is covered for all the major surgical and pathological criteria currently in use.

Validating targets and understanding the biology of newly discovered genes is critical and methods of analyzing cells in vivo and in vitro are also described. Based on these combined approaches, we hope that *Breast Cancer Research Protocols* will contribute to further advances in effective management and therapy of breast cancer in the future.

Susan A. Brooks
Adrian Harris

v

Contents

Preface v

Contributors xi

PART I PREPARATION OF CELL AND TISSUE SAMPLES

1. Breast Tissue Banking: *Collection, Handling, Storage,*
   and Release of Tissue for Breast Cancer Research 3
   Linda Snell and Peter H. Watson

2. Frozen Biopsy Collection and Storage: *Frozen Biopsy Samples* 25
   Russell Leek

3. Serial Biopsies/Fine-Needle Aspirates and Their Assessment 29
   Irene Boeddinghaus and Stephen R. D. Johnson

4. Breast Tissue Microarrays 43
   Robert J. Springall and Cheryl E. Gillett

5. Preparation of Tumor Homogenates for Subsequent Preparation
   of Cytosols, Membrane Fractions, RNA, and DNA 51
   Naomi Robertson and Russell Leek

6. Isolation of RNA From Tumor Samples: *Single-Step Guanidinium*
   Acid–Phenol Method 55
   Naomi Robertson and Russell Leek

7. Isolation of DNA From Tumor Samples 61
   Naomi Robertson and Russell Leek

8. Laser-Assisted Microdissection and Isolation of DNA and RNA 65
   Ulrich Lehmann and Hans Kreipe

PART II MARKERS OF CLINICAL OUTCOME AND PROGNOSIS

9. Traditional and Established Indicators of Prognosis
   and Treatment Success 79
   Derek E. Roskell and Ian D. Buley

10. Sentinel Lymph Node Biopsy in Breast Cancer 91
    Celia Chao and Kelly M. McMasters

11. Pathological Evaluation of Axillary Sentinel Lymph Nodes
    in Breast Cancer 113
    Michael Z. Gilcrease and Aysegul Sahin

12. Measurement of Estrogen Receptor Status by Immunocytochemistry
    in Paraffin Wax Sections 127
    Bharat Jasani, Anthony Douglas-Jones, Anthony Rhodes,
    Susan Wozniak, Peter J. Barrett-Lee, Julia Gee,
    and Robert Nicholson

13. Markers of Apoptosis 147
    Fazlul H. Sarkar and Yiwei Li

14. Quantitative Angiogenesis in Breast Cancer 161
    Stephen B. Fox

PART III ANALYSIS OF TUMOR-DERIVED PROTEINS AND ANTIGENS

15. Immunohistochemistry 191
    Cheryl E. Gillett

16. Detection of Aberrant Glycosylation in Breast Cancer
    Using Lectin Histochemistry 201
    Tracey M. Carter and Susan A. Brooks

17. SDS-PAGE and Western Blotting to Detect Proteins
    and Glycoproteins of Interest in Breast Cancer Research 217
    Chloe Osborne and Susan A. Brooks

18. Breast Cancer Proteomics Using Two-Dimensional Electrophoresis:
    Studying the Breast Cancer Proteome 231
    Miriam V. Dwek and Sarah L. Rawlings

19. Procedures for the Quantitative Protein Determination
    of Urokinase and Its Inhibitor, PAI-1, in Human Breast Cancer
    Tissue Extracts by ELISA 245
    Manfred Schmitt, Alexandra S. Sturmheit, Anita Welk,
    Christel Schnelldorfer, and Nadia Harbeck

PART IV ANALYSIS OF GENES AND GENE EXPRESSION IN TUMOR SPECIMENS

20. Fluorescence *In Situ* Hybridization and Comparative Genomic
    Hybridization 269
    Patricia Gorman and Rebecca Roylance

21. Fluorescence *In Situ* Hybridization Assessment of c-*myc* Gene
    Amplification in Breast Tumor Tissues 297
    Jan K. Blancato, Mary Steele Williams, and Robert B. Dickson

22. Detection of *HER2* Gene Amplification by Fluorescence *In Situ*
    Hybridization in Breast Cancer 309
    John M. S. Bartlett and Amanda Forsyth

23. *In Situ* Hybridization Combined With Immunohistochemistry
    to Localize Gene Expression 323
    Rosemary Jeffery, Toby Hunt, and Richard Poulsom

24. Quantitation of RNA by Ribonuclease Protection Assay 347
    John W. Moore
25. Identification of Steroid Hormone-Regulated Genes
        in Breast Cancer 363
    Bruce R. Westley and Felicity E. B. May
26. Sequencing of the Tumor Suppressor Gene *TP 53* 389
    Barbro Linderholm, Torbjörn Norberg, and Jonas Bergh
27. Expression Profiling Using cDNA Microarrays 403
    Chris Jones, Peter Simpson, Alan Mackay, and Sunil R. Lakhani
28. Gene Expression Analysis Using Filter cDNA Microarrays 415
    Peter Simpson, Chris Jones, Alan Mackay, and Sunil R. Lakhani

PART V STUDYING CANCER CELL BEHAVIOR IN VITRO AND IN VIVO
29. Methods to Analyze the Effects of the Urokinase System
        on Cancer Cell Adhesion, Proliferation, Migration,
        and Signal Transduction Events 427
    *Ute Reuning, Manfred Schmitt, Birgit Luber, Veronika Beck,
        and Viktor Magdolen*
30. Phospho-Specific Antibodies as a Tool to Study In Vivo Regulation
        of BRCA1 After DNA Damage 441
    Kum Kum Khanna, Magtouf Gatei, and Gordon Tribbick
31. Models of Hormone Resistance In Vitro and In Vivo 453
    Jennifer MacGregor Schafer and V. Craig Jordan
32. Generation of Genetically Modified Embryonic Stem Cells
        for the Development of Knockout Mouse Animal Model Systems 465
    *Stephen D. Robinson, Stephen Wilson,
        and Kairbaan M. Hodivala-Dilke*
33. In Vivo Xenograft Models of Breast Cancer Metastasis 479
    Ursula Valentiner, Susan A. Brooks, and Udo Schumacher
34. Neoadjuvant Endocrine Therapy Models 489
    Juliette Murray, William R. Miller, and J. Michael Dixon
35. Primary Mouse Endothelial Cell Culture for Assays of Angiogenesis ... 503
    Louise E. Reynolds and Kairbaan M. Hodivala-Dilke
Index 511

Contributors

PETER J. BARRETT-LEE • *Oncology Unit, Velindre NHS Trust, Cardiff, UK*

JOHN M. S. BARTLETT • *Division of Cancer Sciences and Molecular Pathology, University Department of Surgery, Endocrine Cancer Group and HER2 Reference Laboratory, University of Glasgow, Glasgow Royal Infirmary, Glasgow, UK*

VERONIKA BECK • *Clinical Research Unit, Department of Obstetrics and Gynaecology, Technical University of Munich, Munich, Germany*

JONAS BERGH • *Radiumhemmet, Karolinska Institute and Hospital, Stockholm, Sweden*

JAN K. BLANCATO • *Institute for Molecular and Human Genetics, Georgetown University Medical Center, Washington, DC*

IRENE BOEDDINGHAUS • *Cape Town, South Africa*

SUSAN A. BROOKS • *School of Biological and Molecular Sciences, Oxford Brookes University, Headington, Oxford, UK*

IAN D. BULEY • *Department of Cellular Pathology, The John Radcliffe Hospital, Oxford, UK*

TRACEY M. CARTER • *School of Biological and Molecular Sciences, Oxford Brookes University, Headington, Oxford, UK*

CELIA CHAO • *Division of Surgical Oncology, Department of Surgery, University of Texas Medical Branch, Galveston, TX*

ROBERT B. DICKSON • *Institute for Molecular and Human Genetics, Georgetown University Medical Center, Washington DC*

J. MICHAEL DIXON • *Edinburgh Breast Unit, Western General Hospital, Edinburgh, UK*

ANTHONY DOUGLAS-JONES • *Department of Pathology, University of Wales College of Medicine, Cardiff, UK*

MIRIAM V. DWEK • *Department of Applied and Molecular Biosciences, School of Biosciences, University of Westminster, London, UK*

AMANDA FORSYTH • *Division of Cancer Sciences and Molecular Pathology, University Department of Surgery, Endocrine Cancer Group and HER2 Reference Laboratory, University of Glasgow, Glasgow Royal Infirmary, Glasgow, UK*

STEPHEN B. FOX • *Nuffield Department of Clinical Laboratory Sciences, University of Oxford, John Radcliffe Hospital, Oxford, UK*

MAGTOUF GATEI • *Signal Transduction Laboratory, Cancer and Cell Biology Division, The Queensland Institute of Medical Research, Queensland, Australia*

JULIA GEE • *Tenovus Institute of Cancer Research, Welsh School of Pharmacy, University College Cardiff, Cardiff, UK*

MICHAEL Z. GILCREASE • *Division of Pathology and Laboratory Medicine, Department of Pathology, University of Texas M. D. Anderson Cancer Center, Houston, TX*

CHERYL E. GILLETT • *Hedley Atkins/Cancer Research UK Breast Pathology Laboratory, Guy's Hospital, London, UK*

PATRICIA GORMAN • *Molecular and Population Genetics Laboratory, London Research Institute, Cancer Research UK, London, UK*

NADIA HARBECK • *Clinical Research Unit, Department of Obstetrics and Gynaecology, Technical University of Munich, Munich, Germany*

ADRIAN HARRIS • *Medical Oncology Unit, The Churchill Hospital, Headington, Oxford, UK*

KAIRBAAN M. HODIVALA-DILKE • *Cell Adhesion and Disease Laboratory, Department of Tumour Biology, Cancer Research UK, John Vane Science Centre, Barts and The London School of Medicine and Dentistry, Charterhouse Square, London, UK*

TOBY HUNT • *London Research Institute, Cancer Research UK, London, UK*

BHARAT JASANI • *Department of Pathology, University of Wales College of Medicine, Cardiff, UK*

ROSEMARY JEFFERY • *Cancer Research UK, London Research Institute, London, UK*

STEPHEN R. D. JOHNSON • *Academic Department of Biochemistry and Department of Medicine, Royal Marsden Hospital, London, UK*

CHRIS JONES • *The Breakthrough Toby Robins Breast Research Centre at the Institute of Cancer Research, Chester Beatty Laboratories, London, UK*

V. CRAIG JORDAN • *Breast Cancer Research Program, Fox Chase Cancer Center, Philadelphia, PA*

KUM KUM KHANNA • *Signal Transduction Laboratory, Cancer and Cell Biology Division, The Queensland Institute of Medical Research, Queensland, Australia*

HANS KREIPE • *Institute of Pathology, Medizinische Hochschule Hannover, Hannover, Germany*

SUNIL R. LAKHANI • *The Breakthrough Toby Robins Breast Research Centre at the Institute of Cancer Research, Chester Beatty Laboratories, London, UK*

RUSSELL LEEK • *University of Oxford Medical Sciences Division, Cancer Research UK Tumour Pathology Group, The John Radcliffe Hospital, Oxford, UK*

ULRICH LEHMANN • *Institute of Pathology, Medizinische Hochschule Hannover, Hannover, Germany*

YIWEI LI • *Department of Pathology, Karmanos Cancer Institute, Wayne State University School of Medicine, Detroit, MI*

BARBRO LINDERHOLM • *Radiumhemmet, Karolinska Institute and Hospital, Stockholm, Sweden*

BIRGIT LUBER • *Institute of Pathology, Technical University of Munich, Munich, Germany*

ALAN MACKAY • *The Breakthrough Toby Robins Breast Research Centre at the Institute of Cancer Research, Chester Beatty Laboratories, London, UK*

VIKTOR MAGDOLEN • *Clinical Research Unit, Department of Obstetrics and Gynaecology, Technical University of Munich, Munich, Germany*

FELICITY E. B. MAY • *The University of Newcastle upon Tyne, Northern Institute for Cancer Research, Medical School, Framlington Place, Newcastle upon Tyne, UK*

KELLY M. MCMASTERS • *Department of Surgery, Division of Surgical Oncology, University of Louisville, Louisville, KY*

WILLIAM R. MILLER • *Edinburgh Breast Unit, Research Group, Paderewski Building, Western General Hospital, Edinburgh, UK*

JOHN W. MOORE • *Molecular Oncology Laboratories, Cancer Research UK, Weatherall Institute of Molecular Medicine, John Radcliffe Hospital, Oxford, UK*

JULIETTE MURRAY • *Edinburgh Breast Unit, Western General Hospital, Edinburgh, UK*

ROBERT NICHOLSON • *Tenovus Institute of Cancer Research, Welsh School of Pharmacy, University College Cardiff, Cardiff, UK*

TORBJÖRN NORBERG • *Meadowland Business Partners AB, Uppsala, Sweden*

CHLOE OSBORNE • *Department of Physiology, University of Birmingham Medical School, Birmingham, UK*

RICHARD POULSOM • *London Research Institute, Cancer Research UK, London, UK*

SARAH L. RAWLINGS • *Breast Cancer Research Group, Department of Surgery, Royal Free and University College London Medical School, London, UK*

UTE REUNING • *Clinical Research Unit, Department of Obstetrics and Gynaecology, Technical University of Munich, Munich, Germany*

LOUISE E. REYNOLDS • *Department of Tumour Biology, Cell Adhesion and Disease Laboratory, Cancer Research UK, John Vane Science Centre, Barts and The London School of Medicine and Dentistry, Charterhouse Square, London, UK*

ANTHONY RHODES • *Faculty of Applied Sciences, University of West England, Frenchay Campus, Bristol, UK*

NAOMI ROBERTSON • *Cancer Research UK Molecular Oncology Laboratories, Weatherall Institute of Molecular Medicine, The John Radcliffe Hospital, Oxford, UK*

STEPHEN D. ROBINSON • *Cell Adhesion and Disease Laboratory, Cancer Research UK, St. Thomas' Hospital, London, UK*

pathology examination (e.g., margin assessment), as well as changing the "ethical landscape."

1.2. Types of Tissue Collections

Tissues for research are generally collected through one of three distinct mechanisms:

1. Hospital-based clinical archives.
2. Research study collections.
3. Tumor banks *(1)*.

A "clinical archive" comprises the tissues in clinical pathology departments. Together with the associated clinical patient records, these serve as the basis for many research projects. However, access to, and study of, such material is limited by the ability to efficiently select appropriate samples and cases by research criteria, the restricted nature of the tissue processing, the lack of standardization of pathology reporting, and poor linkage between specimens and patient-related outcome data, as well as case-by-case conflicts with clinical priorities. A "research study collection" comprises a tissue dataset collected either directly at the time of surgery or through the pathology department. These tissue resources are usually designed to answer a specific research question and therefore do not need to consider a design to facilitate other applications or to incorporate the costs and capacity to release material to others. A "tumor bank" or "tissue resource" is similar to a research collection and usually comprises unused tissues left over after pathological examination of surgical specimens. However, extra care in the processing and characterization of the tissues and the associated pathological and linked clinical patient data creates a dataset that is organized in such a way as to facilitate multiuser access and support for different types of research studies. The tissues may include both tumor and adjacent normal tissues, and also blood samples, and may be associated with a spectrum of information obtained by analysis at the time of processing into the bank. This information may encompass the composition (histology) and the tissue alterations that reflect the type and stage of disease (pathology), issues covered in Chapter 9, as well as clinical information about the patient, the initial treatment, and over time, the response to treatment and ensuing state of health.

A tumor bank can efficiently address the limitations of other tissue resources through a dedicated management, processing, storage, retrieval, and release structure, to provide selected and preassembled material and data for research and discovery. Tumor banks thus accelerate and improve the quality of cancer research, are cost-effective, and stimulate investment of focused clinical expertise that benefits research. This chapter will specifically describe the design and detailed operation of the Manitoba Breast Tumor Bank (MBTB), based on accumulated experience over almost 10 yr in handling of breast tissues for research *(2)*.

1.3. Overview of the MBTB

Cases are collected by the MBTB directly from pathology departments and via the provincial steroid receptor laboratory and processed to allow the MBTB to offer a range of cases in different categories (*see* **Notes 1** and **2**) with differing extents of associated data for different types of research question. An electronic "tissue database" is maintained on microcomputer (utilizing the software Microsoft Access) and includes full interpretation of each tissue block stored in the MBTB (e.g., tumor type, grade, cellularity, composition) derived from assessment of an hematoxylin and eosin (H&E) section from each paraffin block. A "clinical database" is also maintained separately, which incorporates demographic and clinical data with baseline staging/prognostic information and diagnosis, staging, primary treatment, follow-up, and outcome data. Active follow-up is initiated by a computerized schedule and through annual review, faxed questionnaires, and direct telephone contact with the primary physician.

Frozen tissue samples are obtained and processed by the MBTB to produce several matching "mirror image" paraffin and frozen tissue blocks. This allows interpretation of the pathology and tissue composition in high-quality H&E-stained paraffin sections, which is essential for accurate distinction between subtle lesions and tumor grading (which is often not feasible in frozen sections). These paraffin or corresponding frozen blocks can then be re-sectioned when required to provide thin sections for release for individual projects and to provide appropriate tissues for a variety of molecular studies.

The MBTB is located within the Department of Pathology and Cancer Care Manitoba. Within the accepted physical and established legal and confidential bounds of practice in these locations, the database is managed only by the MBTB personnel. Freezers ($-70°C$) have local and external alarms to allow continuous monitoring and dedicated CO_2 cylinder-based backup systems. These systems are tested and a crisis-response protocol is reviewed biannually. The MBTB operation is monitored through a regular process of internal evaluation and biannual audit of the tissue and computer databases. A histological quality assessment of nuclear morphology is used to rank all cases, as we have found this relates to RNA quality determined by reverse transcription polymerase chain reaction (RT-PCR) assay. We have formally tested RNA extracted from frozen sections that have been used, stored, and reused several years later by RT-PCR, finding no deterioration within our oldest stored tissues (approx 10 yr) or within frozen tumor blocks sectioned previously over 2 yr.

The MBTB now contains over 4500 fully processed cases and many further samples collected and partially processed in reserve to maintain the "stocks." The MBTB has provided support to researchers for more than 50 projects conducted in research laboratories across North America and in Europe during the past 10 yr. The total aggregate of cases utilized and sections released in support of these projects is more than 7000 cases and 70,000 tissue sections.

The protocols for procurement, processing, storage, and release of tissue and data are described in detail in the following sections.

2. Materials

2.1. Supplies

1. Omnisette® tissue cassettes; tissue cassettes (Fisher Scientific), standard size with lid; histology capsules to carry tissue and label from fixation through processing, embedding, and storage.
2. 2-mL Outside-thread, flat-bottom cryovials (Nalgene) for frozen tissue sample storage.
3. Scalpel handle no. 4 with no. 22 blades, and a larger trimming knife and disposable blades.
4. 3×1-in. microscope slides, frosted on one end (Fisher Scientific), and electrostatically charged SuperfrostPlus® (Fisher Scientific).
5. Glass no. 1 cover slips, 22×22 and 22×30 mm and larger, if necessary (Fisher Scientific).
6. 1.5 and 2 mL microcentrifuge tubes (Seal-Riteä®, Mandel), autoclaved before use.
7. Fine permanent markers for labeling; Staedtler, for cryovials; and lead pencils or solvent-resistant markers (Securline® Precision Dynamics Corp; Fisher Scientific), for cassette and microscope slide labeling.
8. 5-in. Serrated tip forceps. Fine-to-medium paintbrushes or orange sticks are useful for manipulating frozen and paraffin sections.
9. Steel microtome knives (Leica), C profile, 12–16 cm long, for frozen and paraffin sectioning. An alternate option is to use a disposable blade system.
10. Slide racks and dishes for drying and staining tissue slides.
11. Coplin jars, (Scienceware®; Fisher Scientific), polypropylene with screw cap; small staining jars used for rapid staining of frozen sections for microdissection.
12. Slide trays, cardboard, to hold slides while drying after cover slipping.
13. Microscope slide storage system.
14. Metal freezer racks (ThermoForma), with 2-in. cardboard boxes for 2-mL cryovial storage.
15. Paraffin block drawer storage system.
16. Plastic slide mailers, to hold five slides, to safely ship prepared tissue sections on glass slides.
17. 11.5×5-in. honing plates (Leica, no. 14041819971), for Reichert microtome knife sharpener Model 903, to sharpen steel knives with fine and coarse abrasives.

18. Safety supplies: Sharps containers, disposable gloves, autoclave bags for tissue and contaminated paper, countertop mats, chlorine bleach surface disinfectant, absolute ethanol, and Cryofect (Leica) for cryotome disinfection.

2.2. Reagents and Solutions

1. 10% Neutral buffered formalin (Fisher Scientific), ready to use. This routine fixative is recommended and used for most tissues.
2. Modified Harris hematoxylin: used as a routine stain for tissue sections along with a counterstain, eosin Y *(3)*. To make:
   - 10 g of hematoxylin certified biological stain (CI 75290, Fisher); 100 mL of 100% ethanol; 200 g of aluminum ammonium sulfate ($AlNH_4[SO_4]_2$); 2 L of distilled water; 1 g of sodium iodate ($NaIO_3$) powder; and 80 mL of glacial acetic acid, CH_3COOH.
   - Using mild heat, dissolve hematoxylin in ethanol and, separately, in a large beaker, dissolve the aluminum ammonium sulfate in 2 L of distilled water with the aid of mild heat. Remove from heat and mix the two solutions. Allow the solution to cool to room temperature and add the sodium iodate. Place on a magnetic stirrer for 1 h, and then add glacial acetic acid. Mix and store in a brown bottle. Filter before each use and discard when solution no longer turns bright blue when a few drops are added to alkaline water or nuclear staining becomes brownish blue.
3. 0.2% Eosin Y, certified biological stain, CI 45380 in 95% ethanol, counterstain.
4. Diethylpyrocarbonate ([DEPC]; Sigma), used to destroy ribonucleases. To make, add 1 mL DEPC to 9 mL absolute ethanol. Add this to 1 L of distilled water or phosphate-buffered saline (PBS, final concentration is 0.1%) and mix by inverting. Loosen cap slightly and leave under the fume hood overnight or at least 12 h before autoclaving. DEPC cannot be used with Tris-HCl buffers. (**Caution!** Wear gloves and prepare under the fume hood. DEPC is a potential carcinogen *[3]*.)
5. DEPC-treated PBS. To make, dissolve 8 g of KCl, 1.44 g of Na_2HPO_4, and 0.24 g of KH_2PO_4 in 800 mL of distilled water. Adjust pH to 7.4 with HCl. Add water to make volume up to 990 mL and then add 10 mL of 1% DEPC. Mix well by inverting bottle and let stand at room temperature overnight. The next day, autoclave for 20 min at 15 lb/sq on liquid cycle. Store at room temperature. Wear gloves to avoid ribonuclease contamination of salts, glassware, or solutions *(3)*.
6. 4% Paraformaldehyde in PBS. To make, add 40 g of paraformaldehyde to 1 L of DEPC-treated PBS. Heat the solution on a stirrer under the fume hood at 80°C until completely dissolved. After cooling, add 5 mL of sterile 1 *M* magnesium chloride ($MgCl_2$), filter, and store at 4°C for up to 3 wk. Wear gloves to avoid ribonuclease contamination *(3)*.
7. Permount® (Fisher Scientific), commercially available cover slip mounting medium.
8. Histological-grade acetone (CH_3COCH_3), preferred fixative for frozen section immunohistochemistry (IHC).

9. 2% Alcian blue certified biological stain or Cobalt blue (commercially available at art stores), and 2% of mercurochrome used for tissue orientation and to indicate the block face during the paraffin embedding procedure.
10. Gelatin (Mallinckrodt), added to tissue-sectioning bath and allowed to dissolve in distilled water for 30–45 min at 40–45°C prior to routine sectioning. **Note:** gelatin is only added to the tissue bath when noncoated slides are being used.
11. Cryomatrix (Shandon): an inert, commercially available, frozen-specimen-embedding medium, used to mount frozen tissue on pegs for sectioning.
12. RNase Away® (Molecular Bioproducts), commercially available from Fisher Scientific and used to remove ribonucleases (RNases) from the tissue bath walls or other instruments that cannot be autoclaved when carrying out paraffin sectioning for RNA/RNA ISH.
13. Cryofect (Leica) cryotome disinfectant.
14. Microtome knife sharpening compounds, Buehler micropolish, 1-m a-alumina, Buehler Metadi® fluid (Tech-Met Canada), and Leica coarse abrasive. Sharpening times for coarse and fine abrasive will depend on the type of sharpener and honing plate used.
15. 3–4 kg of dry ice is required for overnight frozen tissue shipments up to 24-h in duration.
16. Liquid nitrogen/tank to snap freeze fresh tissue collected in cryovials.
17. 70 and 95% of absolute and graded ethanol; both are used during staining procedures, and 70% is used to store tissue after formalin fixation.

2.3. Resources

The functional space and equipment required for the operation of the MBTB is detailed below. In addition, a tissue-processing machine and embedding center are utilized within the clinical Department of Pathology, Health Sciences Centre.

2.3.1. Tissue Processing Room

The bulk of tissue preparation and handling occurs in the tissue processing room (approx 144 ft^2). It is equipped with two manual rotary microtomes for paraffin sectioning (a Leica Jung RM 2035 and a Shandon 325 Finesse) with accompanying tissue-flotation baths, and two cryotomes for frozen sectioning (both Leica, CM3000 and CM3500). The cryostats also provide cold working space during sorting and banking frozen tissue. Other components of the tissue processing room include a dissecting microscope for tissue section microdissection and a Reichert microtome knife sharpener.

2.3.2. Freezer Room

Three 17-ft^3, ultralow, upright freezers provide sufficient space for a collection of 4500 specimens and additional shelf space for sorting, compiling case sets for release, and temporary storage of unprocessed material. Not only is adequate space provided here (approx 144 ft^2), but the heat and noise generated by the equipment are restricted to this area. Bench space is conveniently located near the freezers to organize racks and boxes during sample retrieval and filing.

2.3.3. Research Laboratory

A molecular biology-capable research laboratory must be affiliated with, and available to undertake, RNA extraction and RT-PCR setup, and in a separate area to undertake PCR and electrophoresis and visualization of PCR products. This is necessary for ongoing quality control.

2.3.4. Slide Reading Room

This room (approx 100 ft^2) holds an H&E histological slide filing system for slides derived from every tissue block. It should be recognized that each case will generate up to three paraffin tissue blocks, each with a reference H&E slide, and also several additional reference paraffin and frozen tissue block H&E slides cut for review, as the content of the cross section of each block may need to be confirmed as it is utilized. A typical case may be therefore associated with 10 or more H&E slides. A double-headed light microscope is also located here to study the slides and document pathological information on each case. A microcomputer containing the tissue database is also located in this room for direct entry of information and reference while reviewing slides.

2.3.5. Clinical Database Room

The clinical database and associated paper files containing clinical reports are compiled and maintained on-site within a dedicated space (approx 100 ft^2) within the provincial cancer registry for each breast cancer case that the MBTB receives.

2.3.6. Computers

The MBTB databases require several microcomputers to facilitate data entry and review of the tissue database while retrieving or storing tissue in the processing and slide reading rooms. The MBTB is equipped with four networked microcomputers (Pentium machines, running the Windows operating system and the database software Microsoft Access).

3. Methods
3.1. Collection and Processing

The MBTB collects fresh breast tissue specimens (immediately after surgery) directly from the local hospital department and frozen specimens from other pathology departments in the city. The following protocol will describe how tissue samples are obtained and processed. Fresh samples from the local center and frozen samples arriving from outside are prepared and handled in a similar fashion (*see* **Fig. 1**).

1. As soon as possible after completion of surgery and removal of tissue from the surgical field, the specimen is placed in a plastic bag within the operating room (OR) and then immersed in a mixture of crushed ice and saline. The OR staff records the time of surgery, the time at which the tissue is excised, and the time at which the specimen is placed on ice.

2. The OR pages the MBTB, and the sample is picked up and transported to the pathology cutting room.

3. If the specimen and tumor are small or the lesion is not easily discernable, all tissue is required for routine histology, and no tissue can be granted to the MBTB without compromising the patient diagnosis. This assessment is made on gross examination by a pathologist unconnected with the MBTB. If there is tissue available, portions are immediately excised and given to the attending MBTB technologist to prepare for fixation and/or freezing (*see* **Notes 3** and **4**). At outside centers, tissue selected for the MBTB is rapidly frozen in a plastic bag and couriered to the MBTB (*see* **Note 5**).

4. Where feasible, the sampling of a breast case for the MBTB includes tissue pieces from multiple sites: tumor, normal breast, normal lymph node, and metastatic lymph nodes. Depending on the nature of the specimen, some tissue types will not be available (for example, earlier diagnosis has led to a decline in the proportion of cases with grossly detectable lymph node metastasis, and smaller excisional biopsies often preclude sampling from surrounding normal breast tissue without compromising assessment of surgical margins).

5. Once processed, each case comprises multiple matching or mirror image frozen and paraffin block pairs, averaging three pairs per case, depending on the size of available tissue. Each pair is labeled in sequence (A, B, C, etc.) along with the year and an identifying case or pathology number, e.g., 02-1234A (for the tumor block), 02-1234B (for the normal breast tissue block), and 02-1234C (normal lymph node block).

6. In order to obtain adequate tissue for both the paraffin and frozen blocks, each fragment of tissue should be trimmed to no less than 4 mm thick before it is bisected. Otherwise, it becomes technically difficult to produce two uniform blocks with sufficient sample in each. The fragment of tissue destined to become the frozen tissue block should be up to 15 mm long and no more than 10 mm wide to accommodate the diameter of the cryovial. Most standard histological cassettes will accommodate this size easily, but the fragment of tissue destined to become the paraffin tissue block should not exceed 3 mm in thickness to ensure quick penetration of the fixative.

7. To ensure accurate tissue orientation, the tissue sample edge is marked with Alcian blue or Cobalt blue dye using an orange stick, before halving. This dye will adhere to the tissue and be microscopically visible at a point on the outer

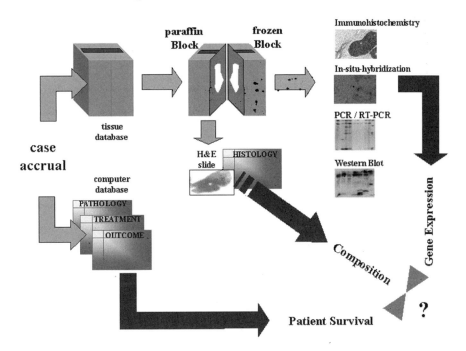

Fig. 1. Overview of Manitoba Breast Tumor Bank. Case accrual triggers collection of data and entry for storage and retrieval into a computerized database. The corresponding tissue is collected and processed to create mirror image paraffin and frozen tissue blocks. This is done by inking the outside and cut surfaces with blue and red inks that facilitate easy reorientation of blocks. The paraffin blocks yield high-quality paraffin sections for analysis of histological and regional composition (which is also stored in the computer database) and for guiding microdissection of frozen tissue. Both paraffin and frozen block formats are necessary to yield tissue sections for a range of assays, including those requiring extraction of nucleic acids or proteins or those based on direct tissue analysis with probes or antibodies. Investigators can then integrate gene expression data acquired in different ways from analysis of adjacent sections and directly with the tissue composition and with clinical data to answer a range of research questions.

edge of the sample. After slicing the tissue at right angles to the line of the blue dye, the exposed and opposing tissue faces are painted with Mercurochrome. Identification of the mirror image face is important when orientating the specimen during embedding and sectioning (**Fig. 1**).

8. Place one half in a cryovial, maintaining the inked face flat, close and snap freeze in liquid nitrogen, and store in the −70°C ultralow freezer. Also, avoid squeezing too much sample into the cryovial, because the flat sectioning surface or face will be folded up and frozen in that orientation. Place the other half flat in a process-

ing cassette ink side up and immerse in 10% neutral buffered formalin for 18–24 h before submitting to routine histological paraffin processing and embedding (**Notes 6** and **7**).

9. Automatic tissue processors have standardized overnight protocols. The processing fluids are exchanged at predetermined time intervals from fixation, through dehydration in graded ethanols, 70, 95 (two changes), and 100% (two changes), clearing in xylene (two changes), and infiltration in paraffin wax (two changes). A constant vacuum in the tissue well speeds the processing time and ensures complete infiltration with paraffin wax by the end of the process.

10. After completion of processing, the labeled cassettes are opened at the embedding center and the tissue removed and placed with the inked side down in an appropriately sized heated mold. The mold is partially filled with molten paraffin while a dissecting needle holds the specimen to the bottom, where it is secured by quickly cooling the base (**Notes 8** and **9**). The labeled portion of the cassette is placed on top, and the mold is filled to the top with more paraffin wax. The blocks are set on the cooling area of the embedding center for 30 min and then removed from the mold. They are now ready to be sectioned.

11. Two H&E-stained slides are then made, one for the MBTB and one for the hospital records. The routine thickness of tissue sections is 5–7 mm. Sections are cut with a steel knife or disposable blade, mounted on plain glass slides, and dried for 1 h at 55°C or overnight at 37°C. Once dry, the tissue sections are stained with H&E and cover-slipped. A more detailed procedure for sectioning is found in **Subheading 3.4.**

12. H&E staining *(3)*. Paraffin sections are transferred through the following solutions and reagents using staining dishes with glass or metal slide racks. Frozen sections begin with a water rinse after fixation and proceeding at **step 7**.

   a. Deparaffinize slides in two changes of xylene for 2 min each.
   b. Hydrate through graded alcohols.
   c. 100% Ethanol, two changes, 2 min each.
   d. 95% Ethanol, two changes, 2 min each.
   e. 70% Ethanol, 2 min.
   f. Wash for 5 min in tap water.
   g. Immerse in Harris hematoxylin (filtered before use), 4 min.
   h. Destain in 1% HCl in 70% ethanol, five to seven dips.
   i. Blue in Scott's tap water (four to five drops of strong ammonia in 250 mL water), 2 min.
   j. Wash for 5 min in tap water.
   k. Rinse in 95% ethanol.
   l. Stain for 2 min in 0.2% eosin Y in 95% ethanol. (**Note:** if staining is pale, add two to three drops of HCl to the eosin Y and restain.)
   m. Destain in 70 and 95% ethanol, 15 and 20 dips, respectively.
   n. Dehydrate in 100% ethanol, two changes, 2 min each.
   o. Clear in xylene, two changes, 2 min each.
   p. Mount using a cover slip with Permount and allow to dry for 2–3 wk before filing.

13. Staining results. The nuclei are deep blue; cytoplasm and connective tissue are shades of pink.
14. Each pathology chit is completed with block acquisition information and filed. The patient's name, pathology number, blocks acquired, and collection times are recorded in a confidential log book, and each case is given a unique MBTB number that renders the case anonymous from the original patient and clinical record.
15. Reading and the compiling the information from each slide are done later, and the information gathered is entered into the computer database.
16. To ensure security, uniformity, and consistency in handling, which includes sectioning, labeling, filing, and retrieval of cases, a limited number of individuals are responsible for handling the MBTB material.

3.2. Storage

1. Paraffin blocks are stored at room temperature in storage drawers and arranged in order by MBTB number.
2. Cryovials of frozen blocks are placed in 2-in. cardboard storage boxes (holding 81 vials each) and stored numerically by MBTB number. Metal racks hold 20 2-in. boxes and assist in separating tissue categories.
3. Posted on the outside of each freezer is a template of the shelves and racks displaying the contents, making storage and retrieval more efficient.
4. The freezer temperature is monitored by an external alarm system connected to 24-h monitoring stations staffed by the campus police and maintenance engineers. A protocol and phone numbers to contact MBTB personnel are in place in the case of a breakdown and, in addition, are posted on each freezer.
5. In the event of freezer breakdown, or power outage, a CO_2 backup system has been installed on each freezer. This comprises a CO_2 cylinder attached via a regulator to an electronic monitor system installed on the freezer. In the event of a freezer failure, a single CO_2 cylinder will maintain tissue temperature below $-20°C$ for approx 15 h per 50-lb cylinder. CO_2 is injected into the freezer when the temperature rises above $-60°C$.
6. Organizing alternate freezer space ahead of time and having a refrigeration company with 24-h service can save undue stress and valuable time.

3.3. Release

Tissue is released in the form of multiple paraffin or frozen sections that can be used for RNA, DNA, and protein extraction as well as for direct tissue-based assays such as IHC and RNA:RNA *in situ* hybridization (ISH). In order to utilize this valuable resource efficiently, standard sectioning and extraction protocols have been modified to successfully extract nucleic acids and proteins in sufficient quantities from small numbers of sections to be able to complete common assays, such as PCR *(4)*, RT-PCR *(5)*, subtraction hybridization *(6)*, and Western blotting *(7)*, while minimizing the amount of tissue necessary. This ensures rationing of the tissue blocks associated with each case for multiple assays and projects and maintenance of block orientation. The cryotome and microtome sectioning procedures for frozen and paraffin, respectively, will be described first, followed by individual details of the various experimental protocols involved in preparing tissue for the extraction of RNA, DNA, and protein, and sections for IHC and ISH.

3.3.1. General Sectioning Protocol for Frozen Tissue

1. A detailed procedure of frozen tissue sectioning can be found in a histology textbook *(3)*, and only a brief description is provided here. For extraction for RT-PCR *(4,5)*, *see* **Notes 10–14**.
2. The frozen tissue vials are transferred to the cryotome, where section preparation is done at –30°C, the temperature recommended for breast tissue.
3. The frozen block is securely mounted, inked (red) side up, on a specimen disc with mounting medium (Cryomount), inserted into the specimen head, and orientated so that the block face is parallel to the knife-edge.
4. The block face is advanced slowly, adjusting and readjusting the tilt of the tissue face until it is very close and parallel to the knife-edge. When a partial section appears, it will indicate how much adjusting still needs to be done before attaining the whole block face. Readjust as necessary. Taking too many partial sections can waste and distort the face of the tissue block.
5. Apply the antiroll plate to the knife and adjust its position (slightly above the knife-edge) until sections slide under and lie flat against the knife surface. For 5-μm sections, optimum alignment is critical in producing quality sections, and a description of this precise adjustment is provided with each cryotome.
6. Set the section thickness at 5 μm for IHC or ISH and 20 μm for extraction samples.
7. Section and collect multiple tissue sections in precooled microfuge tubes or individual sections on electrostatically charged slides (Superfrost Plus). Sections can be mounted on room-temperature slides by inverting the slide at a slight angle over the section as it lies on the knife back. The section will be attracted to the slide and adhere to it.
8. When the sectioning is done, the tissue block is removed quickly and carefully from the specimen disc with a scalpel blade, and excess mounting medium is trimmed from around the sample before returning it to the original storage vial.
9. The cryovials and microfuge tubes are transported back to the –70°C ultralow freezer, in convenient freezer cubes designed for 2-mL cryovials or microfuge tubes. Frozen sections on slides not requiring a fixation step can go directly into sealed, precooled plastic slide boxes or slide mailers sealed with Parafilm for freezer storage. For ISH fixation, *see* **Subheading 3.4.5.**

3.3.2. General Sectioning Protocol for Paraffin Block Tissue

A detailed procedure of paraffin tissue sectioning can be found in a histology textbook, and only a brief description is provided here (*see* **Notes 15–17**).

1. Fill a tissue-sectioning bath with distilled water and set at 40–45°C. For routine H&E staining, add approx 0.1–0.2 mg gelatin and allow the bath to warm. If

sections are being prepared for IHC or ISH, add nothing to the water.

2. Precool paraffin blocks to be sectioned on a tray of ice. This will facilitate sectioning of especially fatty tissue like breast tissue.
3. Using a steel microtome knife or disposable blade (each have an individual holder), set the clearance angle at 0–2° and the section setting at the desired thickness: 5–7 μm for histological sections and 20 μm for extraction purposes.
4. Attach the sample/cassette to the holder on the microtome, loosen the knife holder to bring the knife within 3 or 4 mm of the block face and tighten. Follow by making the block face parallel to the knife-edge, using the *x*/*y* orientation mechanism on the block holder.
5. Advance the block gradually using the coarse adjustment knob, while simultaneously rotating the hand wheel for each advance until tissue sections are produced. As with the frozen blocks, ensure block alignment is precise; readjust as needed so as not to remove and waste too many partial sections.
6. As the block is sectioned, it will produce a "ribbon" of attached tissue sections, which are transferred to the water bath and stretched out to remove wrinkles. Individual sections are mounted from the water bath onto microscope slides and transferred to slide racks to dry. Discard sections with wrinkles, folds, or knife marks, and always allow time for the sections to stretch and flatten before mounting.
7. For 20-μm sections, the water bath is unnecessary, and the individual sections go directly into microfuge tubes ready for extraction.
8. Dry paraffin sections at 37°C overnight for IHC, or approx 55°C for 1 h for routine staining.
9. The sections are stored for shipping in slide mailers.

3.3.3. Preparation of Frozen Tissue Sections for IHC

1. Set the section thickness at 4–5 μm.
2. Cut and mount the sections on room-temperature charged microscope slides (Superfrost Plus).
3. Place the slides in a rack, and allow the sections to dry overnight at room temperature on the bench.
4. The next day, fix in cold acetone for 10 min and leave to dry for about 30 min.
5. Package in slide mailers sealed with Parafilm and store at –20°C in airtight plastic bags.
6. After shipping at room temperature and receipt of the tissue slides (approx 24 h duration), they should again be stored at —20°C or stained immediately. Always bring slide mailers from the freezer to room temperature before opening and staining.

3.3.4. Preparation of Paraffin Tissue Sections for IHC

1. Prepare a distilled water bath set at 42–45°C, with no additives.
2. Section paraffin blocks at 5 μm and mount on charged SuperfrostPlus slides.
3. Dry at 37°C overnight.
4. Store in slide mailers to ship.
5. Slides for IHC should be shipped as soon as possible, because antigen staining

can be affected with time. The elapsed time from sectioning to shipping and receipt of slides is 3–4 d, and this should be taken into consideration with each experiment.

3.3.5. Preparation of Frozen Tissue Sections for ISH

1. Avoid RNases by wearing gloves and changing them frequently.
2. Section at 5–7 μm using SuperfrostPlus slides to mount sections (**Note 18**).
3. Allow sections to dry about 1 min, and immerse in 4% paraformaldehyde, in PBS, pH 7.4, for 20 min.
4. Rinse in two changes of PBS for 2 min each.
5. Dehydrate in 70, 95, and 100% (two changes) for 2 min each.
6. Dry briefly, and place in slide mailers and seal. Place mailers in an airtight plastic bag to keep dry.
7. Store at –70°C.
8. After shipping via overnight delivery on dry ice, slides should be stored at –70°C and brought to room temperature prior to opening sealed mailers to prevent condensation from forming on the sections.

3.3.6. Preparation of Paraffin Tissue Sections for ISH

1. Prepare a tissue bath by wiping with a product like RNase Away to remove RNases, and rinse with DEPC-treated water.
2. Fill bath with DEPC-treated distilled water and warm to 42–45°C.
3. Do not section or touch slides without gloves. Change gloves frequently throughout sectioning.
4. Precool paraffin blocks in an ice tray to make sectioning easier.
5. Cut sections at 5 μm and allow stretching on the water in the tissue bath until all wrinkles have disappeared. Creases will produce signal artifacts (**Note 18**).
6. Place sections on SuperfrostPlus slides and dry at 37°C.
7. Store slides in mailers.

3.3.7. Microdissection Procedure

A manual procedure to microdissect frozen sections of breast tumor tissue was devised to ensure that specific, histologically defined cell populations can be isolated by reference to sections from the corresponding mirror image paraffin block *(5)*. This procedure is still applicable for isolation of large regions of tissue sections and complements more recent microdissection methods based on laser-guided dissection.

1. Wear gloves and change them often throughout the procedure.
2. Before sectioning, several plain slides are prepared with a small central mound of 1% agarose made in DEPC-treated distilled water. The agarose is applied with a sterile Pasteur pipet in the middle of the slide covering an area sufficient to place a section. It is allowed to solidify and cool. The prepared slides will be workable for approx 1 h before the agarose starts to shrink.

3. Sterile 1.5-mL microfuge tubes are labeled and kept on ice ready for the dissected samples.
4. Coplin jars of staining solutions, hematoxylin and 1% eosin Y, plus DEPC-treated distilled water for rinses are set up for rapid staining as follows:
a. Hematoxylin (filtered), 30 s.
b. DEPC water, rinse off excess stain.
c. 0.2% Eosin Y in 95% ethanol, 15 s.
d. DEPC water, two changes to rinse off excess stain.
e. Dissect section while wet.
5. The selected frozen blocks are chosen beforehand according to information obtained from review of the matching H&E-stained paraffin tissue sections. The H&E slides are kept nearby during dissection for confirmation of cell populations and as a guide in locating the cells of interest.
6. The first section from the frozen block is cut at 5–7 μm, fixed, and stained to confirm and provide an H&E-stained sample for reference. Following this, single 10-μm sections are cut and placed on the agarose, usually one per slide.
7. A section is captured on the agarose by inverting the slide over the tissue section and lightly touching the section as it lies flat against the knife surface. If too much pressure is applied to the section, the agarose can stick to the knife and rip the section.
8. Allow the section to adhere to the agarose for a few seconds before immersing in the staining solutions. Some sections will fall off during staining, and these need to be left longer in the solution in order to adhere before staining.
9. After staining, the back of the slide is wiped dry and placed on the dissection microscope platform, where it is dissected while still wet using a fine needle and/ or scalpel blade. The microdissection is done at a magnification of ×160.
10. As soon as the area of cells of interest is teased from the section, it is placed at the bottom of the microfuge tube on ice.
11. Several sections (approx 10–20) depending on the size of the dissecting area, may be required for ample RNA extraction.
12. As soon as possible after dissection, the tubes are centrifuged briefly to pellet the small pieces and stored at –70°C.
13. A modified extraction protocol using scaled down quantities of TriReagent and other reagents are used to extract RNA from these minute amounts of tissue.

3.3.8. Packaging and Shipping Tissue

Human tissue is a potential biohazard and requires special handling at all times, especially during shipping *(8)*. Regulations have been put in place to protect handlers and to ensure that samples are secure, eliminating or minimizing contamination in the event of accidents in transit. In addition, dry ice for frozen tissue shipments via cargo aircraft is considered a hazardous commodity, prohibited by some handlers, and therefore requiring special documentation. Human breast tissue is therefore also considered as a potential biohazard, but unless a specific sample contains a known infectious element, it is best categorized on the waybill as a "biosample, noninfectious, and nonhazardous." The following is a description providing the handling and packaging procedures for frozen tissue in microfuge tubes and paraffin or frozen sections on glass slides.

1. Frozen tissue for extraction purposes must be secured in spill-proof screw-cap vials or tight snap caps like microfuge tubes.
2. These tubes are placed in another container, either a plastic bag or box that will contain any spillage if a tube leaks.
3. For frozen shipments, a 1.5- to 2-in.-thick Styrofoam box, with inside measurements 6 × 8 × 9 in., requires 3–4 kg dry ice, with the top taped securely and the samples positioned in the middle of the dry ice, nearer to the bottom. The Styrofoam box and contents are also placed into a second outer cardboard box, which is secured with packing tape. Note that dry ice is a "class 9 dangerous good" set out by the Transportation of Dangerous Goods Act and a parallel governing body, the International Air Transport Association. A dry ice label and waybill attached to the outside of the box must state the class and weight of the dry ice.
4. Shipping fragile glass slides of paraffin sections is best done using hard plastic slide mailers, placing these filled mailers inside a small box, and then into a larger one surrounded by Styrofoam chips or bubble wrap.
5. Documentation on the waybill includes date of shipment, weight and class of dangerous goods (e.g., 3 kg of dry ice, UN1845, CLS 9,111,904), sender's account number (set up by the carrier), sender's and consignee's address (including room number, postal code, and telephone number), and a description of material being shipped (note below), billing information, the sender's signature, and a release signature by the sender and courier at the time of pickup. The waybill is attached to the top outside of the box in a plastic window, and a carbon copy is left with the sender.
6. Dry ice shipments are best packed in the afternoon for pickup by the courier at 4 or 5 PM for overnight delivery.
7. For continuity, all MBTB shipments, whether on dry ice, are sent priority overnight, and the consignee is notified of the next-day delivery in advance along with the waybill number for tracing purposes.
8. The frozen tissue shipments described are for those within North America, from Canada to the United States. For overseas shipments, the shipping time is extended to approx 4 d, requiring the use of special liquid nitrogen spill-proof containers.

3.4. Inventory of Frozen and Paraffin Blocks and Slides

1. To maintain order and correct any recording errors, a complete inventory of matching blocks and accompanying H&E slides should be done periodically.
2. A hard copy of the database is checked against the inventory and notations made as necessary.
3. Any H&E slides missing or needing repair can also be replaced at this time.

For assistance, a table of used frozen and paraffin blocks are kept.

4. Because tissue is used over time, leaving spaces especially in cryovial storage boxes, inventory can be a time to move samples, concentrating them in fewer boxes. Paraffin block files can also be adjusted and compacted.

5. If blocks have been exhausted, the H&E slide is maintained, but a small colored label is applied to it, indicating whether the paraffin or frozen or both blocks have been used.

3.5. Ethical Issues and Mechanisms for Access

In a typical hospital pathology department practice, surgical tissue is collected and processed into paraffin blocks, and unprocessed tissue is discarded. After initial diagnosis, the processed tissue blocks and clinical data are typically stored by name and/or pathology case number to allow easy retrieval of cases for review. Access to this resource for both clinical and research application is managed by specialist physicians (pathologists) who make professional judgments as to the appropriate use. This is a role that is fundamental to the clinical discipline of pathology. Although these judgments are made with respect to, and in accordance with, clinical knowledge and professional conscience, judgments are hard to assess from other perspectives, as they are not always systematically documented or available for external review.

A tumor bank offers a mechanism that improves this historical process for research access, by ensuring wider peer review for appropriate use and documentation of access. A tumor bank also refines the value, and facilitates the effective use of, tissues and associated clinical pathology data. A tumor bank can utilize excess tissues (that are otherwise disposed of), process these into a format (matched paraffin and frozen blocks) that is more suitable for research assays, and store these in a format that allows easy retrieval for research applications (e.g., by pathology diagnosis and tissue content rather than name or health care identifier).

The tumor bank should exist within, and be governed by, the accepted confidential bounds of clinical practice. In the MBTB, cases are stored and released under anonymous MBTB numbers that are only linked through a computer database to clinical identifiers. The MBTB number is linked to the clinical pathology number within the tissue database and to the oncology number within the separate clinical database. Both tissue and clinical databases reside within secured and password-protected microcomputer databases in the respective clinical departments and are not Web-accessible.

On the research interface, cases are accessible only through application to the MBTB through a formal mechanism and review. Cases are provided on this research interface only in response to anonymous selection criteria (e.g., diagnostic categories) and are released only as sets of cases, each under an anonymous MBTB number, and cannot be practically linked to the patient. The integrity of the insulation resides with the MBTB director, who is a clinical pathologist, and this integrity is open to review by appropriate clinical and research regulatory bodies. In Canada, a tumor bank must be approved by the institutional ethics review board and all studies supported by the bank must conform to the relevant provincial laws *(9)* governing use of tissue and information. In Manitoba, this is the Personal Health and Information Act *(10)*, the National Tri-Council Policy for Ethical Conduct for Research Involving Humans *(11)*, and must conform to the Canadian Association of Pathologists, Guidelines for the Ethical Use of Human Tissue in Research *(12)*. Further information concerning international legal norms on the protection of personal information in health research is also available *(13)*.

Studies supported by the MBTB encompass questions related to basic cell biology and markers of diagnosis and tumor progression. Studies that encompass questions related to genetic risk are not considered. Investigators are then provided with a complete set of anonymous "cases," each designated under a unique MBTB number. Each set typically comprises 100 cases, and each case will typically comprise 1–10 thin (5 μm) tissue sections mounted on glass slides or placed in a tube to facilitate gel-based and section-based assays performed in parallel *(11)*, information about the content of the tissue (such as proportion of tumor and normal cells), information about the classification and diagnosis of the tumor (e.g., tumor type, grade, and size, and presense of associated nodal metastasis), and in some sets, generic information about the type of therapy (e.g., radiation/hormone/chemotherapy) and clinical status of the disease after years of follow-up. Users and the projects that use the facility fall into three general categories:

1. Projects initiated by local researchers in Manitoba.
2. Projects initiated by external academic users (e.g., elsewhere in Canada or in the United States or Europe).
3. Industry-affiliated research users.

Access to the MBTB involves three phases:

1. Formal applications for access are invited quarterly and are required for all categories of user. The application form includes a detailed outline of the investigator curriculum vitae, sources of funding, description of study, techniques to be used, statistical justification, and the type and extent of data (histological, pathological, and clinical) requested. Applications are reviewed by an MBTB application review panel that comprises several individuals selected to encompass a spectrum of clinical, pathological, health records, and scientific expertise. Criteria for review include the background and credentials of the investigator, evidence of peer reviewed, and preferably, national funding, high scientific quality,

and merit. Projects are rated as supportable, supportable with reservations, or unsupportable.

2. All applicants are notified, and those that are supportable are asked to provide institutional and investigator signatures and commitment to the terms of support (which include conditions on the secondary use of materials provided) and documentation of appropriate institutional research ethics board approval for the project. No clinical or demographic information is released that concerns patient or family history or treatment center, as this might compromise anonymity. The MBTB panel considers ethical and confidentiality issues in all cases, in particular with respect to appropriate justification and equitable use of a rare resource donated by patients. However, in accordance with national and local ethics policies with respect to medical research, all applications must be accompanied by documentation of approval of the appropriate research ethics board.

3. Prior to release of study materials, the director then enters into discussion with all users to refine project details, such as specific pathology and histology selection criteria, types of cases available, and assay protocols, to maximize efficient use of invaluable tissue samples. All users are then sent a small test batch (three to five cases) of tissues in the appropriate assay format (e.g., sections in tubes or on coated slides, etc.) to test courier mail "connections" (especially for frozen tissue sent on dry ice) and capability of the laboratory to successfully conduct their assays on MBTB material (i.e., the challenge of small-scale sections and different fixation protocols that may very occasionally influence antibody performance). Only after confirmation of successful receipt and performance of the relevant assay(s) on MBTB material is the study set finally sectioned and released in batches.

4. Notes

1. Using our histological assessment of quality control, approx 80% of all cases accrued have very good preservation with nuclear morphology preserved (rank 3), approx 17% have acceptable nuclear morphology preservation such that distinction of mitoses and tumor grading is possible (rank 2), and approx 3% have poor nuclear preservation such that tumor grading is not possible.

2. The cases are divided on accrual into A, B, C, and D categories. This organizes the quality and type of tissue held in the MBTB, and facilitates selection of appropriate cases for different research projects. Each category of material is described here:

   a. A category. This category of high-quality tissue is collected and frozen very quickly after surgery, and comprises samples of more than one tissue region— tumor, normal, normal lymph node, and metastatic lymph node—where available. The collection protocol includes transport on ice from the operating room to pathology department, and each specimen is associated with a record of the times of start and end of surgery, tissue on ice, and tissue into freezer to provide a measure of tissue quality for consideration when assessing RNA or proteins with short half-lives.

b. B category. This material originates in hospitals within the city and comprises unused primary tumor material from tissue sent to the provincial steroid receptor assay laboratory. Although mostly rapidly frozen and stored at –70°C and transported by courier in dry ice, the transport conditions are not controlled, and the tissue has been handled and sectioned in the clinical laboratory, and there are no recorded times related to collection. In common with the A category cases, these are associated with full clinical and follow-up data.

c. C category. This material is the same as the B category material, but mostly originates at more distant centers within the city and province. Some of this material is also transported frozen over longer distances (approx 200 km) and some on wet ice. These cases are associated with baseline pathology and clinical data, but no treatment or outcome data. This tissue thus provides an efficient resource for comparison of gene expression within regions and components of primary tumors, assays based on DNA protein assessment, and trial experiments and saves the other, more valuable cases from depletion.

d. D category. Despite improvements in early detection, occasional cases are large specimens and after processing the standard number of tissue blocks (up to three matching paraffin and frozen blocks), there remains excess material. This material is stored as intact tissue fragments in 15-mL cryovials. These cases serve as a resource for occasional projects that require large amounts of material, usually for biochemical assays.

3. During processing, multiple cases are transferred to the –30°C cryotome, and each one is cut and halved quickly to avoid thawing. Dry ice can help, but this also makes the tissue very hard and difficult to cut without causing fractures. It is preferred to cut the piece as quickly as possible with a scalpel or larger trimming knife, returning the excess tissue and frozen section to the cryotome while the tissue for the paraffin block is prepared for fixation.

4. Cryovials are labeled and precooled in the cryotome.

5. Prefrozen tissue samples for the MBTB are stored at the outside hospital or emergency room lab until a sufficient quantity accumulates to transport.

6. The tissue cassettes are immersed immediately in 10% neutral buffered formalin for 18–24 h, transferred to 70% ethanol, and stored until a sufficient number of cassettes are ready for embedding. The batch is then taken to the hospital tissue processor, where it is programmed to begin at 70% ethanol.

7. Disinfect the cryotome and accessories with Cryofect or absolute ethanol after sectioning or manipulation of the tissue.

8. An important reminder: treat human tissue as a potential biohazard—wear gloves and wash hands frequently. Autoclave waste tissue, gloves, and counter protectors after use. When done, clean and disinfect the work area.

9. Two necessary embedding issues to keep in mind: keep the tissues warm prior to placing them in the mold. If cool, they may not meld with the added paraffin and pop out of the block during sectioning. Be sure that the inked face is entirely flat against the bottom of the mold, because it is this face that will be sectioned and stained.

10. It has been determined that 5–20 10-μm sections from a tumor block will provide sufficient RNA (approx 5–10 mg) for several RT-PCR experiments. In addition, about twice as many sections are required to obtain enough extract from normal breast tissue blocks. For protein analysis, approximately double the number of sections is needed compared to RNA or DNA extraction. **Note:** this amount varies from case to case depending on fat content and block face size.

11. Wear gloves and change them often. The tissue is a potential biohazard, and when handling tubes for RNA extraction, it is important to eliminate possible sources of RNase contamination.

12. Set the cryostat at –30°C and keep labeled tubes, forceps, tube rack, and a fine brush to clean the knife-edge in it.

13. Several sections are cut one after the other and allowed to accumulate under the antiroll plate. A predetermined number of 20-μm sections are placed in cooled, prelabeled 1.5-mL microfuge tubes and stored in the ultralow freezer. To pick up the sections, use cold forceps and tease them off the bottom of the tube. Holding the tube by the cap minimizes the amount of heat transferred to the body of the tube. Do not allow sections to thaw at any point in the procedure.

14. Extraction is done directly in this tube using a product called TriReagent or Trizol. Detailed protocols that come with these reagents are modified, using less reagent for the small tissue amounts of 5–10 sections.

15. Paraffin and frozen blocks of breast tumor tissue can contain a great deal of fat, making sectioning more difficult than tumor only. **Hints:** make the paraffin block colder using a spray coolant, keep on ice longer, set the cryotome at –35°C, change the speed of sectioning through the block, and clean the built-up fat on the knife-edge using absolute alcohol. For paraffin blocks, use xylene to clean fat and paraffin from the knife-edge.

16. Keep blocks and slides in ascending numerical order, lessening the chance of placing the wrong section on the wrong slide. It also assists label making and subsequent filing.

17. At the end of sectioning or staining, correct labeling can be cross-checked by viewing the sections on the slide and comparing with the block face.

18. For ISH, well-stretched, flat sections are important in avoiding artifacts. The radioactive probe will bind to folds and wrinkles.

Acknowledgments

The MBTB was established with funding from the National Cancer Institute of Canada and is now supported in part by the Manitoba Institute of Cell Ciology; Cancer Care Manitoba; the Department of Pathology, University of Manitoba; and the Guardian Angels, Winnipeg.

References

1. Watson, P. H. (1999) Tumor tissue and clinical databanks—a review of the importance, role and future of tumor banks. *Cancer Strategy* **6,** 1–6.

2. Watson, P. H., Snell, L., and Parisien, M. (1996) The NCIC-Manitoba Breast Tumor Bank: a resource for applied cancer research. *CMAJ* **155,** 281–283.
3. Humason, G. L. (1967) *Animal Tissue Techniques, 2nd Ed.* W.H. Freeman and Company, San Francisco, CA.
4. Watson. P., Safneck, R., Le, K., Dubik, D., and Shiu, R. (1993) Relationship of c-myc amplification to progression of breast cancer from in-situ to invasive tumor and lymph node metastasis. *J. Natl. Cancer Inst.* **85,** 902–907.
5. Hiller, T., Snell, L., and Watson, P. H. (1996) Microdissection RT-PCR analysis of gene expression in pathologically defined frozen tissue sections. *Biotechniques* **21,** 38–44.
6. Leygue, E. R., Watson, P. H., and Murphy, L. C. (1996) Identification of differentially expressed genes using minute amounts of RNA. *Biotechniques* **21,** 1008–1012.
7. Leygue, E., Snell, L., Dotzlaw, H., et al. (2000) Lumican and decorin are differentially expressed in human breast carcinoma. *J. Pathology* **192,** 313–320.
8. Noble, M. A. (1994) Understanding transportation of infectious materials inside Canada—1994. *CACMID Newsl.* **9,** 8–12.
9. http://www.cihr-irsc.gc.ca/publications/ethics/privacy/compendium_e.pdf.
10. http://www.gov.mb.ca/health/legislation/Summary_Researchers.pdf.
11. http://www.nserc.ca/programs/ethics/english/policy.htm.
12. http://www.cap.medical.org.
13. http://www.cihr-irsc.gc.ca/publications/ethics/protection_pi_e.pdf.
14. Al-Haddad, S., Zhang, Z., Leygue, E., et al. (1999) The role of psoriasin (S100A7) in invasive breast cancer. *Am. J. Pathol.* **155,** 2057–2066.

2

Frozen Biopsy Collection and Storage

Frozen Biopsy Samples

Russell Leek

Summary

This chapter describes some simple standard operating procedures for the regular collection of samples from surgical resections and their rapid preservation by freezing for long-term cryogenic storage.

Key Words: Biopsy collection; cryogenic preservation; inventory control.

1. Introduction

When collecting frozen human tissue of any type, the aim is to freeze the specimen in as short a period as possible following excision from the patient. In order to expedite this process, it is necessary to have an organizational structure in place to coordinate the people involved in chain linking the operating theater to the specimen. If biopsy collection is organized via anything apart from an *ad hoc* basis, then the regular cooperation of a host of health care professionals must be sought after and agreed on in advance. The cooperation of clinical staff is an absolute requirement for the smooth running of a regular biopsy collection service. Ideally, surgeons and pathologists should be consulted in advance, and a standard operating procedure should be agreed that does not interfere with the normal clinical routine (*see* **Note 1**).

Ideally, from the research laboratory side, it is desirable to have a dedicated technician available to collect specimens, as they come through the pathology reception at any time during reasonable working hours. If this person is allocated a hospital pager or mobile phone, then he or she is able to respond very quickly. Subsequent to tissue excision from the patient in the operating theater, the sequence of events should be as follows:

From: *Methods in Molecular Medicine, Vol. 120: Breast Cancer Research Protocols*
Edited by: S. A. Brooks and A. L. Harris © Humana Press Inc., Totowa, NJ

1. Biopsy is removed from patient.
2. Biopsy arrives at pathology laboratory.
3. Duty medical laboratory scientific officer calls for pathologist and biopsy collection research technician.
4. Pathologist dissects clinical samples from biopsy and supplies research technician with sample for cryogenic storage.
5. Research technician freezes sample in liquid nitrogen immediately (in the laboratory), and records details of the biopsy for inventory control.

Following this sequence, it should be possible to snap freeze a sample within 35 min of its excision. This is desirable, because experimentation has revealed that after 35 min, RNA degradation is rapid. This is especially important now, as many subsequent procedures involve the preparation of RNA from frozen material for the analysis of gene expression using systems such as microarrays.

1.1. Preparation

To support the short time frame necessary to freeze biopsies rapidly, a certain amount of preparation is valuable. In addition to gaining the cooperation of the professional staff involved and having an allocated "on-call" research technician, it is useful to have a biopsy collection kit that can be "grabbed on the run." Such a kit should contain, as a minimum, the items listed in **Subheading 2.**

2. Materials

2.1. Biopsy Collection Kit Contents

1. Portable cryovessels containing liquid nitrogen.
2. Portable insulated box for dry ice.
3. Scalpel blades and handles (or disposable scalpels).
4. Plastic forceps.
5. Disposable gloves.
6. Cryovials to store tissue.
7. Indelible marker pen to write on cryovials (the ink must be able to withstand freezing to $-180°C$).
8. Pen.
9. Record book.
10. Protective eye shields.

3. Methods

As a priority, the pathologist will take whatever is deemed necessary for clinical diagnosis. Tissue for research may only ever be considered if there is sufficient material remaining following this primary objective. Material available for research should be divided between several cryotubes, so that back-ups are available in the future. This should be done at this point to reduce the number of future freeze–thaw cycles when samples are split. There are a number of ways to freeze tissue samples, but the most effective and rapid way of snap freezing is to cut the biopsy into small pieces roughly 5 mm square, which are frozen directly by being held in liquid nitrogen, using a pair of long plastic forceps. The frozen piece is then placed immediately into a prelabeled tube (which has been precooled on dry ice) and stored temporarily on dry ice before being transported to the cryostorage unit (*see* **Note 2**).

When collecting biopsies, it is useful to consider their future use. If the sample is going to be used in its entirety, it is acceptable to freeze it directly in the tube (before closing the cap). If the sample is going to be split later, blocks should be frozen and placed in the tube separately, so they can be split without thawing. If the block is to be used for cryostat sectioning, it is worthwhile cutting the tissue into square blocks before freezing, so that it can be sectioned easily. It is also possible at this stage to mark the faces of the block with colored inks for orientation purposes.

It is also advisable to remember that it may be useful to have additional specimens of associated normal tissue as well as, for example, in the case of tumor specimens, samples of involved lymph nodes, or other metastases, where possible. These should be collected before the biopsy is preserved in fixative.

In order to preserve the patient's anonymity, it is useful to assign each new specimen an inventory number that can be tracked back to the patient. A single inventory number is a convenient way of labeling a tube without having too much information written on what is sometimes a very small label. The inventory number, pathology number, and hospital number may be written in the record book, which is kept in a secure place. This information may also be stored in a secure database as long as all of the conditions of the Data Protection Act (in the United Kingdom) are adhered to.

3.1. Long-Term Specimen Storage

The preferred method for long-term storage of frozen biopsies is in the vapor phase of liquid nitrogen at a temperature of less than −160°C. It is recommended that samples not be stored in the liquid phase in sealed tubes, as the tubes might explode when removed and the samples begin to thaw. Alternatively, storage in a −80°C freezer is acceptable and does not result in RNA degradation. A normal, −40°C freezer is unsuitable for storage of tissue specimens.

If important samples are to be stored on a long-term basis, it is advisable to keep duplicate samples in separate storage facilities, preferably in separate buildings.

3.2. Inventory Control

When embarking on a tissue collection project, some thought should be given to an inventory control system. This is an absolute necessity if the goal is to collect a tissue bank over a long period. New specimens in an inventory should be assigned a coordinate in the storage bank. The nature of this coordinate depends on the storage system used, but would usually follow a sequential alphanumeric format. For example, in a circular liquid nitrogen vessel containing six triangular stacks of draws, a specimen in stack 4 in the fifth drawer down at position 27 could be assigned a coordinate of 4-5-27. This coordinate may then be entered against the specimen's inventory number in the catalog, so that it can be retrieved rapidly in the future. Small catalogs may be kept as written records, but for larger catalogs, it is advantageous to keep this information on a computerized database (such as Microsoft Access [Windows] or FileMaker Pro [Apple Macintosh]). When samples are recorded on a relational database, it is much easier to link them to other information about the biopsy, patient, and data generated from experimental work on the sample.

4. Notes

1. It may also be necessary to have the informed consent of the patient concerned that tissue be stored for research purposes.
2. It is inadvisable to place cryovials directly into the liquid phase of liquid nitrogen with the cap on, because they can explode when they are removed. Cryovials can only be stored in the liquid phase if they are first wrapped in cryoflex tubing.

3

Serial Biopsies/Fine-Needle Aspirates and Their Assessment

Irene Boeddinghaus and Stephen R. D. Johnson

Summary

Taking a series of repeat biopsies or fine needle aspirates of a tumor during the course of therapy can provide information about treatment-induced changes in tumor biomarkers and help monitor patient response to adjuvant therapy. It is hoped that analysis of biomarkers in serial biopsies will also further our understanding of the molecular mechanisms that determine a tumor's response or resistance to therapy, may facilitate investigation of molecular biology of tumor response, and may provide useful information informing the development of new drugs for breast cancer therapy. In this chapter, practical, clinical considerations in the taking of repeat biopsies are considered and protocols for the taking of fine needle aspirates and core-cut/trucut biopsies are detailed. Their assessment for biomarkers indicative of cellular proliferation, apoptosis, and endocrine response/resistance such as estrogen and progesterone receptor status, HER2 and epidermal growth factor receptor are considered.

Key Words: Serial biopsies, serial fine needle aspirates, FNA, Ki67, TUNEL, ER, PR, EGFR, HER2.

1. Introduction

1.1. Clinical Utility of Serial Biopsies

In breast cancer, the characterization of treatment-induced changes in various tumor biomarkers has been studied in an attempt to further our understanding of the molecular mechanisms that determine a tumor's response or resistance to therapy. For example, the taking of serial biopsies before and during a course of treatment has been investigated to see whether changes in cell proliferation and cell death (apoptosis) correlate with clinical outcome. A decrease in cell proliferation as measured by Ki67 staining in serial fine-needle aspirate (FNA) biopsies taken after 14 or 21 d of tamoxifen therapy has been shown to correlate with clinical response in patients with primary breast cancer (1). Likewise, apoptosis has been shown to increase significantly 24 h after the

From: *Methods in Molecular Medicine, Vol. 120: Breast Cancer Research Protocols*
Edited by: S. A. Brooks and A. L. Harris © Humana Press Inc., Totowa, NJ

start of cytotoxic chemotherapy *(2)*, although subsequently, a substantial decrease in apoptotic index remained 3 mo after the commencement of chemotherapy *(3)*. In patients treated with chemoendocrine treatment, those patients in whom a tumor continued to show a relatively high proliferation and apoptotic index after 3 mo of treatment were less likely to show a clinical response to treatment *(4)*. Whereas there appears to be a relationship of apoptosis induction with response to chemotherapy, as yet, no such clear or consistent relationship has been demonstrated between endocrine therapy and changes in the apoptotic index. The ultimate value of these "intermediate markers" would be to allow early intervention, which may change the course of the clinical outcome; for example, identification of nonresponders to therapy, where an early change in treatment may be indicated. However, so far the variability in individual measurements and lack of correlation of some biomarkers with clinical outcome has prevented this from happening.

Serial tumor biopsies may also facilitate investigation of the molecular biology of tumor response. For example, reliable monoclonal antibodies (MAbs) to intracellular protein kinases implicated in progression of the cell cycle are now available and could be used to study these pathways in treated clinical samples or experimental models. In a hormone-dependent breast cancer xenograft model, an overall marked reduction in levels of cyclin D1 (which regulates progression through the G1 phase of the cell cycle) was seen after estrogen deprivation, with the changes starting as early as 1 d after therapy *(5)*. Similarly, $p27^{Kip1}$, a cyclin-dependent kinase inhibitor, increased markedly after 1 d, with maximal changes by day 3. It is notable that these changes occurred before any measurable decrease in cell proliferation (Ki67), perhaps indicating that in the future, early measurement of cell cycle regulators may predict subsequent changes in proliferation and/or apoptosis and ultimately, tumor growth.

Finally, changes in intermediate biomarkers as determined by serial biopsy may be helpful in the field of drug development. Whereas rigorously validated markers are always preferable, less-developed markers may nonetheless be useful indices during the clinical development of new drugs. This is particularly relevant for many of the new biologically based agents, such as signal transduction inhibitors, cell cycle modulators, or angiogenesis inhibitors. Whereas such data may not be used currently as surrogate end points for clinical effectiveness (as far as the regulatory authorities are concerned), they may be of considerable value in assessing the prospects for any new drug.

Variability in expression of any particular biomarker within and among patients is important to establish before any studies of change in expression with treatment over time are conducted. This allows the subsequent application of biomarker measurements in an individual to be made with a known confidence in its predictability, subsequently permitting the powering of any clinical trials in which the intermediate biomarker might form an important end point for the study. The availability of such data in relation to cell proliferation, apoptosis, and hormone-dependent protein expression was an integral part of the early clinical evaluation of several new hormonal agents including raloxifene, idoxifene, and fulvestrant *(6–8)*.

1.2. Clinical Scenario

The majority of repeat biopsy assessments take place in the early breast cancer setting, in association with primary (neoadjuvant) systemic treatment. Here, analysis of observed biological changes is more readily interpretable as a direct effect of treatment, where correlations can be made with changes in primary tumor size (i.e., clinical response). Likewise, any resistance to treatment can be inferred if lack of change in expression of a given biomarker correlates with no change (or, indeed, any increase) in tumor size. Where therapeutic agents are already known to be active, patients may derive clinical benefit by receiving systemic drug treatment in the preoperative neoadjuvant setting, in the form of tumor downstaging, allowing less radical surgery. In cases where clinical activity of any new agent is less well documented, but safety is already established from clinical trials in the advanced breast cancer setting, patients may be given a short course of treatment lasting between 1 and 3 wk, during the period between initial diagnosis and surgery. By definition, adjuvant treatment after surgery for early breast cancer does not allow for repeat sampling, as tumor burden is extremely low or nonexistent. However, patients with locally advanced primary breast cancer are also suitable for serial biopsies. Patients with metastatic disease may also be suitable for repeat sampling if they have accessible sites, such as skin nodules or lymph nodes, but here, issues may become clouded by questions of tumor heterozygocity and acquisition of multiple resistance mechanisms. The majority of practical concerns relate to the procedure, such as tumor size and suitability for repeat biopsy, accessibility of disease site, general patient fitness (e.g., anticoagulation), and patient consent, especially for repeated biopsies that are primarily for research purposes alone, with no necessary direct clinical benefit to the patient.

1.3. Timing

The optimal timing of serial biopsies used to investigate breast cancer is not always clear. Most analyses looking at the effects of cytotoxic therapy are now carried out on 24-h repeat biopsies, as indicated from a seminal paper showing an increase in apoptosis 24 h after infusion of a first cytotoxic chemotherapeutic regime *(2)*. Some current work is focusing on triplets of pre-, 24-h, and 21-d samples in an effort to detect resistant tissue that may contribute to the development of metastatic disease *(9)*. Biopsies taken much further into the course than this are often so difficult, given that an appreciable percentage of patients have such good initial responses, that the tumor may become difficult to detect and biopsy. Furthermore, following cytotoxic chemotherapy, necrotic and fibrotic changes may start to dominate the histological analysis of the tumor. It is fair to say that these times were chosen for practical reasons only (patients often staying in the hospital overnight for their first course of chemotherapy, and thus being available 24 h later, and once again coming in for cycle 2 on day 21), and as such, may not have maximal biological significance.

Repeat biopsies on patients on endocrine treatment are conventionally taken upon completion of 3 or 4 mo of therapy, although some researchers are analyzing intermediate samples taken at 2 wk. These times are also arbitrarily chosen, endocrine treatment being thought to work mainly by cytostatic means.

There are three types of repeat analyses used: FNA biopsy, core-cut/Trucut biopsy, and incision/excision biopsy.

2. Materials

2.1. FNA Biopsy

1. 23-Gage needle (Oncotech, Irvine, CA).
2. 7-mL Evacuated container (Exetainer; Labco, High Wycombe, UK) or 10-mL syringe.
3. Minimal essential medium (MEM) with phenol red and 25 mM 4-2-hydroxyethyl-1-piperazineethanesulfonic acid (HEPES) buffer (Invitrogen Life Technologies, Buckinghamshire, UK).
4. Alcohol swabs for cleaning.
5. Gauze swabs.
6. Adhesive plaster.
7. 1% Lignocaine (optional) (**Note:** confirm that patient is not allergic to lignocaine.)
8. 25-Gage needle and 5-mL syringe.
9. Sterile gloves.
10. Liquid nitrogen if snap-frozen aliquot is required.
11. Nunc® cryotube (Nalgene, Denmark).

2.2. Core-Cut/Trucut Biopsy

This technique should only be carried out by an appropriately qualified medical practitioner and absolutely requires local anesthesia. Tumors 2 cm along their smallest diameter can generally be biopsied easily with practice. Smaller tumors can be successfully sampled under ultrasound guidance.

1. 1% Lignocaine hydrochloride.
2. 5-mL Syringe.

3. 25-Gage needle.
4. 21-Gage needle.
5. Alcohol for cleaning.
6. Size-10 disposable scalpel (Swann-Morton, Sheffield, UK).
7. 14-Gage × 9-cm disposable biopsy needle (Allegiance Healthcare, McGaw Park, IL).
8. Sterile gauze swabs.
9. Adhesive bandage.
10. Sterile gloves.
11. Formalin-containing specimen bottle/liquid nitrogen and Nunc collection tube.

2.3. Excision/Incision Biopsy

This is a surgical procedure, usually undertaken by a surgeon under local anesthetic. A piece of tumor, usually at least 0.5 cm × 0.5 cm, is taken and placed in either liquid nitrogen or formalin.

2.4. Materials for Slide Preparation

1. FNA sample in suspension (*see* **Subheading 3.3.1.**).
2. Hematocounter and cover slip.
3. Shandon cytospin machine with clip holder, filter paper, and cytospin chamber.
4. 6–12 APES-coated slides (Superfrost® Plus; Merck UK, Lutterworth, UK).
5. Diamond marker pencil.
6. May–Grunwald–Giemsa stain.

3. Methods
3.1. FNA Biopsy

1. Place patient in the supine position on the examining couch, with the tumor exposed in the optimal position. This often requires the patient to roll partially on her side or to put her hands under her head.
2. Clean the area with an alcohol swab and allow it to dry.
3. If lignocaine is to be used, draw up 1–2 mL with a 25-gage needle into a 5-mL syringe and inject a small bleb directly under the epidermis only, so as not to compromise sample collection (*see* **Note 1**).
4. If using a needle and syringe to biopsy, break the air lock on the syringe by expelling the air present in the syringe and attach the needle. Then withdraw back to have 1 cc of air in the syringe.
5. Insert the needle into the tumor (identifiable by a "gritty" feeling under the needle; the site of the tumor is often deeper than expected), and stabilize the tumor between the second and third fingers of the opposite hand. While stabilizing the tumor, pull back on the syringe, using the second finger of the hand holding the syringe, and direct the needle/syringe ±1 cm into the tumor, with the thumb and third finger. Pass the needle back and forth, deliberately but gently, five to six times in differing directions while maintaining traction on the syringe and stabilizing the tumor. There is no need to stab the tumor (*see* **Note 2**).

6. Release traction on the syringe *before* removing the needle/syringe.
7. Apply pressure to the area to minimize bruising. It is very important to minimize hematomata, as bruising makes repeat biopsies difficult and leads to inaccurate tumor sizing.
8. Aspirate 3 mL of the MEM/HEPES medium into the syringe, thereby dispersing the cells in suspension.
9. If snap-frozen material is required, remove an aliquot into a Nunc tube and snap freeze in liquid nitrogen as soon as possible.
10. FNA biopsies generally do not require dressings, but if the puncture wound continues to bleed, dress with an ordinary adhesive plaster.

3.2. Core-Cut/Trucut Biopsy

1. Place patient in the supine position on the examining couch, with the tumor exposed in the optimal position. This often requires the patient to roll partially on her side or to put her hands under her heads.
2. Clean the area with alcohol.
3. Draw up 2–5 mL of 1% lignocaine in a syringe (*see* **Note 3**).
4. Anesthetize the area. Most breast tumors lack pain receptors, but in a few instances, it may be necessary to anesthetize the tumor itself.
5. Make a 0.5-cm incision through the skin and subcutaneous tissue with the scalpel at the position at which the Trucut needle is to be inserted.
6. Prime the Trucut needle by pulling back twice as directed.
7. Insert needle into skin incision and advance until the outer edge of the tumor is felt as an area of gritty tissue; this is generally deeper than it appears. Fix the tumor relative to the breast by holding in place and fire the Trucut needle (*see* **Note 4**).
8. Withdraw Trucut needle and open to reveal specimen. Press firmly on biopsy site with gauze swabs for at least 5 min to minimize bruising. Occasionally, an arteriole might be transected. This bleeding responds to prolonged (±10 min) application of firm pressure and pressure bandaging. It is important to minimize hematomata, as bruising makes repeat biopsies difficult and leads to inaccurate tumor sizing.
9. Gently dislodge specimen with a needle tip into formalin (*see* **Note 5**) or Nunc tube. For snap freezing, drop Nunc tube into liquid nitrogen as soon as possible to preserve RNA.
10. Repeat Trucut procedure at least twice to maximize tumor collection and adequate tumor representation.
11. When finished, clean incision with alcohol and cover with adhesive bandage.
12. Exclude pneumothorax before discharging the patient. Advise patient to apply pressure in the event of bleeding, and that once the local anesthetic wears off, to take a mild analgesic.
13. Repeat/serial samples can usually be taken from the same place, if no excessive bruising has occurred at the site.

3.3. Sample Preparation

3.3.1. FNA Biopsy

The majority of repeat analyses are carried out on samples that have been transferred onto 3-aminopropyltriethoxysilane (APES)-coated slides by means of cytospinning. In general, FNA samples that are transferred directly from the syringe onto a slide and air-dried or fixed are not suitable for serial analyses, as the quantity of material obtained is not sufficient to allow multiple slides to be prepared from the material. Therefore, FNA samples are suspended in medium and transferred onto slides by means of cytospinning.

3.4. Slide Preparation Method

1. Assess the cellularity of the cell suspension by staining 10 μL of the sample with an equal volume of Trypan blue.
2. Aspirate sample using a 20-μL Gilson's pipet and place on hematocounter.
3. Apply cover slip to hematocounter.
4. Place hematocounter under light microscope and count all nine visible squares at a magnification of ×40.
5. Take the average number of cells per square and multiply by 10^4 for the estimated number of cells per milliliter of sample.
6. Discard acellular samples.
7. If there are less than 10,000 cells/mL, 300-μL aliquots will be required. If more than 10,000 cells/mL, aliquots of 100 μL will be required.
8. Set up cytospin: first the clip holder, then APES-coated slide, then filter paper, then cytospin chamber.
9. Pipet sample (100- or 300-μL aliquot as in **step 7**) into Shandon cytospin chamber and centrifuge at 500 rpm for 5 min.
10. Undo clip holder and separate slide with cytospin from clip holder and filter paper. Draw around the cytospin (on the back of the slide) with the diamond pencil.
11. Stain one slide with May–Grunwald–Giemsa (by inserting slide into stain diluted 1× for 30 s, and then air-dry) for cytodiagnosis, air-dry the remaining slides, and store packed in a slide box at −80°C for immunocytochemical analysis.

3.5. Analyses Undertaken With Each Type

3.5.1. Formalin-Fixed Samples

The majority of analyses carried out today can be done on formalin-fixed, paraffin wax-embedded samples (as described in Chapter 1, regarding general tissue handling and storage for details of this technique). This includes markers of cell proliferation (such as Ki67), markers of apoptosis (such as terminal deoxynucleotidyl transferase-mediated dUTP-biotin nick end labeling [TUNEL]/*in situ* end labeling [ISEL]), steroid hormone receptor measurement, and tyrosine kinase growth receptor measurement, e.g., c-ERBb1 and c-ERBb12. More-recent applications include construction of tissue arrays (*see* Chapter 4) (not to be confused with cDNA microarray, using mRNA derived from frozen tissue, *see* Chapters 27 and 28).

3.5.2. Snap-Frozen Samples

Before reliable, specific antibodies for estrogen receptor (ER), progesterone receptor (PgR), and MIB-1 became available, analyses for these factors could only be carried out on frozen samples. However, these techniques have in general been superseded by immunohistochemical methods, which are far easier to carry out, and have been shown to correlate well with the old, semiquantitative methods of analysis. However, frozen samples have become very important again with the advent of cDNA microarray technique (*ssee* Chapters 27 and 28).

3.5.3. Analyses

Once serial samples have been taken by any of the above mechanisms, they may be analyzed. A number of basic principles apply. A series of samples, taken from the same patient at different times, should be stained together in the same batch. They should be scored together, if possible, on the same occasion. They should be scored blind of treatment/time and should be scored by the same person. This minimizes avoidable error. However, the overall variability of this approach remains high, with paired core biopsies taken at the same time, from the same primary breast carcinoma giving a mean ± SD of the difference being 33 ± 16% for Ki67 and 38 ± 22% for apoptosis, respectively (*3*). In essence, this means that for an individual tumor, respective values must differ by at least 50% between two measurements for this difference to be considered statistically significant. Only like techniques should be compared (although, often, Trucut samples are compared with final excision samples). FNA, Trucut, and incision/excision biopsies all lend themselves to the following investigations. In general, cytospin preparations do not require microwaving for antigen retrieval.

3.6. Indices of Tumor Growth

3.6.1. Proliferation

Currently, this is most commonly assessed by immunohistochemical/immunocytochemical utilization of the MIB-1 MAb raised against a recombinant part of the Ki67 epitope (*10*) (*see* Chapter 15). The Ki67 antibody itself reacts with nuclear cell proliferation associated nonhistone proteins of 395 and 345 kDa, which are present in all active parts of the cell cycle (excluding G0 [*11*]). Immunohistochemical staining of frozen breast cancer sections with the Ki67 antibody has been shown to correlate with other established methods for determining proliferation, including flow cytometric measurement of S-phase fraction *(12)*, mitotic count *(13)*, and thymidine-labeling index. More recently, the technique of antigen retrieval by means of microwaving has allowed this technique to be applied successfully to paraffin-embedded samples *(14)*.

For FNA analyses, 100 cells per cytospin slide (provided the cell morphology is intact) has been accepted as sufficient *(1)*. A 90% cell loss during the cytospin process is to be expected. For Trucut and incision/excision biopsies, at least 1000 cells need to be counted *(3)*.

3.6.2. Apoptosis

There is no definitive method for generating an accurate, reproducible, and quantitative measure of cells undergoing apoptosis relative to their counterparts in malignant tissue in order to generate an apoptotic index. Methods include electron microscopy, light microscopy, ISEL and TUNEL, and flow cytometry (*see* Chapter 13). In paraffin-embedded sections, the TUNEL assay, which is based on incorporating biotinylated deoxyuridine at 3'-OH DNA strand breaks utilizing binding with terminal deoynucleotidyl transferase, has proven popular because of the availability of a kit form. An important point is that the necrotic cells, too, generate strand breaks that label positively; therefore, in paraffin-embedded tissues, concomitant morphological assessment is needed when analyzing the tissues. The low level of apoptotic bodies seen in histological samples indicates that at least 3000 cells must be counted.

The TUNEL technique together with flow cytometry may be used for FNA analyses *(15)*, but positively labeling necrotic cells cannot be visually distinguished, and the cutoff taken to define apoptotic and nonapoptotic cells without visual confirmation is unreliable. Cytospin preparations are not suitable for the determination of apoptotic indices because of the high degree of cell loss during preparation. In general, FNA biopsies are not ideal for measuring changes in apoptosis, and indirect measures, such as changes in the levels of the apoptosis regulatory genes *bcl-2* and *bax*, are preferable *(9)*.

3.6.3. Indices of Response/Resistance

Indices of endocrine responsiveness, such as ER (*see* Chapter 12), PgR, and presenilin 2, as well as endocrine resistance—for example, HER2 and epidermal growth factor receptor—are also easily measured in serial biopsies. However the majority of studies that have looked for changes have seen little or no alteration in these indices *(16–18)*, although a decrease in ER and rise in PgR after 14 d of primary tamoxifen therapy that was related to subsequent response has been reported *(1)*. In general, these markers are most commonly used as predictors of response or resistance to cytotoxic or endocrine therapy.

3.6.4. Future Applications

No single tumor marker has yet been shown to possess a sufficient predictive value to render it clinically useful. To achieve a greater predictive value, multiple markers need to be examined and correlated with the response of tumor cells to therapy. The development of cDNA microarray technology has provided such an opportunity. With this technology, it has been possible to identify new classes in breast cancer according to their gene expression patterns and link them with distinct clinical outcomes (19,20). The details of the techniques used are not within the scope of this chapter (but they are described in Chapters 27 and 28), but rely on the successful extraction of RNA from a biopsy, the creation of labeled cDNA from the RNA by reverse transcription-polymerase chain reaction, and the hybridization of the experimental cDNA with a known reference cDNA template (differentially labeled, usually with, e.g., a different-colored label). The annealing of the two strands then creates a hybridized profile that can be read from the relative labeling by means of a confocal microscope (i.e., genes from the experimental sample that match the reference sample are read as one color, but those that are proportionally increased/decreased are read as a different color). Thus, an immense number of genes may be examined simultaneously.

This technique holds out a great deal of promise. There are a number of limiting factors though: it is difficult to obtain adequate amounts of RNA (approx 0.5 μm of RNA) from FNA samples. Without amplification, approximately only 15% of FNA biopsies yield an adequate amount of material (21). However, after amplifying total RNA, at least one group of researchers has been able to identify candidate gene expression profiles that might distinguish tumors with complete response to cytotoxic chemotherapy from those that do not respond (22). Trucut and incision/excision biopsies (as well as FNA biopsies) have had to be stored in liquid nitrogen in order to preserve RNA, a major limiting factor. Recently, an approach to tissue handling by storage in the commercially available RNA*later*® (which does not require snap freezing and allows both the preservation of tissue architecture, as well as RNA preservation), has been developed (23). The hope is that this will facilitate the prospective collection of serial biopsies in large, international trials, which can then be analyzed by means of microarray for alterations in patterns of expression of multiple genes.

Finally, once potentially relevant cancer markers have been isolated by genomic or proteomic analysis, their diagnostic, prognostic, and therapeutic values can be evaluated by means of tissue microarray (tissue chips). These systems consist of small cylindrical section (600 μm in diameter, 5 μm thick) acquired from formalin-fixed tissues and arrayed on a glass slide and are described in Chapter 4. Typical tissue microarrays contain 500–1000 sections.

They are used in large-scale screening of tissue specimens for detection of DNA, RNA, and protein targets *(24)*. Provided at least two samples are tested, these small areas of sections give an adequate representation of the whole *(25)*, at least for ER, PgR, and HER2. Other markers still require validation. Within time, it is likely that these new techniques will become mainstays of serial biopsy assessment.

4. Notes

1. Local anesthesia is not absolutely necessary for FNA biopsy. Many patients find it a relatively atraumatic technique, although a not-insignificant minority find it very painful, and any anxious patient should be offered local anesthesia.
2. This is a difficult technique, which requires some practice (preferably, not initially on a patient) to perfect. In order to minimize cell loss and facilitate multiple sequential FNA samples, a technique using a 23-gage needle attached to a 7-mL vacuum bottle has been developed: insert needle into tumor and attach vacuum bottle. Because there is a vacuum, there is no need to exert traction, so merely pass the needle/bottle back and forth through the tumor. Remove the bottle *before* removing the needle from the tumor to preserve the vacuum in the bottle, and then insert the needle into the MEM/HEPES mixture, reattach the vacuum bottle, and allow the vacuum to draw up 3 mL of medium.
3. 2% Lignocaine may be used, but this concentration is not necessary and means that a smaller volume can be used, which can be a problem when a large area needs to be anesthetized.
4. Aim Trucut needle as parallel as possible to the ribcage so as to minimize the risk of pneumothorax.
5. There is no guaranteed method of telling if a biopsy specimen contains tumor material. Generally, if the specimen sinks in formalin, it is likely to contain tumor material, but this is not certain.

References

1. Makris, A., Powles, T. J., Allred, D. C., et al. (1998) Changes in hormone receptors and proliferation markers in tamoxifen treated breast cancer patients and the relationship with response. *Breast Cancer Res. Treat.* **48,** 11–20.
2. Ellis, P. A., Smith, I. E., McCarthy, K., Detre, S., Salter, J., and Dowsett, M. (1997) Preoperative chemotherapy induces apoptosis in early breast cancer. *Lancet* **349,** 849.
3. Ellis, P. A., Smith, I. E., Detre, S., et al. (1998) Reduced apoptosis and proliferation and increased Bcl-2 in residual breast cancer following preoperative chemotherapy. *Breast Cancer Res. Treat.* **48,** 107–116.
4. Wu, J., Ellis, P. A., Makris, A., Gregory, R. K., Powles, T. J., and Dowsett, M. (1996) Differences in ER, Ki67 and BCl2 expression in primary human breast cancer before and after treatment with neoadjuvant chemoendocrine therapy. *Breast Cancer Res. Treat.* **40,** 240.

5. Detre, S., Salter, J., Barnes, D. M., et al. (1999) Time-related effects of estrogen withdrawal on proliferation- and cell death-related events in MCF-7 xenografts. *Int. J. Cancer.* **81,** 309–113.

6. DeFriend, D. J., Howell, A., Nicholson, R. I., et al. (1994) Investigation of a new pure antiestrogen (ICI 182780) in women with primary breast cancer. *Cancer Res.* **54,** 408–414.

7. Dowsett, M., Dixon, J. M., Horgan, K., Salter, J., Hills, M., and Harvey, E. (2000) Antiproliferative effects of idoxifene in a placebo-controlled trial in primary human breast cancer. *Clin. Cancer Res.* **6,** 2260–2267.

8. Dowsett, M., Bundred, N. J., Decensi, A., et al. (2001) Effect of raloxifene on breast cancer cell Ki67 and apoptosis: a double-blind, placebo-controlled, randomized clinical trial in postmenopausal patients. *Cancer Epidemiol. Biomarkers Prev.* **10,** 961–966.

9. Chang, J., Powles, T. J., Allred, D. C., et al. (1999) Biologic markers as predictors of clinical outcome from systemic therapy for primary operable breast cancer. *J. Clin. Oncol.* **17,** 3058–3063.

10. Cattoretti, G., Becker, M. H., Key, G., et al. (1992) Monoclonal antibodies against recombinant parts of the Ki-67 antigen (MIB 1 and MIB 3) detect proliferating cells in microwave-processed formalin-fixed paraffin sections. *J. Pathol.* **168,** 357–363.

11. Gerdes, J., Schwab, U., Lemke, H., and Stein, H. (1983) Production of a mouse monoclonal antibody reactive with a human nuclear antigen associated with cell proliferation. *Int. J. Cancer* **31,** 13–20.

12. Walker, R. A. and Camplejohn, R. S. (1988) Comparison of monoclonal antibody Ki-67 reactivity with grade and DNA flow cytometry of breast carcinomas. *Br. J. Cancer* **57,** 281–283.

13. Isola, J., Kallioniemi, O. P., Korte, J. M., et al. (1990) Steroid receptors and Ki-67 reactivity in ovarian cancer and in normal ovary: correlation with DNA flow cytometry, biochemical receptor assay, and patient survival. *J. Pathol.* **162,** 295–301.

14. Pinder, S. E., Wencyk, P., Sibbering, D. M., et al. (1995) Assessment of the new proliferation marker MIB1 in breast carcinoma using image analysis: associations with other prognostic factors and survival. *Br. J. Cancer* **71,** 146–149.

15. Dowsett, M., Detre, S., Ormerod, M. G., et al. (1998) Analysis and sorting of apoptotic cells from fine-needle aspirates of excised human primary breast carcinomas. *Cytometry* **32,** 291–300.

16. Bottini, A., Berruti, A., Bersiga, A., et al. (1996) Effect of neoadjuvant chemotherapy on Ki67 labelling index, c-erbB-2 expression and steroid hormone receptor status in human breast tumours. *Anticancer Res.* **16,** 3105–3110.

17. Daidone, M. G., Silvestrini, R., Luisi, A., et al. (1995) Changes in biological markers after primary chemotherapy for breast cancers. *Int. J. Cancer* **61,** 301–35.

18. Frassoldati, A., Adami, F., Banzi, C., Criscuolo, M., Piccinini, L., and Silingardi, V. (1997) Changes of biological features in breast cancer cells determined by primary chemotherapy. *Breast Cancer Res. Treat.* **44,** 185–192.

19. Gruvberger, S., Ringner, M., Chen, Y., et al. (2001) Estrogen receptor status in breast cancer is associated with remarkably distinct gene expression patterns. *Cancer Res.* **61,** 5979–5984.
20. Sorlie, T., Perou, C. M., Tibshirani, R., et al. (2001) Gene expression patterns of breast carcinomas distinguish tumor subclasses with clinical implications. *Proc. Natl. Acad. Sci. USA.* **98,** 10,869–10,874.
21. Assersohn, L., Gangi, L., Zhao, Y., et al. (2002) The feasibility of using fine needle aspiration from primary breast cancers for cDNA microarray analyses. *Clin. Cancer Res.* **8,** 794–801.
22. Sotiriou, C., Powles, T. J., Dowsett, M., et al. (2002) Gene expression profiles derived from fine needle aspiration correlate with response to systemic chemotherapy in breast cancer. *Breast Cancer Res.* **4,** R:3.
23. Ellis, M., Davis, N., Coop, A., et al. (2002) Development and validation of a method for using breast core needle biopsies for gene expression microarray analyses. *Clin. Cancer Res.* **8,** 1155–1166.
24. Horvath, L. and Henshall, S. (2001) The application of tissue microarrays to cancer research. *Pathology* **33,** 125–129.
25. Camp, R. L., Charette, L. A., and Rimm, D. L. (2000) Validation of tissue microarray technology in breast carcinoma. *Lab. Invest.* **80,** 1943–1949.

4

Breast Tissue Microarrays

Robert J. Springall and Cheryl E. Gillett

Summary

Tissue microarrays have been used effectively to study representative tissue from large groups of patients, with minimal technical and reagent costs. The construction of these arrays may appear complex, but with the use of a semiautomated tissue arrayer and a degree of manual dexterity, symmetrical, high-density arrays can be produced. Here, we highlight where problems in the construction, cutting, and evaluation of tissue microarrays can occur and how these can be prevented.

Key Words: Tissue microarrays; breast; technique; high-throughput; donor-block; recipient-block.

1. Introduction

1.1. Background

The development and application of tissue microarray (TMA) technology has been rapid since the initial concept was brought to our attention less than 7 yr ago *(1)*. The original multiblock, used by many immunohistochemists to test out new antibodies, usually contained up to about eight pieces of tissue; however, this has been taken to another level with the advent of TMAs.

The idea of using TMAs is to have a system in which a particular molecule of interest can be evaluated in a large number of different tissues but with minimal use of reagents and technical time—a high-throughput facility. The volume of data already published is testament to the value of using this approach.

A paraffin wax TMA is a block containing multiple plugs of tissue that have been removed, or "cored," from different whole or donor paraffin-wax blocks (often those used for diagnosis). Whereas it is possible to make TMAs manually, there are automated and semiautomated methods available. These enable a core of tissue to be removed from the donor block and immediately placed in

From: *Methods in Molecular Medicine, Vol. 120: Breast Cancer Research Protocols*
Edited by: S. A. Brooks and A. L. Harris © Humana Press Inc., Totowa, NJ

a premade hole in the array or recipient block, creating a symmetrical array. The manual tissue arrayer (MTA)-1 from Beecher Instruments (Sun Prairie, WI) was the first generally available and continues, along with the more sophisticated MTA-2, to be a popular choice.

1.2. TMA Core Size

A TMA can be designed to have different numbers of tissue cores and is dependent on the diameter of the tissue core required. If a 0.6-mm core is used, then the array can consist of up to 1000 cores, whereas, if a larger, 1.5-mm is used, then the array is reduced to 84 cores. There has been considerable debate over the most appropriate diameter of the sampling core and how representative this is of the tissue, but this is, of course, related to its degree of heterogeneity *(2,3)*. Potential problems associated with heterogeneity can be overcome in some respects by having more than one core of tissue from the donor block in each TMA. However, the literature shows that even a single 0.6-mm core can be representative in 95–97% of cases, although this does depend on the expression profile of the molecule being assessed *(4)*.

1.3. TMA Type

Before TMAs are constructed, thought must be given to what material is to be used. This might seem obvious, but the TMA must reflect the focus of the study. For example, with breast tissue, it may be appropriate to have TMAs of consecutive tumor cases if prognostic studies are the main theme of research. Other options might be to classify by histological type/grade, by type of adjuvant treatment, or by disease progression when tissue from normal, primary tumor, and subsequent metastases are included in the array. TMAs specifically for testing new antibodies or probes may also be prepared that consist of a mixture of different benign and malignant breast pathologies.

1.4. Advantages of TMAs

The TMA is not only of value in allowing large numbers of tissue to be assessed using very few sections. Fewer sections mean that the costs associated with the purchase of reagents and in particular, technical time, can be reduced considerably (duplicate samples from 400 whole sections can be reduced to 10 TMA sections). Another advantage is consistency in assay. For example, if the sections are being used with immunohistochemistry (*see* Chapter 15), then all "staining" can be done in a single run, negating any interbatch variability.

TMA can be used with any technique applicable to paraffin wax material. It has a use with immunohistochemistry (*see* Chapter 15), *in situ* hybridization, and fluorescence *in situ* hybridization (*see* Chapters 20, 22, and 23) *(5,6)*. Some groups have even developed frozen tissue TMAs (cryoarrays), using optimal cutting temperature compound to create an array "block," thus overcoming the problems associated with loss of antigenicity and RNA detection in paraffin wax material *(7,8)*.

1.5. TMA Assessment

Accurate documentation of the location of the cores within the TMA is paramount, and it is advisable to either purchase or devise a computer template that can be used when the TMA is being constructed and to assist with subsequent analysis. As the TMA has a symmetrical appearance, it is vital that it always be oriented in the same way, preferably when the section is picked up onto the slide. Ideally, a control core of easily identifiable material should be placed in one corner of the array, or alternatively, orientation cores may be placed outside the main array. Whichever method is chosen should be employed consistently.

TMAs are examined by initially locating the "control" core and traversing the slide by either column or row. If the array is not completely in line on the slide, gridlines may be drawn on the cover slip to aid assessment and to avoid skipping misaligned cores.

There is now TMA evaluation software available for image analysis systems, which "superimpose" a grid over the section. This allows the system to recognize that a core is missing or folded but is still dependent on the reasonably accurate alignment of the section on the slide.

2. Materials

2.1. Identifying Donor Tissue

1. Hematoxylin and eosin (H&E)-stained sections and corresponding wax-embedded tissue blocks.

2.2. Preparation of Recipient Block

1. Paraffin wax.
2. 37 × 24-mm metal-base mold.
3. Plastic tissue cassette.

2.3. Tissue Arrayer

Many laboratories use one of the specifically designed arrayers from Beecher Instruments. The size of punch is dependent on the heterogeneity of the tissue being sampled. For breast tissue work, punches ranging between 0.6 and 1.5 mm in diameter have been used. A 1.5-mm punch gives good representation of tumor tissue.

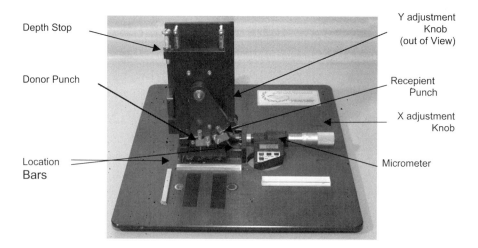

Fig. 1. Manual Tissue Arrayer-1 (Beecher Instruments).

3. Methods
3.1. Identifying Donor Tissue

1. For each case, retrieve the H&E-stained sections from files to determine which block(s) contains(s) the most representative area of tissue.
2. Using the H&E staining as a guide, retrieve the "best" tumor block from files, taking into account tumor size and block thickness (*see* **Note 1**). For small or heterogeneous tumors, the most appropriate areas should be marked on the cover slip to aid location on the donor block.

3.2. Preparation of Recipient Block

1. Create the array or recipient block simply by pouring molten wax into a large, metal-base mold (37 × 24 mm), clearly labeled with a plastic tissue cassette (*see* **Note 2**).

3.3. Tissue Arrayer

Figure 1 shows an annotated illustration of the Beecher MTA-1.

1. Screw the recipient block into the tissue arrayer metal holder, making sure the block is perfectly level and taking care not to overtighten, as this may cause the block to crack.
2. Position the block in its holder against the location bars and make certain it is securely held in position by the magnets (**Fig. 2A**).
3. Align the right-sided, smaller recipient punch to a corner of the block using the X and Y adjustment knobs. The first hole should be at least 4 mm from the long and short edges of the block.

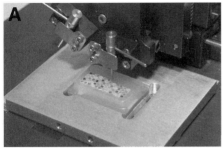

Alignment of recipient punch on array block

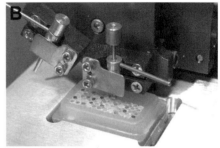

Punch lowered to cut core of wax

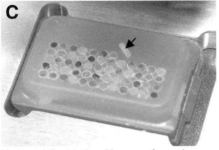

New recipient hole with core of wax (arrowed)

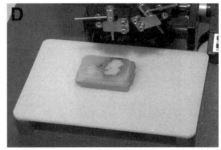

Positioning of donor-bridge and block above recipient block

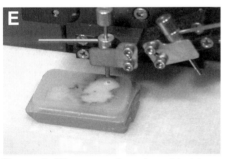

Removal of tissue core from donor block

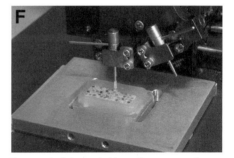

Removal of donor-bridge allows core of tissue to be lowered driectly into recipient hole

Fig. 2. Tissue microarray production.

4. At this point, set the micrometers to "0."
5. Adjust the depth stop so a core of approx 4–5 mm is removed.
6. Push the punch down until the correct depth is reached and rotate the punch to assist the removal of the core. Release the pressure, and the springs will remove the punch from the block (*see* **Fig. 2B**).
7. Using the stylet, push out the core of wax and dispose (*see* **Fig. 2C**).

8. Flick the punch turret to the left so that the slightly larger donor punch is in the vertical position.

9. Place the donor block bridge and the block to be cored over the recipient block and holder.

10. Referring to the H&E stained reference slide, align the corresponding tissue block so that the selected area is directly below the donor punch (*see* **Fig. 2D**).

11. Holding the block firmly, push the punch into the block to a depth of 4–5 mm. (**Note:** the depth stop cannot be used at this stage). Again, rotate the punch to assist the removal of the tissue (*see* **Fig. 2E**).

12. Release the punch from the block and remove the block bridge and donor block.

13. Push the punch down until it is just above the recipient block, and then push the stylet down so that the core of tissue enters the hole created by the smaller punch (*see* **Fig. 2F**).

14. Ensure that the core is firmly pushed to bottom of hole (*see* **Note 2**).

15. Carefully record the identifying number of the block cored on a designated tissue array template.

16. Move the turret along the long axis, using the X coarse feed knob to a distance of 0.250 mm on the micrometer.

17. Repeat **steps 9–18** until a row of cores has been inserted into the recipient block.

18. Move the turret; using the Y coarse feed 0.250 mm on the micrometer and continue coring back along the block as before.

19. Continue inserting tissue cores in this way until the block is full. Make certain that one of the corners has a core that is not breast tissue for orientation purposes. The block may have a domed appearance at this stage.

20. Remove block from holder and heat block in a 60°C oven for 3 min. This melts the wax slightly between the tissue core and donor block, allowing them to amalgamate into a single block when the wax cools.

21. While the wax is still soft, firmly press a glass slide against the block surface to flatten it and fix the cores of tissue in the block.

22. Sections can be cut from the block in the standard way (*see* **Note 3**). Initially, an H&E-stained section should be done to ensure that all cores appear (*see* **Fig. 3**).

23. The type of slide used to pick up the array section will depend on the subsequent technique.

4. Notes

1. A new H&E-stained section may need to be cut from a block if further sections have been cut and the block face no longer closely resembles the original H&E-stained section.

2. The pressure of the punch going into the recipient block can cause the wax to crack (particularly at the edges) or fall off. This damage can be minimized if the recipient block is discarded if there are any imperfections in it before "coring" and also by making sure that the back of the cassette is filled with wax to give additional support.

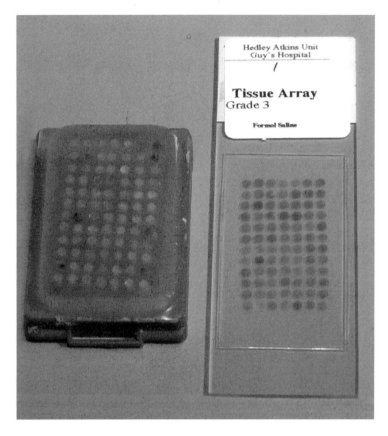

Fig. 3. Tissue microarray with corresponding H&E staining.

3. If the tissue in the donor block is very thin, then cores of tissue can be stacked on top of each other in the recipient block.
4. Occasionally, individual cores will curl before floating out on a water bath. However, this should not be a problem to an experienced microtomist, who would ensure that the block is very cold and a new blade is used.

References

1. Kononen, J., Bubendorf, L., Kallioniemi, A., et al. (1998) Tumour microarrays for high-throughput molecular profiling of tumor specimens. *Nat. Med.* **4,** 844–847.
2. Gillett, C. E., Springall, R. J., Barnes, D. M., and Hanby, A. M. (2000) Multiple tissue core arrays in histopathology research: a validation study. *J. Pathol.* **192,** 549–553.
3. Camp, R. L., Charette, L. A., and Rimm, D. L. (2000) Validation of tissue microarray technology in breast carcinoma. *Lab. Invest.* **80,** 1943–1949.

4. Zhang, D., Salto-Tellez, M., Putti, T. C., Do, E., and Koay, E. S. (2003) Reliability of tissue microarrays in detecting protein expression and gene amplification in breast cancer. *Mod. Pathol.* **16,** 79–84.
5. Anderson, C. L., Hostetter, G., Grigoryan, A., Sauter, G., and Kallioniemi, A. (2001) Improved procedure for fluorescence in situ hybridization on tissue microarrays. *Cytometry* **45,** 83–86.
6. Nocito, A., Kononen, J., Kallioniemi, O. P., and Sauter, G. (2001) Tissue microarrays (TMAs) for high-throughput molecular pathology research. *Int. J. Cancer* **94,** 1–5.
7. Hoos, A. and Cordon-Cardo, C. (2001) Tissue microarray profiling of cancer specimens and cell lines: opportunities and limitations. *Lab. Invest.* **81,** 1331–1338.
8. Fejzo, M. S. and Slamon, D. J. (2001) Frozen tumor tissue microarray technology for analysis of tumor RNA, DNA, and proteins. *Am. J. Pathol.* **159,** 1645–1650.

5

Preparation of Tumor Homogenates for Subsequent Preparation of Cytosols, Membrane Fractions, RNA, and DNA

Naomi Robertson and Russell Leek

Summary

This chapter outlines methods for the preparation of several different cellular fractions from whole samples of tumor and normal tissue.

Key Words: Cytosol; membrane fraction; tumor homogenate; HEPES.

1. Introduction

This protocol enables the investigator to prepare several different cellular fractions from a single tumor sample (or corresponding normal tissue). This is particularly important if tumor samples are small or difficult to obtain in large numbers.

If an RNA sample is to be prepared from a tumor homogenate, it is very important to take appropriate precautions at the start of this procedure to avoid contamination by ribonucleases (*see* Chapter 6 for details).

2. Materials

1 Stock 4-2-hydroxyethyl-1-piperazineethanesulfonic acid (HEPES) and ethylenediaminetetraacetic acid ([EDTA] HE) buffer: 20 mM of HEPES and 1.5 mM of EDTA. Add 1.5 mL of 0.5 M EDTA and 100 mL of 5X HEPES (100 mM) to a 500-mL measuring cylinder. Add enough distilled water to make 500 mL. Store at room temperature (remains stable for months.) Add the following to 50 mL of stock HE buffer: 0.5 mL of benzamidine (50 mM), 0.5 mL of phenylmethyl-sulphonyl fluoride (50 mM), and 50 μL of ovomucoid (1 mg/mL). Prepare on the day needed and keep on ice.

From: *Methods in Molecular Medicine, Vol. 120: Breast Cancer Research Protocols*
Edited by: S. A. Brooks and A. L. Harris © Humana Press Inc., Totowa, NJ

2. Dithiothreitol. Dissolve in distilled water to give 200 mM (100X stock solution). Aliquot into 2-mL Eppendorf tubes and store at –20°C.
3. Benzamidine. 50 mM solution in 100% ethanol. Store at –20°C.
4. Phenylmethylsulfonyl fluoride. 50 mM solution in 100% ethanol. Store at –20°C.
5. Ovomucoid (trypsin inhibitor). Prepare 1 mg/mL in distilled water, aliquot into Eppendorf tubes, and store at –20°C.
6. Tris-buffered saline. 100 mM of Tris-HCl (pH 7.5), 0.9% (150 mM) of NaCl. Store up to several months at 4°C.
7. Pestle and mortar.
8. Liquid nitrogen.
9. Scalpel.
10. Fine forceps.
11. Tissue homogenizer (Ultra Turrax or Polytron).

3. Methods

1. Carry out all procedures on ice.
2. Remove tumor vial from liquid nitrogen and place contents in Petri dish (*see* **Note 1**). Allow frozen sample to warm up slightly (20–30 s at room temperature) to make cutting easier. Hold the sample with forceps and chop up as small as possible using a scalpel.
3. Chill the pestle and mortar with liquid nitrogen. Transfer the chopped tissue into the chilled mortar using the scalpel. Add liquid nitrogen to the mortar to refreeze the chopped tissue. Crush to a powder-like consistency with the pestle, holding a paper towel above the mortar to prevent loss of sample (*see* **Note 2**).
4. Divide the frozen powder into two roughly equal piles. Dispense one into a preweighed, 50-mL Falcon tube and immediately reweigh the tube. Calculate the weight of the pulverized sample and add 20 volumes of cold HE buffer (or 4 mL, if the tumor weight is 0.2 g or less). Shake to disperse the contents. This sample may be processed further to extract DNA, cytosols, and membranes.
5. The other pile of crushed tumor may be dispensed into another 50-mL Falcon tube containing an appropriate volume of denaturing solution (*see* **step 8**). Shake to disperse. This sample can be processed further to extract RNA.
6. Samples in HE buffer: wash the homogenizer twice with distilled water before initial homogenization and between each sample. Homogenize samples on ice with a 10-s burst using an Ultra Turrax (or Polytron), and then allow 60 s of cooling. Repeat twice.
7. Centrifuge the homogenates in HE buffer at 1800g at 2°C for 10 min. Remove the supernatant into ultracentrifuge tubes using disposable transfer pipettes, taking care to avoid any floating lipid. Take up the pellet (largely containing nuclei and cellular debris) in a small volúme of HE buffer and store at –80°C or below. This sample may be further processed to yield DNA.
8. The cytosols and membranes are then separated by ultracentrifugation. Balance pairs of tubes by weighing (add HE buffer to tubes, if necessary). The supernatant is centrifuged at 100,000g) for 44 min at 4°C.

9. The supernatant (cytosol preparation) is transferred into a 14-mL Falcon tube, avoiding any floating lipid. Add 100% dithiothretol concentrate to cystol to give a final concentration of 2 mM. Cytosol samples should be stored at –80°C or below. (These samples are suitable for measurement of estrogen receptor by enzyme-linked immunosorbent assay.)

10. The membrane fraction (pellet after ultracentrifugation) is resuspended in either 1 or 1.5 mL (depending on size of pellet) of cold Tris-buffered saline. Resuspension is made complete by homogenization in a glass–glass homogenizer. Transfer final sample into cryovials and store at –80°C or below.

4. Notes

1. Larger tumor samples can be quite difficult to remove from cryovials while still frozen. Brief warming of the vial in your hand will normally allow the outer portion of the sample to thaw sufficiently to permit forceps to be slid into the vial. Gentle twisting of the forceps should then enable removal of the sample.

2. It is important at this stage that the chopped tissue is frozen, as this will help the formation of a fine powder and minimize degradation of proteins. However, tumor samples vary greatly in their consistency and the ease at which this can be achieved. Some pieces may be extremely hard to crush because of calcification and will have a tendency to fly out of the mortar if it is not covered.

6

Isolation of RNA From Tumor Samples

Single-Step Guanidinium Acid–Phenol Method

Naomi Robertson and Russell Leek

Summary

The guanidinium acid–phenol method of RNA extraction is relatively fast (4 h) and is useful for the processing of large numbers of samples, without the need for ultracentrifugation. This protocol produces total RNA that includes ribosomal, transfer, and messenger RNA.

This high-quality RNA is suitable for Northern blot analysis, dot-blot hybridization, poly (A) RNA selection, in vitro translation, cDNA library construction, reverse transcriptase-polymerase chain reaction, ribonuclease protection assay, and primer extension experiments.

Key Words: RNA isolation; guanidinium acid–phenol; total RNA.

1. Introduction

This single-step method isolates undegraded RNA from tissues (or cells) in 4 h. It can be used to process a large number of samples, without the need for ultracentrifugation *(1,2)*. It is based on the property of RNA to remain water soluble in a solution containing 4 *M* of guanidinium thiocyanate (pH 4.0) in the presence of a phenol/chloroform organic phase. In acidic conditions such as these, most proteins and small fragments of DNA (50 bases to 10 kb) are in the organic phase, whereas larger fragments of DNA and some proteins remain in the interphase.

This protocol produces total RNA, which contains ribosomal RNA, messenger RNA (mRNA), and transfer RNA (if purified mRNA is required another technique must be used). Isolation of intact RNA is critical for the conversion of mRNA to complementary DNA and ultimately, for the identification of protein-coding genes. High-quality intact RNA can be used for various molecular biology purposes, including Northern blot analysis, dot-blot hybridization, poly (A) RNA selection, in vitro translation, complementary DNA library construc-

From: *Methods in Molecular Medicine, Vol. 120: Breast Cancer Research Protocols*
Edited by: S. A. Brooks and A. L. Harris © Humana Press Inc., Totowa, NJ

tion (described in Chapters 27 and 28), reverse transcriptase-polymerase chain reaction, ribonuclease protection assay (described in Chapter 24), and primer extension experiments.

The main reason for failure in any attempt to produce RNA is contamination by ribonuclease. Most ribonucleases are very stable and active enzymes that require no cofactors to function and a small amount of RNase in an RNA preparation will create a real problem. Therefore, it is very important to take appropriate precautions in order to avoid contamination (*see* **Subheading 2.**). Wear gloves at all times when working with RNA solutions, as hands are a likely source of ribonuclease contamination.

2. Materials

1. Glassware/ceramics: double wrap in foil and bake at 300°C for 4 h.
2. Plastics are assumed to be free from contamination if taken straight from the package and are untouched by human hands. NaOH can be used to decontaminate effectively other plastics/materials. Soak apparatus in NaOH solution (40 g/L) overnight, and then rinse very thoroughly several times with deionized water to remove any traces.
3. Solutions: water or salt solutions used in RNA preparation should be treated with the chemical diethylpyrocarbonate (DEPC). This chemical inactivates ribonucleases by covalent modification. However, solutions containing Tris-HCl cannot be effectively treated with DEPC, as Tris-HCl will react with and inactivate it. Add 0.2 mL of DEPC to 100 mL of solution to be treated. Shake vigorously to get the DEPC into solution. Autoclave the solution to inactivate the remaining DEPC (*see* **Note 1**).
4. Denaturing solution: dissolve 250 g guanidinium thiocyanate in 293 mL of distilled water. Add 17.6 mL of 0.75 M sodium citrate (pH 7.0), heat gently, and stir while adding 26.4 mL of 10% sarcosyl. This solution can be stored in the dark at 4°C for up to 3 mo. On the day of the experiment, add 360 µL of 2-mercaptoethanol to 50 mL of the above solution.
5. 2 M Sodium acetate: add 16.42 g of sodium acetate (anhydrous) to 40 mL of water and 35 mL of glacial acetic acid. Adjust the pH of the solution to 4.0 with glacial acetic acid and increase the final volume to 100 mL with distilled water.
6. Water-saturated phenol:dissolve 100 g phenol crystals in water at 60–65°C. Aspirate the upper water phase and store up to 1 mo at 4°C. **Caution:** phenol is a poison and causes burns. It should be disposed of appropriately.
7. Chloroform.
8. Isopropanol (propan-2-ol).
9. 70% Ethanol (made with DEPC water).
10. Electrophoresis-grade agarose.
11. 1X Tris-borate–ethylenediaminetetraacetic acid ([EDTA] TBE).10X TBE stock: 108 g of Tris base, 55 g of boric acid, 40 mL of 0.5 M EDTA (pH 8.0), water to 1 L.
12. Ethidium bromide (**Caution:** ethidium bromide is toxic, handle with care).

13. Ficoll EDTA (10X stock): 20 g of Ficoll, 1 g of sodium dodecyl sulfate , 25 g of bromophenol blue, 20 mL of 0.5 *M* EDTA [pH 8.09], water to 100 mL.
14. 70% Ethylhydroxide.
15. 1% Agarose gel: dissolve 0.6 g agarose in TBE and add 0.5 μg ethidium bromide per milliliter of gel.
16. Ficoll-EDTA loading dye for agarose electrophoresis: 10X stock: 20 g Ficoll, 1 g of SDS, 25 g of bromophenol blue, 20 mL of 0.5 *M* EDTA (pH 8.0), and water to make up to 100 mL.

3. Methods

Always wear gloves. Keep samples on ice whenever possible.

1. Transfer approx 1 g of pulverized tissue to a 50-mL Falcon tube containing 10 mL ice-cold denaturing solution and homogenize using three 10-s bursts with an Ultra-Turrax® T-25 homogenizer while tube is in a container of ice (*see* **Note 2**), waiting 60 s between each burst. Wash the homogenizer twice with distilled water and once with denaturing solution before initial homogenization and between samples. After use, wash homogenizer twice with water and once with methanol.
2. Add 1 mL 2 *M* sodium acetate (pH 4.0) to the tumor homogenates in denaturing solution and mix.
3. Add 10 mL phenol (in fume hood) and mix.
4. Add 2 mL chloroform (in fume hood) and vortex for 15–20 s. Leave on ice for 15 min (avoid keeping samples in denaturing solution for more than 30 min in total).
5. Transfer to sterile, disposable, round-bottomed polypropylene tubes with caps. Centrifuge for 15 min at 20,000*g* at 2°C. Transfer carefully the upper aqueous phase containing the RNA to a new tube and note volume. Avoid transferring any of the interphase (*see* **Note 3**). Add equal volume of isopropanol and mix.
6. Incubate for 1 h at –20°C.
7. Centrifuge as in **step 5**. Discard supernatant.
8. Add 3 mL denaturing solution and 3 mL isopropanol. Mix and incubate for 1 h at –20°C (*see* **Note 4**).
9. Centrifuge. Discard supernatant.
10. Add 6 mL of 70% ethyl hydroxide and mix. Centrifuge.
11. Remove all but 1 mL of ethyl hydroxide. Resuspend pellet and transfer to an Eppendorf tube. Spin down in refrigerated microfuge (or cold room) at 21,000*g* for 2 min.
12. Remove remaining ethanol with pipet tip. If necessary, spin again and remove final drop with a P2/P20 pipet tip.
13. Air-dry RNA pellets (*see* **Note 5**). Redissolve in DEPC water (approx 50–100 μL, but vary according to pellet size).
14. Determining RNA concentration and purity. Using a spectrophotometer, measure the optical density at 260 and 280 nm by diluting a small sample of RNA in DEPC

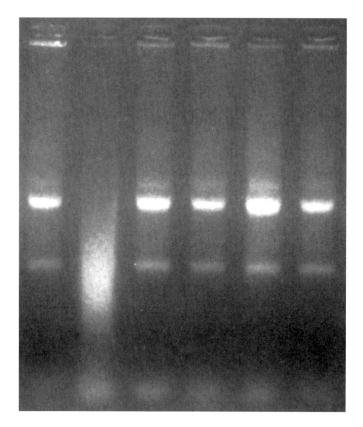

Fig. 1. Isolation of RNA from tumor samples, confirmation of RNA integrity. This is a photograph of an agarose gel demonstrating the two bands corresponding to the 28S and 18S ribosomes, and the 4S to 5S band containing a mix of transfer RNA and 5S ribosomal RNA. The sample in lane 2 has degraded and shows characteristic smearing.

water. For RNA, an optical density at 260 nm = concentration of 40 µg/mL. Therefore, optical density at 260 nm × 40 × dilution factor = concentration of RNA in µg/mL. Ideally, the concentration should be around 1 µg/µL. The absorbance ratio at A_{260}/A_{280} gives an indication of the purity of the RNA (ideally, 1.6–2.0).

15. Integrity of the isolated RNA can be checked by agarose gel electrophoresis (**Fig. 1**). Separation of 2 µg of RNA sample on a 1% agarose gel containing ethidium bromide should yield three definite bands: the 28S (4.7 kb) and 18S (1.9 kb) ribosomal RNA, and 4S to 5S (0.10–0.15 kb) RNA containing a mix of transfer RNA and 5S ribosomal RNA. Degraded RNA will appear as a smear (*see* **Note 6**). Prepare a 1% agarose gel in TBE, adding 0.5 µg ethidium bromide per milliliter of gel. (This intercalates with RNA and will allow visualization of the RNA under ultraviolet light.) Add 2 µg of RNA to 20 µL of DEPC water. Add 4 µL of Ficoll-EDTA loading dye to each sample. Run gel at 80 V for approx 2 h.

16. RNA samples can be stored at –70°C, or in liquid nitrogen, for several years without degradation of RNA. Repeated freezing and thawing of samples is not recommended, although the RNA should remain robust as long as it does not become contaminated on thawing.

4. Notes

1. Many investigators keep the solutions that they use for RNA work completely separate to ensure that they do not become contaminated by "dirty" pipets.
2. Use approx 1 mL of denaturing solution for every 100 mg of tissue. Complete homogenization of the sample is crucial to obtain a large amount of high-quality RNA that is free from proteins and DNA contaminants. Once homogenized, it is possible to store samples in this form in a –80°C freezer for processing at a later date.
3. Most proteins and small fragments of DNA (50 bases to 10 kb) will be found in the organic phase, whereas larger ones and some proteins remain in the interphase.
4. Samples may be left for several days at the –20°C steps.
5. Air-dry pellets. Do not use a speed vacuum for drying the pellet. Leaving the tube open on the bench for 10 min is normally sufficient. Do not let the pellet dry out completely, as this will decrease its solubility; however, remove as much ethanol as possible.
6. The single-step guanidinium acid–phenol method has become the basis for numerous commercial reagents claiming to isolate total RNA from various tissues and cells in 1–4 h, using a single solution of phenol, guanidinium thiocyanate, buffer, and detergents. We have used TRI Reagent (product number T9424; Sigma-Aldrich, Dorsett, UK) and found comparable RNA yields and purity to that obtained using this method.

References

1. Chomczynski, P. and Sacchi, N. (1987) Single-step method of RNA isolation by acid guanidinium thiocyanate-phenol-chloroform extraction. *Anal. Biochem.* **162,** 156–159.
2. Kingston, R. E., Chomczynski, P., and Sacchi, N. (1991) Guanidinium methods for total RNA preparation, in *Current Protocols in Molecular Biology* (Ausubel, F. M., Brent, R., Kingston, R. E., et al., eds.) Wiley, New York, NY, (Suppl 14), pp. 4.2.1–4.2.8.

7

Isolation of DNA From Tumor Samples

Naomi Robertson and Russell Leek

Summary

A method for producing high-molecular-weight DNA from pulverized tissue, nuclear fractions, or cultured cells. This isolation method relies on the powerful proteolytic activity of proteinase K combined with the denaturing ability of the ionic detergent sodium dodecyl sulfate. Ethylenediaminetetraacetic acid is included in the lysis buffer to inhibit DNases.

Key Words: DNA isolation; pulverized tissue; nuclear fractions; proteinase K; SDS.

1. Introduction

This method is suitable for preparing DNA from cultured cells, pulverized tissue or from a "nuclei" fraction prepared as described in Chapter 5.

There are a number of different procedures for the preparation of high-molecular-weight genomic DNA. They all rely on some form of cell lysis, followed by deproteination and recovery of DNA. The isolation procedure described here is relatively brief and relies on the powerful proteolytic activity of proteinase K combined with the denaturing ability of the ionic detergent sodium dodecyl sulfate (SDS). Ethylenediaminetetraacetic acid (EDTA) is included in the lysis buffer to inhibit DNases.

2. Materials

1. Lysis buffer: 10 mM Tris-HCl (pH 8.0), 100 mM EDTA (pH 8.0), 0.5% SDS.
2. DNase-free RNase A.
3. Proteinase K.
4. Phenol.
5. Phenol/chloroform/isoamyl alcohol mixture (25:24:1).
6. Chloroform/isoamyl alcohol (25:1).
7. 3 M Sodium acetate (pH 5.2).
8. 100% Ethanol.

From: *Methods in Molecular Medicine, Vol. 120: Breast Cancer Research Protocols*
Edited by: S. A. Brooks and A. L. Harris © Humana Press Inc., Totowa, NJ

9. 70% Ethanol.
10. Tris-HCl/EDTA buffer: 10 m*M* Tris-HCl (pH 7.4, 7.5, or 8.0), 1 m*M* EDTA (pH 8.0).
11. Ficoll EDTA (10X stock): 20 g of Ficoll, 1 g of SDS, 25 g of bromophenol blue, 20 mL of 0.5 M EDTA (pH 8.0), water to make 100 mL.
12. Agarose gel for electrophoresis: 0.3% agarose in Tris-borate/EDTA (0.2 g agarose in 60 mL of Tris-borate/EDTA), add 0.5 μg ethidium bomide per milliliter of gel.

3. Methods

1. Resuspend pulverized tissue or "nuclei" pellet in approx 10X the volume of lysis buffer.
2. Add DNase-free RNase A to a final concentration of 20 μg/mL, followed by incubation at 37°C for 30 min.
3. Add proteinase K to a final concentration of 100 μg/mL and incubate overnight at 37°C.
4. Add an equal volume of phenol and gently extract by inverting the tube several times (do *not* vortex). Centrifuge the mixture at 800*g* for 10 min.
5. Remove the aqueous phase and add to it an equal volume of phenol/chloroform/ isoamyl alcohol mixture (25:24:1). Gently extract as in **step 4** and centrifuge at 800*g* for 10 min (*see* **Note 1**).
6. Repeat **step 5**.
7. Aspirate the aqueous phase and add 1/10 the volume of 3 *M* of sodium acetate (pH 5.2) and 2.5X the volume of ice-cold 100% ethanol (calculated after the salt addition; *see* **Note 2**).
8. Freeze at −20°C overnight.
9. The following day, centrifuge the solution at 800*g* for 10 min and wash the resulting precipitate in 70% ethanol (*see* **Note 3**).
10. Air-dry the pellet for 10 min at room temperature.
11. Resuspend the DNA pellet in 20–50 μL of water and quantify spectrophotometri- cally. Alternatively, dissolve in Tris-HCl/EDTA buffer, pH 8.0, if it is going to be stored indefinitely. DNA will remain stable at 4°C for an indefinite period (*see* **Note 4**).
12. Determining DNA concentration and purity: using a spectrophotometer, measure the optical density at 260 and 280 nm by diluting a small sample of DNA in water. For DNA, an optical density at 260 nm equates to a concentration of 50 μg/mL. Therefore, optical density at 260 nm × 50× dilution factor = concen- tration of DNA in μg/mL.
13. Agarose gel electrophoresis can be used to check for the presence of high- molecular-weight DNA. Prepare a 0.3% agarose gel in Tris-borate/EDTA, add- ing 0.5 μg of ethidium bromide per milliliter of gel. Add 1 μg of DNA to 20 μL water. Add 4 μL of Ficoll EDTA loading dye to each sample. Running a sample of λDNA at the same time will enable some estimate of size of the DNA obtained (*see* **Note 5**). Run gel at approx 1 V/cm for approx 2 h.

4. Notes

1. Failure of the organic phase to separate cleanly from the aqueous phase is generally because of a very high concentration of DNA and/or cellular debris in the aqueous phase. Dilution with more lysis buffer and re-extraction may solve this.

2. After the addition of the sodium acetate/ethanol mix, the DNA should precipitate in long, stringy fibers. If there is no precipitate or if the precipitate is flocculent, the DNA is either degraded or not purified away from the cellular debris. This may be because of improper handling of the tissue before digestion or too much tissue in the lysis step.

3. It is very important to rinse the pellet well at this stage to remove residual salt and phenol. In addition, the DNA pellet will not stick well to the walls of the tube after the 70% ethanol wash, and care must be taken to avoid aspirating the pellet out of the tube.

4 Large quantities of DNA may require vortexing and brief heating (5 min at 65°C) to resuspend. High-molecular-weight genomic DNA may require one to several days to dissolve and should be shaken gently (not vortexed) to avoid shearing, particularly if it is to be used for applications requiring high-molecular-weight DNA. Gentle shaking on a rotating platform or a rocking apparatus is recommended.

5. Molecular-weight markers. Among the samples loaded onto a gel, at least one lane should contain a series of DNA fragments of known sizes to allow estimation of the approximate size of unknown DNA fragments. The most commonly used molecular-weight markers are restriction digests of phage λDNA or, for smaller fragments, the plasmid pBR322. Many commercial preparations of molecular-weight markers are also available. These products usually cover a wide range of DNA sizes.

8

Laser-Assisted Microdissection and Isolation of DNA and RNA

Ulrich Lehmann and Hans Kreipe

Summary

One of the major challenges in molecular analysis of breast cancer specimens is tissue heterogeneity. The admixture of contaminating bystander cells might distort the results of quantitative molecular analyses. Therefore, pure tumor cell populations have to be isolated in order to obtain reliable molecular data.

In this chapter, we present protocols for the laser-assisted microdissection of breast cancer tissue sections (using a laser microdissection microscope from P.A.L.M.®, Bernried, Germany) and the subsequent isolation of genomic DNA or total RNA. The protocols presented in here have been used in our laboratory for the exact quantification of gene copy numbers in intraductal and invasive tumor cells and for the quantitative assessment of promoter hypermethylation during breast cancer progression.

We have added some guidelines for the organization of the laser-microdissection and polymerase chain reaction laboratory, which prevent crosscontamination of samples and carry-over contamination because of polymerase chain reaction products.

Key Words: Laser-assisted microdissection; gene amplification; promoter hypermethylation; paraffin-embedded tissue; nucleic acid isolation.

1. Introduction

One of the most demanding methodological problems in the analysis of tissue biopsies is tissue heterogeneity. For example, a resection specimen of breast tissue infiltrated by a malignant tumor contains at least eight (and often, nine) different cell types:

1. Fat cells in the adipose tissue.
2. Normal breast epithelium in the branching ducts.
3. Myoepithelial cells.
4. Fibroblasts in the connective tissue.
5. Endothelial cells lining the blood vessels.

From: *Methods in Molecular Medicine, Vol. 120: Breast Cancer Research Protocols*
Edited by: S. A. Brooks and A. L. Harris © Humana Press Inc., Totowa, NJ

Table 1
Overview of Systems Available for the Laser-Assisted
Dissection of Histological Sections or Cytospin Preparations

Arcturus	www.arctur.com
Bio-Rad Laboratories	www.microscopy.bio-rad.com
Cell Robotics	www.cellrobotics.com
Eppendorf	www.eppendorf.com
Leica Microsystems	www.leica-microsystems.com
MMI AG	www.molecular-machines.com
P.A.L.M.	www.palm-microlaser.com
Nikon AG	www.nikonusa.com

6. Leukocytes infiltrating the cancerous tissue.
7. Preinvasive intraductal carcinoma cells.
8. Invasive carcinoma cells.
9. Premalignant epithelial cells (e.g., atypical hyperplasia).

Frequently, the cells of interest constitute only a minor fraction of the whole biopsy and are not recognized macroscopically. Thus, any extract derived from a tissue biopsy constitutes a complex mixture of cellular components of different cell types.

In order to get meaningful molecular data, especially in a cell-specific and quantitative manner, it is necessary to isolate the cells of interest in a pure, homogenous form. The most convenient tool for isolating morphologically defined, pure cell populations from complex tissues is laser-assisted microdissection *(1,2)*. This technology allows the isolation of single cells or groups of cells from complex tissues, thereby enabling the subsequent molecular analysis of pure and morphologically defined cell populations and eliminating all distortions because of bystander cells. The basic principle of this technology is to cut out the cells of interest from histological sections with the help of a laser beam and to separate the dissected cells from the surrounding tissue. **Figure 1** illustrates the isolation of a single epithelial duct from a breast biopsy using laser-assisted microdissection. The elimination of contaminating bystander cells as lymphocytes, fibroblasts, or endothelial cells, which may mask molecular alterations in the cells of interest, enables the subsequent acquisition of exact quantitative molecular data.

The immunohistochemical staining before laser-assisted microdissection *(3)* permits the molecular analysis on the DNA and/or RNA level of cells which have been characterized phenotypically on the protein level.

In general, this sophisticated technology gives the opportunity to identify microscopically what is analyzed subsequently on a molecular level, applying qualitative assays or in exact quantitative terms.

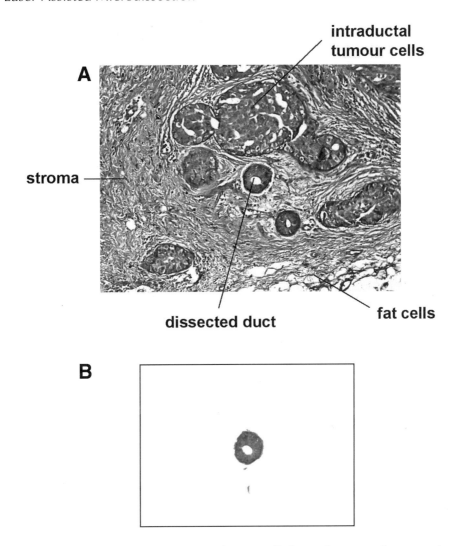

Fig. 1. (**A**) Isolation of pure intraductal tumor cells from a breast carcinoma section. The reduced optical quality is because of the fact that the tissue section is dried and not cover slipped. The dissected duct is already completely separated from the surrounding tissue (methylene blue staining, original magnification ×100). (**B**) Isolated intraductal carcinoma cells in the lid of a reaction tube (original magnification ×200).

Table 1 gives a short list of commercially available microdissection devices currently in use. The interested reader is referred to the specified websites cited in the table for further information. In addition, more- or less-comprehensive lists of references using the different systems are available on the websites of the manufacturers. We have been working with the P.A.L.M. system for several years, and most of the protocols described herein are specifically adapted to this system.

We have used the microdissection methodology in breast cancer research for the exact quantification of gene copy numbers in intraductal and invasive components of breast carcinomas *(4,5)* and for the quantitative assessment of promoter hypermethylation during breast cancer development *(6,7)*. Additional applications include the detection of *in situ* chimerism after organ transplantation *(8)* and messenger RNA quantification in defined cell populations of the bone marrow *(9)*.

1.1. Organization of the Laboratory

The enormous amplification power of polymerase chain reaction (PCR; up to $\times 10^{13}$), which is the basis for the exquisite sensitivity of this technology, also creates a serious problem: risk of contamination because of the introduction of exogenous DNA into the reaction mixture. This problem is especially prevalent in the case of analyzing minute amounts of starting material isolated by laser-assisted microdissection. Because every PCR produces vast amounts of amplifiable molecules (usually much more than 10^9 molecules) that can potentially contaminate subsequent amplifications of the same target sequence, the strict physical separation of the analysis of reaction products (postamplification) from all stages of sample preparation (preamplification) has to be implemented.

For these reasons, strictly enforced guidelines concerning the cleaning of instruments and the handling of samples before and after amplification need to be followed by all personnel involved. We perform all preamplification steps, including the laser-assisted microdissection, in a separate laboratory consisting of two rooms: one for setting up the PCR master mix (a "template-free" room) and the other for preparation of tissue sections, microdissection, nucleic acid extraction, bisulfite treatment, and adding DNA or complimentary DNA to the PCR mixes.

Plastic labware and benches are cleaned using a 3% hypochlorite solution. The PCR products are analyzed in a separate laboratory. Under no circumstances should amplified samples or equipment from this working area be brought back to the pre-PCR area.

The protocols described below for laser-assisted microdissection concentrate on the following steps:

1. Preparation of foil-coated glass slides.
2. Cutting and staining of histological tissue sections.
3. Laser microdissection and specimen recovery.
4. Isolation of DNA and/or RNA from microdissected cells.

2. Materials

The manufacturers or distributors are only specified if reagents or laboratory equipment might be important for the outcome, or if a source might be difficult to identify. All chemicals were purchased in p.a. quality from Merck (Darmstadt, Germany), Roth (Karlsruhe, Germany), or Sigma (Taufkirchen, Germany) and kept strictly separate from the postamplification area in our institute.

1. Glass slides.
2. Cyanoacrylate glue (UHU, Buehl, Germany).
3. Soft brush for sleeking the foil on the glass slides before fixing it with glue.
4. Poly-L-lysine (0.1% aqueous solution; Sigma), stored at 4°C.
5. 1.2-μm-thick polypropylene foil (P.A.L.M.).
6. Xylol-Ersatz, a xylene substitute, which is less toxic and smells less unpleasant (Vogel, Karlsruhe, Germany).
7. Ethanol (100, 96, and 70%).
8. Glass cuvets.
9. ABC Vectastain Kit (Vector Laboratories, Burlingame, CA).
10. Methylene blue (Loeffler's methylene blue; Merck).
11. Methyl green (Merck). **Note:** staining solutions are stored at room temperature in the dark.
12. Liquid wax (MJ Research, Boston, MA).
13. Proteinase K buffer: 50 mM Tris-HCl (pH 8.1), 1 mM of ethylenediaminetetraacetic acid (EDTA), 0.5% Tween-20.
14. Digestion solution: 4 M guanidinium isothiocyanate, 30 mM Tris-HCl (pH 8.0), 0.5% sarcosyl, 0.1 M β-mercaptoethanol.
15. Proteinase K, stock solution: 20 mg/mL in water, aliquots stored at −20°C (Merck).
16. Tris-HCl/EDTA buffer: 10 mM Tris-HCl (pH 8.1), 1 mM EDTA.
17. 26-Gage, 3/8-in., 0.45 × 10 sterile canula, for picking up dissected cells.
18. 0.5-mL Tubes with transparent lid and lowered inner lid, for collecting dissected and catapulted cells (P.A.L.M.).
19. Scissors, for cutting the lids from the reaction tubes.
20. DNase- and RNase-free, aerosol-resistant pipet tips (Sarstedt, Nümbrecht, Germany).
21. Sterile water.
22. 3 M of sodium acetate (pH 7.0) containing 100 μg/mL Dextran T500 (Sigma).
23. Hypochlorite solution (Roth) diluted 1:4 with tap water.
24. PCR bench with ultraviolet lamp, for decontamination of racks and irradiation of polypropylene foil (in-house construction).
25. Refrigerated tabletop centrifuge for 0.2- to 2.0-mL tubes (max. 14,000g).
26. Vortex mixer.
27. 40°C Incubator.
28. Thermoshaker (Eppendorf, Hamburg, Germany).
29. Thermoshaker with heated lid (CLF, Emersacker, Germany).

3. Methods

3.1. Preparation of Foil-Coated Glass Slides

The tissue section which is to be microdissected is not mounted directly onto a glass slide as are all routine histological sections. Instead, the section is mounted on a glass slide coated with very thin foil. This foil serves as a carrier for the tissue and is glued to the glass slide only at the four corners. Therefore, after microdissection, the dissected piece of tissue can be easily removed together with the supporting foil, which is completely inert and does not interfere with any subsequent analysis.

Slides coated with polypropylene foil can be obtained from P.A.L.M., but they are very expensive. We (as do most other people working in the field) buy the foil from P.A.L.M. and prepare the coated slides ourselves. For the coating with poly-L-lysine, a drop of the solution (0.1% in sterile water) is spread over the foil with a sterile pipet tip, carefully avoiding any damage of the very thin foil. (Any leakage underneath the foil might result in problems with P.A.L.M. Laser Pressure Catapulting technology, because the poly-l-lysine will glue the foil to the glass slide.) The foil, pretreated in such a way, is cut in appropriately sized pieces and mounted onto the glass slides. (It is very important to use a very sharp scalpel blade, because anything less than very sharp will destroy the foil instead of cutting it.) Any fold of the foil is removed with a clean soft brush, and it is fixed at the four corners with cyanacrylate glue from UHU (*see* **Note 1**).

After curing overnight, the foil-coated glass slides are irradiated for 45 min with short-wavelength ultraviolet light to destroy all traces of DNA or RNA (*see* **Note 2**).

3.2. Specimen Preparation

3.2.1. Frozen Sections

Snap-frozen biopsies are cut using a standard cryotome and mounted onto slides coated with foil. Because the slides cannot be refrigerated (tissue sections will not adhere to an ice-cold slide), the tissue will thaw immediately upon mounting onto the slide and has to be fixed immediately with absolute ethanol (a few drops). Subsequently, the sections are allowed to dry at room temperature (*see* **Note 3**).

For staining with methylene blue, the dried sections are rehydrated with a drop of sterile water for 30 s. Afterward, the sections are covered with methylene blue solution for 30 s, rinsed twice with sterile water, dehydrated with a drop of absolute ethanol, and allowed to dry at room temperature.

After cutting a biopsy, the cryotome blade and the sample holder is cleaned meticulously before the next biopsy is cut to avoid any crosscontamination.

3.2.2. Paraffin Sections

Formalin-fixed, paraffin-embedded biopsies are cut using a conventional microtome, and sections are mounted on foil-covered slides. To improve the adhesiveness, the slides with sections are incubated for 15 min at 55°C. Then, the sections are deparaffinized and rehydrated using Xylol-Ersatz and ethanol (twice with xylene substitute for 10 min, twice with 100% ethanol for 5 min, twice with 96% ethanol for 5 min, once with 70% ethanol for 5 min, and sterile water for 5 min).

The sections are stained with methylene blue or methyl green (depending on personal preferences and the combination with immunohistochemical stains; *see* **Subheading 3.2.3.**).

3.2.3. Immunohistochemical Stains

For labeling cells with antibodies before microdissection, we use the Vectastain kit from Vector Laboratories. As outlined in **Subheading 2.**, all reagents brought into contact with samples before amplification (pre-PCR) have to be strictly separated from all other reagents used in the laboratory (post-PCR). The great advantage of ready-to-use kits is that the components are free of any potentially contaminating PCR products and completely separated from all reagents normally used in the laboratory. This justifies the higher costs (*see* **Note 4**).

3.3. Microdissection Using the P.A.L.M. Laser Microdissection Microscope

The width of the laser cut can be trimmed by adjusting the laser energy and/ or the focus of the laser. In our setting, the optimal focus for using the ×40 long-distance objective from Zeiss (×40/0.60 Korr ×/0-2) is around 980 (arbitrary units); for using the ×10 objective from Zeiss (×10/0.50 ×/0.17), the optimal value is 680. Depending on the thickness of the section and the tissue type, the energy for cutting is between 920 and 1000 (arbitrary units), for catapulting greater than 1020. The actual numbers for the energy and focus setting may vary for different instruments calibrated and adjusted in a slightly different way (*see* **Note 5**).

For recovery of dissected cells using the Laser Pressure Catapulting technology of the P.A.L.M. system, the 0.5-mL tubes distributed by P.A.L.M. are most suitable because of the lowered inner lid, which shortens the distance the catapulted cells have to fly. In addition, the visibility of the specimens in the transparent lid is quite good. For catapulting a dissected cell or a group of cells, the laser is focused slightly below the section, and the laser energy is increased. A single, short laser impulse is sufficient for catapulting the specimen into the lid of a reaction tube placed directly above the section. The lid of the reaction tube is conveniently positioned in the holder of the micromanipulator (*see* **Note 6**).

Despite having the very sophisticated (and often necessary) Laser Pressure Catapulting technology, we can recover dissected pieces of tissue with a sterile needle if they are large enough. This can be done easily by hand, without any technical support. After some practice, this turns out to be unsurpassed in terms of speed and ease for those working with the laser microscope.

3.4. Isolation of Nucleic Acids

3.4.1. Isolation of DNA

If the sample contains very few cells (1–30), they are lysed in the lid of the reaction tube by adding 10–30 µL Tris/EDTA buffer containing 40 µg proteinase K. The closed tubes are incubated in a small incubator in an inverted position at 45°C overnight. Larger samples of more than approx 50 cells are lysed in proteinase K buffer (*see* **Subheading 2.**) containing 500 µg/mL proteinase K. The samples are incubated in a thermoshaker with a heated lid at 56°C overnight. If several hundred or even thousands of cells are isolated, the samples are lysed in a larger volume of proteinase K buffer (100–300 µL) containing 500 µg/mL proteinase K. The samples are incubated in a vigorously shaking thermoshaker at 56°C overnight. The next day, the lysate is transferred to a new tube (*see* **Note 7**), and the DNA is precipitated by adding sodium acetate (pH 7.0) containing Dextran T500 (Sigma, Taufkirchen, Germany) as a carrier (100 µg/mL) and ethanol. This precipitation step removes contaminating dyes and cell debris almost completely.

3.4.2. Isolation of RNA

3.4.2.1. ISOLATION OF RNA FROM FORMALIN-FIXED, PARAFFIN-EMBEDDED SPECIMENS

For the isolation of RNA from formalin-fixed, paraffin-embedded specimens, we use a protocol described elsewhere in detail *(10)*:

1. The dissected specimens are incubated overnight at 55°C in a vigorously agitating thermoshaker (Eppendorf) in the digestion solution containing 0.5 mg proteinase K (total volume, 100 µL).
2. The lysate extracted with water-saturated phenol and chloroform.
3. The RNA is precipitated from the aqueous phase with isopropanol and glycogen as a carrier.
4. If only a few cells are collected, the lysis buffer (20–50 µL) is directly added to the lid of the reaction tube, and the closed tube is incubated in an inverted position at 45°C overnight (*see* **Note 8**).

3.4.2.2. ISOLATION OF RNA FROM FROZEN BIOPSIES

For the isolation of RNA from frozen biopsies, we use the micro-RNA isolation kit from Stratagene (Heidelberg, Germany), following the manufacturer's instructions.

4. Notes

1. We have tested several glues and tapes, following tips and hints from colleagues, and P.A.L.M. cyanoacrylate glue (two-component glue) turned out to be the best, nearly completely resisting xylene and 100% ethanol. (All other glues or tapes tested dissolved in one of these solvents; even this glue starts dissolving after prolonged incubations of longer than 45 min).

2. It is very important to wait until the glue is completely cured, before ultraviolet irradiation starts, because otherwise, the glue will never cure and will dissolve rapidly in xylene or the xylene substitute used.

3. The embedding medium might interfere with downstream applications. Therefore, we decided to use no embedding medium at all and to freeze the biopsy with a drop of water placed directly onto the sample holder.

4. The in-house setup for detection reagents under PCR contamination-free conditions is only cost-effective if immunostaining for larger microdissection is routinely performed on a large scale. We did not perform a comprehensive comparison of commercially available staining kits; therefore, other kits might work as well.

5. The width of the laser cut depends very much on the thickness of the section and the type of tissue structure that has to be cut (e.g., fat tissue is very easily cut; connective tissue is often quite resistant). That means that the energy sufficient for a fine cut through fat tissue will not be sufficient for cutting connective tissue structures, and the energy adjusted to the latter tissue type will create a quite broad, irregular cut through fat tissue. However, adjustment of the appropriate laser focus and energy has to be learned by trial and error, and the numbers given in the text give only a rough estimation.

6. Dissected cells can also be catapulted into the lid of a reaction tube without changing the focus of the laser but this will create a "bullet hole" in the specimen. This is no problem if larger structures are dissected and the laser bullet hole can be placed in an irrelevant part of the specimen (e.g., the lumen of a vessel dissecting the vessel lining endothelial cells). When dissecting single-cell or very small cell clusters, it is absolutely necessary to change the focus of the laser. This adjustment of the laser focus for catapulting has to be learned by trial and error, and the right adjustment is a delicate balance between the size of the specimen and the laser focus and the laser energy. A tiny drop of liquid wax from MJ Research (Boston, MA) is distributed in the lid of the reaction tube. This wax film ensures that the catapulted specimens will firmly adhere to the lid.

7. The transfer of the lysate of larger groups of cells to a new tube before precipitation is necessary in order to separate the pieces of supporting membranes from the cell lysate. These pieces are isolated together with the dissected cells. They are not lysed, and these pieces interfere physically with precipitation of nucleic acids by preventing the formation of a compact pellet at the bottom of the tube during centrifugation.

8. The average fragment length of DNA or RNA isolated from formalin-fixed biopsies ranges from 200 to 400 bp. Therefore, the PCR products (amplicons) have to be as short as possible in order to achieve maximal amplification efficiency and to reduce the influence of nucleic acid fragmentation because of fixation.

Acknowledgments

The authors would like to thank Oliver Bock, Andreas Pich, and Ulrika Schade for critically reading the manuscript and many helpful hints concerning the practice of microdissection, and Britta Hasemeier for expert assistance in preparing Figure 1. The work of the authors is supported by grants from the Deutsche Forschungsgemeinschaft (DFG Fe 516/1-2) and the Deutsche Krebshilfe (10-1842-Le I).

References

1. Emmert-Buck, M. R., Bonner, R. F., Smith, P. D., et al. (1996) Laser capture microdissection. *Science* **274,** 998–1001.
2. Schütze, K. and Lahr, G. (1998) Identification of expressed genes by laser-mediated manipulation of single cells. *Nat. Biotechnol.* **16,** 737–742.
3. Fend, F., Emmert-Buck, M. R., Chuaqui, R., et al. (1999) Immuno-LCM: laser capture microdissection of immunostained frozen sections for mRNA analysis. *Am. J. Pathol.* **154,** 61–66.
4. Lehmann, U., Glöckner, S., Kleeberger, W., Feist H., von Wasielewski, R., and Kreipe, H. (2000) Detection of gene amplification in archival breast cancer specimens by laser-assisted microdissection and quantitative real-time polymerase chain reaction. *Am. J. Pathol.* **156,** 1855–1864.
5. Glöckner, S., Lehmann, U., Wilke, N., Kleeberger, W., Länger, F., and Kreipe, H. (2001) Amplification of growth regulatory genes in intraductal breast cancer is associated with higher nuclear grade but not with the progression to invasiveness. *Lab. Invest.* **81,** 565–571.
6. Lehmann, U., Hasemeier, B., Lilischkis, R., and Kreipe, H. (2001) Quantitative analysis of promoter hypermethylation in laser-microdissected archival specimens. *Lab. Invest.* **81,** 635–638.
7. Lehmann, U., Länger, F., Feist, H., Glöckner, S., Hasemeier, B., and Kreipe, H. (2002) Quantitative assessment of promoter hypermethylation during breast cancer development. *Am. J. Pathol.* **160,** 605–612.
8. Kleeberger, W., Rothämel, T., Glöckner, S., Flemming, P., Lehmann, U., and Kreipe, H. (2002) High frequency of epithelial chimerism in liver transplants demonstrated by microdissection and STR-analysis. *Hepatology* **35,** 110–116.
9. Bock, O., Schlué, J., Lehmann, U., von Wasielewski, R., Länger, F., and Kreipe, H. (2002) Megakaryocytes from myeloproliferative disorders show enhanced nuclear bFGF expression. *Blood* **100,** 2274–2275.
10. Bock, O., Kreipe, H., and Lehmann, U. (2001) One-step extraction of RNA from decalcified and archival biopsies. *Anal. Biochem.* **295,** 116–117.
11. Simone, N. L., Bonner, R. F., Gillespie, J. W., Emmert-Buck, M. R., and Liotta, L. A. (1998) Laser-capture microdissection: opening the microscopic frontier to molecular analysis. *Trends Genet.* **14,** 272–276.
12. Fink, L., Seeger, W., Ermert, L., et al. (1998) Real-time quantitative RT-PCR after laser-assisted cell picking. *Nat. Med.* **4,** 1329–1333.

13. Luo, L., Salunga, R. C., Guo, H., et al. (1999) Gene expression profiles of laser-captured adjacent neuronal subtypes (published *erratum* appears in *Nat. Med.* [1999] **5**, 355). *Nat. Med.* **5**, 117–122.

14. Walch, A., Specht, K., Smida, J., et al. Tissue microdissection techniques in quantitative genome and gene expression analysis. *Histochem. Cell Biol.* **115**, 269–276.

15. Okuducu, A. F., Hahne, J. C., von Deimling, A., and Wernert, N. (2005) Laser-assisted microdissection, techniques and applications in pathology. *Int. J. Mol. Med.* **15**, 763–769.

Suggested Readings

Emmert-Buck, M. R., Bonner, R. F., Smith, P. D., et al. (1996) Laser capture microdissection. *Science* **274**, 998–1001, and Simone, N. L., Bonner, R. F., Gillespie, J. W., Emmert-Buck, M. R., and Liotta, L. A. (1998) Laser-capture microdissection: opening the microscopic frontier to molecular analysis. *Trends Genet.* **14**, 272–276.

First and comprehensive description of the Acturus system, which is based on different principals for dissection and specimen recovery and a very good early review.

A detailed practical guide introducing the Arcturus system can be found in *Current Protocols of Molecular Biology* (Ausubel et al., eds. Wiley, New York, NY).

Fink, L., Seeger, W., Ermert, L., et al. (1998) Real-time quantitative RT-PCR after laser-assisted cell picking. *Nat. Med.* **4**, 1329–1333.

First description of quantitative mRNA analysis in laser-microdissected cells.

Luo, L., Salunga, R. C., Guo, H., et al. (1999) Gene expression profiles of laser-captured adjacent neuronal subtypes (published *erratum* appears in *Nat. Med.* [1999] **5**, 355). *Nat. Med.* **5**, 117–122.

First description of cDNA array based expression profiling of laser-microdissected cells.

II

Markers of Clinical Outcome and Prognosis

9

Traditional and Established Indicators of Prognosis and Treatment Success

Derek E. Roskell and Ian D. Buley

Summary

The outcome of breast cancer in an individual patient can be predicted by assessing a range of factors relating to the particular cancer. This assessment can be used to select treatments that are most likely to be successful, and to avoid futile or unnecessarily aggressive procedures.

Histopathological examination provides information on most of these factors. The most useful prognostic indicators in standard use are currently tumor stage, tumor grade, completeness of surgical excision, and estogen receptor status.

Key Words: Prognosis; grade; stage; special type; hormone receptors; margins; metastasis lymph nodes.

1. Introduction

From the earliest understanding of breast cancer as a life-threatening disease, it was clear that the outcome was not the same in all cases. Some cancers progressed rapidly from first detection of a lump through to metastasis and death, whereas others followed a more insidious course over many years, with patients often eventually succumbing to another disease altogether.

1.1. Historical Aspects of Prognosis and Treatment

Surgical treatment of breast cancer in the early days of radical mastectomy was aimed largely at curing the disease by cutting it out. This included surgically removing a very large surrounding area of normal tissue in an attempt to remove microscopic traces of the cancer spreading beyond a more obvious mass. Radiotherapy was used to destroy any cancer that could not be removed by surgery. Chemotherapy was a relatively forlorn hope for those with disseminated disease. These three steps of treatment represented three worsening phases of the disease. The use of radiotherapy or chemotherapy was decided

From: *Methods in Molecular Medicine, Vol. 120: Breast Cancer Research Protocols*
Edited by: S. A. Brooks and A. L. Harris © Humana Press Inc., Totowa, NJ

by the behavior of the particular cancer in the individual patient. Put simply, the prognosis was established by how the cancer behaved. If it was difficult to excise and required radiotherapy, it was bad. If it metastasized or recurred locally, it was worse.

1.2. Matching Treatment to an Individual Cancer

Modern treatments for breast cancer use combinations of surgery, radiotherapy, and chemotherapy from the outset, tailoring the treatment chosen to the individual patient and particular cancer. Use of chemotherapy and radiotherapy early in treatment is based on identifying which patients are at risk of local recurrence or metastasis and giving the treatment without waiting for these to occur. More aggressive treatment is used for patients at the highest risk. Conversely, patients whose cancer is not particularly aggressive can avoid the trauma and side effects of unnecessarily extensive intervention. The role of surgery in this context has changed. In some cases, removing the tumor in an attempt at cure can still be considered the main aim. For others, however, the role of surgery is essentially to control the disease locally and to provide a specimen from which the likelihood of local recurrence or metastatic spread can be established. This information is then used to determine the adjuvant therapies that are most likely to succeed in keeping the disease at bay for as long as possible.

2. Standard Prognostic Factors

The factors that need to be assessed to gain a realistic assessment of prognosis are tumor stage (size, invasion of surrounding structures, involvement of lymph nodes, and presence of distant metastasis), including completeness of surgical excision, tumor grade, tumor type, and tumor expression of estrogen receptor. These standard prognostic factors remain the most predictive, though a considerable range of other biological factors provide prognostic data.

3. Assessment of Stage in Breast Cancer

The *stage* of a cancer refers to the degree of spread from the site of origin into surrounding tissue, lymph nodes, or to distant sites. For breast carcinoma, increasing stage (worsening prognosis) follows the size of the primary tumor, the degree of involvement of local lymph nodes, the local invasion of deep muscle of the chest wall, and metastatic spread to distant sites, in ascending order (*see* **Tables 1** and **2**).

3.1. Size of Tumor

First principles would suggest that, even if subsequently completely excised, a larger carcinoma would have had a greater chance of establishing metastatic

Table 1
Summary of Pathological Staging of Breast Cancer

Breast cancer T, N, M categories, and stage groupings

Primary tumor (T)

TX Primary tumor cannot be assessed.

T0 No evidence of primary tumor.

Tis Carcinoma *in situ*; intraductal carcinoma, lobular carcinoma *in situ*, or Paget's disease of the nipple with no associated tumor mass.

T1 Tumor 2 cm or less in greatest dimension.

T2 Tumor more than 2 cm but not more than 5 cm in greatest dimension.

T3 Tumor more than 5 cm in greatest dimension.

T4 Tumor of any size growing into the chest wall or skin.

Regional lymph nodes (N) pathological staging

NX Regional lymph nodes cannot be assessed (for example, removed previously).

N0 Cancer has not spread to regional lymph nodes.

N1 Cancer has spread to one to three axillary lymph node(s) on the same side as the breast cancer and/or in internal mammary nodes with microscopic disease found by sentinel node biopsy but that are not found on imaging studies or by clinical exam. This category includes the situation where only a small cluster of cancer cells is detected.

N2 Cancer has spread to four to nine lymph nodes on the same side as the breast cancer or in internal mammary nodes found by imaging studies or clinical exam in the absence of axillary lymph node metastasis.

N3 Cancer has spread to 10 or more axillary lymph nodes, or in infraclavicular lymph nodes, or in supraclavicular nodes or in internal mammary lymph nodes.

Metastasis (M)

MX Presence of distant spread (metastasis) cannot be assessed.

M0 No distant spread.

M1 Distant spread is present.

Stage groupings

	T	N	M
Stage 0	Tis	N0	M0
Stage I	T1	N0	M0
Stage IIA	T0	N1	M0
	T1	N1	M0
	T2	N0	M0
Stage IIB	T2	N1	M0
	T3	N0	M0
Stage IIIA	T0	N2	M0
	T1	N2	M0

(continued)

Table 1 (*Continued*)
Summary of Pathological Staging of Breast Cancer

Breast cancer T, N, M categories, and stage groupings

	T2	N2	M0
	T3	N1	M0
	T3	N2	M0
Stage IIIB	T4	N0, N1, N2	M0
Stage IIIC	Ant T	N3	M0
Stage IV	Any T	Any N	M1

Adapted from **ref. *1a*.**

Table 2
Breast Cancer Survival by Stage

Stage	5-Yr relative survival rate
0	100%
I	98%
IIA	88%
IIB	76%
IIIA	56%
IIIB	49%
IV	16%

From the American Cancer Society.

deposits than would a small one. This is likely, because the time taken to reach a larger size provides a longer opportunity for the process to occur, and within a larger cancer, there is a greater scope for different subclones of tumor cells to have the aggressive properties required to metastasize. Analyses of large numbers of patients show that size is indeed an independent predictor of both overall survival and recurrence (*1–3*). In the tumor–node–metastasis system, tumor size is described by using the letter T plus a number (1–4): T1, up to 20 mm; T2, up to 50 mm; T3, more than 50 mm; and T4, any size, with direct extension to chest wall or skin. Five-year survival for these groups, in lymph node-negative cases, is approx 98, 88, and 76%, respectively. The size of a tumor should be assessed in three dimensions, with microscopic confirmation of the size of the invasive component, because it is this, and not coexisting *in situ* carcinoma, that determines survival.

3.2. Spread to Lymph Nodes

Most breast cancers that have spread to lymph nodes are found in the ipsilateral axillary nodes. Medial tumors may also spread to the internal mammary chain, and occasionally involvement of infra- or supraclavicular nodes is seen. Histologically determined involvement of lymph nodes is the single most important predictor of disease-free survival and overall survival in breast cancer *(4)*. The prognosis is worse the greater the number of lymph nodes involved. For a cancer less than 2 cm (T1), the presence of 1–3 positive axillary nodes reduces the 5-yr survival rate from 98 to 88%, 4–9 nodes to 56%, and 10 or more nodes to less than 50%. Involvement of nodes higher in the axilla and spread to internal mammary nodes carries a worse prognosis.

3.2.1. Assessment of Sentinel Lymph Nodes and Micrometastases

The lymph node part of the tumor–node–metastasis staging assessment for breast cancer relies on enough nodes being assessed to allow a meaningful count of positive nodes. In principle, the more axillary tissue taken, the greater the number of lymph nodes that can be assessed and the more reliable the prognostic information. This information comes, however, at a cost. Clearance of the axillary contents to retrieve lymph nodes carries a significant risk of the serious complication of lymphedema. When this occurs, the lymphatic drainage of the arm is so compromised that it becomes severely swollen, causing significant discomfort and disability. The risk of this is reduced when less tissue is removed. Alternative approaches to lymph node assessment include axillary node sampling, where a limited number of nodes are removed from the axilla, or by identifying one or two nodes only that are draining the tumor bed, and assessing only those for the presence of metastases. These "sentinel nodes" can be identified by injecting a dye or radioactive marker into the tumor bed at the time of surgery, and locating those nodes to which the marker is first carried. The application of sentinel node biopsy to establishing the prognosis in breast cancer is explored in Chapters 10 and 11.

Histological examination of nodes by examination of 5-μm-thick sections inevitably involves sampling only a small part of the node, and sampling protocols are used to maximize the detection of metastatic disease within the constraints of practicality *(5)*. Immunohistochemistry can also be used to detect small metastases, which might otherwise be undetected. Serial step sectioning and the application of immunohistochemistry can increase the pickup of metastatic disease in apparently node-negative cases by 20%, but the significance of the detection of micrometastases, variably defined as less than 1 or 2 mm in size, remains uncertain *(6)*. Extranodal spread of tumor into surrounding axillary adipose tissue appears to provide little additional prognostic information, except in cases where it occurs when only a few nodes are positive for metastases *(1)*. The presence of invasion into lymphatic channels or blood vessels within the breast can be a surrogate for lymph node involvement where nodes are not available for examination. It also provides prognostic information where nodes are apparently free of disease, both in terms of local recurrence and long-term survival *(7)*.

3.3. Direct Spread Beyond the Breast

Extension of a cancer into the muscle of the chest wall or the skin is usually associated with a large tumor and hence, a poor prognosis. It is also independently predictive of a poor outcome *(8)*. Cancers in men or small-breasted women, and any originating close to the deep fascia, may extend beyond the breast even when the tumor is small. The reasons for a poorer prognosis are many. First, anatomical boundaries may have been breached, so that the carcinoma has reached an area rich in lymphatic vessels, increasing the potential for metastasis. This may explain the poor prognosis associated with invasion of the skin. Spread through fascial boundaries also demonstrates the ability of a carcinoma to destroy tissue, so that any tumor being carried within a blood or lymphatic vessel to a distant site is likely to have the means to get out of the vessel and establish a distant metastasis. Probably the most significant factor, however, is simply the capacity of the tumor to be resected at surgery.

3.4. Metastatic Spread to Distant Sites

The presence of a metastasis beyond the local lymph nodes implies the worst stage (stage IV), regardless of all the other factors discussed above. With this stage, only about 1 in 6 patients will survive 5 yr (16% overall survival).

4. Tumor Grade as a Prognostic Factor

The *grade* of a cancer refers to its perceived aggression, based on its degree of differentiation by morphological assessment. Clearly, the greatest predictor of aggression is behavior, and tumors that are at an advanced stage at presentation would be expected to demonstrate a generally higher grade. However, the grade of a cancer can be assessed independently, so that for any particular stage of disease, a prediction of the prognosis can be made, depending on the grade. Conventionally in cancer biology, low-grade cancers are slower growing and have more resemblance to normal tissue (well differentiated), whereas high-grade cancers are faster growing and poorly differentiated.

4.1. Assessment of Grade in Breast Cancer

In breast cancer, the rate of growth is assessed microscopically by a count of the number of mitotic figures visible in 10 standardized, high-power fields.

Differentiation is assessed by scoring the proportion of the cancer forming recognizable glandular structures, this being a marker of good differentiation. Nuclear pleomorphism is the degree of variation in cancer cell nuclear size and staining characteristics and is scored using standardized definitions. More bizarre and variable nuclei represent greater variation in nucleic acids, with a greater number of mutations and amplifications in the DNA, and greater transcription into RNA, all of which are characteristics of a more aggressive malignancy. The scores for mitotic count, tubules, and nuclear pleomorphism are combined to give the cancer a grade of from 1 to 3, where 3 is the least well differentiated and most aggressive *(5,9)*. Tumor necrosis does not form part of the assessment of grade but is a prognostically unfavorable feature associated with high-grade tumors; it is uncertain whether it is an independent prognostic variable.

4.2. Special Types of Breast Cancer

Grading, as described in **Subheading 4.1.**, gives the most information from the appearance of the cancer, but tumor type also contributes. Adenocarcinoma of the breast can be split into histological subtypes, some of which have prognostic significance. Most breast cancers come into the category of "ductal carcinoma of no special type." Though these cancers can have a wide variety of appearances, their grades are best assessed by using the standard scoring system. The "special types" of breast cancer are largely low-grade carcinomas (grade 1), for which the prognosis is even better than would be expected for a ductal carcinoma of the same grade and stage but of no special type. The two best-characterized special types of breast cancer conveying important prognostic features are tubular and mucinous carcinomas. These are both well-differentiated cancers, the former being made up of infiltrating tubules that closely resemble normal breast ducts, and the latter by scattered clusters of bland epithelium set within copious amounts of extracellular mucin. A tumor is required to show the defined appearances in at least 90% of the tumor mass to be considered a pure special type. Mixed carcinomas show less-extensive special-type differentiation *(5,10)*. Tubular carcinoma in particular is usually a very indolent disease. It is frequently identified in mammographic screening programs and has a particularly favorable prognosis.

5. Expression of Estrogen and Progesterone Receptors

Normal breast tissue expresses estrogen and progesterone receptors to varying degrees, depending on the hormonal pattern of the menstrual cycle or pregnancy. Expression of these receptors by a breast cancer may be seen as a sign of better differentiation, and indeed, it is the lower-grade carcinomas that tend to express them most strongly. Very strong expression of estrogen receptor gives tumor cells a selective advantage, as estrogenic hormones promote tumor growth. Blocking this pathway offers a means of treating the disease, at least in terms of slowing its growth. This can be achieved in several ways, the most direct being to block the receptors with a drug, such as tamoxifen. Other drugs, such as aromatase inhibitors and luteinizing hormone-releasing hormone agonists, decrease endogenous production of estrogens, rendering largely obsolete older treatments such as ovarian ablation or excision *(11)*.

5.1. Prognosis Related to Quantification of Steroid Receptors

Expression of estrogen receptor may be quantified biochemically, usually by using ligand-binding techniques or immunohistochemically. Immunostaining (described in Chapter 12) is now the usual method, and tumors can be scored in terms of the amount of receptor per cell and the proportion of cells expressing it *(12)*. Strongly positive cancers have a 75% likelihood of the outcome being improved by administering an endocrine treatment alongside standard therapies. Endocrine therapies are normally well tolerated, but are not without side effects. Patients whose cancers do not express estrogen or progesterone receptors will not respond to such therapies, and this information can be used to avoid unnecessary treatment.

5.2. Tumor Progression in Grade and Receptor Status

It is common for a cancer to recur after treatment; this can happen while an endocrine treatment, such as tamoxifen, is still being administered. This may be associated with an increase in the cancer grade or with the loss of estrogen and progesterone receptor expression as the carcinoma evolves new clones that are not dependent on hormonal stimulation. Assessment of the presence of steroid receptors is usually undertaken using immunohistochemistry to detect the receptor protein. This may still be detectable even though the cancer is clearly no longer responding to tamoxifen. In such a case, knowing that the receptor is still present, at least in part, can be helpful, as a change of therapy to an aromatase inhibitor may still block the activation of the receptor pathway. Eventually, however, some cancers stop responding to any currently available endocrine treatments.

6. Assessment of the Surgical Margins

It is nearly always the aim of surgery to achieve a clear margin by removing all of the identified primary tumor rather than simply debulking it. Histopathological assessment of the margins of excision is most thorough for small excision specimens, where in "breast conservation surgery," the aim is to remove the carcinoma with the least damaging cosmetic effect on the breast. The techniques involved vary depending on the type of specimen, but may include microscopy of shaves of tissue a few millimeters thick from the cavity created by excision of the tumor. A proportion of cases will require a further excision if microscopic involvement of the margins is found. Intraoperative assessment of margins may be achieved using frozen section histology, but the limited reliability of this method confines its use to special circumstances in most centers. For example, in cases where reconstructive plastic surgery will be carried out at the same time as the cancer is removed, checking the margins during surgery helps avoid the possibility of having a subsequent complicated re-excision operation, which would involve taking apart the reconstruction.

An awareness of the presence of cancer at or close to margins that cannot be excised, such as the chest wall, allows the selection of appropriate radiotherapy.

Achieving a clear surgical margin, proved by histology, has an undoubted beneficial effect on local recurrence rates. Whether it affects overall survival is less clear, as the latter depends more on metastatic spread *(13)*.

7. *In Situ* Carcinoma and Prognosis

In situ *carcinoma* refers to the presence of neoplastic cells within ducts and lobules of the breast, without invasion into the surrounding tissues. Usually, it is a microscopic disease, though it can occasionally present as lumpiness or a mass in the breast. Its prognostic significance depends on the context in which it is seen.

7.1. In Situ *Carcinoma as an Isolated Condition*

In a patient without an invasive breast cancer, the presence of preinvasive *in situ* carcinoma identifies an increased risk of developing an invasive malignancy. The risk is greater depending on the extent of the *in situ* disease, the histological subtype, and, for ductal carcinoma *in situ*, its grade (assessed by nuclear pleomorphism and the presence of necrosis) *(14)*. Ductal carcinoma *in situ* is normally treated by excision of the involved area. This may require mastectomy or local excision with histologically clear margins. Following local excision, there is a role for postoperative radiotherapy and tamoxifen treatment in estrogen receptor-positive *in situ* disease to reduce the incidence of subsequent recurrence of *in situ* carcinoma or invasive disease *(15)*.

7.2. In Situ *Carcinoma-Accompanying Invasive Carcinoma*

In a patient who already has an invasive cancer, the presence of *in situ* carcinoma has slightly different prognostic implications. The risk of developing invasive cancer has already manifested itself. After local excision of an invasive malignancy, the patient is likely to have radiotherapy and endocrine therapy, both of which are used to treat residual *in situ* carcinoma. Nonetheless, *in situ* carcinoma at the surgical margins remains an indicator for an increased risk of local recurrence of infiltrating malignancy, and surgical clearance of both the invasive and *in situ* disease is desirable. Clearly, if the invasive malignancy has already metastasized, then the need for further surgery to re-excise any residual *in situ* carcinoma is less of a priority given the adverse prognosis.

References

1. Fitzgibbons, P. L., Page, D. L., Weaver, D., et al. (2000) Prognostic factors in breast cancer. College of American Pathologists consensus statement 1999. *Arch. Pathol. Lab. Med.* **124,** 966–978.

1a. Sobin, L. H. and Wittekind, C. H., eds. (2002) *TNM Classification of Malignant Tumours, 6th Edition.* Wiley-Liss, New York, NY.

2. Carter, C. L., Allen, C., and Hensen, D. E. (1989) Relation of tumor size, lymph node status and survival in 24,740 breast cancer cases. *Cancer* **63,** 181–187.

3. Hensen, D. E., Ries, L., Freedman, L. S., and Carriaga, M. (1991) Relationship among outcome, stage of disease and histologic grade for 22,616 cases of breast cancer. *Cancer* **68,** 2142–2149.

4. Veronesi, U., Galimberti, V., Zurrida, M., et al. (1993) Prognostic significance of number and level of axillary node metastases in breast cancer. *Breast* **2,** 224–228.

5. National Coordinating Group for Breast Cancer Screening Pathology (2003) *Pathology reporting in breast cancer screening.* NHSBSP Publications, Sheffield, UK.

6. Weaver, D. L. (2003) Sentinel lymph nodes and breast carcinoma. Which micrometastases are clinically significant? *Am. J. Surg. Pathol.* **27,** 842–845.

7. Pinder, S., Ellis, I. O., O'Rourke, S., et al. (1994) Pathological prognostic factors in breast cancer. III. Vascular invasion: relationship with recurrence and survival in a large series with long-term follow-up. *Histopathology* **24,** 41–47.

8. Perrone, F., Carlomagno, C., Lauria, R., et al. (1996) Selecting high-risk early breast cancer patients: what to add to the number of metastatic nodes? *Eur. J. Cancer* **32A,** 41–46.

9. Elston, C. W. and Ellis, I. O. (1991) Pathological prognostic factors in breast cancer. I. The value of histological grade in breast cancer: experience from a large study with long-term follow-up. *Histopathology* **19,** 403–410.

10. Pereira, H., Pinder, S. E., Sibbering, D., M., et al. (1995) Pathological prognostic factors in breast cancer IV: Should you be a typer or a grader? A comparative study of two histological prognostic features in operable breast carcinoma. *Histopathology* **27,** 219–226.

11. Should aromatase inhibitors replace tamoxifen? (2003) *Drug Ther. Bull.* **41,** 57–59.

12. Leake, R., Barnes, D., Pinder, S., et al. (2000) Immunohistochemical detection of steroid receptors in breast cancer: a working protocol. UK Receptor Group, UK NEQAS, The Scottish Breast Cancer Pathology Group, and The Receptor and Biomarker Study Group of the EORTC. *J. Clin. Pathol.* **53,** 634–635.

13. Singletary, S. E. (2002) Surgical margins in patients with early-stage breast cancer treated with breast conservation therapy. *Am. J. Surg.* **184,** 383–393.

14. Jensen, R. A. and Page, D. L. (2003) Ductal carcinoma *in situ* of the breast. Impact of pathology on therapeutic decisions. *Am. J. Surg. Pathol.* **27,** 828–831.

15. Mokbel, K. (2003) Towards optimal management of ductal carcinoma *in situ* of the breast. *Eur. J. Surg. Oncol.* **29,** 191–197.

10

Sentinel Lymph Node Biopsy in Breast Cancer

Celia Chao and Kelly M. McMasters

Summary

Sentinel lymph node biopsy is now a widely accepted method of axillary lymph node staging for invasive breast cancer. This review encompasses the historical perspective of surgical management of the axilla; the data that has emerged over the last decade highlighting the accuracy, safety, and applicability of this procedure; and the technical details necessary to perform this procedure. Successful adaptation of sentinel node biopsy implies that the operator has a high identification rate and a low false-negative rate, as well as the collaborations with the other involved disciplines: pathology, radiology, and nuclear medicine.

Key Words: Breast cancer; axillary nodal staging; sentinel node biopsy.

1. Introduction

Axillary lymph node status is the most powerful predictor of recurrence and survival in breast cancer patients. It remains an essential component of the decision to offer adjuvant therapy. During the last century, experience with axillary dissection has shown that this procedure can result in significant morbidity: pain, paresthesias, seroma, infection, limitation of arm and shoulder motion, lymphedema, and lymphangitis (1,2). The development and adaptation of sentinel lymph node (SLN) biopsy has revolutionized the staging of melanoma and breast cancer. SLN biopsy is a highly accurate technique with minimal morbidity.

2. Historical Perspective

Axillary dissection offers accurate nodal staging, as well as effective regional disease control. Although the therapeutic impact of axillary dissection is unknown, there is substantial evidence that local disease control affects improved survival (3,4). Despite the controversy, experts agree that there is no value in removing normal lymph nodes. Axillary lymph node dissection for

From: *Methods in Molecular Medicine, Vol. 120: Breast Cancer Research Protocols*
Edited by: S. A. Brooks and A. L. Harris © Humana Press Inc., Totowa, NJ

clinically node-negative breast cancer is an elective, or prophylactic, lymph node dissection. Overall, approx 70% of patients with clinically node-negative breast cancer who undergo axillary dissection have negative lymph nodes. If the SLN is negative, the patient can potentially be spared a complete axillary dissection.

Noninvasive methods, such as clinical examination, mammography, ultrasonography, computed tomography, and positron emission tomography to stage the axilla have not been shown to be accurate *(5–7)*. Random sampling of axillary nodes has been suggested but is associated with false-negative rates as high as 40%; likewise, removal of only level I nodes might result in a lower complication rate, but it is associated with a high false-negative rate of 10–15% *(8)*. SLN biopsy is a reliable, minimally invasive alternative to standard level I/II axillary dissection. Because the procedure involves intraoperative lymphatic mapping, a directed assessment of axillary nodes is possible.

The SLN is the first draining lymph node in the axilla to receive lymphatic drainage from the primary breast tumor. If regional metastatic disease should exist, it is the node most likely to contain metastases. As a corollary, if the SLN is negative, then the remainder of the nodal basin will also be negative. Therefore, the SLN should reflect the histopathological status of the entire axilla. In 1992, Morton's group performed SLN biopsy in more than 500 melanoma patients, removing the sentinel node, as well as the remaining regional lymph nodes *(9)*. The pathology of the sentinel node predicted the remaining regional nodal status with 99% accuracy. His pioneering work was validated by studies at other institutions with completion lymphadenectomy and histopathological examination, and with long-term follow-up to identify potential recurrences in undissected nodal basins following a negative sentinel node biopsy *(10–12)*. Similarly, initial experience with SLN biopsy for breast cancer was reported by Giuliano et al. *(13)* using vital blue dye injection; this was validated with histopathological examination of the non-SLNs *(14)*. Krag et al. *(15)* reported a preliminary series of breast cancer SLN biopsies using injection of technetium sulfur colloid with detection using a hand-held γ-probe.

Numerous studies (**Table 1**) have validated the SLN concept and have demonstrated that SLN biopsy can accurately determine axillary nodal status *(13,15–42)*. Acceptable results have been reported by a number of institutions, but there are still questions about the dissemination of this technique into general practice *(43)*. Studies from the University of Louisville have resolved some issues related to the optimal technique for SLN biopsy.

Table 1
Published Experience With Sentinel Lymph Node Biopsy and Completion Axillary Lymph Node Dissection

Study (ref.)	N (Number of patients in study)	Injection technique	TP	FN	ID rate	FN rate
Krag 1993 (*15*)	22	Radioactive colloid alone	7	0	18/22 (81.8%)	0/7 (0%)
Giuliano 1994 (*13*)	174	Blue dye alone	37	5	114/174 (65.5%)	5/42 (11.9%)
Albertini 1996 (*16*)	62	Dual agent	18	0	57/62 (91.9%)	0/18 (0%)
Giuliano 1997 (*17*)	107	Blue dye alone	42	0	100/107 (94%)	0/42 (0%)
Pijpers 1997 (*18*)	37	Radioactive colloid alone	11	0	30/37 (81.1%)	0/11 (0%)
Roumen 1997 (*19*)	83	Radioactive colloid alone	22	1	57/83 (68.7%)	1/23 (4.2%)
Borgstein 1997 (*20*)	25	Dual agent	14	0	25/25 (100%)	0/14 (0%)
Veronesi 1997 (*21*)	163	Dual agent	81	4	160/163 (98.2%)	4/85 (4.7%)
Guenther 1997 (*22*)	45	Blue dye alone	28	3	103/145 (71%)	3/31 (9.7%)
Flett 1998 (*23*)	68	Blue dye alone	15	3	56/68 (82%)	3/18 (16.7%)
Borgstein 1998 (*20*)	104	Radioactive colloid alone	44	1	104/104 (100%)	1/45 (2.2%)
Miner 1998 (*25*)	42	Radioactive colloid alone	6	1	41/42 (97.6%)	1/7 (14.3%)
Krag 1998 (*27*)	443	Radioactive colloid alone	101	13	413/443 (93.2%)	13/114 (11.4%)
Krag 1998 (*28*)	157	Radioactive colloid alone	39	2	119/157 (75.8%)	2/41 (4.9%)
Offoidile 1998 (*29*)	41	Radioactive colloid alone	18	0	40/41 (97.6%)	0/18 (0%)
Snider 1998 (*29*)	80	Radioactive colloid alone	13	1	70/80 (87.5%)	1/14 (7.1%)
Rubio 1998 (*30*)	55	Radioactive colloid alone	15	2	53/55 (96.4%)	2/17 (11.8%)
Barnwell 1998 (*31*)	42	Dual agent	15	0	38/42 (90.5%)	0/15 (0%)
Nwariaku 1998 (*32*)	119	Dual agent	26	1	96/119 (80.7%)	1/27 (3.7%)
O'Hea 1998 (*33*)	59	Dual agent	17	3	55/59 (93.2%)	3/20 (15.0%)
Canavese 1998 (*34*)	100	Dual agent	28	5	96/100 (96.0%)	5/33 (15.2%)
Crossin 1998 (*35*)	50	Radioactive colloid alone	7	1	42/50 (84.0%)	1/8 (12.5%)
Winchester 1999 (*36*)	72	Radioactive colloid alone	35	4	58/72 (80.6%)	4/39 (10.3%)
Bass 1999 (*37*)	186	Dual agent	53	1	173/186 (93.0%)	1/54 (1.9%)

(continued)

Table 1 (*Continued*)
Published Experience With Sentinel Lymph Node Biopsy and Completion Axillary Lymph Node Dissection

Study (ref.)	N (Number of patients in study)	Injection technique	TP	FN	ID rate	FN rate
Veronesi 1999 (*38*)	376	Dual agent	168	12	371/376 (98.7%)	12/180 (6.7%)
Morrow 1999 (**39**)	139	Dual agent	28	4	110/139 (79.1%)	4/32 (12.5%)
Kern 1999 (*40*)	40	Blue dye alone	15	0	39/40 (97.5%)	0/15 (0%)
Tafra 2001 (*41*)	535	Dual agent	122	18	446/535 (87.1%)	18/140 (12.9%)
McMasters 2001 (**42**)	2121	Dual agent	625	55	1957/2121 (92.3%)	55/680 (8.1%)

TP, true-positive result; FN, false-negative result; ID, identification.
False-negative rate = false-negative results ÷ positive axillary lymph nodes = FN/(FN + TP).
Only patients in whom sentinel lymph node biopsy was followed by completion axillary dissection are included.
(Adapted, with permission, from **ref. 42.**)

3. Definitions

There are two critical parameters of successful SLN biopsy: the SLN identification rate and the false-negative rate. The *SLN identification rate* is the frequency of finding and removing a sentinel node. When a sentinel node cannot be identified, a standard level I/II axillary dissection must be performed. The *false-negative rate (44)* is the proportion of patients with positive lymph nodes who are incorrectly staged by the SLN biopsy procedure. It is the number of patients with false-negative events divided by all positive cases (true positives and false negatives). Suppose a surgeon performs 100 SLN biopsies for breast cancer, followed by completion level I/II axillary dissection. Of the 100 patients, 75 had negative axillary lymph nodes and 25 had positive nodes. There were only three false-negative events—three patients in whom the sentinel node was negative, but other nodes in the axillary dissection proved to have metastases. One might calculate the false-negative rate as 3/100 or 3%. The true denominator, however, is the number of patients with positive lymph nodes, such that 3/25, or 12%, is the correct false-negative rate. The false-negative rate represents the percentage of patients with nodal metastases that would be understaged with SLN biopsy. It is difficult to determine an acceptable rate for false-negative results. For example, a standard axillary dissection removes level I and II lymph nodes and we accept a 2–3% false-negative rate with this procedure because of potential disease remaining in the level III nodes. Level III nodes are not generally removed for standard breast cancer staging because of the increased risk of lymphedema. Therefore, we accept a small false-negative rate ($\leq 5\%$) in order to spare the majority of true negative patients the morbidity of a full level I and II axillary dissection.

4. Pathological Examination of the Sentinel Node

When a pathologist is presented with the few nodes most likely to harbor regional metastases, a detailed and focused histological assessment is possible. Such intense analysis makes it possible to detect occult nodal metastases more frequently than with routine axillary dissection; indeed, SLN biopsy may be even more sensitive than the standard axillary dissection. That is, routine histological examination of an axillary dissection typically involves bisecting the lymph nodes then sectioning and staining each half with hematoxylin and eosin (H&E) to search for tumor cells. Only a small area of the lymph node is ever examined. SLN biopsy allows for identification of the node most likely to harbor metastases.

By performing serial sections, a more thorough examination of the nodal specimen is possible. Serial sectioning in combination with immunohistochemical staining for cytokeratins, increases the sensitivity of sentinel node biopsy for detection of metastatic disease *(44)*. The sentinel node biopsy identifies the nodes that should be subject to closer scrutiny because such a focused examination would be cost-prohibitive and time-consuming to perform on the entire contents of an axillary dissection. (Methodology for pathological assessment of the SLN is the subject of Chapter 11.)

5. Establishing a Successful SLN Program

Implementation of this technology requires the cooperative efforts of multiple disciplines. The "team" must meet and agree on a protocol: how to perform injections, how to dispose of radioactive waste, what type of radionuclide to use, and what SLN pathology protocol to adapt. In addition to the surgeons and the operating room staff, it is necessary to involve colleagues from the departments of radiology, nuclear medicine, pathology, and anesthesiology.

6. Operative Technique

6.1. Patient Eligibility

SLN biopsy is most appropriate for patients with T1 and T2 breast cancers (tumor size <5 cm) without palpable nodal metastases (clinical N0) (*see* Chapter 9, **Subheading 3.**). Although SLN biopsy appears accurate for T3N0 tumors, it must be recognized that up to 75% of these patients have nodal metastases *(45,46)*. SLN biopsy is certainly applicable for patients undergoing either breast-conserving surgery or mastectomy. It can be performed accurately either after excisional breast biopsy or needle biopsy has been performed. The procedure is most appropriate for biopsy-proven invasive cancer. Cases of ductal carcinoma *in situ* (**Fig. 1**), which may be preoperatively understaged, are an exception to this rule *(47)*. Contraindications include pregnancy, palpable axillary nodal metastases, preoperative chemotherapy or radiation therapy, multifocal breast cancers, hypersensitivity to either blue dye or technetium sulfur colloid, and prior major breast or axillary operations that could interfere with lymphatic drainage *(44)*. Although a potential role for SLN biopsy in axillary nodal staging prior to neoadjuvant therapy in patients attempting to downstage their tumors and attempt breast conservation surgery, performing a SLN biopsy after neoadjuvant therapy outside of a clinical trial should be considered controversial *(48)*.

6.2. Dual-Agent Injection Technique

Intraoperative lymphatic mapping using vital blue dye, radioactive colloid, or a combination of both, is performed to identify the sentinel node. We advocate the use of dual-agent injection in order to facilitate sentinel node localization. The combination of the two techniques—visualization of the blue dye and intraoperative γ-probe detection—provides overlapping and complementary ability to discriminate sentinel nodes. Some sentinel nodes may be blue-stained

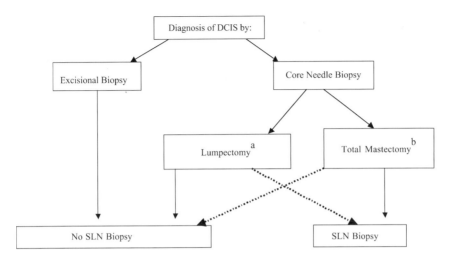

Fig. 1. Sentinel lymph node (SLN) biopsy for ductal carcinoma *in situ*. [a]For patients with a high risk of invasive tumors SLN biopsy performed at the same time as lumpectomy is warranted. [b]For patients with low risk of invasive tumor (low-grade ductal *carcinoma in situ*), small area of microcalcifications, no palpable mass, and no nodular density on mamogram or ultrasound. SLN biopsy may not be warranted. (Adapted with permission from ref. *47*.)

but not radioactive ("blue, not hot") and others may be radioactive but without blue-dye staining ("hot, not blue"), but the majority of sentinel nodes will be both "blue" and "hot."

The current evidence from the largest prospective, multi-institutional study for SLN biopsy in breast cancer seems to suggest that injection of vital blue dye plus radioactive colloid provides more accurate nodal staging than the use of either agent alone *(49–51)*. From a recent analysis of our data *(49)*, it is clear that the SLN identification rate and false-negative rate are optimized using both radioactive colloid and blue dye for lymphatic mapping (**Table 2**). The use of the dual-agent technique is also associated with a greater mean number of sentinel nodes removed. **Table 3** shows that the increased ability to identify multiple nodes, when present, may account for the lower false-negative rate *(50)*.

We recommend preoperative dermal radioactive colloid injection using 0.5 mCi of 0.2-μ technetium-99 sulfur colloid in a volume of 0.2–0.5 cc at least 30 min prior to operation. The use of filtered or unfiltered colloid has been shown to be equivalent in terms of identification rates and false-negative rates. Equal injections are made into the dermis using a tuberculin syringe and a 25- to 30-gage needle (raising a wheal) immediately anterior (superficial) to the tumor site using four to five separate injections (**Fig. 1**). The use of routine

Table 2
Results of Sentinel Lymph Node Biopsy
by Injection Technique in a Large, Multi-Institutional Study

Injection technique[a]	SLN identified (%)	Mean # of SLNs removed	Overall accuracy	False-negative rate
Single agent	86%	1.50	95.7%	11.8%
Dual agent	90%	2.10[b]	98.2%	5.8%[c]
All techniques	88%	1.95	97.5%	7.2%

[a]Single-agent technique includes patients undergoing sentinel node biopsy with blue dye injection alone or with radioactive colloid injection alone. Dual-agent injection refers to the use of both blue dye and radioactive colloid injection techniques.
[b]$p < 0.0001$ vs single-agent injection, analysis of variance.
[c]$p < 0.05$ vs single-agent injection, Fisher's Exact Test.
SLN, sentinel lymph nodes. (Adapted with permission from **ref. 49**.)

Table 3
Impact of Number of Sentinel Nodes Removed
on the False-Negative Rate: Results From a Large, Multi-Institutional Study

No. of SLNs removed	No. of Patients with SLN identified	No. of Patients with true-positive SLN	No. of Patients with false-negative SLN	False-negative rate
One	537	132	22	14.3%
Two or more	750	223	10	4.3%[a]

[a]$p = 0.0004$, χ-square.
(Adapted with permission from **ref. 50**.)

lymphoscintigraphy has been shown to be neither necessary nor helpful in SLN biopsy for breast cancer (*52*).

Injection in the areolar border has become popular in recent years (*53–55*). Embryologically, all the lymphatic drainage of the breast converges in the peri- or subareolar plexus of lymphatics. Therefore, injection of the areola will accurately reflect the drainage of tumors in any part if the breast. This technique has been advocated for patients with multicentric or multifocal breast cancer (*56*). As with other techniques, this technique is acceptable as long as acceptable identification (>90%) and false-negative rates (≤5%) can be achieved in the hands of the operating surgeon.

Following radioactive colloid injection, the patient is taken to the operating room. For patient comfort, we perform almost all of SLN biopsies under general anesthesia, although it is possible to use local anesthesia. Patients should be counseled preoperatively that the blue dye injection will impart a change to the color of their urine, and that there is a small chance of allergic reaction to the dye (approx 1 in 10,000). Adverse reactions to vital blue dye are rare, but anaphylactic reactions have been documented *(57)*. Allergic reaction to the blue dye may manifest as blue-colored hives *(58)*.

Patients will occasionally have a noticeably blue tattoo on the skin after the procedure. They should be told that this color will fade and disappear with time. The anesthesiologist should be aware that pseudohypoxia is often seen intraoperatively as a result of the blue dye, which interferes with the pulse oximeter readings giving a falsely decreased oxygen saturation. The use of radioactive colloid is safe, and numerous reports have documented the relatively low amount of radiation exposure associated with its use *(59,60)*.

Before prepping and draping the patient, Lymphazurin™ (1% isosulfan blue) dye is injected peritumorally, with care being taken to disperse the dye around the tumor. A 5-min massage of the area following blue dye injection helps to stimulate lymphatic uptake toward the axilla *(61)*. Peritumoral injection of isosulfan blue dye is performed by injecting 1 cc in each of four corners around the tumor, with the final 1 cc injected superficial to the tumor (between the tumor and the skin). For palpable tumors, the injection is easily accomplished. For nonpalpable tumors, the injection is guided by ultrasound or by judging the depth and direction of the imbedded wire following standard needle localization. It is helpful for the radiologist to mark on the skin anterior to the tumor with an indelible marker at the time of needle localization. We do not recommend injecting all of the blue dye or radioactive colloid down the localization needle, as this does not disperse the blue dye well, and it may concentrate the dye deep within the breast tissue. For patients who previously have undergone excisional biopsy, injection should be made around the biopsy cavity, avoiding the seroma cavity.

Many centers perform peritumoral injection of both blue dye and radioactive colloid. However, peritumoral injection of radioactive colloid results in a large zone of diffusion that can obscure the objective of locating the axillary SLNs, especially for upper outer quadrant tumors. This is often noted to be the "shine-through" effect: background radiation from the primary tumor site interfering with detection of axillary SLNs; some centers use a sterile lead shield to block the radioactive interference from the upper outer quadrant of the breast. Furthermore, peritumoral injection results in relatively little uptake of the tracer from the breast tissue compared with dermal injection. The data from the University of Louisville Breast Cancer SLN Study indicate that dermal injection of radioactive colloid significantly improves sentinel node identification rate and minimizes the false-negative rate *(42)*. For instance, dermal injection of radioactive colloid is associated with sentinel nodes that are five- to sevenfold more radioactive, or "hot," than with the peritumoral injection method (**Table 4**). The dermal injection technique offers easier and quicker

Table 4
Results of Sentinel Lymph Node Biopsy Based on Radioactive Colloid Injection Technique

Radioactive colloid injection technique	SLN ID rate[a]	False-negative rate[b]	Transcutaneous-to-final-background-count ratio	Ex vivo-to-final-background-count ratio
Peritumoral	89.9%	8.3%	51	113
Subdermal	95.3%[c]	7.8%	126	550
Dermal	98.0%[d,e]	6.5%	239[f]	859[g]

[a]$p < 0.0001$, significant difference among peritumoral, subdermal, dermal, and blue dye alone groups, χ^2.

[b]No significant differences among peritumoral, subdermal, dermal, and blue dye alone groups, χ^2.

[c]$p = 0.0037$ vs peritumoral injection, χ^2.

[d]$p < 0.0001$ vs peritumoral injection, χ^2.

[e]$p = 0.026$ vs subdermal injection, χ^2.

[f]$p < 0.0001$, compared to peritumoral injection.

[g]$p < 0.0001$, compared to peritumoral injection.

The transcutaneous-to-final background count ratio is measured by the hand-held γ-probe: the ratio of the transcutaneous counts per s of the most radioactive, or "hottest" sentinel lymph node (SLN) in the axilla to the final background count after removal of all SLN.

The ex vivo-to-final background count ratio is measured as the ex vivo counts per s of the hottest SLN divided by the final background counts after removal of all SLN.

(Adapted with permission from **ref. 42**.)

labeling and identification of the sentinel node, more reliable transcutaneous localization with the hand-held γ-counter, and less "shine-through" effect. When the dermal injection is used, the skin overlying the tumor can be retracted medially, away from the axilla, in order to facilitate γ-probe detection.

For beginners, we recommend that the entire arm be prepped and draped into the operative field. This allows for mobility of the arm and offers potentially easier access to the sentinel node(s). The hand-held γ-counter is used to identify the location of the sentinel node transcutaneously, and a 3- to 4-cm incision is made in line with the usual axillary dissection incision. The localization of the "hot spot" allows for the planning of a small incision over the suspected site of the SLN. If a "hot spot" is not identified, a curved transverse incision in the lower axilla just below the hairline provides excellent exposure. After dissecting through the subcutaneous tissue, the clavipectoral fascia is divided to gain exposure to the axillary contents. The γ-counter is then used to pinpoint the location of the SLN. As the dissection continues, the signal from the probe should increase in intensity (**Fig. 2**). If there is difficulty in identify-

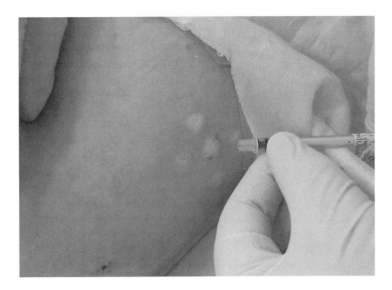

Fig. 2. Dermal injection of radioactive colloid is performed by raising a wheal in skin superficial to the tumor site.

ing a sentinel node, the clavipectoral fascia along the lateral border of the pectoralis major and minor muscles should be divided to gain easy access to the entire axilla *(37)*. This is accomplished by moving the arm (which has been incorporated in the sterile field) medially to facilitate exposure of levels II and III.

Using a combination of the visualization of blue dye in the afferent lymphatics and lymph nodes themselves, as well as γ-probe counts, the sentinel node is localized (**Figs. 3** and **4**). Care should be taken not to disrupt the capsule of the lymph node. Hemoclips are used for hemostasis, as well as to clip the afferent lymphatic channels. Meticulous clipping of the lymphatics will prevent postoperative lymphocoele formation. This is important because a closed suction drain is not placed for SLN biopsy. The sentinel node is removed, ex vivo radioactive counts are obtained, and the node may be sent to pathology for frozen section analysis (*see* **Subheading 6.3.**). The background radioactivity in the axilla is then checked. Based on results from the University of Louisville Breast Cancer SLN Study, false-negative rates are lowest if all blue nodes and nodes greater than 10% of the ex vivo count of the hottest SLN are harvested *(62)*. That is, if there is focal activity of 10% or greater of the ex vivo counts of the hottest sentinel node (**Fig. 5**), a diligent search should be made for another sentinel node. Hence, this is referred to as the "10% rule."

All blue nodes should be removed regardless of radioactivity because blue dye staining indicates a direct lymphatic pathway from the tumor to the node.

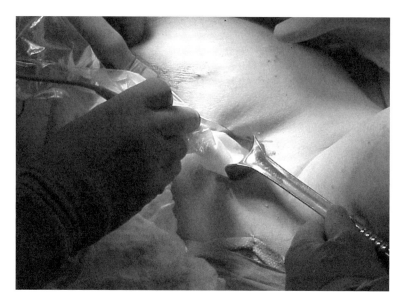

Fig. 3. The hand-held γ-probe is used to pinpoint the location of the sentinel node within the axilla.

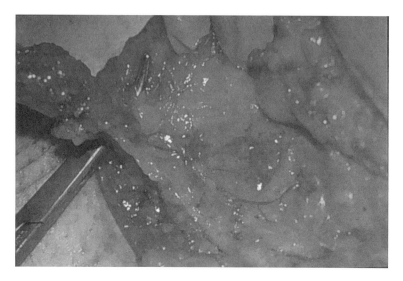

Fig. 4. A blue-stained afferent lymphatic channel can be found leading to a sentinel node.

Usually the hottest nodes are also blue, indicating that both techniques identify the same sentinel node. In fact, the γ-probe can actually help identify blue nodes. After removal of blue and/or hot nodes, palpation of the surgical bed for

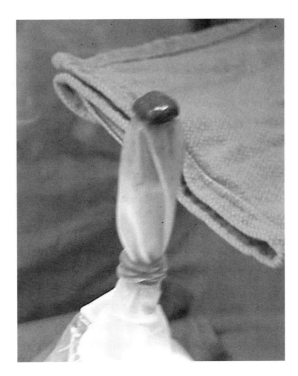

Fig. 5. The node is place on the γ- probe to obtain the ex vivo radioactive count. The "10% rule:" for example, if the highest reading ("hottest node") recorded is 7099 counts per second, then any additional sentinel lymph node with counts greater than 710 (10% of the hottest node) should be removed.

enlarged, firm, or otherwise suspicious lymph nodes should be performed. A pathological lymph node may not be hot or blue for two reasons: the lymph node is completely replaced with tumor and the lymphatics are "blocked" from uptake of any tracer, and unexplainable false-negative results do occur.

A tumor-positive, non-hot or non-blue node should still be considered a "sentinel" node because it accurately staged the axilla of that patient. If no sentinel nodes can be identified, then a default level I/II axillary dissection must be performed. On average, two to three sentinel nodes are removed per case.

Hot spots in the internal mammary chain and the supraclavicular region may be seen if a preoperative lymphoscintigram is obtained. We do not recommend dissection of these lymph nodes because traditional staging of breast cancer on which adjuvant therapy is based has been by evaluating the axillary nodes. The number of cases in which the internal mammary nodes are positive for tumor whereas the axillary nodes are negative, and in which therapeutic decisions would be impacted by the knowledge of a positive internal mammary node, is very small.

Table 5
Frozen Section Analysis of Breast Cancer:
Review of the Literature

Author	No. of axillae	No. of pts	False-negative[a]	Accuracy	FNPV
Hingston/Flett *(64)*	92	97	11%	95%	4%
Turner[b] *(65)*	—	278	26.3%	93.2%	8.4%
Veronesi[c] *(66)*	—	119	5.5%	97%	4.5%
Zurrida *(67)*	—	192	32%	86%	19%
Canavese *(34)*	—	96	27%	91%	12%
van Diest *(68)*	74	54	13%	95%	6.5%
Rahusen *(69)*	106	100	43%	84%	20%
Weiser *(70)*	—	890	42%	89%	12.7%
Chao *(63)*	203	200	32.1%	92.6	10.2%

[a]False-negative (FN) rate = 1-sensitivity

Note: the FN rate in this context relates to the pathological concordance between the sentinel lymph node (LN) frozen section result compared with the permanent section results.

[b]Includes frozen section and imprint cytology.

[c]Includes a 50-min intraoperative evaluation involving 30 sections. Previous 192 patients *(68)* had only three sections of half the LN examined and as FN rate of 32.1%.

FNPV, false-negative predictive value: risk of incorrect staging at the time of frozen section; complement to the negative predictive value (NPV) or 1-NPV; pts, patients.

(Adapted with permission from **ref. *63*.**)

SLN biopsy is followed by either breast-conserving surgery or mastectomy. If mastectomy is planned, it is helpful to perform the sentinel node biopsy first by opening a small portion of the axillary portion of the mastectomy incision prior to raising the flaps. Depending on the tumor location, raising the entire superior flap may result in blue dye spillage into the axilla, which can make it difficult to identify the sentinel node.

6.3. Histopathological Evaluation and Frozen-Section Analysis of the Sentinel Node

Based on studies of specimens and radioactivity, it is not necessary to quarantine the specimens *(60)*. Some authors advocate frozen section of the sentinel node, whereas other institutions never use frozen section because of the issue of sampling error in this setting (**Table 5**). The decision to incorporate frozen-section evaluation into one's program depends on the comfort level of the pathologist and surgeon. Patients are informed preoperatively that frozen section analysis will miss some positive sentinel nodes, and that the final analysis may change. **Table 6** shows that the sensitivity of frozen-section analysis decreases with micrometastatic deposits, defined as 2 mm or less of tumor in the sentinel node.

Table 6
Size of Sentinel Lymph Node Metastasis Impacts on Frozen Section Results

SLN frozen section result	N	Size (cm) of SLN metastasis[a] (Mean ± SD)	% SLN micrometastasis[b] (≤2 mm)
False-negative	17	0.16 ± 0.07	94%
True-positive	29	0.62 ± 0.61	21%

[a]Student's t-test: $p = 0.0032$.
[b]Fisher's Exact Test; $p < 0.0001$.
(Adapted with permission from **ref. 63**).

The nodes should be examined by H&E staining at a minimum of 2-mm intervals. This type of processing ("bread loafing") increases the detection of micrometastases. By directing the pathologist to the node most likely harboring regional metastases, SLN biopsy directs a more focused histological examination with multiple sections. As a result, this more intensive pathological evaluation detects occult nodal metastases more frequently than routine axillary dissection. If there is a positive sentinel node found on completion of frozen-section examination, then this is an indication for complete axillary dissection under the same anesthetic setting. If frozen section is not used, then the patient can return to the operating room (1 or 2 wk later) for completion of level I/II node dissection after final sections have been confirmed to be tumor-positive. Typical pathological handling of the completion axillary lymph nodes include bisecting each node in the specimen and staining with H&E only.

The routine use of immunohistochemistry (IHC) in addition to serial sections for the detection of occult micrometastases is hotly debated. The American College of Pathology has recommended against routine cytokeratin IHC analysis of sentinel nodes *(72)*. Because the prognostic significance of such micrometastases is unproven, this information should not be used for clinical decision making. Two prospective trials, the American College of Surgeons Oncology Group Z0010 and the NSABP (National Surgical Adjuvant Breast and Bowel Project) B-32 will evaluate the significance of SLN micrometastases detected by IHC for patients with invasive cancer. Until the results of these studies suggest otherwise, IHC for routine evaluation of SLN should be considered investigational. Should we aggressively treat patients with cytokeratin positive sentinel nodes without H&E correlation? "Upstaging" patients by IHC staining outside of a controlled clinical trial is discouraged.

6.4. Surgeon Experience

Unless specially trained in this procedure in a formal setting, all surgeons must climb the learning curve and begin to learn this procedure by offering

Table 7
Impact of Surgeon Experience
on Sentinel Lymph Node Identification and False-Negative Rates

No. of cases performed	No. of patients	No. of surgeons	SLN ID rate	FN rate
1–20	1817	226	91.7%	9.0%
>20	331	28	96.7%[a]	1.9%[b]

[a]$p = 0.0015$.
[b]$p = 0.014$ vs 1–20 cases, χ^2
SLN, sentinel lymph node; ID, identification; FN, false negative.
(Adapted with permission from **ref. 51**.)

sentinel node biopsy with planned backup axillary dissection. This will allow for the individual surgeon to calculate his/her own identification and false-negative rates. Surgeons who wish to adopt this technology must ensure that in their own hands, a false-negative rate of less than or equal to 5% and an identification rate of 90% or higher are achieved. As shown in **Table 7**, the false-negative rate significantly decreased from 9 to 1.9% when 20 cases or less were compared to more than 20 cases. It must be emphasized however, that false-negative results and nonidentification of the sentinel node can occur even after appropriate surgical training. Patients must be told of the small risk of a false-negative result and balance this against the benefits of a less invasive procedure. If staged to be sentinel node-negative, the patient may have a small life-time risk of axillary recurrence owing to the potential of a false-negative result.

7. Clinical Implications

If, in fact, SLN biopsy with diligent pathological examination identifies a population of "true" lymph node-negative patients, these patients may not require adjuvant therapy at all. The challenge that lies ahead is not only to more accurately identify those women with micrometastatic nodal disease who need additional therapy, but to determine if some subsets of node-negative women can safely avoid adjuvant therapy.

Our tolerance for accepting false-negative results may differ for certain subsets of women with breast cancer *(44)*. For example, when the risk of axillary lymph node metastases is very low (e.g., T1a tumors), we might accept a higher false-negative rate, because the risk of nodal metastases is generally less than 10 to 15% *(72)*. Even if the false-negative rate for sentinel node biopsy was 10%, only about one patient in 100 would be understaged. An equally valid and alternative argument is that patients with very early breast cancer are precisely the ones for whom we cannot accept a high false-negative rate, because the finding of a positive lymph node would most dramatically alter the postoperative therapy.

Finally, sentinel node technology identifies a subpopulation of patients with very small nodal metastasis. Previous to this procedure, these patients would have been pathological stage N0. The "Will Rogers Phenomenon" (illustrated by the concept of "stage migration") will predict that the prognosis of both node-negative and node-positive patients will improve.

8. Conclusions

High success rates of this technology have been reported, and its dissemination into general surgery practice is occurring at a rapid pace in order to meet patient demand for this procedure. Implementation of SLN biopsy requires multidisciplinary cooperation and must be tempered with high standards of quality control. Ongoing studies, such as the American College of Surgeons Oncology Group Trials Z0010 and Z0011, and the NSABP trial B-32 should provide answers to many of the remaining questions.

References

1. Petrek, J. A. and Heelan, M. C. (1998) Incidence of breast carcinoma-related lymphedema. *Cancer* **83,** 2776–2781.
2. Velanovich , V. and Szymanski, W. (1999) Quality of life of breast cancer patients with lymphedema. *Am. J. Surg.* **177,** 184–188.
3. Sosa, J. A., Diener-West, M., Gusev, Y., et al. (1998) Assocation between extent of axillary lymph node dissection and survival in patients with stage I breast cancer. *Ann. Surg. Oncol.* **5,** 140–149.
4. Cabanes, P. A., Salmon, R. J., Vilcoq, J. R., et al. (1992) Value of axillary dissection in addition to lumpectomy and radiotherapy in early breast cancer. *Lancet* **339,** 1245–1248.
5. Noguchi, M., Ohta, N., Thomas, M., et al. (1993) Clinical and biological prediction of axillary and internal mammary lymph node metastases in breast cancer. *Surg. Oncol.* **2,** 51–58.
6. De Freitas, R., Costa, M. V. and Schneider, S. V. (1991) Accuracy of ultrasound and clinical examination in the diagnosis of axillary lymph node metastases in breast cancer. *Eur. J. Surg. Oncol.* **17,** 240–244.
7. Nieweg, O. E., Kim, E. E., Wong, W. H., et al. (1993) Positron emission tomography with fluorine-18-deoxyglucose in the detection and staging of breast cancer. *Cancer* **71,** 3920–3925.
8. Davies, G. C., Millis, R. R. and Hayward, J. L. (1980) Assessment of axillary lymph node status. *Ann. Surg.* **192,** 148–151.
9. Morton, D. L., Wen, D. R., Wong, J. H., et al. (1992) Technical details of intraoperative lymphatic mapping for early stage melanoma. *Arch. Surg.* **127,** 392–399.
10. Morton, D. L., Wen, D. R., Foshag, L. J., et al. (1993) Intraoperative lymphatic mapping and selective cervical lymphadenectomy for early-stage melanomas of the head and neck. *J. Clin. Oncol.* **11,** 1751–1756.
11. Gershenwald, J. E., Colome, M. I., Lee, J. E., et al. (1998) Patterns of recurrence following a negative sentinel lymph node biopsy in 243 patients with stage I or II melanoma. *J. Clin. Oncol.* **16,** 2253–2260.

12. Ramnath, E. M., Kamath, D., Brobeil, A., et al. (1997) Lymphatic mapping for melanoma: Long term results of regional nodal sampling with radioguided surgery. *Cancer Control* **4,** 483–490.
13. Giuliano, A. E., Kirgan, D. M., Guenther, J. M., and Morton, D. L. (1994) Lymphatic mapping and sentinel lymphadenectomy for breast cancer. *Ann. Surg.* **220,** 391–401.
14. Turner, R. R., Ollila, D. W., Krasne, D. L., and Giuliano A. E. (1997) Histopathologic validation of the sentinel lymph node hypothesis for breast carcinoma. *Ann. Surg.* **226,** 271–278.
15. Krag, D. N., Weaver, D. L., Alex, J. C., and Fairbanks, J. T. (1993) Surgical resection and radiolocalization of the sentinel lymph node in breast cancer using a gamma probe. *Surg. Oncol.* **2,** 335–340.
16. Albertini, J. J., Lyman, G. H., Cox, C., et al. (1996) Lymphatic mapping and sentinel node biopsy in the patient with breast cancer. *JAMA.* **276,** 1818–1822.
17. Giuliano, A. E., Jones, R. C., Brennan. M., et al. (1997) Sentinel lymphadenectomy in breast cancer. *J. Clin. Oncol.* **15,** 2345–2350.
18. Pijpers, R., Meijer, S., Hoekstra, O. S., et al. (1997) Impact of lymphoscintigraphy on sentinel node identification with technetium 99-m colloidal albumin in breast cancer. *J. Nucl. Med.* **38,** 366–368.
19. Roumen, R. M. H., Valkenburg, J. G .M., and Geuskens, L. M. (1997) Lymphoscintigraphy and feasibility of sentinel node biopsy in 83 patients with primary breast cancer. *Eur. J. Surg. Oncol.* **23,** 495–502.
20. Borgstein, P. J., Meijer, S., and Pijpers, R. (1997) Intradermal blue dye to identify sentinel lymph node in breast cancer (research letter). *Lancet* **349,** 1668–1669.
21. Veronesi, U., Paganelli, G., Galimberti, V., et al. (1997) Sentinel-node biopsy to avoid axillary dissection in breast cancer with clinically negative lymph-nodes. *Lancet* **349,** 1864–1867.
22. Guenther, J. M., Krishnamoorthy, M., and Tan, L. R.. (1997) Sentinel lymphadenectomy for breast cancer in a community managed care setting. *Cancer J. Sci. Am.* **3,** 336–340.
23. Flett, M. M., Going, J. J., Stanton, P. D., and Cooke, T. G. (1998) Sentinel node localization in patients with breast cancer. *Br. J. Surg.* **85,** 991–992.
24. Borgstein, P. J., Pijpers, R., Comans, E. F., vanDiest, P. J., Boom, R. P., and Meijer, S. (1998) Sentinel lymph node biopsy in breast cancer: Guidelines and pitfalls of lymphoscintigraphy and gamma probe detection. *J. Am. Coll. Surg.* **186,** 275–283.
25. Miner, T. J., Shriver, C. D., Jaques, D. P., Maniscalco-Theberge, M. E., and Krag, D. N. (1998) Ultrasonographically guided injection improves localization of the radiolabeled SLN in breast cancer. *Ann. Surg. Oncol.* **5,** 315–321.
26. Krag, D., Weaver, D., Ashikaga, T., et al. (1998) The SLN in breast cancer: A multicenter validation study. *N. Engl. J. Med.* **339,** 941–946.
27. Krag, D. N., Ashikaga, T., Harlow, S. P., and Weaver, D. L. (1998) Development of sentinel node targeting technique in breast cancer patients. *Breast Journal* **4,** 67–74.

28. Offodile, R, Hoh, C., Barsky, S. H., et al. (1998) Minimally invasive breast carcinoma staging using lymphatic mapping with radiolabelled dextran. *Cancer* **82,** 1704–1708.

29. Snider, H., Kowlatshahi, K., Fan, M., Bridger, W. M., Rayudu, G., and Oleske, D. (1998) Sentinel node biopsy in the staging of breast cancer. *Am. J. Surg.* **176,** 305–310.

30. Rubio, I. T., Korourian, S., Cowan, C., et al. (1998) SLN biopsy for staging breast cancer. *Am. J. Surg.* **176,** 532–537.

31. Barnwell, J. M. Arredondo, M. A., Kollmorgen, D., et al. (1988) Sentinel node biopsy in breast cancer. *Ann. Surg. Oncol.* **5,** 126–130.

32. Nwariaku, F. E., Euhus, D. M., Beitsch, P. D., et al. (1998) SLN biopsy, an alternative to elective axillary dissection for breast cancer. *Am. J. Surg.* **176,** 529–531.

33. O'Hea, B. J., Hill, A. D. K., El-Shirbiny, A. M., et al. (1998) SLN biopsy in breast cancer: Initial experience at Memorial Sloan-Kettering Cancer Center. *J. Am. Coll. Surg.* **186,** 423–427.

34. Canavese, G., Gipponi, M., Catturich, A., et al. (1998) SLN mapping opens a new perspective in the surgical management of early-stage breast cancer: A combined approach with vital blue dye lymphatic mapping and radioguided surgery. *Semin. Surg. Oncol.* **15,** 272–277.

35. Crossin, J. A., Johnson, A. C., Stewart, P. B., and Turner, W. W. (1998) Gamma probe-guided resection of the SLN in breast cancer. *Am. Surg.* **64,** 666–669.

36. Winchester, D. J., Sener, S. F., Winchester, D. P., et al. (1999) Sentinel lymphadenectomy for breast cancer: Experience with 180 consecutive patients: efficacy of filtered technetium 99m sulphur colloid with overnight migration time. *J. Am. Coll. Surg.* **188,** 597–603.

37. Bass, S. S., Cox, C. E., Ku, N. N., et al. (1999) The role of SLN biopsy in breast cancer. *J. Am. Coll. Surg.* **189,** 184–194.

38. Veronesi, U., Paganelli, G., Viale, G., et al. (1999) SLN biopsy and axillary dissection in breast cancer: results in a large series. *J. Natl. Cancer Inst.* **91,** 368–373.

39. Morrow, M., Rademaker, A. W., Bethke, K. P., et al. (1999) Learning sentinel node biopsy: Results of a prospective randomized trial of two techniques. *Surgery* **126,** 714–720.

40. Kern K. A. (1999) SLN mapping in breast cancer using subareolar blue dye. *J. Am. Coll. Surg.* **189,** 539–545.

41. Tafra, L., Lannin, D. R., Swanson, M. S., et al. (2001) Multicenter trial of sentinel node biopsy for breast cancer using both technetium sulfur colloid and isosulfan blue dye. *Ann. Surg.* **233,** 51–59.

42. McMasters, K. M., Wong, S. L., Martin, R. C. G., et al. (2001) Dermal injection of radioactive colloid is superior to peritumoral injection for breast cancer SLN biopsy: Results of a multi-institutional study. *Ann. Surg.* **233,** 676–687.

43. Lucci, Jr. A., Kelemen, P. R., Miller, III. C., et al. (2001) National practice patterns of SLN dissection for breast cancer. *J. Am. Coll. Surg.* **192,** 452–458.

44. McMasters, K. M., Giuliano, A. E., Ross, M. I., et al. (1998) SLN biopsy for breast cancer: Not yet the standard of care. *N. Engl. J. Med.* **339,** 990–995.

45. Silverstein, M. J., Gierson, E. D., Waisman, J. R, Colburn, W. J., and Gamagami, P. (1995) Predicting axillary node positivity in patients with invasive carcinoma of the breast by using a combination of T category and palpability. *J. Am. Coll. Surg.* **180,** 700–704.
46. Wong, S. L., Edwards, M. J., Chao, C., et al. (2001) Predicting the status of nonsentinel axillary nodes: a multicenter study. *Arch. Surg.* **136,** 563–568.
47. McMasters, K. M., Chao, C., Wong. S. L., et al. (2002) SLN biopsy in patients with ductal carcinoma-in-situ: a proposal. *Cancer* **95,** 15–50.
48. Nason, K. S., Anderson, B. O., Byrd, D. R., et al. (2000) Increased false negative SLN biopsy rates after preoperative chemotherapy for invasive breast cancer. *Cancer* **89,** 2187–2194.
49. McMasters, K. M., Tuttle, T. M., Carlson, D. J., et al. (2000) SLN biopsy for breast cancer: A suitable alternative to routine axillary dissection in multi-institutional practice when optimal technique is used. *J. Clin. Oncol.* **18,** 2560–2566.
50. Wong, S. L., Edwards, M. J., Tuttle, T. M., et al. (2001) SLN biopsy for breast cancer: Impact of the number of sentinel nodes removed on the false negative rate. *J. Am. Coll. Surg.* **193,** 684–691.
51. McMasters, K. M., Wong, S. L., Chao, C., et al. (2001) Defining the optimal surgeon experience for breast cancer sentinel lymph node (SLN) biopsy: a model for implementation of new surgical techniques. *Ann. Surg.* **234,** 292–300.
52. McMasters, K. M, Wong, S. L., Tuttle, T. M., et al. (2000) Preoperative lymphoscintigraphy for breast cancer does not improve the ability to identify axillary SLNs. *Ann. Surg.* **231,** 724–731.
53. Klimberg, V. S., Rubio, I. T., Henry, R. et al. (1999) Subareolar versus peritumoral injection for location of the SLN. *Ann. Surg.* **229,** 860–865.
54. Borgstein, P. J., Meijer, S., Pijpers, R. J., et al. (2000) Functional lymphatic anatomy for sentinel node biopsy in breast cancer: echoes from the past and the periareolar blue method. *Ann. Surg.* **232,** 81–89.
55. Kern, K. A. (1999) SLN mapping in breast cancer using subareolar injection of blue dye. *J. Am. Coll. Surg.* **189,** 539–545.
56. Schrenk, P. and Wayand, E. (2001) Sentinel node biopsy in axillary lymph node staging for patients with multicentric breast cancer. *Lancet* **357,** 122.
57. Woltsche-Kahr, I., Komericki, P., Kranke, B., et al. (2000) Anapylactic shock following peritumoral injection of patent blue in SLN biopsy procedure. *Eur. J. Surg. Oncol.* **26,** 313–314.
58. Sadiq, T. S., Burns, W. W., Taber, D. J., et al. (2001) Blue urticaria: a previously unreported adverse event associated with isosulfan blue. *Arch. Surg.* **136,** 1433–1435.
59. Stratmann, S. L., McCarty, T. M. and Kuhn, J. A. (1999) Radiation safety with breast sentinel node biopsy. *Am. J. Surg.* **178,** 454–457.
60. Schwartz, G. F., Guiliano, A. E. and Veronesi, U. (2002) Proceedings of the consensus conference on the role of SLN biopsy in carcinoma of the breast. *Cancer* **94,** 2542–2551.
61. Bass, S. S., Cox, C. E., Salud, C. J., et al. (2001) The effects of postinjection massage on the sensitivity of lymphatic mapping in breast cancer. *J. Am. Coll. Surg.* **192,** 9–16.

62. Martin, R. C. G., Edwards, M. J., Wong, S. L., et al. (2000) Practical guidelines for optimal gamma probe detection of SLNs in breast cancer: results of a multi-institutional study. *Surgery* **128,** 139–144.

63. Chao, C., Wong, S. L., Ackermann, D., et al. (2002) Utility of intraoperative frozen section analysis of SLNs in breast cancer. *Am. J. Surg.* **182,** 609–615.

64. Hingston, G. R., Cooke, T. G., Goping, J. J., et al. (1999) Accuracy of intraoperative frozen-section analysis of axillary nodes. *Br. J. Surg.* **86,** 1092.

65. Turner, R. R., Hansen, N. M., Stern, S. L., et al. (1999) Intraoperative examination of the SLN for breast carcinoma staging. *Am. J. Clin. Pathol.* **112,** 627–634.

66. Veronesi, U., Paganelli, G., Galimberti, V. (1999) Sentinel node biopsy and axillary dissection in breast cancer: results in a large series. *J. Natl. Cancer. Instit.* **91,** 368–378.

67. Zurrida, S., Galimberti, V., Orvieto, E., et al. (2000) Radioguided sentinel node biopsy to avoid axillary dissection in breast cancer. *Ann. Surg. Oncol.* **7,** 28–31.

68. van Diest, P. J., Torrenga, H., Corstein, P. J., et al. (1999) Reliability of intraoperative frozen section and imprint cytological investigation of SLNs in breast cancer. *Histopathology* **35,** 14–18.

69. Rahusen, F. D., Pijpers, R., van Diest, P. J., et al. (2000) The implementation of sentinel node biopsy as a routine procedure for patients with breast cancer. *Surgery* **128,** 6–12.

70. Weiser, M. R., Montgomery, L. L,, Susnick, B., et al. (2000) Is routine intraoperative examination of sentinel nodes in breast cancer worthwhile? *Ann. Surg. Oncol.* **7,** 651–655.

71. Hammond, M. E. H., Fitzgibbons, P. L., Compton, C. C., et al. (2000) College of American Pathologists Conference XXXV: solid tumor prognostic factors: which, how, and so what? *Arch. Pathol. Lab. Med.* **124,** 958–965.

72. Mustafa, I. A., Bland, K. I. (1998) Indications for axillary dissection in T1 breast cancer. *Ann. Surg. Oncol.* **5,** 4–8.

11

Pathological Evaluation of Axillary Sentinel Lymph Nodes in Breast Cancer

Michael Z. Gilcrease and Aysegul Sahin

Summary

Nodal staging is the most important prognostic factor in the management of patients with breast cancer. Sentinel lymph node (SLN) procedure enables selective targeting of the first lumph node that drains the tumor when the initial metastases occur. A negative sentinel node predicts the absence of tumor mestastases in the other regional lymph nodes with high accuracy. Thorough histopathological evaluation of SLNs important for accurate assessment. In this chapter, we discuss the histopathological evaluation of SLNs.

Key Words: Sentinel node; breast cancer; pathological evaluation.

1. Introduction

Axillary lymph nodes are the most common sites of metastasis for breast carcinoma, and the presence of axillary lymph node metastases is the most important adverse prognostic factor for invasive breast cancer (1–3). Sentinel lymph node (SLN) biopsy has become a well-established method for staging clinically negative axillary lymph nodes (4–10). The "sentinel" node is the first node that drains a particular anatomic region (5–7). Intraoperative injection of isosulfan blue dye allows the surgeon to identify the axillary SLN by searching for the blue node (4,8–12). Alternatively, local injection of technetium-labeled sulfur colloid allows intraoperative identification of the SLN using a γ-probe (4,9,11–13). (These approaches are described in Chapter 10.) Many studies have shown that the presence of metastatic tumor within the SLN predicts whether additional metastases are present in the remaining regional lymph nodes (5–7,11,12,14–16). Current surgical practice is to forego an axillary lymph node dissection if the axillary SLN is found to be free of tumor.

The initial step in evaluating the SLN is to serially section the node at 2- to 3-mm intervals (17–21). A variety of methods may be used to determine

From: *Methods in Molecular Medicine, Vol. 120: Breast Cancer Research Protocols*
Edited by: S. A. Brooks and A. L. Harris © Humana Press Inc., Totowa, NJ

whether metastatic tumor is present within one or more of the lymph node sections. These include cytological examination of touch imprints *(22–27)*, histological evaluation of frozen *(26–29)* or formalin-fixed, paraffin-embedded tissue sections *(17–21)*, immunohistochemical analysis of tissue sections to detect cells with epithelial antigens *(30–33)*, and reverse transcriptase-polymerase chain reaction assays for detecting tumor cell mRNA *(34–36)*. Because tumor cells are not actually visualized, and no known mRNA is entirely specific for tumor cells, the reverse transcriptase-polymerase chain reaction is not currently used in the clinical setting to detect metastatic tumor in SLN specimens.

The cytological examination of SLN touch imprints is often performed intraoperatively, because the technique is rapid and easy to perform *(22–27)*. A result can be obtained quickly during the operative procedure, and if metastatic tumor is detected, a complete lymph node dissection can be performed immediately. This avoids the cost and morbidity of a second surgical procedure *(28,37)*. Although the method is not as sensitive as histological evaluation of formalin-fixed, paraffin-embedded tissue sections, the tissue is not compromise by the cytological procedure, so the lymph node sections can still be processed subsequently for histological evaluation to check for the possibility of a false-negative cytological result.

The histological evaluation of frozen lymph node sections is also a quick method that can be used intraoperatively to detect metastatic tumor *(26–29)*. Many studies have shown that the sensitivity and specificity of intraoperative SLN evaluation by cytological imprint and frozen-section methods are similar *(26,27,38)*. Frozen sections allow architectural histological features to be evaluated in addition to the cytological characteristics of the tumor cells. The architectural features can be particularly helpful in evaluating low-grade metastases. However, some of the tissue is cut away in the process of preparing frozen histological sections. Depending on the care and skill of the histotechnician, the subsequent evaluation of formalin-fixed, paraffin-embedded tissue sections can be compromised by preparing intraoperative frozen sections.

If intraoperative cytological or frozen-section evaluation is performed and no metastatic tumor is detected, the lymph node sections should be fixed and processed for paraffin embedding. Histological evaluation of formalin-fixed, paraffin-embedded tissue sections is more sensitive than both cytological and frozen-section methods and, thus, remains the definitive method at present for determining whether there is metastatic tumor in the SLN. Histological evaluation of formalin-fixed tissues cannot be done intraoperatively, but if metastatic tumor is detected on the final paraffin sections, the patient can undergo a second operation later to complete the axillary lymph node dissection. Both frozen and formalin-fixed, paraffin-embedded sections are stained with hema-

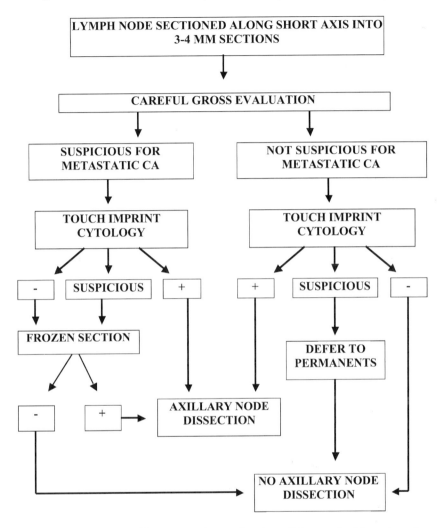

Fig. 1. Algorithm of intraoperative evaluation of the sentinel lymph node.

toxylin and eosin (H&E) for routine evaluation, but this can be supplemented with immunohistochemical staining for epithelial antigens (e.g., cytokeratin, epithelial membrane antigen) to increase the sensitivity for detecting rare metastatic tumor cells *(30–33)*. (The technique of immunohistochemistry is described in Chapter 15.)

This chapter describes the methods used in clinical practice for the cytological and histological evaluation of the axillary SLNs from patients with breast cancer. A suggested algorithm for the intraoperative assessment of the SLN is provided in **Fig. 1.**

2. Materials

2.1. Fresh-Tissue Handling

1. Latex gloves.
2. Cutting board.
3. Scalpel handle and blades.
4. Forceps.
5. Gauze.

2.2. Cytological Touch Imprints

1. Latex gloves.
2. Clean glass slides.
3. Forceps.
4. 95% Ethyl alcohol.
5. Coplin jars.

2.3. Frozen Sections

1. Latex gloves.
2. Large forceps.
3. Isopentane.
4. Liquid nitrogen.
5. Pyrex beaker.
6. Insulated thermos flask.
7. Mounting blocks.
8. Tissue-Tek® optimum cutting temperature (OCT) media (Baxter Diagnostics, McGaw Park, IL).
9. Cryostat microtome.
10. Clean glass slides.

2.4. Paraffin Sections

1. Latex gloves.
2. Embedding cassettes.
3. 10% Neutral buffered formalin 1 part 37% formalin: 9 parts deionized water, 4 g monobasic sodium phosphate, 6.5 g dibasic sodium phosphate.
4. 100% and 95% ethyl alcohol.
5. Alcoholic formalin 10 parts 37% formaldehyde: 65 parts absolute ethyl alcohol:25 parts distilled water.
6. Xylene.
7. Paraplast embedding media (Fisher Scientific).
8. 88% Formic acid.
9. 88% Ammonium hydroxide.
10. Automatic tissue processor (TissueTek VIP™, Sakura Finetek; Shandon Pathcentre® and Shandon Citadel®, Thermo Electron).
11. Embedding center (TissueTek, TEC™, Sakura Finetek; Microm, Microm International, Walldorf, Germany).

12. Paraffin wax dispenser.
13. Embedding forceps.
14. Metal embedding tamp.
15. 24 mm × 20 mm × 5-mm metal embedding molds (Sakura Finetek).
16. Microtome.
17. Flotation water bath.
18. Positively charged glass slides.

2.5. H&E Staining

1. Latex gloves.
2. Staining jars.
3. Slide holders.
4. Xylene.
5. Ethyl alcohol (anhydrous).
6. Hematoxylin 2 (Richard Allen Scientific, Kalamazoo, MI).
7. Eosin Y solution (Richard Allen).
8. Eosin-phloxine solution (Polyscientific, Bay Shore, NY).
9. Clarifier 2 (Richard Allen).
10. Bluing agent (Richard Allen).
11. Permount® mounting medium (Fisher Scientific).
12. Cover slips.

2.6. Immunohistochemical Staining

1. Latex gloves.
2. Humid chamber leveling tray with lid.
3. Staining racks and dishes.
4. Citrate buffer: 0.01 M citrate pH 6.0 containing 0.1% (v/v) Tween-20.
5. Tris-buffered saline (TBS): 0.05 M Tris-HCl and 0.15 M NaCl, pH 7.6.
6. Phosphate-buffered saline: 0.01 M sodium phosphate, 0.89% sodium chloride, pH 7.40 $\pm$ 0.05.
7. Primary anti-cytokeratin antibody.
8. Secondary antibody labeled with biotin.
9. EnVision-HRP-enzyme conjugate (DakoCytomation, Carpenteria, CA).
10. 10% Normal serum in phosphate-buffered saline.
11. Avidin-biotin complex horseradish peroxidase reagent (Vector Laboratories, Burlingame, CA).
12. 3,3'-Diaminobenzidine tetrahydrochloride ([DAB] Sigma, St. Louis, MO) and DAB+ (DakoCytomation).
13. Meyer's hematoxylin counterstain.
14. 6 M Ammonium hydroxide diluted 1:50 in deionized water.
15. 100% Ethanol.
16. Xylene.
17. Permount mounting medium.
18. Cover slips.

3. Methods

3.1. Handling the Lymph Node Tissue

1. Wear latex gloves and observe universal precautions under the assumption that all tissues are potentially infectious.
2. Measure the entire specimen.
3. Dissect the lymph node(s) from the adipose tissue (*see* **Note 1**).
4. Make a small nick in the capsule of nodes smaller than 4 mm to help the fixative penetrate the tissue.
5. For lymph nodes 4 mm or larger, slice each node at 2- to 3-mm intervals (*see* **Note 2**).
6. Evaluate the cut surfaces for areas of nodularity that appear different from the surrounding lymph node tissue. Particular attention should be given to cytological or histological preparations from slices grossly suspicious for involvement by metastatic tumor (*see* **Note 3**).

3.2. Preparation of Intraoperative Cytological Touch Imprints

1. Place up to four slices of lymph node tissue in a linear arrangement so that a glass slide can cover them and overlap the tissue at least 3 mm on all sides.
2. Lay a glass slide on top of the linear arrangement of lymph node slices and press gently (*see* **Note 4**).
3. Immediately place the glass slide in a Coplin jar with 95% ethyl alcohol (*see* **Note 5**).
4. Rinse in tap water, agitating several times.
5. Perform an H&E stain (*see* **Subheading 3.5.**) and compare the amount of lymphoid cells on the slide with the lymph node slices to make sure the cytological imprints are representative (*see* **Note 6**).

3.3. Preparation of Intraoperative Frozen Sections

1. Pour isopentane into a Pyrex beaker and immerse the beaker into an insulated thermos flask containing liquid nitrogen.
2. Place enough OCT embedding medium onto a mounting block to produce a base greater in diameter than the tissue that is to be cut.
3. Using long forceps, immerse the mounting block with the OCT medium into the cooled isopentane for 2 s to allow the medium to adhere to the mounting block.
4. Place one or two slices of lymph node tissue on the OCT base.
5. Immerse the tissue into the cooled isopentane for 10–15 s.
6. Fasten the mounting block to the block holder in the cryostat, and align the blade so that it touches the surface of the tissue.
7. Begin cutting the block until a flat surface is produced across (the) entire portion(s) of tissue.
8. Cut a 5-μm section and touch a glass slide to the section so that the section adheres to the slide.
9. Allow the slide to air dry.

3.4. Preparation of Paraffin-Embedded Tissue Sections

1. Place sections of the entire SLN(s) in embedding cassettes (*see* **Note 7**).
2. Place the cassettes in neutral buffered formalin for 4–24 h.
3. Process the cassettes in an automatic molten tissue processor for dehydration, alcohol clearing, and infiltration with paraffin wax (*see* **Note 8**).
4. Transfer the cassettes into the heated holding area of the embedding center.
5. Dispense molten paraffin wax into a metal embedding mold.
6. Place the mold on the heated platform of the embedding center. Using heated forceps, transfer the lymph node sections from the cassettes into the metal molds filled with melted paraffin wax. Make sure the tissue sections are in the center of the mold with a uniform border of paraffin wax at the periphery.
7. Allow the tissue to settle to the bottom of the mold and move the mold onto the cooling platform.
8. Pick up the metal tamp with forceps and press lightly over the top of the tissue so that the lymph node sections are entirely flat along the bottom of the mold as the paraffin wax cools and solidifies.
9. Place an embedding cassette directly on top of the mold; the open side should face opposite the mold.
10. Fill the space in the cassette with melted paraffin wax.
11. Transfer the mold to the cooling block and allow the paraffin wax to solidify completely.
12. Separate the metal mold from the paraffin-wax block.
13. Place the paraffin-wax block in the block holder of the microtome.
14. Cut 5-µm sections in tandem so that a ribbon forms and float the paraffin wax ribbon onto a flotation water bath.
15. Using a dissecting needle, tease apart the ribbon into separate sections.
16. Place a positively charged glass slide under the lymph node section and lift the section up out of the water onto the slide.
17. Allow the slide to dry thoroughly.

3.5. H&E Staining

1. Place paraffin sections in a 70°C oven for 20 min to start melting the paraffin wax and to evaporate any remaining water on the slide. (Omit **steps 1–3** for frozen sections and cytological preparations.)
2. Pass slides through three sequential Coplin jars of xylene, agitating each slide up and down several times to dissolve all residual paraffin wax and leave only the tissue exposed.
3. Pass slides through two sequential jars of 100% ethyl alcohol, followed by two jars of 95% ethyl alcohol, and then one jar of tap water, agitating each slide several times to gradually hydrate the tissue.
4. Place in hematoxylin 2 for 2 min.
5. Rinse in tap water, agitating each slide several times.
6. Place in Clarifier 2 solution for 15 s.

7. Rinse in tap water, agitating several times.
8. Place in bluing agent for 1 min.
9. Rinse in tap water, agitating several times.
10. Place in eosin Y solution for 30 s.
11. Pass through two sequential jars of 95% ethyl alcohol, then two jars of 100% ethyl alcohol, agitating several times.
12. Pass through three sequential jars of xylene, agitating several times.
13. Place a few drops of xylene on the slide, then add Permount mounting medium and a cover slip.
14. Wipe the sides and back of the slide with gauze.

3.6. Immunohistochemical Staining of Paraffin Sections

1. Place paraffin sections in a 70°C oven for 20 min to start melting the paraffin wax and to evaporate any remaining water on the slide.
2. Pass slides through three sequential Coplin jars of xylene, agitating each slide up and down several times to dissolve all residual paraffin wax and leave only the tissue exposed.
3. Pass slides through two sequential jars of 100% ethyl alcohol, followed by one jar of 95% ethyl alcohol, then one jar of tap water, agitating each slide several times to gradually hydrate the tissue.
4. Place slides in a microwaveable slide tray, and place tray in a microwaveable pressure cooker filled with 1500 mL citrate buffer.
5. Place pressure cooker inside a microwave and heat at max. power (900 W) for 40 min (*see* **Note 9**).
6. Release pressure and allow slides to cool for 30 min.
7. Rinse slides through two jars of Tris-buffered saline.
8. Place slides in another jar with TBS plus 10% normal serum (from the species from which the secondary antibody was generated) for 5 min.
9. Add anti-cytokeratin antibody at recommended dilution and incubate for 2 h at room temperature in a humid chamber (*see* **Note 10**).
10. Wash slides twice in TBS for 3 min each wash, then wash in TBS plus 2% horse serum for 5 min.
11. Add secondary biotinylated antibody and incubate for 30 min at room temperature in a humid chamber.
12. Repeat **step 10**.
13. Mix 10 μL of avidin and 10 μL of biotin-peroxidase (Reagents A and B from the Vector ABC Elite kit; Vector Laboratories) in 1 mL of TBS and incubate for 10 min at room temperature to prepare the ABC complex. Apply 100 μL of the ABC solution to each lymph node section for 30 min at room temperature in a humid chamber.
14. Wash slides three times in TBS for 3 min each wash.
15. Dissolve 20 mg DAB in 100 mL TBS and add 0.01% H_2O_2. Incubate slides in DAB solution for 10–20 min (*see* **Note 11**).
16. Wash slides in TBS.
17. Place in Meyer's hematoxylin for 15 s.

18. Pass through two sequential jars of 95% ethyl alcohol, then two jars of 100% ethyl alcohol, agitating several times.
19. Pass through three sequential jars of xylene, agitating several times.
20. Place a few drops of xylene on the slide, and then add Permount mounting medium and a cover slip.
21. Wipe the sides and bottom of the slide with gauze.

3.7. Immunohistochemical Staining of Frozen Sections

1. Place frozen section slide in a Coplin jar of acetone for 1 min at room temperature.
2. Remove slide and allow to air-dry at room temperature for 15 s.
3. Add anti-cytokeratin antibody at recommended dilution in EnVision antibody diluent and incubate for 3 min on a thermal plate at 37°C.
4. Wash slides in TBS for 10 s at room temperature.
5. Blot the end of the slide on a paper towel to absorb excess liquid.
6. Add Envision-HRP-enzyme conjugate and incubate for 3 min at 37°C.
7. Wash slides in TBS for 10 s at room temperature.
8. Blot the end of the slide on a paper towel to absorb excess liquid.
   Incubate in DAB+ solution for 3 min 37°C.
9. Wash slides in tap water for 10 s at room temperature, followed by a quick dip in distilled water.
10. Place in Meyer's hematoxylin for 15 s.
11. Pass through two sequential jars of 95% ethyl alcohol, then two jars of 100% ethyl alcohol, agitating several times.
12. Pass through three sequential jars of xylene, agitating several times.
13. Place a few drops of xylene on the slide, then add Permount mounting medium and a cover slip.
14. Wipe the sides and bottom of the slide with gauze.

4. Notes

1. The adipose tissue should be gently palpated for lymph nodes. Excess adipose tissue surrounding the lymph node(s) should be carefully trimmed away. The tissue may be placed on a paper towel and gently rubbed until almost all of the fat is rubbed into the paper towel. When all of the fat is rubbed away, the remaining lymph nodes can be readily detected. It is important to remove as much of the fat as possible, because excess fat can interfere with the preparation of cytological imprints and make frozen sections difficult to cut.
2. Although theoretically the same amount of surface area is exposed whether the nodes are cut across the long or the short axis, in practice it is easier to obtain thin sections if the nodes are cut from one pole to the next, perpendicular to the long axis.
3. If frozen sections are performed, the suspicious slice should be frozen separately to be sure that the area in question is appropriately sampled.
4. Although cytological preparations of known tumor samples are usually made by lightly touching a glass slide against the cut surface of the tumor, a more-rigorous method is generally useful in evaluating SLNs. False negatives are usually a

result of inadequate sampling, so a thicker smear is preferable to a sparse preparation when one is trying to identify micrometastatic tumor. A suggested method is to place a glass slide over the lymph node slices and press firmly while rocking in a "see-saw" fashion a few times. It is important to realize that the thicker smears obtained in this manner, although reducing the possibility of a false negative, may cause more difficulty in interpretation, particularly by a pathologist with little experience in the evaluation of touch imprints. Experience in the evaluation of cytological imprints is essential to avoid both false positives and false negatives because of interpretive errors *(24)*.

5. There should be no delay between pressing the slide against the lymph node slices and placing the slide into alcohol. Even minimal air-drying of the slide can introduce drying artifact, making interpretation of the cytological imprint more difficult.

6. Fatty areas may interfere with adherence of cells. Make separate cytological imprints of particularly fatty nodes, or touch fleshy areas separately from the fatty areas. If no tumor cells are identified on cytological imprints from lymph node slices with small nodules or areas suspicious for involvement by metastatic tumor, the cellularity on the slides should be compared to the lymph node slices to make sure that the areas of nodularity have been sampled. In general, cytological imprints should always be compared with the gross tissue slices to make sure that they are representative.

7. Avoid placing large and small slices of tissue together in the same cassette. Small portions of tissue may be lost when the paraffin-wax block is trimmed, or small portions may not be present in the same plane of section as the larger portions. In general, small portions should be placed together in a separate cassette.

8. Automatic tissue processors are recommended. The purpose of tissue processing is to prepare the tissue for sectioning and viewing by light microscopy. After fixation, the tissue must be dehydrated by passing through a series of increasing concentrations of ethyl alcohol. The alcohol must then be cleared with xylene before the tissue can be infiltrated with paraffin wax. Paraffin wax infiltration is necessary before the tissue can be embedded in a block of paraffin, which provides a solid support medium in which the tissue can be sliced.

9. Never allow slides to dry during the antigen-retrieval method.

10. A humid chamber can be prepared by simply placing a wet paper towel in the bottom of chamber.

11. The reaction product is dark brown. Use a known positive control and monitor the development using a microscope to determine the appropriate time to obtain the desired intensity of staining with DAB.

References

1. Ferguson, D. J., Meier P., Karrison T., et al. (1982) Staging of breast cancer and survival rates: an assessment based on 50 years of experience with radical mastectomy. *JAMA* **248,** 1337–1341.

2. Fisher E. R., Anderson S., Redmond C., and Fisher B. (1993) Pathologic findings from the National Surgical Adjuvant Breast Project Protocol B-06: 10-year pathologic and clinical prognostic discriminations. *Cancer* **71**, 2507–2514.
3. Veronesi, U., Rilke, F., Luini, A., et al. (1993) Prognostic significance of number and level of axillary nodal metastases in breast cancer. *Breast* **2**, 224–228.
4. Krag, D. N., Weaver, D. L., Alex, J. C., et al. (1993) Surgical resection and radiolocalization of the sentinel lymph node in breast cancer using a gamma probe. *Surg. Oncol.* **2**, 335–340.
5. Giuliano, A. E., Kirgan, D. M., Guenther, J. M., and Morton, D. L. (1994) Lymphatic mapping and sentinel lymphadenectomy for breast cancer. *Ann. Surg.* **220**, 391–401.
6. Giuliano, A. E., Dale, P. S., Turner, R. R., et al. (1995) Improved axillary staging of breast cancer with sentinel lymphadenectomy. *Ann. Surg.* **222**, 394–401.
7. Giuliano, A. E., Jones, R. C., Brennan, M., and Statman, R. (1997) Sentinel lymphadenectomy in breast cancer. *J. Clin. Oncol.* **15**, 2345–2350.
8. Reintgen, D., Giuliano, R., and Cox, C. E. (2000) Sentinel node biopsy in breast cancer: an overview. *Breast J.* **6**, 299–305.
9. Hsueh, E. C., Turner, R. R., Giuliano, A. E. (2001) Lymphoscintigraphy and lymphatic mapping for identification of sentinel lymph nodes. *World J. Surg.* **25**, 794–797.
10. Weaver, D. L. (2001) Sentinel lymph node biopsy in breast cancer: creating controversy and defining new standards. *Adv. Anat. Pathol.* **8**, 65–73.
11. Canavese, G., Gipponi, M., Catturich, A., et al. (1998) Sentinel lymph node mapping opens a new perspective in the surgical management of early-stage breast cancer: a combined approach with vital blue dye lymphatic mapping and radioguided surgery. *Semin. Surg. Oncol.* **15**, 272–277.
12. Rubio, I. T. and Klimberg, V. S. (2001) Techniques of sentinel lymph node biopsy. *Semin. Surg. Oncol.* **20**, 214–223.
13. Borgstein, P. J., Pijpers, R., Comans, E. F., et al. (1998) Sentinel lymph node biopsy in breast cancer: guidelines and pitfalls of lymphoscintigraphy and gamma probe detection. *J. Am. Coll. Surg.* **186**, 275–283.
14 Veronesi, U., Paganelli, G., Galimberti, V., et al. (1997) Sentinel node biopsy to avoid axillary dissection in breast cancer with clinically negative nodes. *Lancet* **349**, 1864–1867.
15. Krag, D., Weaver, D., Ashikaga, T., et al. (1998) The sentinel node in breast cancer: a multicenter validation study. *N. Engl. J. Med.* **339**, 941–946.
16. Imoto, S., Hasebe, T. (1999) Initial experience with sentinel node biopsy in breast cancer at the National Cancer Center Hospital East. *Jpn. J. Clin. Oncol.* **29**, 11–15.
16. Weaver, D. L., Krag, D. N., Ashikaga, T., et al. (2000) Pathologic analysis of sentinel and nonsentinel lymph nodes in breast carcinoma: a multicenter study. *Cancer* **88**, 1099–1107.
17. Cibull, M. L. (1999) Handling sentinel lymph node biopsy specimens. *Arch. Pathol. Lab. Med.* **123**, 620–621.

18. Fitzgibbons, P. L., Page, D. L., Weaver, D., et al. (1999) Prognostic factors in Breast Cancer, College of American Pathologists Consensus Statement, 1999. *Arch. Path. Lab. Med.* **124,** 966–978.
19. Meyer, J. S. (1998) Sentinel lymph node biopsy: strategies for pathologic examination of the specimen. *J. Surg. Oncol.* **69,** 212–218.
20. Liberman, L. (2000) Pathologic analysis of sentinel lymph nodes in breast carcinoma. *Cancer* **88,** 971–977.
21. Rubio, I. T., Korourian, S., Cowan, C., Krag, D. N., Colvert, M., and Klimberg, S. (1998) Use of touch preps for intraoperative diagnosis of sentinel lymph node metastases in breast cancer. *Ann. Surg. Oncol.* **5,** 689–694.
22. Ku, N. N. K., Ahmad, N., Smith, P. V., et al. (1997) Intraoperative imprint cytology of sentinel lymph nodes in breast cancer. *Acta Cytol.* **41,** 1606–1607.
23. Molyneux, A. J., Atanoos, R. L., and Coghill, S. B. (1997) The value of lymph node imprint cytodiagnosis: an assessment of interobserver agreement and diagnostic accuracy. *Cytopathology* **8,** 256–264.
24. Ratanawichitrasin, A., Biscott, C. V., Levy, L., Crowe, J. P. (1999) Touch imprint cytological analysis of sentinel lymph nodes for detecting axillary metastases in patients with breast cancer. *Br. J. Surg.* **86,** 1346–1348.
25. Motomura, K., Inaji, H., Komoike, Y., et al. (2000) Intraoperative sentinel lymph node examination by imprint cytology and frozen sectioning during breast surgery. *Br. J. Surg.* **87,** 597–501.
26. van Diest, P. J., Torrenga, H., Borgstein, P. J., et al. (1999) Reliability of intraoperative frozen section and imprint cytological investigation of sentinel lymph nodes in breast cancer. *Histopathology* **35,** 14–18.
27. Viale, G., Bosari, S., Mazzarol, G., et al. (1999) Intraoperative examination of axillary sentinel lymph nodes in breast carcinoma patients. *Cancer* **85,** 2433–2438.
28. Weiser, M. R., Montgomery, L. L., Sunsnik, B., et al. (2000) Is routine intraoperative frozen-section examination of sentinel lymph nodes in breast cancer worthwhile? *Ann. Surg. Oncol.* **7,** 651–655.
29. Dogliani, C., Dell'Orto, P., Zanetti, G., et al. (1990) Cytokeratin-immunoreactive cells of human lymph nodes and spleen in normal and pathological conditions. An immunocytochemical study. *Virchows Arch. A Pathol. Anat. Histopathol.* **416,** 479–490.
30. Chilosi, M., Lestoni, M., Pedron, S., et al. (1994) A rapid immunostaining method for frozen sections. *Biotech. Histochem.* **69,** 235–239.
31 Ahmed, N., Ku, N. N., Nicosia, S. V., et al. (1998) Evaluation of sentinel lymph node imprints in breast cancer: role of intraoperative immunostaining in breast cancer staging. *Acta Cytol.* **42,** 1218.
32 Cote, R. J., Peterson, H. F., Chaiwan, B., et al. (1999) Role of immunohistochemical detection of lymph node metastases in management of breast cancer. *Lancet* **354,** 896–900.
33. Noguchi, S., Aihara, T., Nakamori, S., et al. (1994) The detection of breast carcinoma micrometastases in axillary lymph nodes by means of reverse transcriptase-polymerase chain reaction. *Cancer* **74,** 1595–1600.

34. Mori, M., Mimori, K., Inoue, H., et al. (1995) Detection of cancer micrometastases in lymph nodes by reverse transcriptase-polymerase chain reaction. *Cancer Res.* **55,** 3417–3420.
35. Bostick, P. J., Huynh, K. T., Sarantou, T., et al. (1998) Detection of metastases in sentinel lymph nodes of breast cancer patients by multiple RT-PCR. *Int. J. Cancer* **79,** 645–651.
36. Turner, R. R., Ollila, D. W., Stern, S., and Giuliano, A. E. (1999) Optimal histopathologic examination of the sentinel lymph node for breast carcinoma staging. *Am. J. Surg. Pathol.* **23,** 263–267.
37. Turner, R. R. and Giuliano, A. E. (1998) Intraoperative pathologic examination of the sentinel lymph node. *Ann. Surg. Oncol.* **5,** 670–672.

12

Measurement of Estrogen Receptor Status by Immunocytochemistry in Paraffin Wax Sections

Bharat Jasani, Anthony Douglas-Jones, Anthony Rhodes, Susan Wozniak, Peter J. Barrett-Lee, Julie Gee, and Robert Nicholson

Summary

The estrogen receptor (ER) status and, to a lesser extent, progesterone receptor status have been recommended by recently published guidelines as important for routine prognostic and predictive evaluation of breast cancer.

Although the clinical utility of ER status has been largely validated using biochemical ligand-binding assays such as the dextran-coated, charcoal ligand-binding assay, there has been the need to develop the ER immunocytochemical assay as a more accurate and practical alternative. In particular, ER status as determined on paraffin sections by immunocytochemical assay has been shown to be superior to the ligand-binding assay for predicting response to adjuvant endocrine therapy in breast cancer.

The success of the paraffin-section assay is founded on two principles. The first relates to the advent of the heat-mediated, antigen-retrieval technique capable of restoring ER and progesterone receptor antigenicity in routinely prepared diagnostic formalin-fixed, paraffin-embedded tissue sections. The second is associated with the capacity for this substrate to provide more reliable and reproducible semiquantitative assessment of ER status in morphologically better-preserved tissue used routinely for histopathological diagnosis.

The aim of this chapter is to describe the methodology currently used for optimal reproducible demonstration, scoring, and assessment of ER status in paraffin wax-embedded tissue sections in relation to the management of breast cancer in a routine or clinical-trial setting.

Key Words: Estrogen receptor assay; ER; immunohistochemistry; ER-ICA; breast cancer predictive marking.

1. Introduction

The estrogen receptor (ER) status and, to a lesser extent, progesterone receptor (PR) status have been recommended by recently published guidelines as important for routine prognostic and predictive evaluation of breast cancer.

From: *Methods in Molecular Medicine, Vol. 120: Breast Cancer Research Protocols*
Edited by: S. A. Brooks and A. L. Harris © Humana Press Inc., Totowa, NJ

Although the clinical utility of ER status has been largely validated using biochemical ligand-binding assays such as the dextran-coated, charcoal ligand-binding assay (DCCA), there has been the need to develop the ER immunocytochemical assay (ER-ICA) as a more accurate and practical alternative for the following reasons.

The biochemical assay is not only technically demanding, time-consuming, and carries the risk of using radioactivity, but it also requires the availability of relatively large amount of immediately frozen tumor tissue for reliable results. It has also proved to have a relatively low predictive index. Thus, only 55–60% of ER-DCCA-positive tumor patients appear to respond to endocrine treatment, and approx 10% of ER-DCCA-negative patients show a significant response as well.

The above discrepancies have been attributed to a combination of two or more of the following:

1. The unavoidable contamination of the sample by benign epithelium and connective tissue surrounding the tumor.
2. Potential nonspecific binding of the ligand.
3. Lack of detection of ER already occupied by endogenous estrogen or tamoxifen in some patients.
4. The intrinsic failure of the assay to account for cell-to-cell variation of ER concentration.
5. Inaccuracy of measurement on low-cellularity tumors.

The potential for immunocytochemical assays to overcome these drawbacks has led to the development of ER-ICA and PR-ICA. These were initially designed to work only in appropriately fixed, freshly frozen tissue sections. However, because of the logistical difficulty of obtaining good-quality, freshly frozen tissue on a routine basis, newer, more practical assays based on the use of readily available paraffin-embedded tissue sections have been developed. Recently, ER status as determined on paraffin sections by ICA has also been shown to be superior to the ligand-binding assays for predicting response to adjuvant endocrine therapy in breast cancer *(3)*.

The success of the paraffin-section assay is founded on two principles. The first relates to the advent of the heat-mediated, antigen-retrieval technique capable of restoring ER and PR antigenicity in routinely prepared diagnostic formalin-fixed, paraffin-embedded tissue sections. The second is associated with the capacity for this substrate to provide more reliable and reproducible semiquantitative assessment of ER status in morphologically better-preserved tissue used routinely for histopathological diagnosis.

The aim of this chapter is to describe the methodology currently used for optimal reproducible demonstration, scoring, and assessment of ER status in paraffin wax-embedded tissue sections in relation to the management of breast cancer in a routine or clinical-trial setting. The demonstration and assessment of PR status is conducted along identical lines, and for the sake of brevity and for maintaining the focus on ER (which is the main marker used), information relating to PR-ICA will not be considered further. For a broader understanding of immunocytochemical procedures, the reader is referred to a recent excellent text on the subject by Polak and Van Noorden *(4)*, and in Chapter 15.

1.1. Immunocytochemical Demonstration of ER

Immunocytochemical demonstration of ER in breast cancer, like any other immunocytochemical marker, involves a multistep procedure that follows three sequential phases of tissue handling: preanalysis, analysis, and postanalysis, respectively. The methodological approach and the rationale adopted for each step involved are described in **Subheadings 1.1.1–1.1.16**. The protocols for ER demonstration and assessment are summarized in **Sections 3.1.** and **3.2.**, respectively.

1.1.1. Preanalysis

This phase of analysis involves a series of steps extending from the initial collection or reception of the breast tumor tissue specimen from the surgical theater unit to its sectioning and adherence onto glass slides.

1.1.2. Tissue Fixation

The majority of breast tumor tissue specimens are received as either needle biopsies for diagnosis or wide local excision and mastectomy for treatment. Each specimen is given a unique case identification number. The specimens are then immediately immersed in a fixative, if not already received treated with it from the theater. After a few hours of fixation, the larger lumpectomy and mastectomy specimens are sliced open at approx 1-cm intervals, with paper wicks inserted between the slices to allow free and even penetration of the fixative. Fixation is allowed to proceed in 2–10 × tissue volume of the fixative solution at room temperature for 12–24 h (i.e., overnight) to allow for the relatively slow penetration rate (approx 10 mm/24 h) and crosslinking reaction of formalin.

For optimum fixation, an isotonic solution of phosphate-buffered formalin (4% final formaldehyde concentration) is recommended. Nonbuffered 10% formal saline or acidified formalin-fixed tissue with the aid of appropriate level of antigen retrieval is also able to provide satisfactory results *(5)*.

Immediate and adequate fixation of the surgically removed tissue should be aimed for in every case to ensure optimum preservation of its antigenicity and morphology. In reality, however, for some specimens, there may be unavoidable delays in fixation because of delayed transportation of the tissue from the theater to the laboratory. In addition, some of the larger specimens may be fixed without slicing, which delays penetration of the fixative to the center of the tumor tissue. Fixation issues should not be a problem for core biopsy material, which is usually fixed immediately after its removal in the clinic and for which the overall fixation distance is quite small.

1.1.3. Tissue Processing and Embedding

The small biopsy tissue is wrapped in paper (to avoid its loss during processing) and encased in a plastic embedding cassette. The use of dyes to mark the small biopsies should be avoided, as they may interfere with the analysis. From larger specimens, representative tissue blocks measuring approx 1 × 1 × 0.5 cm thick are cut to include tumor tissue together with an edge of surrounding normal breast tissue. The blocked tissue is then taken through a series of alcohol-followed-by-xylene changes, and then infiltrated with paraffin wax, all in an automated tissue processor.

1.1.4. Paraffin Section Preparation

Glass slides either coated with a suitable adhesive (e.g., TESPA; Sigma, St. Louis, MO) or with electrostatically charged surfaces (e.g., SuperFrost® Plus) are used to ensure firm and flat adherence of the sections. The section thickness is set at 3–5 μm. Serial sections are cut and mounted onto the slide in an orderly fashion in the same orientation and position. The sections are allowed to dry overnight at 60°C (overnight at 37°C is preferred by some laboratories in an attempt to preserve greater levels of antigen). Sections can be stored at room temperature and should be used or discarded ideally within 2–3 mo, as there is evidence for gradual loss in antigenicity with long-term storage.

It is noteworthy that ER, like many other antigens, is less significantly affected by the differences in tissue processing and embedding protocols than it is by the differences in the fixation regimens applied.

1.1.5. Analysis

This phase involves the steps extending from dewaxing of sections and their pretreatment through to their immunostaining and final mounting for viewing using the microscope.

1.1.6. Section Dewaxing and Antigen Retrieval

Dewaxing is conducted in a series of a minimum of two xylene changes (each at least 2 min long), followed by five absolute alcohol changes (each least 5 min long). The sections are then treated with endogenous peroxidase blocking solution (0.5% [v/v] H_2O_2 in absolute methanol) for 15 min, and washed in running tap water for a minimum of 10 min. The slides are then transferred to preheated antigen-retrieval medium (e.g., 10 mM ethylene-diaminetetraacetic acid [EDTA] solution adjusted to pH 7.0 with concentrated NaOH solution) treated in a microwave (800 W) for 25 min. The sections are then allowed to cool for 5 min before washing them in running tap water for 5 min; they are then transferred first to distilled water, then to wash buffer.

1.1.7. Immunostaining Procedure

Antigen-retrieved sections are removed from the tap water and transferred to the wash buffer and equilibrated for 10 min. Slides are removed and immunostained either manually or in an automated immunostainer, using the staining protocol summarized in **Subheading 3.1.**

For routine immunostaining of ER, the immunoperoxidase method is by far the most widely used technique. It involves five sequential steps:

1. Application of primary antibody.
2. Addition of secondary detection reagent(s).
3. Enzyme-product generation and deposition.
4. Hematoxylin counter-staining.
5. Permanent mounting of the stained section under a cover slip.

For the primary antibody reagent, commercially available monoclonal antibodies with proven high specificity and sensitivity should be used. Likewise, commercially prepared secondary detection reagents and substrate development systems giving the highest detection power should be used. The counter-staining should be of just-sufficient intensity and clarity to reveal all the nucleated cells, without masking the specific nuclear staining.

Automated immunostaining should be used in preference to the manual method for applying the antibody and enzyme substrate reagents for analysis of large numbers of samples for routine diagnostic purposes.

1.1.8. Postanalysis

This phase involves the steps from the mounting of the slides, labeling with the relevant protocol and patient information, and submission of the slides for microscopic viewing for ensuring good internal and external quality assurance (EQA). It is followed by interpretation of the morphological distribution of the immunostaining and its semiquantitative assessment and the final reporting of these results, as described next.

1.1.9. Assessment of the ER Status

The tumor section is scanned using a microscope at low power (×4 objective) to identify the character and the layout of the tumor and background breast tissue components and to assess the overall intensity and distribution of the specific nuclear staining. The background normal-appearing breast lobular epithelium is checked as positive internal control. Within the tumor, the *in situ* and the invasive components are separately assessed. Any staining clearly visible at this power is recorded to be strong and is given a "+++" rating. The tissue is then scanned sequentially at ×10, ×20, and ×40 objective settings, and the staining becoming clearly visible at each of these powers is rated to be of moderate (++), weak (+), and borderline (±) intensity level, respectively. The overall extent of staining (i.e., inclusive of all intensities of staining visible) is then estimated and rated to be either less than 10, 11–25, 26–50, 51–75, or more than 75%, respectively. A note is made of the distribution of the overall staining, and it is rated as negative, focal, multifocal, diffuse, or heterogeneous (i.e., a combination of the latter variety). Any artifactual or nonspecific form of staining (e.g., patchy, uneven, and/or cytoplasmic staining) is also recorded. These observations and comments are recorded in the ER score sheet illustrated in **Table 1**.

1.1.10. Reporting of ER Status

Interpretation of individual case related results should always be preceded by a careful assessment of the quality of external and internal positive control tissues.

For the external control tissue, a composite block of tumors with known ER status of negative, weak, and strong intensity of staining should tested with each batch of analysis. The internal control assessment should relate to normal-appearing background breast tissue included in the block representative of the test tumor tissue. If the control results are of satisfactory quality with respect to the specificity and sensitivity of immunostaining, one should proceed to assess the batch-related results. It is important to record the external control results obtained for every batch analyzed for retrospective review of the results for auditing purposes as well as for troubleshooting for any occasional intractable technical problems.

A composite block of three breast cancer or cell line blocks representative of ER negative, weak-positive, and strong-positive status is included with each batch of staining. The results of this block are cataloged with respect to the extent, intensity, and distribution of staining obtained for the tumor cell and background breast epithelial components, respectively. Provided these results are of satisfactory quality for all three of tumors in the external control, the analysis of the individual tumor case included in the batch is conducted.

The typical results obtained for the ER-strong, ER-weak/-moderate, and ER-negative controls are shown in **Fig. 1A–D**. The staining of normal breast epithelium in close proximity to the tumor is used as internal positive control.

Table 1
Estrogen Receptor Immunocytochemistry Score Sheet

1. Background breast
2. *In situ* cancer component
3. Invasive cancer component
4. Overall receptor status

Reporting Status

1. Ready for reporting
2. Refer to specialist pathologist for advice on histological identification of tumor cells
3. Repeat study to exclude false-negative result or other technical artifacts
4. Undertake further studies on alternative tissue block
5. Any other additional work

This is particularly useful for judging and verifying an ER-negative as illustrated in **Fig. 1A**.

The assessment of ER status of a tumor is based on scoring of the of specific nuclear staining in terms of its extent (i.e., percentage of positive cells recorded in categories of <10, between 10 and 25, 25–50, 50–75, and >75%) and intensity (categorized as: ± or borderline, + or weak, ++ or moderate, +++ or strong), as well as its overall pattern of expression (e.g., focal, multifocal, diffuse; homogenous or heterogeneous) using the hematoxylin-counterstained normal and tumor cells as the backdrop. The levels of staining obtained for *in situ* vs invasive components vs background breast epithelium should be recorded separately for comparison. These overall results should be reported formally as illustrated in **Table 2**, with the tumor ER status summarized as positive or negative, together a statement about the grade of the positivity recorded (i.e., weak, moderate, or strong).

For the purposes of some oncology clinics, as well as for clinical trials and research projects, it may be necessary to provide the results according to certain established methods of scoring such as the "quick" score or on a continuous (rather than categorical) scale such as histological (H) scores. These are described in **Subheading 3.2.**

1.1.11. Clinical Significance and Reliability of ER Status

The value of the ER assay in breast cancer management is ultimately related to the power with which it is able to predict the responsiveness of the individual breast cancer to adjuvant antiestrogen therapy.

In general, if ER status is either negative (i.e., <10% ±) or borderline positive (i.e., 10–25% ±), the benefits of tamoxifen are expected to be very small,

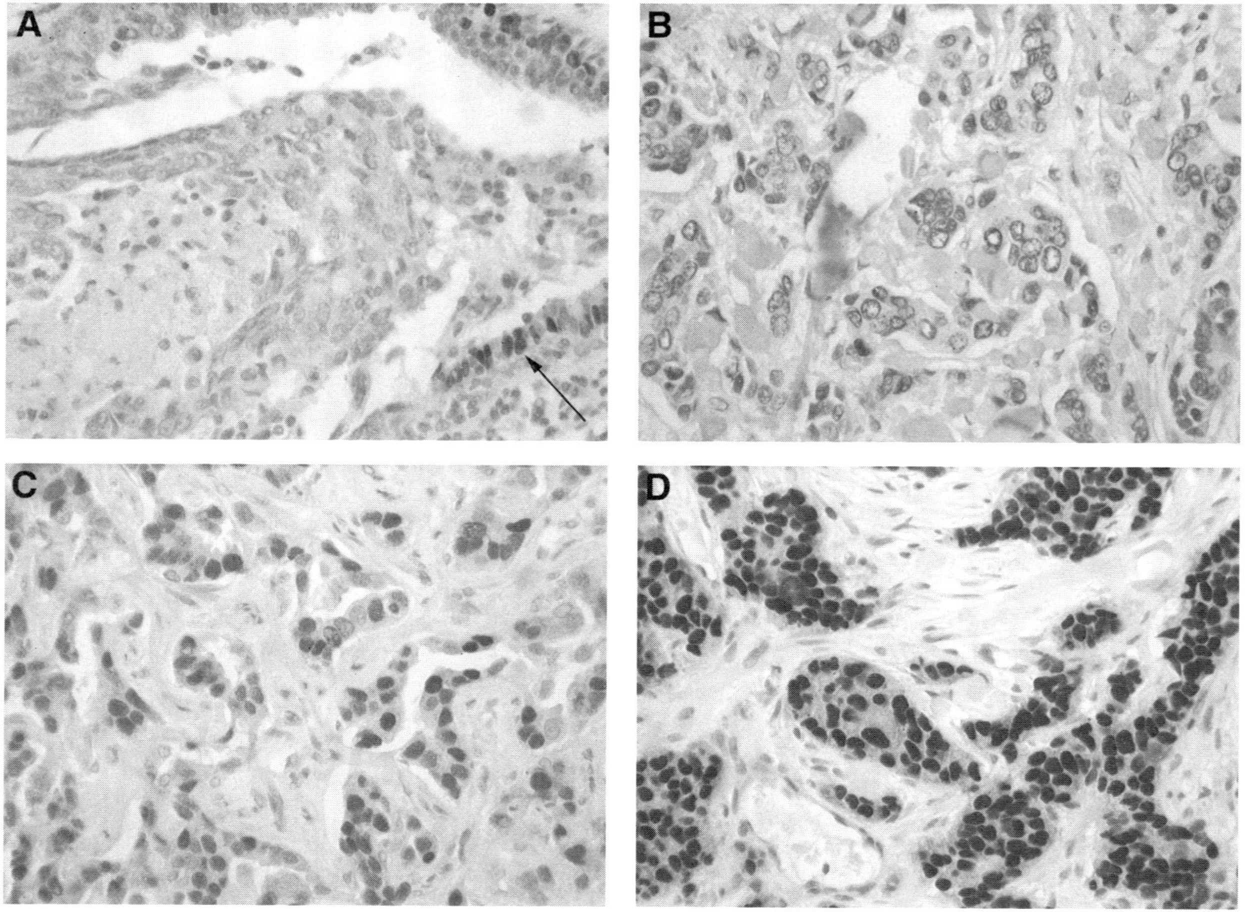

Fig. 1. Illustrations of different grades of ER immunostaining.

Table 2
Estrogen Receptor Immunocytochemistry Report

(Hospital/block no. XXXX/XX)
Percentage positive nuclei, intensity of staining

1	Background breast:	75–100%, +/++ /+++[a]
2	*In situ* component:	Negative
3	Invasive component:	Negative
4.	Overall status:	Estrogen receptor/negative

Estrogen receptor-negative tumor

[a]+, weak staining intensity; ++, moderate staining intensity; +++, strong staining intensity.

and chemotherapy, if appropriate, should be considered as an early option. Tumors with weak-to-moderate grades of ER staining (i.e., 25–50% + to ++) are expected to have moderate levels of response to tamoxifen, whereas those with moderate-to-strong levels of ER staining (50–100% ++ to +++) are likely to benefit significantly. These categories of results may also have value in breast cancer prognostication, treatment of metastatic disease, and entry of breast cancer patients into clinical trials *(6)*.

Several biological factors have been suggested to be associated with endocrine response including protein expression induced by estrogens, such pS2 *(7,8)*. Endocrine failure is also correlated with the expression of positive growth factor receptors such as epidermal growth factor-receptor and c-erbB-2 or HER-2 *(9–11)*. None of these markers is routinely employed, because their results do not appear to add to the predictive power of ER status alone in multivariate analysis. This is partly because epidermal growth factor-receptor- and c-erbB-2-positive tumors are mainly ER-negative, and pS2-positive tumors are invariably ER-positive.

1.1.12. Reproducibility and Accuracy of ER/PR Status Assessment

The reliability of ER status as a predictive marker is inherently limited by the subjective and qualitative nature of the microscopic assessment involved. Nevertheless, for the extremes of results (i.e., tumors that are ER-/PR-negative or uniformly strongly positive), the subjectivity and the lack of a quantitative index are unlikely to affect the accuracy of the assay.

The critical area of difficulty is that of defining the intermediate grades of staining both accurately and reproducibly. This is because immunocytochemically demonstrated ER positivity is ultimately expected to reflect a continuum of ER content, correlating ultimately with the level of the clinical response. A reliable scoring system is seen to be one that provides as complete and objective a description of the staining distribution and intensity and the overall pattern of expression in any given case. From this, a conclusion about the ER status is drawn that is likely to reflect the clinical responsiveness of the tumor as accurately as possible. A scoring system of this type has been adopted in the University Hospital of Wales, Cardiff, for the past 4 yr.

1.1.13. Role of Image Analysis

A number of image analytical methods have been developed for quantitative analysis of ER nuclear positivity for research purposes. These include the SAMBA 200 cell image processor (Thomson TITN, Grenoble, France) utilized by Charpin et al. *(12)* and Cohen et al. *(13)*, the microTICAS image analysis system (developed by Dr. L. Wied, University of Chicago) used by Franklin et al. *(14)*, and the CAS 200 (Cell Analysis Systems, Elmhurst, IL) and Biocom 500 (Biocom, Les Ulis, France) systems applied by El-Badawy et al. *(15)* and Rostagno et al. *(16)*, respectively.

These systems are targeted at estimating percentage of ER-positive cells as well as their average intensity of staining. The accuracy of the image analysis is dependent on the number of images analyzed and the capacity of the operator to identify and electronically separate tumor cells from neighboring background breast epithelial cells. The approach has the capacity to delineate intercell and intratumor heterogeneity in a biological and therapeutically meaningful way *(13)*. The main problem with these systems for their application on a routine basis on large numbers of breast cancers is that they are semi-interactive, involving a procedure that is time-consuming and labor-intensive for each slide.

Some of the labor intensity is relieved by adoption of a novel approach called the Automated Cellular Imaging System developed by Chroma Vision Medical Systems (San Juan Capistrano, CA) *(17)*. This is capable of reading the entire stained tissue section or cell preparation on a stand-alone basis for the purpose of detecting, counting, and classifying cells of clinical interest according to three-dimensional color-intensity measurement and morphometric characterization. The data are downloaded on to disks to be read by the reporting pathology staff member at his/her own workstation, capable of reading, analyzing, and issuing an automatic and photomicrographically illustrated report on an individual case basis.

1.1.14. Role of Automated Immunostaining

The advent of automation in immunostaining procedure has brought in the advantage of greater reproducibility and faster and greater workload throughput.

There are essentially two types of automated immunostaining platforms available on the market that are depicted as either "open" or "closed." The closed variety has been developed by primarily by Ventana Research (San

Mateo, CA), and their FDA-approved BenchMark system is an example of it. The system is fully bar code-operated and entirely closed to any outside interference. The only steps involving the operator are the loading on of paraffin wax-embedded slides, off-loading, and cover slipping of fully immunostained and counterstained slides at the end of the set run. The open system is used with the DakoCytomation Autostainer and the Menarini (UK) Optimax. Both of these allow the operator to follow a variety of immunostaining protocols of their own choice, if they are programmable on the machine. Both systems offer reliable platforms for ER and PR immunostaining.

1.1.15. Role of Quality Assurance and Validation

Stringent internal and EQA exercises are essential for ensuring reproducible and accurate output from routinely applied ER-ICA. To monitor quality inclusion of receptor-negative, receptor-poor, and receptor-rich invasive breast carcinomas as controls is mandatory in every batch of analysis conducted. Cell line blocks may provide standardized, readily available control material in the future. The simple use of a single strong-positive control may mask subtle reduction in sensitivity from run to run, leading to unrecognized false-negative results. The inclusion of normal background breast tissue as an internal positive control in every test section is equally important, because a negative result may be because of unexpected technical mishaps, which may arise even when using automated immunostaining protocols. This is particularly important in the analysis of core biopsy material in which there may be no background. Negative core assays without internal control should be repeated with external positive tissue placed on the same slide if possible.

In addition to the regular use of internal and external controls, the ER-ICA should be regularly tested against samples supplied by an EQA scheme. This is to ensure the accuracy of the assay and eliminate the possibility that its sensitivity may be set overall either too high or too low, resulting in either overscoring or underscoring of ER-positive or -negative cases with respect to the rates expected from nationally or internationally established trends (*18–20*).

1.1.16. Conclusion and Future Needs

The ultimate value of an ER-ICA is based on the accuracy with which the results obtained are able to predict the responsiveness to antiestrogen treatment in any given patient. This chapter has described a methodological approach to achieve reliable ER status assessment in individual cases. The use of ER-ICA directed at paraffin-embedded sections, however, needs to be performed with an automated immunostainer, and the staining resulting from it analyzed with a sophisticated image analysis system to produce technically the most reliable results. Nevertheless, whereas the results of ER-ICA have been shown to correlate well with those of DCCA, the assay has been available for too short a time to yield sufficient follow-up data to clinically validate its predictive value. However, the hope is that that future studies will confirm the ability of this practical and reproducible assay to predict responsiveness to hormone-based treatment and provide prognostic information in individual patients *(3)*.

2. Materials

1. General-purpose solvents (xylene and alcohol) are used for dewaxing the sections; care should be taken to make sure that the final treatment is given in a fresh change of solvent. These are also used for dehydrating and clearing the stained sections.
2. Antigen-retrieval solution is prepared using 37.2 g EDTA (code ED2SS, Sigma) dissolved in 10 L distilled water, together with 3.2 g of NaOH pellets, and stirred for 2 h at room temperature, with adjustment of the pH to 7.0, using concentrated sodium hydroxide (drop-wise). The antigen retrieval is conducted in a microwave oven or a pressure cooker, using an optimized number of slides per batch. The antigen-retrieval solution should be applied in sufficient quantities to allow an adequate depth of fluid above the slides to ensure uniform treatment.
3. Wash buffer (ChemMate™ S3006; DakoCytomation, Cambridgeshire, UK).
4. Commercially available endogenous peroxidase blocking agent (S2023, DakoCytomation or methanol/H_2O_2 solution/283.2 mL methanol and 4.8 mL H_2O_2) could be used before or after the addition of the primary antibody to remove any endogenous peroxidatic activity.
5. Optimal dilution of primary antibody (Novocastra ER 6F11) should be prepared using commercially available antibody diluent (S2022, DakoCytomation). The optimal dilution should be determined using known ER-strong, ER-weak, and ER-negative breast cancer control sections.
6. Detection kit reagents (ChemMate K5001, DakoCytomation) should applied according to the manufacturer's recommendations in either an automated stainer or using a manual mode.
7. Diaminobenzidine (DAB) disposable cartridges are used for disposing DAB waste.
8. Hematoxylin is used as a counterstain.
9. DPX, which is a mixture of distyrene (a polystyrene), tricresyl phosphate (a plasticizer) and xylene, is used as the preferred mounting medium.
10. Standard cover slips.

3. Methods

3.1. ER Staining

ER immunostaining should be conducted in batches of slides and ideally, using an automated immunostainer. The protocol described here is adaptable to both the manual and automated modes of staining

1. Dewax slides with sequential xylene (two 5-min changes), followed by alcohol (five 1-min changes).
2. Wash sections well in running tap water for at least 5 min.
3. Microwave the sections in a plastic rack placed inside 600 mL of preheated 10 mM EDTA solution, pH 7.0, at full power (800 W) for 25 min, followed by a 5-min standing time, ensuring no drying out of the sections at any stage.
4. Transfer the rack to a sink filled with running tap water and wash for a maximum of 5 min, followed by a rinse in distilled water, and then immersion into wash buffer until ready for immunostaining.
5. Treat with endogenous peroxidase blocking agent solution for 5 min, or methanol/H_2O_2 solution for 15 min to block endogenous peroxidase activity.
6. If required, apply PAP pen to the top and bottom and the side edges of the slides.
7. Apply sequentially the following immunoreagents either manually or by placing the slides in the automated immunostainer, at their respective working dilutions for the specified times at ambient temperature.
   a. Primary anti-ER antibody (Novocastra ER 6F11), 45 min.
   b. Secondary detection kit reagents (ChemMate S3006, DakoCytomation) according to the manufacturer's instructions, 30 min each reagent.
   c. Develop DAB color reaction for more than 10 min.
   d. Rinse in running tap water to remove the excess substrate solution.
   e. Lightly counterstain with hematoxylin.
   f. Take through a reversed series of alcohol and xylene changes.
   g. Mount the sections under glass cover slips using a permanent mounting medium.
   h. Label the slide with the corresponding case number and abbreviated reagent treatment profile.

3.2. Assessment of Immunostaining Score

Assessment of ER positivity using biochemical assays produces a numerical result and the cutoff point between ER positivity and ER negativity has been set at 20 fmol/g of protein. Histological examination of breast carcinoma sections stained for ER show variation in the intensity and distribution of nuclear positivity associated with the tumor nuclei. Thus, in a case it might be observed that clusters of tumor nuclei showing moderate (2+ more readily visible at medium power)-to-strong (3+ readily visible at low power) positivity might lie next to tumor cell nuclei showing either no immunopositivity, very faint (1±, i.e., just visible at the highest power), or weak (1+, most readily visible at high power) nuclear positivity. It seems likely that a tumor in which all (100%) nuclei show strong (3+) nuclear positivity is more likely to respond to antiestrogen treatment than a tumor in which a smaller proportion (e.g., 10–25%) of nuclei are weakly (1+) positive, although both may be classified as ER-positive. A number of scoring systems for assessing the intensity and distribution of ER positivity have therefore been developed. In routine practice, the assessment should be quick, easy to apply, and reproducible. The simplest, most widely used approach is to designate a tumor as positive if there is nuclear staining of any intensity is visible in more than 10% of the tumor cells. The most elaborate system is the H score method, in which the percentage of tumor nuclei showing positivity is assessed at high power, and within the positive group, the percentage of nuclei showing strong, moderate, and weak positivity is systematically estimated. For any particular field, the percentage showing weak (1+) positivity is multiplied by 1, the percentage showing moderate (2+) positivity is multiplied by 2, and the percentage showing strong (3+) positivity is multiplied by 3. These three products are then added to give an aggregate score out of a theoretical maximum of 300. The scoring process is performed in three high-power fields in different areas of the tumor, and the mean of the three fields is calculated. This method attempts to take into account the range of intensity and distribution of nuclear positivity, but it is slow and laborious to perform on large numbers of cases in routine practice. The semiautomated image analysis packages such as Chroma Vision have been developed to automate aspects of the H scoring system. However, to achieve optimal results with these automated systems, it is necessary to adjust the staining protocols according to the manufacturers' instructions. The distribution of the tumor staining may be more quickly assessed simply by scoring the percentage of positivity associated with any level of intensity as indicated below:

1. Zero: negative.
2. 1–25% of tumor area.
3. 26–50% of tumor area.
4. 50–75% of tumor area.
5. Greater than 75% of tumor area.

Similarly, intensity may be scored as:

1. Zero: negative.
2. Weak: readily visible only at high power.
3. Moderate: readily visible at medium power.
4. Strong: clearly visible at low power.

The score for distribution and the score for intensity can be multiplied to give an "immunoreactive score" out of a total of 12 or added up to give a quick score, with a range of 0–7. The methods of assessment have been compared on a group of cases of breast cancer treated with tamoxifen in which outcome was known (*21*), yielding good correlation with outcome whatever method was used. It is noteworthy that the quick score method correlated most closely with the time to progression in Cox multivariate analysis. No scoring method has been universally adopted, but if intensity and distribution are both to be taken into account for an easy and rapid assessment applicable to routine practice, the quick score method appears to the most attractive. This method has there-fore been recommended for routine diagnostic assessment of ER status in breast cancer *(22)*. It is likely that in the future, automated image analysis systems will be developed to assay immunohistochemical preparations automatically to provide objective numerical data.

4. Notes

1. Barrett-Lee, P., Nicholson, R., and McClelland, R. (unpublished data). In view of the prospective nature of a recent adjuvant breast cancer trial, preliminary work was done to consider the potential influence a number of factors might have on staining quality before beginning the full staining analysis of sections. Of particular concern was the potential for variance in staining quality, which might arise from the necessity of using long-term stored, previously sectioned material obtained from multiple centers. In order to study these effects on ER expression, an ICA-QA study was performed, particularly as the ER antigen is recognized as being heat-labile and therefore potentially sensitive to storage-induced deterioration. Forty-six paraffin blocks, from which sections had already been cut and stored, were randomly selected from five UK hospitals and recalled to the Tenovus (Institute of Cancer Research, Welsh School of Pharmacy, University College, Cardiff) laboratory. Fresh sections were cut, and these were stained in parallel with their previously cut-and-stored (for periods of between 49 and 150 wk) coun-terparts using the well-documented and validated 1D-5 (antibody) ER-ICA method for use with paraffin-embedded material. Staining was semiquantified using our established combination staining intensity and overall percentage posi-tivity H score procedure *(12)*.

   H scores of 5 or more and 300 or less were considered to be ER-positive and those of less than 5 ER-negative. Of the 46, 33 were classified as ER-positive (H scores: 5, 300) for both freshly cut and stored samples. Two cases from the freshly cut and stained group were also classified as ER-positive, but their counterparts were ER-negative (H score: <5). Eleven samples were classified as ER-negative in both. The McNemar test for matched samples confirmed the good overall agreement between statuses, confirming that the two datasets were not statistically different ($p = 0.500$). Comparison of differences in H-score datasets showed that freshly cut blocks often had scores higher than the previously cut samples (Wilcoxon rank sum test, $p < 0.005$) and that the longer the storage time the greater the difference (Wilcoxon rank sum test, $p < 0.005$), but this latter effect was not linear (Spearman's rank correlation, $p = 0.243$).

   Bland–Altman agreement between the results of the freshly cut and stored sections was assessed and showed that recently cut blocks had higher H scores than the stored sections (mean: 32.13, SD: 42.95). The limits of agreement were −53.17 to 117.43, i.e., freshly cut blocks may have H scores of 53 below or 117 above stored material. Comparison of differences in H score using Wilcoxon tests showed that freshly cut blocks often had scores higher than the previously cut samples ($p < 0.005$), thus supporting the results of the Bland–Altman analysis, and that the longer the storage time the greater the difference in H score ($p < 0.005$). An analysis for assessing agreement between established and new clinical measurement techniques confirmed the wide range of variations between data pairs observed; however, it also showed that despite this, only the two cases identified by status change had differences outside of the accepted ±2 SD range for levels of agreement.

In conclusion, 33 of 46 blocks (72%) were classified as ER-positive for both freshly cut and stored samples, and eleven (24%) of samples were classified as ER-negative in both. Two cases from the freshly cut and stained group were classified as ER-positive, but their stored counterparts were ER-negative (**Table 3**). This preliminary QA study confirms that, although there is some loss of ER antigenicity with time deriving from long-term storage of sectioned paraffin material, this loss is unlikely to significantly affect the population ER status characteristics for the overall study.

2. The results of a recent questionnaire survey have shown that the time and temperature of antigen retrieval to be the single most important determinant of the reproducible high quality of ER staining achieved by the "expert" compared to other participant laboratories *(23)*. A higher proportion of the expert laboratories were observed to use pressure cookers for antigen retrieval in contrast to microwave ovens used by the other participating laboratories. Probably the most salient difference between the pressure cooker and the majority of other heating appliances used for antigen retrieval, including the microwave oven, is the maximum temperature reached during heating. Pressure-cooking results in temperatures of 115°C or higher (referred to as "super heating"), whereas the microwave oven does not raise the temperature of an aqueous buffer above 100°C, although this temperature is reached more quickly *(23)*. Recent studies have shown a consistent correlation between antigen-retrieval time and the temperature required to achieve optimal immunohistochemistry results, with longer antigen-retrieval times being required for lower temperatures and vice versa *(24–29)*. As temperatures significantly higher than 100°C cannot be achieved with the standard microwave oven, extension of the heating time seems to be the only practical way of increasing the efficiency of antigen retrieval with this piece of equipment. Poor staining for ER has been shown to be because of a too-short microwave heating time for the max. temperature maintained during the antigen retrieval step, with extension of the heating time (+5, +10, or +15 min), resulting in significant improvement on the same cases by a group of laboratories participating in national external quality assessment *(19)*. Antigen-retrieval time was found to be the main limiting factor, resulting in weak staining in this study. Change of primary antibody conditions with or without extended antigen retrieval failed to produce any significant improvement when compared to the baseline. Microwave oven antigen-retrieval heating time was investigated irrespective of which buffer or its pH value used by the participants. Though 79% of laboratories used

Table 3
Results of the Estrogen Receptor Quality Assurance Program in the Adjuvant Breast Cancer Trial

ER status according to H-score results	Number of stored sections (%)	Number of freshly cut sections (%)
ER-positive	33 (72)	35 (76)
ER-negative	13 (28)	11 (24)
Total	46	46

H-score results, histological-score results; ER, estrogen receptor.

a standard citrate buffer at pH 6.0–6.2, improvement was seen with increasing antigen-retrieval time regardless of the type of buffer or its pH. Consequently, laboratories obtaining weak staining for ER at assessment and using a standard microwave oven are recommended either to switch to the use of pressure-cooking antigen retrieval, as prevalently used by the expert centers, or to extend the microwave heating time by increments of 5 min until optimal staining is achieved. This is evident when the maximal numbers of invasive tumor nuclei are reliably demonstrated with the maximal staining intensity. Excessive microwave heating beyond this point is apparent by a fall in staining intensity and clarity, very poor nuclear morphology, or nonspecific nuclear staining of lymphocytes and fibroblasts. The use of a microwave oven with a relatively high power output, as used by laboratories in the study (mean value: 800 W, 95% CI: 760–840), is recommended. In addition, the reproducibility of the staining using the same heating time is assisted by a rotating stage in the microwave oven to help to prevent development of hot and cold spots, and keeping the microwave oven contents (buffer container and volume, number of slides) constant between runs, as this greatly influences the heating efficiency of the microwave oven *(28)*.

Using the Cardiff scoring system, a survey conducted on 1500 consecutive cases analyzed over the past 2 yr, the average rates of negative and strongly positive tumors observed over four 6-mo intervals have been recorded to be 9% (range: 4.5–16.9%) and 56.4% (range: 36.4–67.0%), respectively. On this basis, 25–40% of cases have proved to have intermediate grade of ER staining. Although the semiquantitative approach adopted by us provides a flexible and clinically relevant basis for assessing the ER status, it requires great stringency and skills of interpretation on part of an operator experienced in breast histopathology. There is therefore a need for adopting computer-assisted image analysis packages to reduce senior staff commitment. To get the best value out of image analysis, it is important that the immunostaining procedure is rendered reproducible through use of an automated immunostainer, and that the overall procedure is regulated by stringent internal and external quality controls and assessments.

Recent surveys conducted by us and others have indicated that whereas the majority of laboratories have little trouble in demonstrating ER- or PR-rich tumors, significant numbers of laboratories have in the past produced false-negative results on receptor-poor tumors circulated by an EQA scheme *(18–20,23)*. In our experience, false-positive results are less common, are usually the result of application of the primary antibody at a too-high concentration, and are frequently accompanied by nonspecific staining of lymphocytes and connective tissue elements in the test material or external controls). In addition, the pattern of nuclear staining in normal glands should usually be of single, scattered cells surrounded by receptor-negative cells *(30)*. ER-positive cells in normal lobules are reported to account for 4–15% of the epithelial population *(6,31,32)*. Consequently, if on examination of the normal glands and lobules, all the nuclei are stained and the examination is accompanied by staining of lymphocytes and stromal cells, false-positive nuclear staining is likely to have occurred in the invasive tumor, and the staining should be rejected.

References

1. Blamey, R. W. (2002) EUSOMA Guidelines on endocrine therapy of breast cancer. *Eur. J. Cancer* **38,** 615–634.
2. McCarty, K. S., Miller, L. S., Cox, E. B., et al. (1985) Estrogen receptor analyses. *Arch. Pathol. Lab. Med.* **109,** 716–721.
3. Harvey, J. M., Clark, G. M., Osborne, C. K., and Allred, D. C. (1999) Estrogen receptor status by immunohistochemistry is superior to the ligand binding assay for predicting response to adjuvant endocrine therapy in breast cancer. *J. Clin. Oncol.* **17,** 1474–1481.
4. Polak, J. M. and Van Noorden, S. (2003) *Introduction to Immunocytochemistry, 3rd Edition.* BIOS Scientific Publishers, Oxford, UK.
5. Williams, J. H., Mepham, B. L., and Wright, D. H. (1997) Tissue preparation for immunocytochemistry. *J. Clin. Pathol.* **50,** 422–428.
6. Williams, G., Anderson, E., Howell, A., et al. (1991) Oral contraceptive (OCP) use increases proliferation and decreases oestrogen receptor content of epithelial cells in the normal human breast. *Int. J. Cancer.* **48,** 206–210.
7. Henry, J. A., Piggott, N. H., Mallick, U. K., et al. (1991) PNR-2/pS2 immunohistochemical staining in breast cancer: correlation with prognostic factors and endocrine response. *Br. J. Cancer* **63,** 615–622.
8. Schwartz, L. H., Koemer, F. C., Edgerton, S. M., et al. (1991) PS2 expression and response to hormonal therapy in patients with advanced breast cancer. *Cancer Res.* **51,** 624–628.
9. Nicholson, R. I., McClelland, R. A., Gee, J. M., et al. (1994) Epidermal growth factor expression in breast cancer: association with response to endocrine therapy. *Breast Cancer Res. Treat.* **29,** 117–125.
10. Carlomagno, C., Perrone, F., Gallo, C., et al. (1996) C-erbB-2 overexpression decreases the benefit of adjuvant tamoxifen in early stage breast cancer without axillary lymph node metastases. *J. Clin. Oncol.* **14,** 2702–2708.
11. Elledge, R. M., Green, S., Ciocca, D., et al. (1998) HER-2 expression and response to tamoxifen in estrogen receptor positive breast cancer: a Southwest Oncology Group Study. *Clin. Cancer Res.* **4,** 7–12.

12. Charpin, C., Martin, P-M., Jacquemier, J., et al. (1986) Estrogen receptor immunocytochemical assay (ER-ICA): computerized image analysis system, immunoelectron microscopy, and comparisons with estradiol binding assays in 115 breast carcinomas. *Cancer Res.* **46(Suppl 8),** 4271s–4277s.

13. Cohen, O., Brugal, G., Seigneurin, D., et al. (1988) Image cytometry of estrogen receptors in breast carcinomas. *Cytometry* **9,** 579–587.

14. Franklin, W. A., Bibbo, M., Doria, M. I., et al. (1987) Quantitation of estrogen receptor content and Ki-67 staining in breast carcinoma by the microTICAS image analysis system. *Anal. Quant. Cytol. Histol.* **9,** 279–286.

15. El-Badawy, N., Cohen, C., Derose, P. B., et al. (1991) Immunohistochemical progesterone receptor assay. Measurement by image analysis. *Am. J. Clin. Pathol.* **96,** 704–710.

16. Rostagno, P., Birtwisle, I., Ettore, F., et al. (1994) Immunohistochemical determination of nuclear antigens by color image analysis: application for labelling index, estrogen and progesterone receptor status in breast cancer. *Anal. Cell. Pathol.* **7,** 275–287.

17. MacGrogan, G., Mauriac, L., Durand, M., et al. (1996) Primary chemotherapy in breast invasive carcinoma: predictive value of the immunohistochemical detection of hormonal receptors, p53, c-erbB-2, MiB1, pS2 and GST pi. *Br. J. Cancer* **74,** 1458–1465.

18. Rhodes, A., Jasani, B., Balaton, A. J., et al. (2000) Frequency of oestrogen and progesterone receptor positivity by immunohistochemical analysis in 7,016 breast carcinomas: correlation with patient age, assay sensitivity, threshold value and mammographic screening. *J. Clin. Pathol.* **53,** 688–696.

19. Rhodes, A., Jasani, B., Barnes, D. M., et al. (2000) Reliability of immunohistochemical demonstration of oestrogen receptors in routine practice: inter-laboratory variance in the sensitivity of detection and evaluation of scoring systems. *J. Clin. Pathol.* **53,** 125–130.

20. Rhodes, A., Jasani, B., Balaton, A. J., et al. (2000) Immunohistochemical demonstration of oestrogen and progesterone receptors: correlation of standards achieved on "in house" tumours with that achieved on external quality assessment material in over 150 laboratories from 26 countries. *J. Clin. Pathol.* **53,** 292–301.

21. Barnes, D. M., Harris, W. H., Smith, P., et al. (1996) Immunohistochemical determination of estrogen receptor: comparison of different methods of assessment of staining and correlation with clinical outcome of breast cancer patients. *Br. J. Cancer* **74,** 1445–1451.

22. Leake, R., Barnes, D., Pinder, S., et al. (2000) Immunohistochemical detection of steroid receptors in breast cancer: a working group protocol. *J. Clin. Path.* **53,** 634–635.

23. Rhodes, A., Jasani, B., Balaton, A. J., et al. (2001) Study of interlaboratory reliability and reproducibility of estrogen and progesterone receptor assays in Europe: documentation of poor reliability and identification of insufficient microwave antigen retrieval time as a major contributory element of unreliable assays. *Am. J. Clin. Pathol.* **115,** 44–58.

24. Suurmeijer, A. J. H. and Boon, M. E. (1999) Pretreatment in a high-pressure microwave processor for MIB1 immunostaining of cytological smears and paraf-

fin tissue sections to visualize the various phases of the mitotic cycle. *J. Histo-chem. Cytochem.* **47,** 1015–1020.

25. Lucasssen, P. J., Ravid, R., Gonatas, N. K., et al. (1993) Activation of the human supraoptic and paraventricular nucleus neurons with ageing and in Alzieheimer's disease as judged from increasing size of the Golgi apparatus. *Brain Res.* **632,** 105–113.

26. Kawai, K., Serizawa, A., Hamana, T., et al. (1994) Heat-induced antigen retrieval of proliferating cell nuclear antigen and p53 protein in formalin-fixed, paraffin-embedded sections. *Pathol. Int.* **44,** 759–764.

27. Pileri, S. A., Roncador, G., Ceccarelli, C., et al. (1997) Antigen retrieval techniques in immunohistochemistry: comparison of different methods. *J. Pathol.* **183,** 116–123.

28. Shi, S. R., Cote, R. J., Yang, C., et al. (1996) Development of an optimal protocol for antigen retrieval: a 'test battery' approach exemplified with reference to the staining of retinoblastoma protein (pRB) in formalin fixed paraffin sections. *J. Pathol.* **179,** 347–352.

29. Shi, S. R., Cote, R. J., Chaiwun, B., et al. (1998) Standardisation of immunohistochemistry based antigen retrieval technique for routine formalin-fixed tissue sections. *Appl. Immunohistochem.* **6,** 89–96.

30. Shoker, B. S., Jarvis, C., Sibson, D. R., Walker, C., and Sloane, J. P. (1999) Oestrogen receptor expression in the normal and pre-cancerous breast. *J. Pathol.* **188,** 237–244.

31. Peterson, O. W., Hoyer, P. E., and van Deurs, B. (1987) Frequency and distribution of estrogen receptor-positive cells in normal, non-lactating human breast tissue. *Cancer Res.* **47,** 5748–5751.

32. Clark, R. B., Howell, A., Potten, C. S., and Anderson, E. (1997) Dissociation between steroid receptor expression and cell proliferation in the human breast. *Cancer Res.* **57,** 4987–4999.

13

Markers of Apoptosis

Fazlul H. Sarkar and Yiwei Li

Summary

Apoptosis is a physiological process that occurs in cells during development and normal cellular processes. The useless, unwanted, or damaged cells die during the apoptotic process. However, if signals instructing cells to carry out apoptosis are lost, a variety of malignant disorders may result. Normal mammary gland development is controlled by a balance between cell proliferation and apoptosis, and the balance is important for normal mammary gland differentiation. The formation of breast cancer will happen as soon as the balance is upset by carcinogens. The uncontrolled cell proliferation and the reduced levels of apoptosis will result in cancer growth. It is useful to detect apoptosis in breast cancer to determine the malignancy of the cancer. It is also important to measure the apoptosis index in breast cancer or other cancers treated with anticancer agents to verify the effect of the anticancer agent. In this chapter, we provide detailed protocols of commonly used apoptosis assays, including DNA ladder formation, enzyme-linked immunosorbent assay for histone/DNA fragment, poly-ADP-ribose-polymerase cleavage assay, and terminal deoxynucleotidyl transferase-mediated dUTP nick-end-labeling assay.

Key Words: Apoptosis; DNA fragment; histone; PARP; TUNEL.

1. Introduction

Apoptosis, also known as programmed cell death, is a physiological process that occurs in cells during development and normal cellular processes. It refers to an orderly sequence of responses to biochemical or physical signals to maintain cellular homeostasis. The useless, unwanted, or damaged cells die during apoptotic process. It has been reported that cells altered beyond repair by normal mechanisms or cells that have completed their programmed biological function begin the apoptosis process. *(1)* Apoptosis can be initiated by cell signals and induced via the stimulation of several different cell surface receptors (e.g., Fas) in association with caspase activation *(2,3)*. The activation of caspases (cysteinyl-aspartate-specific proteinases), a family of intracellular

From: *Methods in Molecular Medicine, Vol. 120: Breast Cancer Research Protocols*
Edited by: S. A. Brooks and A. L. Harris © Humana Press Inc., Totowa, NJ

cysteine proteases, plays important roles in the initiation of apoptosis and activation of sequential apoptotic processes *(4–7)*. Poly-ADP-ribose-polymerase (PARP), a 116-kDa protein that binds specifically at DNA strand breaks, is a substrate for certain caspases (e.g., caspases 3 and 7). The activated caspases cleave PARP into two fragments during early stages of apoptosis; thus, the cleavage of PARP serves as an early marker of apoptosis *(8,9)*. It has been reported that some important genes including, for example, *Bcl-2*, *Bax*, and *p53*, are critically involved in the apoptotic processes *(10–12)*. During the apoptotic process, another important response of cells is activation of an endogenous Ca^{2+}- and Mg^{2+}-dependent nuclear endonuclease *(13,14)*. In the human chromosome, histone and DNA strand tightly combine to form nucleosomal units, and each unit includes approx 180–200 bp DNA and histone protein. When apoptosis occurs, the activated endonuclease selectively cleaves DNA at sites located between nucleosomal units (linker DNA), generating typically approx 180–200 bp $\times$ n DNA fragments with histone *(15)*. During apoptosis, mitochondrial permeability is also altered, and apoptosis-specific protease activators are released from mitochondria. Cytochrome C and other activators are released into the cytoplasm and promote caspase activation *(2,6,16)*, resulting in the sequential biological reaction and the morphological features of apoptosis. These features include chromatin aggregation, nuclear and cytoplasmic condensation, and partition of cytoplasm and nucleus into membrane bound-vesicles known as apoptotic bodies. In vivo, these apoptotic bodies are rapidly recognized and phagocytized by either macrophages or adjacent epithelial cells. In this way, the unwanted or damaged cells are eliminated to maintain the normal physiological process.

However, if signals instructing cells to carry out apoptosis are lost, a variety of malignant disorders may result. Normal mammary gland development is controlled by a balance between cell proliferation and apoptosis; and the balance is important for normal mammary gland differentiation *(17)*. The formation of breast cancer will happen as soon as the balance is upset by carcinogens *(18)*. The uncontrolled cell proliferation will result in cancer growth. However, there is growing evidence that tumor growth is not just because of uncontrolled proliferation but also because of reduced levels of apoptosis *(18,19)*. In cancer, not enough cells die, resulting in uncontrolled cancer growth, invasion, and metastasis. It is now generally accepted that inhibition of apoptosis plays an important role in the carcinogenic process. Studies of breast cancer specimens have demonstrated that apoptosis is related to the biological behaviors of breast cancer *(20,21)*.

It is useful to detect apoptosis in breast cancer to determine the malignancy of the cancer. It is also important to measure the apoptosis index in breast cancer or other cancers treated with anticancer agents to verify the effect of the

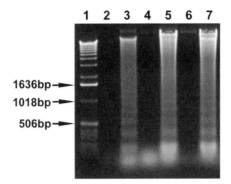

Fig. 1. DNA ladder formation in PC3 prostate cancer cells treated with genistein. Lane 1: DNA marker. Lanes 2, 4, and 6: days 1, 2, and 3 PC3 control cells. Lanes 3, 5, and 7: PC3 cells treated with 50 μ*M* genistein for 1, 2, and 3 d, showing clear characteristic DNA ladder.

anticancer agents. Apoptosis can be detected in breast cancer by apoptosis assays, which encompass several markers of apoptosis. As mentioned above, the apoptotic process begins with a sequential activation of proteases including caspases, which cleave PARP into two fragments. Thus, the activation of caspases and the cleavage of PARP serve as the early markers of apoptosis. After serial activation of various enzymes, the activated endonuclease cleaves DNA strands between nucleosomal units, resulting in the formation of DNA/ histone fragments. The DNA/histone fragments migrate into the cytoplasm; the fragments are another important marker of apoptosis. Once DNA strands are cleaved by endonuclease during the apoptotic process, they can be detected by terminal deoxynucleotidyl transferase (TdT)-mediated dUTP nick-end-labeling (TUNEL) assay no matter if they remain in the nucleus or migrate to the cytoplasm, and serve as another marker of apoptosis as described on the following page.

The cytoplasmic fragments of DNA/histone may be assayed either by DNA ladder formation revealed in agarose gel electrophoresis or histone/DNA enzyme-linked immunosorbent assay (ELISA). The cytoplasmic DNA fragments after gel electrophoresis show a characteristic pattern, with the 180–200-bp multiples as "rungs" of the ladder (**Fig. 1**), clearly demonstrating the formation of apoptosis. ELISA analysis for histone/DNA fragment provides a quantitative value for apoptotic cells (**Fig. 2**). This assay is based on the quantitative sandwich immunoassay principle, using two antibodies directed against histone and DNA to detect the cleaved nucleosomes. After immobilizing antihistone antibody, histone/DNA fragment, and peroxidase-conjugated anti-DNA antibody, the amount of histone/DNA fragments can be determined pho-

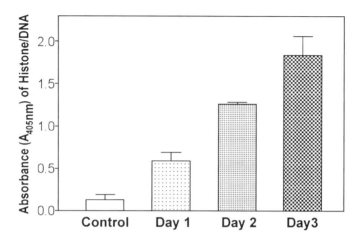

Fig. 2. Detection of histone/DNA fragments in PC3 prostate cancer cells treated with genistein using enzyme-linked immunosorbent assay. Control: untreated PC3 cells. Day 1, 2, and 3: PC3 cells treated with 50 μ*M* genistein for 1, 2, and 3 d, showing increase in absorbance at 405 nm.

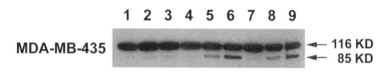

Fig. 3. Poly-ADP-ribose-polymerase (PARP) cleavage assay for MDA-MB-435 breast cancer cells treated with genistein. Lanes 1, 4, and 7: day 1, 2, and 3 MDA-MB-435 control cells. Lanes 2, 5, and 8: MDA-MB-435 cells treated with 30 μ*M* genistein for 1, 2, and 3 d. Lanes 3, 6, and 9: MDA-MB-435 cells treated with 50 μ*M* genistein for 1, 2, and 3 d. PARP of 116 kDa were cleaved to 85- and 31 kDa fragments. The anti-PARP antibody recognized 116- and 85-kDa PARP.

tometrically with peroxidase substrate 2,2'-azino-di-3-ethylbenzthiazoline sulfonate (ABTS). The activation of caspases cleaves its substrate PARP, a 116-kDa protein, to fragments of approx 85 and 31 kDa. The cleaved PARP fragments can be detected with the anti-PARP antibody, which recognizes 116- and 85-kDa PARP. Hence, the activation of caspases and cleavage of PARP can be assayed by Western blot analysis with anti-PARP antibody (**Fig. 3**). The cleaved DNA strand in cells can be detected by TUNEL assay. TUNEL assay utilizes the property of terminal deoxynucleotidyl transferase to add fluorescent- or biotin-labeled dUTP to the free 3'-hydroxyl end of cleaved DNA strand, enabling the detection of apoptotic cells (**Fig. 4**). It provides *in situ* apoptotic information without destroying the structure of tissue. Here, we provide a detailed

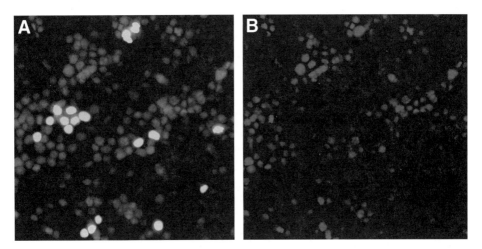

Fig. 4. Terminal deoxynucleotidyl transferase-mediated dUTP nick-end-labeling assay for PC3 prostate cancer cells. (**A**) Apoptotic cells show strong green fluorescence. (**B**) All cells stained with phosphatidylinositol show strong red fluorescence.

protocol for commonly used apoptosis assays, including DNA ladder formation, ELISA for histone/DNA fragment, PARP cleavage assay, and TUNEL assay.

2. Materials

2.1. DNA Ladder Assay

1. 1 *M* Tris-HCl, pH 8.0. Prepare 100 mL. Autoclave and store at room temperature. It remains stable for at least 6 mo.
2. 0.5 *M* Ethylenediaminetetraacetic acid (EDTA), pH 8.0. Prepare 100 mL. Autoclave and store it at room temperature. It remains stable for at least 6 mo (*see* **Notes 1** and **2**).
3. Lysis buffer: 0.2% Triton X-100, 10 m*M* Tris-HCl, 1 m*M* EDTA, pH 8.0. Prepare 10 mL and store it at 4°C. It remains stable for 1 wk.
4. 0.5 µg/µL DNase-free RNase (cat. no.1119915; Roche, Indianapolis, IN). Store at –20°C.
5. 20% Sodium dodecyl sulfide (SDS). Prepare 100 mL. (**Caution:** Use a mask when weighing SDS.) Do not autoclave it. Store it at room temperature. It remains stable for 1 yr.
6. Proteinase K (20 mg/mL): Dissolve proteinase K (cat. no. 25530-015; Invitrogen, Carlsbad, CA) in dH$_2$O. Store at –20°C in 0.5-mL aliquots.
7. 5 *M* NaCl. Prepare 100 mL. Autoclave and store it at room temperature. It remains stable for at least 6 mo.
8. Tris-HCl/EDTA (TE) buffer: 10 m*M* Tris-HCl, 1 m*M* EDTA, pH 8.0. Prepare 10 mL. Autoclave and store it room temperature. It remains stable for 6 mo.

9   Phenol. Equilibrate 100 mL of phenol four times with equal volumes of TE buffer and cover it with small mount of TE buffer. Store in the dark at 4°C.

10. Phenol/chloroform/isoamyl alcohol (50:49:1 v/v/v). Prepare freshly 10 mL of phenol/chloroform/isoamyl alcohol (50:49:1 v/v/v).

11. Isopropanol (cat. no. A416-4; Fisher, Fair Lawn, NJ).

12. 70% Ethanol. Prepare 100 mL of 70% ethanol. Store at 4°C.

13. 50X Tris-EDTA/glacial acetic acid (TAE). Prepare 100 mL of 50X TAE by combining 24.2 g of Tris-HCl base, 10 mL of 0.5 M EDTA (pH 8.0), and 5.71 mL of glacial acetic acid. Autoclave and store at room temperature. It remains stable for 6 mo.

14. Loading buffer: 50% glycerol in 1X TAE. Prepare 10 mL and store at 4°C.

15. 1.5% Agarose gel. Melt agarose in 1X TAE. Cast into electrophoresis equipment.

16. 10 mg/mL ethidium bromide. For staining DNA in gel, final concentration of ethidium bromide is 0.5 µg/mL. (**Caution:** Wear gloves when handling ethidium bromide, because ethidium bromide is a powerful mutagen.)

2.2. ELISA

1. Incubation buffer (cat. no. 1544675, Roche).

2. Sample preparation for ELISA. Prepare freshly by diluting 25 µL of sample in 225 µL of incubation buffer.

3. Streptavidin-coated microtiter plate, 96-well plate modules and frame (cat. no.1544675, Roche).

4. Coating buffer (cat. no. 1544675, Roche).

5. Biotin-labeled antihistone antibody (cat. no. 1544675, Roche).

6. Coating solution. Dilute one part of concentrated coating buffer with nine parts of dH$_2$O. Shortly before use, dilute one part of biotin-labeled antihistone antibody with nine parts of diluted coating buffer.

7. Washing buffer (cat. no. 1544675, Roche).

8. Washing solution. Dilute one part of concentrated washing buffer with nine parts of dH$_2$O and mix thoroughly. Store at 4°C. It remains stable for 2 mo.

9. Peroxidase conjugated anti-DNA antibody (cat. no. 1544675, Roche).

10. Conjugate solution. Dilute one part of peroxidase conjugated anti-DNA antibody with nine parts of incubation buffer.

11. Substrate buffer (cat. no. 1544675, Roche).

12. ABTS substrate tablet (cat. no. 1544675, Roche).

13. Substrate solution. Dissolve ABTS substrate tablet in total volume of substrate buffer. Store in the dark at 4°C. It remains stable for at least 1 mo.

2.3. PARP Assay

1. Phosphate-buffered saline (PBS), pH 7.4. Prepare 200 mL of PBS by dissolving 1 tablet of PBS tablet (cat. no. P4417; Sigma, St. Louis, MO) in 200 mL of dH$_2$O. Autoclave and store it 4°C. It stable for 6 mo.

2. 20 mM Tris-HCl. Prepare 100 mL. Autoclave and store at 4°C. It remains stable for 6 mo.

3. 1 M Sodium chloride. Prepare 100 mL. Autoclave and store at 4°C. It remains stable for 6 mo.
4. 150 mM Sodium pyrophosphate. Prepare 50 mL. Store at 4°C. It remains stable for 6 mo.
5. 500 mM Sodium fluoride. Prepare 10 mL. Store at 4°C. It remains stable for 6 mo.
6. 1 M Sodium orthovandate. Prepare 10 mL. Store at 4°C. It remains stable for 6 mo.
7. 50 mM Iodoacetic acid. Prepare 10 mL. Store at 4°C. It remains stable for 6 mo.
8. 1 mM Zinc chloride. Prepare 10 mL. Store at 4°C. It remains stable for 6 mo.
9. 100 mM Phenlymethylsulfonyl fluoride. Prepare 2 mL. Store at –20°C in 0.5-mL aliquots. It remains stable for at least 6 mo.
10. Lysis buffer. Prepare freshly 5 mL: 10 mM Tris-HCl, 50 mM sodium chloride, 30 mM sodium pyrophosphate, 50 mM sodium fluoride, 100 mM sodium orthovandate, 2 mM iodoacetic acid, 5 µM zinc chloride, 1 mM phenlymethyl-sulfonyl fluoride, and 0.5% Triton X-100 for PARP protein extraction.
11. BCA protein assay reagent (cat. no. 23227; Pierce, Rockford, IL)
12. 1.0-mm Thick, 10 × 10-cm plastic gel casting cassettes.
13. 30% Acrylamide/*bis*-acrylamide stock (37.5:1 [v/v], cat. no. A3699, Sigma).
14. Separating gel buffer: 1 M Tris-HCl, pH 8.8. Prepare 100 mL.
15. Stacking gel buffer: 375 mM Tris-HCl, pH 6.8. Prepare 100 mL. Autoclave and store at room temperature. It remains stable for at least 6 mo.
16. 20% SDS. Prepare 100 mL. (**Caution:** Use a mask when weighing SDS.) Do not autoclave it. Store at room temperature. It remains stable for 1 yr.
17. 10% Ammonium persulfate (APS). Prepare freshly 1–3 mL, depending on the number of gels to be prepared.
18. N,N,N',N'-tetramethylethylenediamine (TEMED; cat. no. T8133, Sigma). Store it in the dark at 4°C.
19. 2X Sample buffer: 62.5 mM Tris-HCl (pH 6.8), 2% SDS, 20% glycerol, 0.01% bromophenol blue, and 4% β-mercaptoethanol. Prepare 10 mL and store at room temperature. It remains stable for 2 wk.
20. Protein Ladder BenchMark (cat. no. 10748-010; Invitrogen, Carlsbad, CA)
21. Running buffer: 25 mM Tris-base, 192 mM glycine, 0.1% SDS, pH 8.3. The pH should be correct without adjusting. Prepare 1 L and store at room temperature. It remains stable for 6 mo.
22. Transfer buffer: 25 mM Tris-base, 192 mM glycine, 20% methanol. Prepare 1 L and store at 4°C. It remains stable for 6 mo.
23. Tris-base/Tween-20 (TBS/T). Prepare TBS (20 mM Tris-base, 137 mM NaCl, pH 7.6) supplemented with 0.1% Tween-20. Store at room temperature. It remains stable for 6 mo.
24. 7.5 and 5% nonfat dry milk in TBS/T. Prepare freshly 10 mL of 7.5 and 5% nonfat dry milk in TBS/T.
25. Mouse monoclonal anti-PARP primary antibody (cat. no. SA-250; Biomol, Plymouth Meeting, PA).

26. Horseradish peroxidase-conjugated goat anti-mouse secondary antibody (cat. no. 170-6516; Bio-Rad, Hercules, CA).
27. Luminol/Enhancer Solution and Stable Peroxide Solution (SuperSignal West Pico Chemiluminescent Substrate, cat. no. 34080, Pierce).

2.4. TUNEL Assay

1. Poly-L-lysine-coated microscope slides. Apply 50–100 mL of 0.1% (w/v) poly-L-lysine (cat. no. P8920, Sigma) to the surface of sterile glass microscope slides. Spread evenly over the slides. Air-dry the slides for 1 h and store at 4°C for up to 1 wk.
2. PBS, pH 7.4. Prepare 200 mL of PBS by dissolving 1 tablet of PBS tablet (cat. no. P4417, Sigma) in 200 mL of deionized H_2O. Autoclave and store at 4°C. It remains stable for 6 mo.
3. 4% Formaldehyde/PBS, pH 7.4. Prepare 4% formaldehyde/PBS immediately before use. Combine 70 mL of PBS and 25 mL of 16% methanol-free formaldehyde (cat. no. 44124-4, Sigma). Adjust pH to 7.4 with 1 N NaOH.
4. 0.2% Triton X-100/PBS. Prepare freshly 100 mL.
5. DNase I buffer: 40 mM Tris-HCl (pH 7.9), 10 mM NaCl, 6 mM MgCl$_2$, 10 mM CaCl$_2$. Prepare 1 mL.
6. DNase I (cat. no. 18047-019, Invitrogen). The final working concentration of DNase I in buffer is 0.5–1 mg/mL.
7. Equilibration buffer: 200 mM potassium cacodylate (pH 6.6), 25 mM Tris-HCl (pH 6.6), 0.2 mM DTT, 0.25 mg/mL BSA, and 2.5 mM cobalt chloride. (**Caution:** Potassium cacodylate [dimethylarsinic acid] is a mild irritant. Wear gloves and safety glasses to avoid skin and eye contact.) Prepare 10 mL and store at –20°C. Alternatively, order from Clontech (cat. no. K2024-1; Palo Alto, CA).
8. 20X sodium chloride–sodium citrate (SSC) buffer: 3 M NaCl, 300 mM sodium-citrate. Prepare 100 mL. Autoclave and store at room temperature. It remains stable for at least 6 mo.
9. 2X SSC. Prepare before use 100 mL of 2X SSC by diluting 20X SSC in dH$_2$O.
10. Nucleotide mix (cat. no. K2024-1, Clontech).
11. TdT Terminal transferase (cat. no. K2024-1, Clontech).
12. Propidium iodide/PBS (PI/PBS): dissolve 10 mg of propidium iodide (cat. no. P4170, Sigma) in 10 mL of PBS to make stock solution (1 mg/mL). Store in the dark at 4°C. Before use, prepare 100 mL of working solution (10 ng/mL).
13. Anti-fade reagent (cat. no. S7461; Molecular Probes, Eugene, OR).

3. Methods
3.1. DNA Ladder Assay

1. Culture cells in 100-mm cell culture dish. Treat the cells with an agent that induces apoptosis.
2. Collect medium with floating cells and centrifuge at 1000g for 5 min.
3. Trypsinize the adherent cells and centrifuge at 1000g for 5 min.

4. Resuspend the adherent and floating cell pellet in 300 µL lysis buffer and centrifuge for 15 min at 13,800*g*.
5. Transfer the supernatant (containing cytoplasmic DNA/histone fragment) to an Eppendorf tube. Add 15 µL RNase (0.5 µg/µL) to the tube. Incubate at 37°C for 1 h.
6. Add 20 µL of 20% SDS, 8 µL of proteinase K (20 mg/mL), and 25 µL of 5 *M* NaCl to the tube. Incubate at 37°C for 30 min.
7. Add 370 µL of phenol to the tube, mix, and centrifuge for 10 min at 13,000*g*.
8. Transfer the upper phase of liquid to an Eppendorf tube. Add equal volume of phenol/chloroform/isoamyl alcohol (50:49:1 [v/v/v]) to the tube, mix, and centrifuge for 10 min at 13,000*g*.
9. Transfer the upper phase of liquid to an Eppendorf tube. Add the equal volume of isopropanol and place it at –20°C overnight (*see* **Note 3**).
10. Centrifuge at 13,000*g* for 20 min at 4°C.
11. Wash the pellet with 70% ethanol and centrifuge at 13,000*g* for 10 min at 4°C.
12. Dry the pellet briefly. Resuspend the pellet in 10 µL of TE buffer, and then add 2 µL of loading buffer.
13. Prepare 1.5% agarose gel.
14. Load the samples and DNA marker onto agarose gel wells.
15. Electrophorese the samples and DNA marker on the 1.5% agarose gel in 1X TAE. Stain the gel with ethidium bromide (0.5 µg/mL) and photograph using UV transilluminator.

3.2. ELISA for Histone/DNA Fragment

1. Culture cells in 60-mm cell culture dish. Treat the cells with an agent that induces apoptosis.
2. Collect medium with floating cells and centrifuge at 1000*g* for 5 min.
3. Trypsinize the adherent cells and centrifuge at 1000*g* for 5 min.
4. Resuspend the adherent and floating cell pellet in 5 mL culture medium and count the cell number.
5. Transfer 5×10^4 cells into Eppendorf tube and centrifuge at 1000*g* for 5 min.
6. Discard the supernatant, resuspend the cell pellet with 500 µL incubation buffer, mix thoroughly, and incubate the sample for 30 min at room temperature to lyse the cells.
7. Centrifuge the lysate at 20,000*g* for 10 min and remove 400 µL of the supernatant (containing cytoplasmic histone/DNA fragments) to a new tube. Store the sample at –20°C (*see* **Note 4**).
8. Pipet 100 µL coating solution (biotin-labeled antihistone antibody) into each well of the microtiter plate (MTP). Cover MTP tightly with the adhesive cover foil and incubate for 1 h at room temperature (alternatively, overnight at 2–8°C).
9. Remove coating solution thoroughly. Pipet 200 µL incubation buffer into each well of the MTP. Cover MTP tightly with the adhesive cover foil and incubate for 30 min at 15–25°C.
10. Remove solution thoroughly, rinse wells three times with 250 µL washing solution per well, and remove washing solution thoroughly.

11. Dilute 25-µL sample from **step 7** in 225 µL incubation buffer and pipet 100 µL of diluted sample solution into each well of the MTP. Cover MTP tightly with the adhesive cover foil and incubate at 15–25°C for 90 min and wash as described in **step 9**.

12. Pipet 100 µL of peroxidase-conjugated anti-DNA antibody into each well of the MTP. Cover MTP tightly with the adhesive cover foil and incubate for 90 min at room temperature and wash as described in **step 9**.

13. Pipet 100 µL of substrate solution into each well of the MTP and incubate on a plate shaker at 250 rpm for 10–20 min until the color development is sufficient for a photometric analysis.

14. Mix the content of the wells by careful tapping at the MTP edges and measure at 405 nm in a microplate reader (cat. no. 170-6850, Bio-Rad).

3.3. PARP Assay

1. Culture cells in 60- or 100-mm cell culture dish. Treat the cells with an agent that induces apoptosis.

2. Scrape the cells off the plate and transfer cells and media to a 15-mL tube.

3. Centrifuge at 3000g for 3 min and aspirate medium from tube.

4. Add 6 mL of ice-cold PBS to the cell pellet, and resuspend the cell pellet.

5. Centrifuge at 3000g for 3 min and discard the supernatant.

6. Add 50 µL (for 60-mm plate, adjust the volume according to the cell number) or 100 µL (for 100-mm plate) of lysis buffer, mix, and leave on ice for 30 min. Vortex vigorously every 10 min.

7. Centrifuge at 12,000g for 20 min. Transfer the supernatant to a new Eppendorf tube.

8. Use BCA protein assay reagent kit (Pierce) to quantify the protein (*see* **Note 5**).

9. Prepare 10% separating gel. For four small gels (10 × 10 cm), mix 6.87 mL of dH$_2$O, 8.33 mL of 30% acrylamide/*bis*-acrylamide stock, 9.38 mL of 1 M Tris-HCl (pH 8.8), 0.25 mL of 10% SDS, and 125 µL of 10% APS.

10. Prepare 4% stacking gel. For four small gels, mix 6.45 mL of dH$_2$O, 1.65 mL of 30% acrylamide/*bis*-acrylamide stock, 4.2 mL of 375 mM Tris-HCl (pH 6.8), 0.125 mL of 10% SDS, and 62.5 µL of 10% APS.

11. Add 12.5 µL of TEMED to the separating gel solution and swirl the solution. Immediately pipet 5.8 mL of separating gel solution into each cassette, avoiding the formation of bubbles.

12. Carefully overlay the separating gel solution with dH$_2$O up to the top of the cassette. Do not disturb the surface of the separating gel solution.

13. Let the gel polymerize for at least 1 h at room temperature.

14. Decant the overlay water from the separating gel. Add 12.5 µL of TEMED to the stacking gel solution and swirl the solution. Immediately pipet the solution onto the top of the separating gel until it reaches the top of cassette.

15. Insert the combs into the liquid stacking gel. Let the gel polymerize at room temperature, about 30–60 min (*see* **Note 6**).

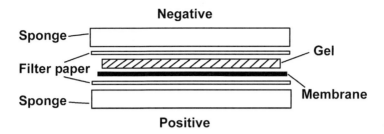

Fig. 5. Sandwich order for Western blot transfer.

16. Take 50 μg protein for each lane for running through 10% SDS-polyacrylamide gel. Add equal volume of 2X sample buffer to each sample. Boil the samples for 5 min.

17. Load samples and 8 μL BenchMark (Invitrogen) in wells of 10% SDS-polyacrylamide gel.

18. Run the gel in 1X running buffer at 120 V until the marker dye reaches the bottom of the gel.

19. Cut off the stacking gel. Soak nitrocellulose membrane (cat. no. 10439396; Schleicher & Schuell, Keene, NH) in dH$_2$O and then in transfer buffer. Soak filter paper and sponge in transfer buffer.

20. Make transfer sandwich (*see* **Fig. 5**).

21. Transfer proteins to membrane at 100 V for 2–3 h (using Bio-Rad Mini Trans Blot or equivalent apparatus).

22. Block the membrane with 7.5% nonfat dry milk in TBS/T at room temperature for 1 h, with rocking (5 mL each membrane).

23. Discard the solution and incubate the membrane in anti-PARP primary antibody (primary antibody in 5 mL of TBS/T with 5% nonfat dry milk), with rocking, overnight at 4°C or at room temperature for 1 h.

24. Wash the membrane in TBS/T three times for 15 min each at room temperature, with rocking.

25. Incubate the membrane with horseradish peroxidase-conjugated secondary antibody (in 5 mL of TBS/T with 5% nonfat dry milk) at room temperature for 1 h, with rocking.

26. Wash the membrane with TBS/T three times for 10 min each at room temperature, with rocking.

27. Mix equal volume (approx 2 mL, 0.125 mL/cm^2) of Luminol/Enhancer Solution and Stable Peroxide Solution (SuperSignal West Pico Chemiluminescent Substrate, Pierce).

28. Place the membrane in a flat position. Do not let it dry. Add the mixed substrate solution to the membrane and incubate for 5 min. Make sure to cover the membrane completely.

29. Take the membrane out. Wrap with plastic membrane. Expose it to X-ray film for 1 min. Develop the film. Adjust subsequent exposure time (from 10 s up to 24 h) as necessary.

3.4. TUNEL Assay

1. Grow cells on poly-L-lysine-coated slides prepared before cell culture.
2. Induce apoptosis in the cells using an agent that induces apoptosis.
3. Following induction, wash slides twice by dipping slides in a jar containing PBS.
4. Immerse slides in a jar containing fresh 4% formaldehyde/PBS at 4°C for 25 min to fix the cells. The fixed cells can be stored in 70% ethanol at –20°C for up to 2 wk.
5. Wash the slides twice by immersing the slides in a jar containing fresh PBS for 5 min at room temperature.
6. Immerse the slides in prechilled 0.2% Triton X-100/PBS to permeabilize the cells. Incubate for 5 min on ice.
7. Prepare a positive control:
   a. Add 100 µL of DNase I Buffer to the portion where the cells grow on the slide.
   b. Incubate at room temperature for 5 min.
   c. Tap the slide gently to remove the liquid.
   d. Add 100 µL of DNase I Buffer containing 0.5–1 mg/mL DNase.
   e. Incubate at room temperature for 10 min.
   f. Gently tap the slide to remove the liquid.
   g. Immerse three to four times in dH$_2$O.
8. Immerse slides twice in fresh PBS for 5 min at room temperature.
9. Remove slides from PBS and tap gently to remove excess liquid.
10. Cover the cells in 100 µL of equilibration buffer and gently place a piece of plastic cover slip on top of the cells to evenly spread the liquid. Equilibrate at room temperature for 10 min.
11. Prepare TdT incubation buffer for samples. For one reaction, mix 45 µL of equilibration buffer, 5 µL of nucleotide mix, and 1 µL of TdT enzyme. Protect TdT incubation buffer from light. Keep on ice at all times.
12. Remove the plastic cover slip, gently tap the slides to remove excess liquid, and add 50 µL of TdT incubation buffer onto the cells over an approx 5-cm^2 area. Gently place a piece of plastic cover slip on top of the cells to spread evenly the liquid. (If performing a TdT-minus negative control, add 50 µL of TdT-minus control incubation buffer that omits the TdT enzyme.)
13. Place the slides in a dark, humidified 37°C incubator for 60 min.
14. Immerse slides in 2X SSC to terminate the tailing reaction. Incubate at room temperature for 15 min.
15. Wash slides twice by immersing in PBS for 5 min at room temperature.
16. Stain the cells with PI by incubating slides in fresh PI/PBS at room temperature for 5–10 min.
17. Wash the cells three times by immersing the slides in dH$_2$O and incubate at room temperature for 5 min.
18. Add a drop of Anti-Fade Solution and cover the slide with a glass cover slip. The sealed slides can be stored overnight at 4°C in the dark.
19. View slides as soon as possible. Apoptotic cells will exhibit strong, green fluorescence using a standard fluorescence filter set (520 ± 20 nm). All cells stained with phosphatidylinositol exhibit strong red fluorescence when viewed at higher than 620 nm.

4. Notes

1. When making 0.5 M EDTA, the disodium salt of EDTA will not go into solution until the pH of the solution is adjusted to approx 8.0 by the addition of NaOH. Slowly add NaOH solution to the EDTA solution while monitoring the pH of the solution.
2. Alternately, the sample can be placed at −70°C for 2 to 3 h.
3. For best results, the samples can only be stored at −20°C for 2 d. Longer storage will decrease the sensitivity of the assay.
4. After quantifying the proteins, the samples can be aliquoted and stored at −70°C for at least 6 mo. Avoid repeated freezing and thawing.
5. It is also convenient to prepare the gels in advance, because the polymerized acrylamide gels can be stored at 4°C for 1 mo.

References

1. Gulbins, E., Jekle, A., Ferlinz, K., Grassme, H., and Lang, F. (2000) Physiology of apoptosis. *Am. J. Physiol Renal Physiol.* **279,** 605–615.
2. Zhou, Z., Sun, X., and Kang, Y. J. (2001) Ethanol-induced apoptosis in mouse liver: Fas- and cytochrome c-mediated caspase-3 activation pathway. *Am. J. Pathol.* **159,** 329–338.
3. Suzuki, A., Tsutomi, Y., Akahane, K., Araki, T., and Miura, M. (1998) Resistance to Fas-mediated apoptosis: activation of caspase 3 is regulated by cell cycle regulator p21WAF1 and IAP gene family ILP. *Oncogene* **17,** 931–939.
4. Chlichlia, K., Peter, M. E., Rocha, M., et al. (1998) Caspase activation is required for nitric oxide-mediated, CD95(APO-1/Fas)-dependent and independent apoptosis in human neoplastic lymphoid cells. *Blood* **91,** 4311–4320.
5. Zheng, T. S., Schlosser, S. F., Dao, T., et al. (1998) Caspase-3 controls both cytoplasmic and nuclear events associated with Fas-mediated apoptosis in vivo. *Proc. Natl. Acad. Sci. USA* **95,** 13,618–13,623.
6. Guo, Y., Srinivasula, S. M., Druilhe, A., Fernandes-Alnemri, T., and Alnemri, E. S. (2002) Caspase-2 induces apoptosis by releasing proapoptotic proteins from mitochondria. *J. Biol. Chem.* **277,** 13,430–13,437.
7. Paroni, G., Henderson, C., Schneider, C., and Brancolini, C. (2002) Caspase-2 can trigger cytochrome C release and apoptosis from the nucleus. *J. Biol. Chem.* **277,** 15,147–15,161.
8. Boulares, A. H., Yakovlev, A. G., Ivanova, et al. (1999) Role of poly(ADP-ribose) polymerase (PARP) cleavage in apoptosis. Caspase 3-resistant PARP mutant increases rates of apoptosis in transfected cells. *J. Biol. Chem.* **274,** 22,932–22,940.
9. Simbulan-Rosenthal, C. M., Rosenthal, D. S., Iyer, S., Boulares, H., and Smulson, M. E. (1999) Involvement of PARP and poly(ADP-ribosyl)ation in the early stages of apoptosis and DNA replication. *Mol. Cell Biochem.* **193,** 137–148.
10. Crompton, M. (2000) Bax, Bid and the permeabilization of the mitochondrial outer membrane in apoptosis. *Curr. Opin. Cell Biol.* **12,** 414–419.
11. Schuler, M. and Green, D. R. (2001) Mechanisms of p53-dependent apoptosis. *Biochem. Soc. Trans.* **29,** 684–688.

12. Bruckheimer, E. M., Cho, S. H., Sarkiss, M., Herrmann, J., and McDonnell, T. J. (1998) The Bcl-2 gene family and apoptosis. *Adv. Biochem. Eng. Biotechnol.* **62,** 75–105.
13. Boulares, A. H., Zoltoski, A. J., Contreras, F. J., Yakovlev, A. G., Yoshihara, K., and Smulson, M. E. (2002) Regulation of DNAS1L3 endonuclease activity by poly(ADP-ribosyl)ation during etoposide-induced apoptosis. Role of poly(ADP-ribose) polymerase-1 cleavage in endonuclease activation. *J. Biol. Chem.* **277,** 372–378.
14. Yakovlev, A. G., Wang, G., Stoica, B. A., et al. (2000) A role of the Ca^{2+}/Mg^{2+} -dependent endonuclease in apoptosis and its inhibition by poly(ADP-ribose) polymerase. *J. Biol. Chem.* **275,** 21,302–21,308.
15. Walker, P. R. and Sikorska, M. (1997) New aspects of the mechanism of DNA fragmentation in apoptosis. *Biochem. Cell Biol.* **75,** 287–299.
16. Brenner, C., Marzo, I., and Kroemer, G. (1998) A revolution in apoptosis: from a nucleocentric to a mitochondriocentric perspective. *Exp. Gerontol.* **33,** 543–553.
17. Strange, R., Metcalfe, T., Thackray, L., Dang, M. (2001) Apoptosis in normal and neoplastic mammary gland development. *Microsc. Res. Tech.* **52,** 171–181.
18. Kumar, R., Vadlamudi, R. K., and Adam, L. (2000) Apoptosis in mammary gland and cancer. *Endocr. Relat. Cancer* **7,** 257–269.
19. Parton, M., Dowsett, M., and Smith, I. (2001) Studies of apoptosis in breast cancer. *BMJ* **322,** 1528–1532.
20. Bucci, B., Carico, E., Rinaldi, A., et al. (2001) Biological indicators of aggressiveness in T1 ductal invasive breast cancer. *Anticancer Res.* **21,** 2949–2955.
21. Lipponen, P. (1999) Apoptosis in breast cancer: relationship with other pathological parameters. *Endocr. Relat. Cancer* **6,** 13–16.

14

Quantitative Angiogenesis in Breast Cancer

Stephen B. Fox

Summary

Over the last few years, great advances in our understanding in tumor neovascularization have emerged, with several new mechanisms of neovascularization being proposed. Solid tumors establish a vasculature through angiogenesis, vasculogenesis, vascular remodeling, co-option, and possibly also intussusception and vascular mimicry. Quantitative measurements of the tumor vasculature have generally measured the number of microvessels, highlighted using immunohistochemistry and antibodies to factor VIII-related antigen at high power over a defined field area. The generation of more sensitive and specific markers—in particular antibodies to CD34—together with the use of a Chalkley eyepiece graticule have improved the objectivity of the assessment of tumor vascularity. The protocol for this is discussed, with several variations such as vascular grade, microvessel density, and the alterations required for the assessment of vascularity in *in situ* breast disease. Also outlined are potential other measures of the angiogenic activity of breast tumors including the use of angiogenic factors and their receptors, endothelial cell proliferation, vessel maturation index, cell adhesion molecules, proteolytic enzymes, and the recently identified hypoxic markers.

Key Words: Angiogenesis; microvessel density; vascular grading; Chalkley counting; *in situ* breast disease.

1. Introduction
1.1. Background and Scope of This Chapter

Over the last few years, great advances in our understanding of tumor neovascularization have emerged, with several new mechanisms of neovascularization being proposed. The concept that Judah Folkman presented that tumors are angiogenesis-dependent *(1)* may no longer hold for all tumor types. Indeed, a so-called nonangiogenic phenotype of lung cancer has been reported. *(2)*. In this pattern, tumor cells fill the existing lung alveolar spaces, entrapping themselves within the alveolar septa, utilizing the blood vessels, but without concomitant destruction that is seen in sprouting angiogenesis.

From: *Methods in Molecular Medicine, Vol. 120: Breast Cancer Research Protocols*
Edited by: S. A. Brooks and A. L. Harris © Humana Press Inc., Totowa, NJ

Thus, unlike many solid tumors, which are more vascular than their normal tissue counterpart, these nonangiogenic tumors, have the same structure and number of vessels as normal lung. Similarly, "co-option" of normal blood vessels without an angiogenic response has been described in animal models of brain tumors *(3,4)*. In these circumstances, continued tumor growth in the absence of angiogenesis resulted in hypoxia, necrosis, and tumor death from the lack of a blood supply, which nonetheless was soon followed by a robust angiogenic response and tumor recrudescence. The co-option model is probably not limited to model systems, because a similar mechanism of vascularization of hepatic metastases has been reported *(5)*.

Although angiogenesis is likely to be the primary process in the neovascularization of most tumors through their development, alternative processes, such as those that occur in the embryo, such as vasculogenesis, are also likely to contribute. Thus, using a variety of elegant experimental techniques, it has been shown that endothelial cells from circulating precursors or mobilized from the bone marrow by tumor-derived growth factors lodge in the cancer vasculature and enhance tumor neovascularization through more conventional angiogenesis *(6–9)*. An alternative mechanism for the establishment of a tumor blood supply is that of intussusception. This refers to the growth and insertion of columns of tumor cells into vessels splitting the lumen, thus dividing it into one or more channels. Unlike conventional sprouting angiogenesis, endothelial cell proliferation is not a feature *(10,11)*.

The concept of using a quantitative method for measuring angiogenesis in tissue sections was originally recognized by Folkman and colleagues as having a potentially important role in predicting tumor behavior and therefore altering patient management. They therefore developed a microscopic angiogenesis grading system, designated the "MAGS score," measuring vessel number, endothelial cell hyperplasia, and cytology in tinctorially stained tissue sections *(12,13)*. The thought was that this would be a highly objective measure of tumor vascularity that would give useful data on the relationship with clinicopathological characteristics and help in the testing antiangiogenic therapies. Unfortunately, although it was possible to classify tumors into "endothelial poor" or "rich," the tools available at that time did not adequately allow discrimination between more-subtle tumor differences. Nevertheless, quantitative measures of tumor angiogenesis were revived in the 1980s, with the advent of nonspecific endothelial markers *(14,15)*. However, it has been only in the last 10 yr, with the advent of more specific endothelial markers that could be used in archival formalin-fixed, paraffin-embedded biopsies, that rigorous quantitation studies have been able to be performed.

Most of these studies have measured only the number of immunohistochemically highlighted microvessels in tissue sections. However, with our broadening knowledge of the processes involved in tumor angiogenesis, other measures of endothelial or capillary activation or differentiation phenotypes, including vascular maturation, proliferation, protease production, adhesion molecule, and growth factor receptor expression, have been investigated as other potential useful adjuncts to microvessel number.

Most early studies that investigated microvessel quantitation employed a method based on that developed by Folkman and colleagues *(16)*. Most studies pertain to female breast cancer, but there is evidence that microvessel density also gives prognostic information in male breast cancer *(17)*. Tumor blood vessels are immunohistochemically highlighted, and the number of microvessels are then quantified in the most-vascular area (the so-called "hot spots") of the tumor. Although many of these studies showed that an increased microvessel density was a powerful prognostic tool in many human tumor types including breast cancer (reviewed in **ref. *18***), because of limitations in capillary identification and quantitation, many investigators have been unable to confirm these findings *(19–30)*. This chapter will briefly discuss the considerations in quantifying tumor angiogenesis in tissue sections and give the current optimal protocol for assessment. Other candidate techniques that have potential for the future are outlined. The reader is also referred to Chapter 35, which covers methodology for in vitro assays of angiogenesis.

It is should be emphasized that time should be devoted to optimizing the immunohistochemical staining procedure, because quality staining with little background greatly facilitates assessment. Many histopathology laboratories are well versed in immunohistochemistry, necessitating only minor adjustments to the preferred immunohistochemical protocol outlined in this chapter. Immunohistochemistry is also the subject of Chapter 15.

1.2. Other Measures of Angiogenesis

The microvessels highlighted by immunohistochemistry in tissue sections are the end result of a dynamic, multistep process. The evolving neovasculature is the result of a complex interplay among extracellular matrix remodeling, endothelial cell migration and proliferation, capillary differentiation, and anastomosis *(31,32)*. Although it may soon be possible to measure these continuous processes in vivo, for human tissues, measurement of molecules involved in these events might be surrogate end points of angiogenesis. Thus, partly because of many of the inherent and methodological difficulties of vascular counts, these alternative strategies for quantifying tumor angiogenesis have also been pursued.

1.2.1. Angiogenic Factors and Receptors

Angiogenesis is the result of the net change in the balance of angiogenic stimulators and inhibitors (i.e., gain of promoters and/or loss of inhibitors). There are now numerous reports documenting upregulation of several angiogenic factors and their receptors at the mRNA and protein level, using a variety of techniques in a range of histological tumor types including breast *(33–40)*. However, only a few have correlated these data to clinicopathological parameters or survival. Some angiogenic factors, such as vascular endothelial growth factor (VEGF)-A, have shown a significant relationship between tumor levels and microvessel density in breast *(41–43)*. Furthermore, some studies have shown tumor VEGF expression levels gave prognostic information in breast carcinomas *(44–49)* that may be improved by combining in a ratio with soluble fms-like tyrosine kinase *(50)*. However, the story is more complex than these single-factor association studies suggest in that there are now four members if the VEGF family, with the *VEGF-A* and *VEGF-B* genes generating additional isoforms to further muddy the waters. There are very few studies in breast tissues examining the different VEGFs *(51)*, and some, but not all, studies have shown associations with clinicopathological factors *(52–54*; unpublished data). It is unknown for human breast tumors what is/are the dominant factor(s) and/ or isoform(s) at different stages of neoplastic progression. Antibodies have been developed that identify the complex of VEGF with its receptor kinase insert domain receptor *(55)* that also may be clinically useful *(56)*.

Similarly, thymidine phosphorylase expression, a migratory rather than mitogenic angiogenic factor, which is expressed in *in situ* and invasive breast cancer *(57)* has also been reported to be associated in some studies with microvessel density *(57,58)* and survival *(59–62)*.

A particular advantage of angiogenic factor measurement in patient sera, urine, or cerebrospinal fluid is the ability to perform serial measurements. Although some of the these studies have shown a relationship between angiogenic factor expression as a measure of tumor angiogenesis and patient survival, none of the current techniques is sensitive or specific enough to use for quantifying tumor angiogenesis. This may be because of differences in handling methodology, because serum VEGF has been shown to increase variably up to 2 h and isolation of supernatant in these investigations varied from immediate to 30 min and at different temperatures *(63)*. Different tumors use different angiogenic factors during the various phases of their development. Breast carcinomas coexpress VEGF and thymidine phosphorylase *(64)*, whereas they are reciprocally expressed in bladder cancers *(65,66)*, and it is more likely that determining specific profiles for individual tumor types might play an increasing role in quantitative tumor angiogenesis. Nevertheless, some sera investigations may also be compromised by the high VEGF levels present in platelets and not reflect tumor-derived VEGF, suggesting plasma measurement may be more accurate *(67)*.

1.2.2. Endothelial Cell Proliferation

It is now possible to measure endothelial cell proliferation in tissue sections, using double immunohistochemistry employed antibodies to proliferation and endothelial markers to discriminate endothelial cells from other tissue elements. We have used combinations of CD31 or CD34 (for endothelium) and BrdU and MIB-1 (as proliferation markers) with good results, but some of the newer cell cycle markers that can also be used on archival tissue such as minichromosome maintenance proteins 2 and 5 may also be of use *(68,69)*. This technique allows simultaneous assessment of tumor and endothelial cell proliferation and may help in stratifying patients for novel therapies.

1.2.3. Vessel Maturation Index

A late event in the establishment of a tumor blood supply that accompanies downregulation of endothelial cell proliferation is pericyte recruitment and secretion of a basement membrane. This basement membrane is irregular and is composed of abnormal ratios of fibronectin, laminin, and collagen, depending on the maturation state of the capillary. Although many studies have documented the heterogeneity, few studies have assessed its significance. Nevertheless, some studies examining the ratio of endothelial cells with a pericyte *(70)* or basement membrane *(71)* cover as a surrogate of vessel maturation have been performed. There is great variation among tumor types *(70)*, but in breast carcinomas, these have shown that the vascular maturation index gives a different measure to that of microvessel density, that there is continual remodeling of vessels in normal breast, and a subset of patients can be identified who have an elevated risk of node recurrence *(71)*. The vascular maturation index may also give more functional information *(71)*.

1.2.4. Cell Adhesion Molecules

Increasing evidence suggests that many of the endothelial cell adhesion molecules (CAMs) of the immunoglobulin, selectin, and integrin superfamilies, which have physiological roles in immune trafficking and tumor metastasis, also play a major role in angiogenesis. Some clinical studies have shown that melanoma patients with upregulated CAMs on endothelium have a significantly worse prognosis and this is validating the interest in CAMs and their cognate ligands in tumor angiogenesis *(72,73)*. Indeed, soluble CAMs are readily identified in sera of cancer-bearing patients, although their relationship to tumor angiogenesis is yet unknown *(74,75)*. Similarly, integrins, including $\beta 3 \, \alpha v$, have also been shown to be upregulated in human breast carcinomas compared to normal or benign breast and might also be a potential surrogate marker for angiogenesis *(76,77)*.

1.2.5. Proteolytic Enzymes

Several studies have demonstrated that proteolytic enzymes, including the plasminogen activators and the matrix metalloproteinases that are important in tumor cell invasion and migration, are also important in angiogenesis *(78–83)*. Although no correlation was observed between microvessel density and both urokinase-type plasminogen activator and plasminogen activator inhibitor type-1 *(84)*, the poor prognosis in tumors *(85–91)* associated with elevated levels of the urokinase-type plasminogen activator system are likely to be partly because of the angiogenic activity of these tumors. Thus, measurement of proteases particularly components of the urokinase system might give some indication of the angiogenic activity of a tumor. Quantification of urokinase and its inhibitor PAI-1 is the subject of Chapter 19.

1.2.6. Hypoxic Markers

Once a tumor vasculature has been established, there is still continued remodeling of vessels. The remodeling process is likely to be related to an exaggerated stress response and therefore, is profoundly influenced by the tumor micro-environment. Hypoxia has been frequently reported despite the increased microvessel density in tumors. The hypoxia may be because of the reduction in blood flow from structural differences in blood vessels *(92,93)*, from the influence of permeability factors such as VEGF-A *(94)*, or, as has been reported in several tumor types, from shunting of blood across the tumor vascular bed *(95)*. In any of these scenarios, tissue hypoxia results in stabilization of the hypoxic inducible factors that mediate transcription of angiogenic pathways, thereby enhancing tumor angiogenesis. A pivotal pathway is the regulation by hypoxia of VEGF through the transcription factor hypoxia-inducible factor (HIF)-1α and -2α. The HIFs binds to the aryl-hydrocarbon nuclear translocator (HIF-1β), which then binds a specific DNA hypoxia-response element, increasing mRNA transcription. Antibodies to both HIFs *(96)* and a downstream gene, carbonic anhydrase IX *(97)*, have been shown to be surrogates of hypoxia *(98)*. Measurement of the factors involved in the regulation of the hypoxic response may be clinically important in breast cancer management *(99,100)*. Nevertheless, these techniques require a degree of quantitation and are currently unsuitable for a general diagnostic pathology laboratory. The presence of a fibrotic focus as a surrogate marker of hypoxia is being examined. This is defined as a scar-like area, consisting of fibroblasts and collagen fibers in the center of an invasive ductal carcinoma of the breast. It was first proposed in 1996 by Hasebe et al. *(101,102)* as an indicator of tumor aggressiveness. The presence of a fibrotic focus is associated with a higher microvessel density *(103)* and more latterly a marker of intratumoral hypoxia. Thus, a fibrotic focus may be a useful surrogate marker of hypoxia-driven, ongoing angiogenesis *(104)*.

1.3. Conclusion

Continuing research into angiogenesis by using quantitative data will not only broaden our understanding of the angiogenic process, but will have several potential clinical applications beyond its use for predicting prognosis. It might help in stratifying patients for cytotoxic therapy, aid monitoring and prediction of their response, and, with the advent of antiangiogenesis and vascular targeting, treatment could be stratified and altered based on these angiogenic measurements (reviewed in **refs. *18*** and ***105***). The next few years will provide the data as to the reliability of quantitation of angiogenesis in tissue sections. During this time, it is also probable that basic research will describe several candidate molecules that might become objective, sensitive, and specific enough to supercede the presently used assays.

2. Materials

2.1. Staining Procedure

1. Adhesive-coated slides (Snowcoat Xtra; Surgipath, UK).
2. Citroclear (HD Supplies, Buckinghamshire, UK) or xylene.
3. Graded alcohols (100% ethanol, 100% ethanol, and 70% ethanol).
4. 0.5% (v/v) H_2O_2 in methanol.
5. Phosphate-buffered saline (PBS), pH 7.4.
6. Anti-CD34 (Q/bend10; Novocastra, UK) primary antibody solution, prepared according to manufacturer's instructions.
7. EnVision or StreptABC detection kits (DakoCytomation, UK). (If using StreptABC kits, biotinylated goat anti-mouse antibody [DakoCytomation] diluted 1:40 in PBS.)
8. Diaminobenzidine (DAB)/H_2O_2 solution: 0.5 mg/mL DAB and 0.03% (v/v) H_2O_2 in PBS.
9. DPX [mixture of distyrene (a polystyrene), tricresyl phosphate (a plasticizer) and xylene] mountant (Raymond A. Lamb, London, UK).

3. Methods

3.1. Staining Procedure

1. Cut 4-μm, formalin-fixed, paraffin-embedded sections of the representative tumor block (*see* **Notes 1** and **2**) onto adhesive-coated slides.
2. Dry at 37°C overnight in an incubator (*see* **Note 3**).
3. Dewax using Citroclear or xylene for 15 min before passing through graded alcohols (100% ethanol, 100% ethanol, and 70% ethanol) into water before placing in PBS for 5 min.

4. If using the StreptABC method (*see* **Note 4**), block endogenous peroxidase by incubating sections in H_2O_2 in methanol for 20 min.
5. Rinse in fresh PBS and apply anti-CD34 primary antibody for 30 min.
6. Wash thoroughly three times, for 5 min each wash in, PBS.
7. If using the EnVision system, follow kit instructions, then proceed to **step 10**. If using the StreptABC system, incubate with biotinylated goat anti-mouse antibody for 30 min, then follow **step 8** and beyond.
8. Wash thoroughly three times, for 5 min each wash, in PBS
9. Incubate with the StreptABC kit streptavidin-biotin-HRP complex (*see* **Note 4**) for 30 min.
10. Wash thoroughly three times, for 5 min each wash, in PBS.
11. Incubate with DAB-H_2O_2 for 10 min.
12. Wash thoroughly three times, for 5 min each wash, in PBS.
13. Rinse in tap water for 2 to 3 min.
14. Dehydrate through graded alcohols to remove water, tap dry, and mount in DPX.
15. Confirm satisfactory staining using normal entrapped vasculature as internal positive control.
16. An optional parallel negative control section using an IgG_1 isotype antibody may also be run.

3.2. Method of Assessment of Invasive Carcinomas

3.2.1. Identification of Hot Spots

The three "hot spot" areas containing the maximum number of *discrete* microvessels should be identified by scanning the entire tumor at low power (×40 and ×100 magnification, **Fig. 1**). This is the most subjective step of the procedure. It has been demonstrated that the experience of the observer determines the success of identifying the relevant hot spots *(106)*. Poor selection will lead, in turn, to an inability to classify patients into different prognostic groups. Therefore, it is recommended that inexperienced observers spend time in a laboratory where a period of training can be undertaken. Ideally, comparisons among hot spots chosen by an experienced investigator and trainee should performed and continued on different series until there is more than 90% agreement. Training can be completed by assessing sections from a series that has already been assessed for prognostic information *(107)*.

Inexperienced observers tend to be drawn to areas with dilated capillaries, generally within the sclerotic body of the tumor. These central fibrotic areas together with necrotic tumor should be ignored. Vascular lumens or the presence of erythrocytes is not a requirement to be considered a countable vessel, and indeed, many of the microvessels have a collapsed configuration. Although the hot-spot areas can occur anywhere within the tumor, they are generally at the tumor periphery, where angiogenesis is most active, making it important to include the normal-tumor interface in the representative area to be assessed.

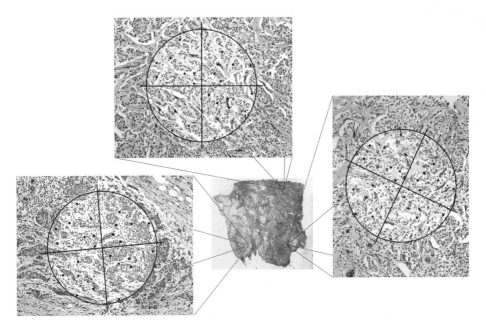

Fig. 1. The section of invasive breast carcinoma is scanned at low power (×40–100 magnification) and the three most-vascular fields that contain the highest number of discrete microvessels are selected. The sclerotic center is avoided.

Vessels outside the tumor margin by one ×200–250 field diameter and immediately adjacent benign breast tissue should not be counted. The procedure should take between 2 and 5 min.

3.2.2. Chalkley Counting

Once selected, a 25-point Chalkley point eyepiece graticule (*see* **Note 5**) *(108)* at ×200–250 should then be oriented over each hot-spot region so that the max. number of graticule points are on or within areas of highlighted vessels (**Fig. 2**). Particular care should be taken in occasional cases where an intense inflammatory cell infiltrate is present, which can obscure the underlying tumor vasculature. The mean of the three Chalkley counts is then generated for each tumor and used for statistical analysis. The procedure takes 2–3 min.

3.2.3. Intratumoral Microvessel Density

For this index, any endothelial cell or endothelial cell cluster separate from adjacent microvessels, tumor cells, or connective tissue elements is considered a countable vessel. Those that appear to be derived from the same vessel, if separate, should also be counted. Again, vessel lumens and erythrocytes are

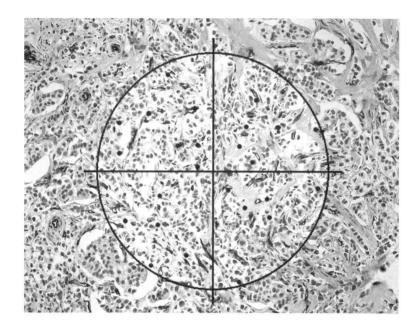

Fig. 2. Areas of tumor containing the highest number of discrete microvessels are examined at high power (×200–250 magnification) and the Chalkley point graticule rotated in the eyepiece so the max. number of graticule points is aligned on or within the vessels, which is then recorded for each area.

not included in the criteria defining a microvessel, but the sclerotic areas usually in the center should be ignored. There is no cutoff for vessel caliber. The procedure takes 3–6 min.

3.3. Method of Assessment of Ductal Carcinoma In Situ

With the advent of screening programs, the number of patients presenting with *in situ* disease is such that this now accounts for 10–25% of breast cancers. Although several new classifications for ductal carcinoma *in situ* (DCIS) have emerged that have attempted to identify those patients at risk of relapse or progression to invasive disease, several investigators have examined the microvessel architecture and number in DCIS. As with normal breast tissues, the stromal tissues are highly vascular. Nevertheless, rather than observing useful differences in microvessel density as with invasive carcinomas, two distinct angiogenic patterns were defined *(109–112)*: type I is a diffuse increase in stromal vascularity between ducts filled with tumor cells (**Fig. 3**), and type II is a dense rim of capillaries immediately adjacent to the duct membrane involved by *in situ* disease (**Fig. 3**). These have been noted to be present alone in 11 and 16%, respectively, of cases and 57 and 62%, respectively, in

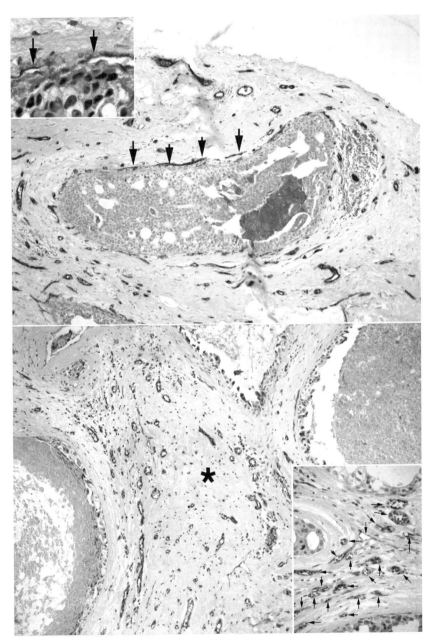

Fig. 3. Type I vascular pattern (top panel) in a low-nuclear-grade ductal carcinoma *in situ*, showing close apposition of microvessels to form a rim around the involved duct (arrows). Type II vascular pattern (lower panel) in a high-nuclear-grade ductal carcinoma *in situ*, showing an increase in the number of microvessels between involved ducts (*see* inset).

total. Studies in *in situ* carcinomas should attempt to define these two patterns, because they are likely to be relevant in that elevated angiogenic factor expression is associated with type II neovascularization *(109)*. A further study using the proportion of involved ducts surrounded by type II vessels has shown an association with aggressive disease *(113)*.

3.4. Assessing Angiogenesis in Tissue Sections

An interesting observation has been reported for aggressive ocular melanomas and ovarian tumors *(114)*, whereby tumor cells themselves rather than endothelium line contain the capillary network conducting the blood supply *(115,116)*. The tumor cells assumed the morphology and phenotype of endothelium, and the process has therefore been termed "vascular mimicry." Although partial lining of the capillary surface by tumor cells has been known for many years and more recently reported in animal models using newer techniques *(117)*, in this author's experience, when using morphology and double immunohistochemistry with cytokeratin and endothelial markers in several tumor types including breast cancer, this does not appear to be a prominent feature (unpublished results). Thus, the majority of the tumor vasculature is lined by endothelial cells expressing a variety of antigenic profiles, depending on the tissue bed or origin. Nevertheless, it has been suggested that certain breast tumor types may display this unusual form of "neovascularization" *(118,119)*.

Because endothelium is highly heterogeneous *(120)*, the choice of antibody profoundly influences the number of microvessels available for assessment. Many, such as those directed to vimentin *(121)*, lectin *(122,123)*, alkaline phosphatase *(14)*, and type IV collagen *(124,125)*, suffer from low specificity and are present on many nonendothelial elements. Others including antibodies to factor VIII-related antigen, the marker used in most studies (reviewed in **ref. *126***) identifies only a proportion of capillaries and also detects lymphatic endothelium. CD34 is now considered the optimal marker for quantitative angiogenic studies in tumors for its robustness and ease of use *(127)* and has superceded CD31 as the endothelial marker of choice for invasive breast disease *(107)*, because many laboratories have had difficulties in antigen retrieval. However, CD34 is also expressed by breast stromal cells, and CD31 or antibodies to factor VIII-related antigen should still be used for studies on ductal carcinoma *in situ* *(110,112,128)*.

Once the tumor vasculature has been immunohistochemically highlighted with CD34, the tumor is scanned to identify angiogenic hot spots. These are the areas of tumor that are counted, beause they are the regions that are likely to be most biologically relevant, derived from tumor clones with the highest angiogenic potential and likelihood of blood dissemination. The number of vessels is then quantified at higher magnification in these regions. Although some breast tumors have a more homogenous vascular profile, those tumors with heterogeneous vascularization have a limited number of hot spots. If too many of these areas are assessed, it is likely that microvessel density would be diluted. Thus, although the number of hot spots counted in studies varies from one to five *(19–21,125,129–133)*, most studies have examined three from a single representative tissue block. This is not just a pragmatic approach, because although there are some data to suggest that there is variation of tumor vascularity among different tumor tissue blocks *(134)*, the use of one tissue block alone for counting is justified by the prevailing evidence that shows a high concordance in vessel number among different blocks *(19,135,136)*. Nevertheless, both the magnification used and its corresponding tumor field area also determine the vessel number derived from each hot spot. A high magnification, which will identify more microvessels by virtue of increased resolution *(137)*, used over a too-small area will always give a high vessel index, whereas a low magnification over a too-large area will dilute out the hot spot. It is therefore recommended that three regions be examined using a microscope magnification of field area of between ×200 and ×400 (corresponds to areas of approx 0.15–0.74 mm^2, depending on the microscope type) *(107,127,138)*.

Although less subjective than identifying angiogenic hot spots *(107,127)*, the process of counting vessels has also resulted in significant variation in published series. The original criteria used by Weidner et al. *(129)* and subsequent studies using microvessel density were that the sclerotic central areas were not counted, and that any highlighted endothelial cell or cluster separate from adjacent endothelial, tumor, or stromal element was considered a countable vessel; vessel lumens or red cells within were not a requirement. It will soon become apparent to any observer that there are differences in interpretation of these criteria, and although consensus agreement by two observers was a requirement, problems have remained. This has been demonstrated in the study of Axelsson et al. *(139)* where the authors, after an initial training period with Weidner *(129)*, who defined the criteria as to what constituted individual microvessels (*see* **Subheading 3.2.2.**), did not observe a correlation between microvessel density and patient survival. Even experienced observers occasionally disagree as to what constitutes a microvessel. To overcome these problems, after selection of each hot spot, a 25-point Chalkley microscope eyepiece graticule *(108)* has been used to quantify tumor angiogenesis (*see* **Subheading 3.**). This gives a measure of the relative area that the vessels cover rather than microvessel density, but there is a strongly significant association between vessel area and number *(138)*. This method is not only objective *(140)*, because no decision is required as to whether adjacent stained structures are separate, but is rapid (2–3 min per section), reproducible, and gives independent prognostic information in breast *(138,141,142)* and bladder *(143)* cancers. Thus, it is currently the preferred method contained in recent multicenter discussion paper *(128)*.

The final consideration in quantifying angiogenesis is the differences in the value used for stratification into different study groups. This alone will result in different conclusions being drawn from the same dataset. Studies have used continuous counts *(144)*; the highest, the mean, and the median *(137)*; tertiles *(138)*; mean count in node-negative patients with recurrence *(145)* or variable cutoffs given as a function of tumor area *(19,129)*; and microscope magnification *(131)*. The median and tertile groups avoid strong assumptions about the relationship between tumor vascularity and other variables including survival and is therefore useful clinically. However, there is some loss of information making it optimal to use continuous data where possible.

3.5. Potential Improvements to Current Methods

3.5.1. Vascular Grading

Quantitation of tumor vascularity by Chalkley counting or microvessel density is still only considered by the College of American Pathologists as a category III marker, that is "factors not sufficiently studied to demonstrate their prognostic value." This author would also add that it is a time-consuming and laborious process, making it unsuitable for use in a routine diagnostic histopathology laboratory. Therefore, to facilitate assessing angiogenesis in tissue sections, akin to semiquantitative tumor grading, a vascular grading based on the subjective appraisal by trained observers over a conference microscope has been assessed (**Fig. 4**). Highly significant relationships between vascular grade and both microvessel density and Chalkley count have been demonstrated, indicating the utility of this methodology in quantitation of the tumor vasculature. However, although the method is reproducible *(146)*, delineating criteria is difficult because of the subjective nature of the assessment and considerable time and quality assurance schemes would be required to align and retain the cutoffs required for multicenter studies. Nevertheless, the overall time savings engendered by this make it an attractive proposition, and although there is some loss of power associated with translation of numerical to categorical data, there is some evidence that this also gives independent prognostic information *(147)*. Further validation in a large series of randomized patients is warranted to determine its prognostic utility before its application can be considered in such studies.

3.5.2. Novel Angiogenic Antigens

Pan-endothelial markers such as CD34 highlight the entire tumor-associated endothelium. An alternative approach is to selectively identify only the

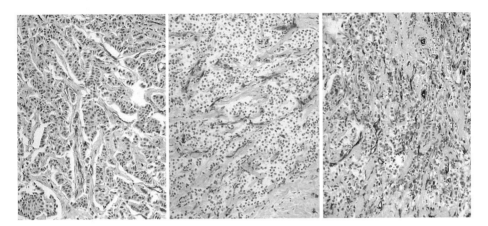

Fig. 4. Examples of vascular grading with increasing vascularity from left to right (left, low-; middle, medium-; and right, high-vascular grade).

vasculature that is undergoing active neovascularization. This might be valuable not only in more accurately quantifying tumor angiogenesis, but it might also have important implications for antivascular and antiangiogenic targeting *(148,149)*. A number of antibodies have been identified that recognize antigens that have been reported to be upregulated in tumor-associated endothelium compared with normal tissues and include EN7/44, CD105, and endosialin. Some, such as CD105 or endoglin, a transforming growth factor-β receptor, have shown an association with prognosis *(132)*. However, there is no body of literature demonstrating their advantages.

3.5.3. Tumor Vascular Architecture

The vascular morphology of tumors is different within tumors of similar and different histological types *(92)*. It has been suggested that particular vascular patterns might both help distinguish benign from malignant lesions *(150,151)* and be a prognostic marker; in ocular melanomas, a closed back-to-back loop vascular pattern was associated with death from metastasis *(152)* and in lung carcinomas, there are distinct patterns of neovascularization including basal, papillary, and diffuse *(2)* as well as nonangiogenic. Their significance may be in their potential to identify patients who will respond differently to anticancer treatments *(2,153,154)*.

3.5.4. Automation

We and others have attempted to automate the counting procedure by using computer image analysis systems *(106,121,123,125,138,155,156)*. These systems have several drawbacks, not including the capital and running costs notwithstanding those shared with manual methods. An endothelial marker that gives sensitive and specific capillary staining is essential to reduce background signal. Although software able to identify hot spots is being developed, full automation will require motorized stages, which are exceedingly time-consuming at additional expense *(157)*. Although partially automated systems with area and shape filters using defined color tolerances are available, most systems are not fully automated, require a high-degree operator interaction, and like manual counting, suffer from observer bias. Currently, a computer image analysis system is more costly, time-consuming, and no more accurate than a trained observer, making it unsuitable for routine diagnostic practice, but it is still commonly used in the research setting *(28,29,158)*.

Nevertheless, data from these studies have demonstrated that most vascular indices including microvessel density, vessel perimeter, and vascular area are significantly correlated, suggesting that they are equivalent indices of angiogenesis *(138)*. Previously, it had been hypothesized that microvessel density might not be the most important vascular parameter, because a large vascular perimeter or area might be better measures of angiogenesis, as it may reflect the functional aspects of endothelial surface and volume of blood available for interaction with the tumor *(138)*.

4. Notes

1. 8-μm Cryostat sections can also be used, but the area of the tumor assessed is smaller and therefore, less representative.
2. The tumor block should be selected by examining hematoxylin and eosin stained slides and should encompass the max. area of the tumor periphery where angiogenesis is most active.
3. If sections continually float off after antigen retrieval, drying at 56°C overnight will increase tissue adherence.
4. If using this methodology in other tissues, such as liver and kidney (which contain high endogenous biotin), the EnVision latex (DakoCytomation) or similar system is preferred to eliminate background staining that will confound assessment.
5. This can be obtained from Graticules, Morley Road, Botany Trading Estate, Tonbridge Wells, Kent, TN9 1ZN, UK. The size of the graticule required will depend on the eyepiece diameter of the microscope lens.

References

1. Folkman, J. (1990) What is the evidence that tumors are angiogenesis dependent? *J. Natl. Cancer Inst.* **82,** 4–6.
2. Pezzella, F., Pastorin, O. U., Tagliabue, E., et al. (1996) Non-small-cell lung carcinoma tumor growth without morphological evidence of neo-angiogenesis. *Am. J. Pathol.* **151,** 1417–1423.
3. Holash, J., Maisonpierre, P. C., Compton, D., et al. (1999) Vessel co-option, regression, and growth in tumors mediated by angiopoietins and VEGF. *Science* **284,** 1994–1998.

4. Holash, J., Wiegand, S. J., and Yancopoulos, G. D. (1999) New model of tumor angiogenesis: dynamic balance between vessel regression and growth mediated by angiopoietins and VEGF. *Oncogene* **18,** 5356–5362.

5. Vermeulen, P. B., Colpaert, C., Salgado, R., et al. (2001) Liver metastases from colorectal adenocarcinomas grow in three patterns with different angiogenesis and desmoplasia. *J. Pathol.* **195,** 336–342.

6. Asahara, T., Masuda, H., Takahashi, T., et al. (1999) Bone marrow origin of endothelial progenitor cells responsible for postnatal vasculogenesis in physiological and pathological neovascularization. *Circ. Res.* **85,** 221–228.

7. Gunsilius, E., Duba, H. C., Petzer, A. L., et al. (2000) Evidence from a leukaemia model for maintenance of vascular endothelium by bone-marrow-derived endothelial cells. *Lancet* **355,** 1688–1691.

8. Rafii, S. (2000) Circulating endothelial precursors: mystery, reality, and promise. *J. Clin. Invest.* **105,** 17–19.

9. Asahara, T., Takahashi, T., Masuda, H., et al. (1999) VEGF contributes to postnatal neovascularization by mobilizing bone marrow-derived endothelial progenitor cells. *EMBO J.* **18,** 3964–3972.

10. Patan, S., Munn, L. L., and Jain, R. K. (1996) Intussusceptive microvascular growth in a human colon adenocarcinoma xenograft: a novel mechanism of tumor angiogenesis. *Microvasc. Res.* **51,** 260–272.

11. Patan, S. (2000) Vasculogenesis and angiogenesis as mechanisms of vascular network formation, growth and remodeling. *J. Neurooncol.* **50,** 1–15.

12. Brem, S., Cotran, R., and Folkman, J. (1972) Tumor angiogenesis: a quantitative method for histological grading. *J. Natl. Cancer Inst.* **48,** 347–356.

13. Porschen, R., Classen, S., Piontek, M., and Borchard, F. (1994) Vascularization of carcinomas of the esophagus and its correlation with tumor proliferation. *Cancer Res.* **54,** 587–591.

14. Mlynek, M., van Beunigen, D., Leder, L-D., and Streffer, C. (1985) Measurement of the grade of vascularisation in histological tumor tissue sections. *Br. J. Cancer* **52,** 945–948.

15. Svrivastava, A., Laidler, P., Davies, R., Horgan, K., and Hughes, L. (1988) The prognostic significance of tumor vascularity in intermediate-thickness (0.76–4.0-mm thick) skin melanoma. *Am. J. Pathol.* **133,** 419–423.

16. Weidner, N., Semple, J. P., Welch, W. R., and Folkman, J. (1991) Tumor angiogenesis and metastasis—correlation in invasive breast carcinoma. *N. Engl. J. Med.* **324,** 1–8.

17. Shpitz, B., Bomstein, Y., Sternberg, A., et al. (2000) Angiogenesis, p53, and c-erbB-2 immunoreactivity and clinicopathological features in male breast cancer. *J. Surg. Oncol.* **75,** 252–257.

18. Fox, S. B., Gasparini, G., and Harris, A. L. (2001) Angiogenesis: pathological, prognostic, and growth-factor pathways and their link to trial design and anticancer drugs. *Lancet Oncol.* **2,** 278–289.

19. Van Hoef, M. E., Knox, W. F., Dhesi, S. S., Howell, A., and Schor, A. M. (1993) Assessment of tumor vascularity as a prognostic factor in lymph node negative invasive breast cancer. *Eur. J. Cancer* **29A,** 1141–1145.

20. Hall, N. R., Fish, D. E., Hunt, N., Goldin, R. D., Guillou, P. J., and Monson, J. R. (1992) Is the relationship between angiogenesis and metastasis in breast cancer real? *Surg. Oncol.* **1,** 223–229.
21. Sightler, H., Borowsky, A., Dupont, W., Page, D., and Jensen, R. (1994) Evaluation of tumor angiogenesis as a prognostic marker in breast cancer. *Lab. Invest.* **70,** 22A (abstract).
22. Siitonen, S., Haapasalo, H., Rantala, I., Helin, H., and Isola, J. (1995) Comparison of different immunohistochemical methods in the assessment of angiogenesis: lack of prognostic value in a group of 77 selected node-negative breast carcinomas. *Mod. Pathol.* **8,** 745–752.
23. Goulding, H., Abdul, R. N., Robertson, J. F., et al. (1995) Assessment of angiogenesis in breast carcinoma: an important factor in prognosis? *Hum. Pathol.* **26,** 1196–1200.
24. Costello, P., McCann, A., Carney, D. N., and Dervan, P. A. (1995) Prognostic significance of microvessel density in lymph node negative breast carcinoma. *Hum. Pathol.* **26,** 1181–1184.
25. Morphopoulos, G., Pearson, M., Ryder, W. D., Howell, A., and Harris, M. (1996) Tumor angiogenesis as a prognostic marker in infiltrating lobular carcinoma of the breast. *J. Pathol.* **180,** 44–49.
26. Tan, P., Cady, B., and Wanner, M. (1997) et al. The cell cycle inhibitor p27 is an independent prognostic marker in small (T1a,b) invasive breast carcinomas. *Cancer Res.* **57,** 1259–1263.
27. Clahsen, P. C., van de Velde, C. J., Duval, C., et al. (1998) p53 protein accumulation and response to adjuvant chemotherapy in premenopausal women with node-negative early breast cancer. *J. Clin. Oncol.* **16,** 470–479.
28. Fridman, V., Humblet, C., Bonjean, K., and Boniver, J. (2000) Assessment of tumor angiogenesis in invasive breast carcinomas: absence of correlation with prognosis and pathological factors. *Virchows Arch.* **437,** 611–617.
29. Lee, J. S., Kim, H. S., Jung, J. J., Kim, Y. B., Park, C. S., and Lee, M. C. (2001) Correlation between angiogenesis, apoptosis and cell proliferation in invasive ductal carcinoma of the breast and their relation to tumor behavior. *Anal. Quant. Cytol. Histol.* **23,** 161–168.
30. Vincent-Salomon, A., Carton, M., Zafrani, B., et al. (2001) Long-term outcome of small size invasive breast carcinomas independent from angiogenesis in a series of 685 cases. *Cancer* **92,** 249–256.
31. Paweletz, N. and Knierim, M. (1989) Tumor-related angiogenesis. *Crit. Rev. Oncol. Hematol.* **9,** 197–242.
32. Blood, C. H. and Zetter, B. R. (1990) Tumor interactions with the vasculature: angiogenesis and tumor metastasis. *Biochim. Biophys. Acta* **1032,** 89–118.
33. Brown, L. F., Berse, B., Jackman, R. W., et al. (1995) Expression of vascular permeability factor (vascular endothelial growth factor) and its receptors in breast cancer. *Hum. Pathol.* **26,** 86–91.
34. Moghaddam, A. and Bicknell, R. (1992) Expression of platelet-derived endothelial cell growth factor in *Escherichia coli* and confirmation of its thymidine phosphorylase activity. *Biochemistry* **31,** 12141–12146.

35. Anandappa, S. Y., Winstanley, J. H., Leinster, S., Green, B., Rudland, P. S., and Barraclough, R. (1994) Comparative expression of fibroblast growth factor mRNAs in benign and malignant breast disease. *Br. J. Cancer* **69**, 772–776.

36. Relf, M., LeJeune, S., Scott, P. A., et al. (1997) Expression of the angiogenic factors vascular endothelial cell growth factor, acidic and basic fibroblast growth factor, tumor growth factor beta-1, platelet-derived endothelial cell growth factor, placenta growth factor, and pleiotrophin in human primary breast cancer and its relation to angiogenesis. *Cancer Res.* **57**, 963–969.

37. Garver, R. J., Radford, D. M., Donis, K. H., Wick, M. R., and Milner, P. G. (1994) Midkine and pleiotrophin expression in normal and malignant breast tissue. *Cancer* **74**, 1584–1590.

38. Smith, K., Fox, S. B., Whitehouse, R., et al. (1999) Upregulation of basic fibroblast growth factor in breast carcinoma and its relationship to vascular density, oestrogen receptor, epidermal growth factor receptor and survival. *Ann. Oncol.* **10**, 707–713.

39. Wong, S. Y., Purdie, A. T., and Han, P. (1992) Thrombospondin and other possible related matrix proteins in malignant and benign breast disease. An immunohistochemical study. *Am. J. Pathol.* **140**, 1473–1482.

40. Visscher, D. W., DeMattia, F., Ottosen, S., Sarkar, F. H., and Crissman, J. D. (1995) Biologic and clinical significance of basic fibroblast growth factor immunostaining in breast carcinoma. *Mod. Pathol.* **8**, 665–670.

41. Toi, M., Kondo, S., Suzuki, H., Yamamoto, Y., et al. (1996) Quantitative analysis of vascular endothelial growth factor in primary breast cancer. *Cancer* **77**, 1101–1106.

42. Lantzsch, T., Hefler, L., Krause, U., et al. (2002) The correlation between immunohistochemically-detected markers of angiogenesis and serum vascular endothelial growth factor in patients with breast cancer. *Anticancer Res.* **22**, 1925–1928.

43. Valkovic, T., Dobrila, F., Melato, M., Sasso, F., Rizzardi, C., and Jonjic, N. (2002) Correlation between vascular endothelial growth factor, angiogenesis, and tumor-associated macrophages in invasive ductal breast carcinoma. *Virchows Arch.* **440**, 583–588.

44. Linderholm, B., Tavelin, B., Grankvist, K., Henriksson, and R. Vascular (1998) Endothelial growth factor is of high prognostic value in node-negative breast carcinoma. *J. Clin. Oncol.* **16**, 3121–3128.

45. Gasparini, G., Toi, M., Gion, M., et al. (1997) Prognostic-significance of vascular endothelial growth-factor protein in node-negative breast-carcinoma. *J. Natl. Cancer Inst.* **89**, 139–147.

46. Obermair, A., Kucera, E., Mayerhofer, K., et al. (1997) Vascular endothelial growth factor (VEGF) in human breast cancer: correlation with disease-free survival. *Int. J. Cancer* **74**, 455–458.

47. Manders, P., Beex, L. V., Tjan-Heijnen, V. C., et al. (2002) The prognostic value of vascular endothelial growth factor in 574 node-negative breast cancer patients who did not receive adjuvant systemic therapy. *Br. J. Cancer* **87**, 772–778.

48. Eppenberger, U., Kueng, W., Schlaeppi, J. M., et al. (1998) Markers of tumor angiogenesis and proteolysis independently define high- and low-risk subsets of node-negative breast cancer patients. *J. Clin. Oncol.* **16,** 3129–3136.
49. Coradini, D., Boracchi, P., Daidone, M. G., et al. (2001) Contribution of vascular endothelial growth factor to the Nottingham prognostic index in node-negative breast cancer. *Br. J. Cancer* **85,** 795–797.
50. Toi, M., Bando, H., Ogawa, T., Muta, M., Hornig, C., and Weich, H. A. (2002) Significance of vascular endothelial growth factor (VEGF)/soluble VEGF receptor-1 relationship in breast cancer. *Int. J. Cancer* **98,** 14–18.
51. Salven, P., Lymboussaki, A., Heikkila, P., et al. (1998) Vascular endothelial growth factors VEGF-B and VEGF-C are expressed in human tumors. *Am. J. Pathol.* **153,** 103–108.
52. Gunningham, S., Currie, M., Cheng, H., et al. (2000) The short form of the alternatively spliced flt-4 but not its ligand VEGF-C is related to lymph node metastasis in human breast cancers. *Clin. Cancer Res.* **6,** 4278–4286.
53. Gunningham, S., Currie, M., Cheng, H., et al. (2000) VEGF-B expression in human breast cancers is associated with positive lymph node status. *J. Pathol.* **193,** 325–332.
54. Kinoshita, J., Kitamura, K., Kabashima, A., Saeki, H., Tanaka, S., and Sugimachi, K. (2001) Clinical significance of vascular endothelial growth factor-C (VEGF-C) in breast cancer. *Breast Cancer Res. Treat.* **66,** 159–164.
55. Brekken, R. A., Huang, X., King, S. W., and Thorpe, P. E. (1998) Vascular endothelial growth factor as a marker of tumor endothelium. *Cancer Res.* **58,** 1952–1959.
56. Giatromanolaki, A., Sivridis, E., Brekken, R., et al. (2001) The angiogenic "vascular endothelial growth factor/flk-1(KDR) receptor" pathway in patients with endometrial carcinoma: prognostic and therapeutic implications. *Cancer* **92,** 2569–2577.
57. Fox, S. B., Westwood, M., Moghaddam, A., et al. (1996) The angiogenic factor platelet-derived endothelial cell growth factor/thymidine phosphorylase is up-regulated in breast cancer epithelium and endothelium. *Br. J. Cancer* **73,** 275–280.
58. Toi, M., Hoshina, S., Taniguchi, T., Yamamoto, Y., Ishitsuka, H., Tominaga, T. (1995) Expression of platelet-derived endothelial cell growth factor/thymidine phosphorylase in human breast cancer. *Int. J. Cancer* **64,** 79–82.
59. Toi, M., Ueno, T., Matsumoto, H., et al. (1999) Significance of thymidine phosphorylase as a marker of protumor monocytes in breast cancer. *Clin. Cancer Res.* **5,** 1131–1137.
60. Yang, Q., Barbareschi, M., Mori, I., et al. (2002) Prognostic value of thymidine phosphorylase expression in breast carcinoma. *Int. J. Cancer* **97,** 512–517.
61. Kanzaki, A., Takebayashi, Y., Bando, H., et al. (2002) Expression of uridine and thymidine phosphorylase genes in human breast carcinoma. *Int. J. Cancer* **97,** 631–635.
62. Nagaoka, H., Iino, Y., Takei, H., and Morishita, Y. (1998) Platelet-derived endothelial cell growth factor/thymidine phosphorylase expression in macro-

phages correlates with tumor angiogenesis and prognosis in invasive breast cancer. *Int. J. Oncol.* **13**, 449–454.

63. Dittadi, R., Meo, S., Fabris, F., et al. (2001) Validation of blood collection procedures for the determination of circulating vascular endothelial growth factor (VEGF) in different blood compartments. *Int. J. Biol. Markers* **16**, 87–96.

64. Toi, M., Yamamoto, Y., Inada, K., et al. (1995) Vascular endothelial growth factor and platelet-derived endothelial growth factor are frequently co-expressed in highly vascularized breast cancer. *Clin. Cancer Res.* **1**, 961–964.

65. O'Brien, T., Fox, S. B., Dickinson, A., et al. (1996) Expression of the angiogenic factor thymidine phosphorylase/platelet derived endothelial cell growth factor in primary bladder cancers. *Cancer Res.* **56**, 4799–4804.

66. O'Brien, T. S., Smith, K., Cranston, D., Fuggle, S., Bicknell, R., and Harris, A. L. (1995) Urinary basic fibroblast growth factor in patients with bladder cancer and benign prostatic hypertrophy. *Br. J. Urol.* **76**, 311–314.

67. Adams, J., Carder, P. J., Downey, S., et al. (2000) Vascular endothelial growth factor (VEGF) in breast cancer: comparison of plasma, serum, and tissue VEGF and microvessel density and effects of tamoxifen. *Cancer Res.* **60**, 2898–2905.

68. Freeman, A., Morris, L. S., Mills, A. D., et al. (1999) Minichromosome maintenance proteins as biological markers of dysplasia and malignancy. *Clin.Cancer Res.* **5**, 2121–2132..

69. Stoeber, K., Swinn, R., Prevost, A. T., et al. (2002) Diagnosis of genito-urinary tract cancer by detection of minichromosome maintenance 5 protein in urine sediments. *J. Natl. Cancer Inst.* **94**, 1071–1079.

70. Eberhard, A., Kahlert, S., Goede, V., Hemmerlein, B., Plate, K. H., and Augustin, H. G. (2000) Heterogeneity of angiogenesis and blood vessel maturation in human tumors: implications for antiangiogenic tumor therapies. *Cancer Res.* **60**, 1388–1393.

71. Kakolyris, S., Fox, S. B., Koukourakis, M., et al. (2000) Relationship of vascular maturation in breast cancer blood vessels to vascular density and metastasis, assessed by expression of a novel basement membrane component, LH39. *Br. J. Cancer* **82**, 844–851.

72. Schadendorf, D., Heidel, J., Gawlik, C., Suter, L., and Czarnetzki, B. M. (1995) Association with clinical outcome of expression of VLA-4 in primary cutaneous malignant melanoma as well as P-selectin and E-selectin on intratumoral vessels. *J. Natl. Cancer Inst.* **87**, 366–371.

73. Kageshita, T., Hamby, C. V., Hirai, S., Kimura, T., Ono, T., and Ferrone, S. (2000) Alpha(v)beta3 expression on blood vessels and melanoma cells in primary lesions: differential association with tumor progression and clinical prognosis. *Cancer Immunol. Immunother.* **49**, 314–318.

74. Kageshita, T., Yoshii, A., Kimura, T., et al. (1993) Clinical relevance of ICAM-1 expression in prmary lesions and serum of patients with malignant melanoma. *Cancer Res.* **53**, 4927–4932.

75. Banks, R. E., Gearing, A. J., Hemingway, I. K., Norfolk, D. R., Perren, T. J., and Selby, P. J. (1993) Circulating intercellular adhesion molecule-1 (ICAM-1),

E-selectin and vascular cell adhesion molecule-1 (VCAM-1) in human malignancies. *Br. J. Cancer* **68,** 122–124.

76. Brooks, P. C., Stromblad, S., Klemke, R., Visscher, D., Sarkar, F. H., and Cheresh, D. A. (1995) Antiintegrin b_3a_v blocks human breast cancer growth and angiogenesis in human skin. *J. Clin. Invest.* **96,** 1815–1822.

77. Gasparini, G., Brooks, P. C., Biganzoli, E., et al. (1998) Vascular integrin alpha(v)beta3: a new prognostic indicator in breast cancer. *Clin. Cancer Res.* **4,** 2625–2634.

78. Pepper, M. S. (2001) Role of the matrix metalloproteinase and plasminogen activator-plasmin systems in angiogenesis. *Arterioscler. Thromb. Vasc. Biol.* **21,** 1104–1117.

79. John, A. and Tuszynski, G. (2001) The role of matrix metalloproteinases in tumor angiogenesis and tumor metastasis. *Pathol. Oncol. Res.* **7,** 14–23.

80. Haas, T. L. and Madri, J. A. (1999) Extracellular matrix-driven matrix metalloproteinase production in endothelial cells: implications for angiogenesis. *Trends Cardiovasc. Med.* **9,** 70–77.

81. Lochter, A. and Bissell, M. J. (1999) An odyssey from breast to bone: multi-step control of mammary metastases and osteolysis by matrix metalloproteinases. *APMIS* **107,** 128–136.

82. Parfyonova, Y. V., Plekhanova, O. S., Tkachuk, V. A. (2002) Plasminogen activators in vascular remodeling and angiogenesis. *Biochemistry (Mosc)* **67,** 119–134.

83. Nielsen, B. S., Sehested, M., Kjeldsen, L., Borregaard, N., Rygaard, J., and Dano, K. (1997) Expression of matrix metalloprotease-9 in vascular pericytes in human breast cancer. *Lab. Invest.* **77,** 345–355.

84. Fox, S. B., Taylor, M., Grondahl-Hansen, J., Kakolyris, S., Gatter, K., and Harris, A. (2001) Plasminogen activator inhibitor-1 as a measure of vascular remodelling in breast cancer. *J. Pathol.* **195,** 236–243.

85. Grøndahl-Hansen, J., Christensen, I. J., Rosenquist, C., et al. (1993) High levels of urokinase-type plasminogen activator and its inhibitor PAI-1 in cytosolic extracts of breast carcinomas are associated with poor prognosis. *Cancer Res.* **53,** 2513–2521.

86. Grøndahl-Hansen, J., Peters, H. A., J, van Putten, W. L., et al. (1995) Prognostic significance of the receptor for urokinase plasminogen activator in breast cancer. *Clin. Cancer Res.* **1,** 1079–1087.

87. Grøndahl-Hansen, J., Hilsenbeck, S. G., Christensen, I. J., Clark, G. M., Osborne, C. K., Brünner, N. (1997) Prognostic significance of PAI-1 and uPA in cytosolic extracts obtained from node-positive breast cancer patients. *Breast Cancer Res. Treat.* **43,** 153–163.

88. Janicke, F., Pache, L., Schmitt, M., et al. (1994) Both the cytosols and detergent extracts of breast cancer tissues are suited to evaluate the prognostic impact of the urokinase-type plasminogen activator and its inhibitor, plasminogen activator inhibitor type 1. *Cancer Res.* **54,** 2527–2530.

89. Foekens, J. A., Look, M. P., Peters, H. A., van Putten, W. L., Portengen, H., Klijn, J. G. (1995) Urokinase-type plasminogen activator and its inhibitor PAI-1:

predictors of poor response to tamoxifen therapy in recurrent breast cancer. *J. Natl. Cancer Inst.* **87**, 751–756.

90. Duffy, M. J. (2002) Urokinase plasminogen activator and its inhibitor, PAI-1, as prognostic markers in breast cancer: from pilot to level 1 evidence studies. *Clin. Chem.* **48**, 1194–1197.

91. Harbeck, N., Schmitt, M., Kates, R. E., et al. (2002) Clinical utility of urokinase-type plasminogen activator and plasminogen activator inhibitor-1 determination in primary breast cancer tissue for individualized therapy concepts. *Clin. Breast Cancer* **3**, 196–200.

92. Warren, B. (1979) The vascular morphology of tumors, in *Tumor Blood Circulation* (Peterson, H., ed.) CRC, Boca Raton, FL, pp. 1–47.

93. Warren, B., Greenblatt, M., and Kommineni, V. (1972) Tumor angiogenesis: ultrastructure of endothelial cells in mitosis. *Br. J. Exp. Path.* **53**, 216–224.

94. Dvorak, H. F., Nagy, J. A., Feng, D., Brown, L. F., and Dvorak, A. M. (1999) Vascular permeability factor/vascular endothelial growth factor and the significance of microvascular hyperpermeability in angiogenesis. *Curr. Top. Microbiol. Immunol.* **237**, 97–132.

95. Vaupel, P., Kallinowski, F., and Okunieff, P. (1989) Blood flow, oxygen and nutrient supply, and metabolic microenvironment of human tumors: a review. *Cancer Res.* **49**, 6449–6465.

96. Talks, K. L., Turley, H., Gatter, K. C., et al. (2000) The expression and distribution of the hypoxia-inducible factors HIF-1alpha and HIF-2alpha in normal human tissues, cancers, and tumor- associated macrophages. *Am. J. Pathol.* **157**, 411–421.

97. Wykoff, C. C., Beasley, N. J., Watson, P. H., et al. (2000) Hypoxia-inducible expression of tumor-associated carbonic anhydrases. *Cancer Res.* **60**, 7075–7083.

98. Loncaster, J. A., Harris, A. L., Davidson, S. E., et al. (2001) Carbonic anhydrase (CA IX) expression, a potential new intrinsic marker of hypoxia: correlations with tumor oxygen measurements and prognosis in locally advanced carcinoma of the cervix. *Cancer Res.* **61**, 6394–6399.

99. Qin, C., Wilson, C., Blancher, C., Taylor, M., Safe, S., and Harris, A. L. (2001) Association of ARNT splice variants with estrogen receptor-negative breast cancer, poor induction of vascular endothelial growth factor under hypoxia, and poor prognosis. Clin *Cancer Res.* **7**, 818–823.

100. Schindl, M., Schoppmann, S. F., Samonigg, H., et al. (2002) Overexpression of hypoxia-inducible factor 1alpha is associated with an unfavorable prognosis in lymph node-positive breast cancer. *Clin. Cancer Res.* **8**, 1831–1837.

101. Hasebe, T., Sasaki, S., Imoto, S., Mukai, K., Yokose, T., and Ochiai, A. (2002) Prognostic significance of fibrotic focus in invasive ductal carcinoma of the breast: a prospective observational study. *Mod. Pathol.* **15**, 502–516.

102. Hasebe, T., Tsuda, H., Hirohashi, S., et al. (1996) Fibrotic focus in invasive ductal carcinoma: an indicator of high tumor aggressiveness. *Jpn. J. Cancer Res.* **87**, 385–394.

103. Jitsuiki, Y., Hasebe, T., Tsuda, H., et al. (1999) Optimizing microvessel counts according to tumor zone in invasive ductal carcinoma of the breast. *Mod. Pathol.* **12**, 492–498.

104. Colpaert, C., Vermeulen, P., Fox, S. B., Harris, A. L., Dirix, L., and van Marck, E. (2003) The presence of a fibrotic focus in invasive breast carcinoma correlates with expression of carbonic anhydrase IX and is a marker of hypoxia and poor prognosis. *Br. Cancer Res. Treat.* **81,** 137–147.

105. Fox, S. B. and Harris, A. (1997) Markers of tumor angiogenesis: clinical applications in prognosis and anti-angiogenic therapy. *Invest. New Drugs* **15,** 15–28.

106. Barbareschi, M., Weidner, N., Gasparini, G., et al. (1995) Microvessel quantitation in breast carcinomas. *Appl. Immunochem.* **3,** 75–84.

107. Vermeulen, P. B., Gasparini, G., Fox, S. B., et al. (1996) Quantification of angiogenesis in solid human tumors: an international consensus on the methodology and criteria of evaluation. *Eur. J. Cancer* **32A,** 2474–2484.

108. Chalkley, H. (1943) Method for the quantative morphological analysis of tissues. *J. Nat. Cancer Inst.* **4,** 47–53.

109. Engels, K., Fox, S. B., Whitehouse, R. M., Gatter, K. C., and Harris, A. L. (1997) Up-regulation of thymidine phosphorylase expression is associated with a discrete pattern of angiogenesis in ductal carcinomas *in situ* of the breast. *J. Pathol.* **182,** 414–420.

110. Guidi, A., Fischer, L., Harris, J., and Schnitt, S. (1994) Microvessel density and distribution in ductal carcinoma *in situ* of the breast. *J. Natl. Cancer Inst.* **86,** 614–619.

111. Ottinetti, A. and Sapino, A. (1988) Morphometric evaluation of microvessels surrounding hyperplastic and neoplastic mammary lesions. *Breast Cancer Res. Treat.* **11,** 241–248.

112. Lee, A. H., Happerfield, L. C., Bobrow, L. G., and Millis, R. R. (1997) Angiogenesis and inflammation in ductal carcinoma in situ of the breast. *J. Pathol.* **181,** 200–206.

113. Heffelfinger, S., Yassin, R., Miller, M., and Lower, E. (1996) Vascularity of proliferative breast disease and carcinoma *in situ* correlates with histological features. *Clin. Cancer Res.* **2,** 1873–1878.

114. Sood, A. K., Seftor, E. A., Fletcher, M. S., et al. (2001) Molecular determinants of ovarian cancer plasticity. *Am. J. Pathol.* **158,** 1279–1288.

115. Folberg, R., Hendrix, M. J., and Maniotis, A. J. (2000) Vasculogenic mimicry and tumor angiogenesis. *Am. J. Pathol.* **156,** 361–381.

116. McDonald, D. M., Munn, L., and Jain, R. K. (2000) Vasculogenic mimicry: how convincing, how novel, and how significant? *Am. J. Pathol.* **156,** 383–388.

117. Chang, Y. S., di Tomaso, E., McDonald, D. M., Jones, R., Jain, R. K., and Munn, L. L. (2000) Mosaic blood vessels in tumors: frequency of cancer cells in contact with flowing blood. *Proc. Natl. Acad. Sci. U. S. A.* **97,** 14608–14613.

118. Shirakawa, K., Wakasugi, H., Heike, Y., et al. (2002) Vasculogenic mimicry and pseudo-comedo formation in breast cancer. *Int. J. Cancer* **99,** 821–828.

119. Shirakawa, K., Tsuda, H., Heike, Y., et al. (2001) Absence of endothelial cells, central necrosis, and fibrosis are associated with aggressive inflammatory breast cancer. *Cancer Res.* **61,** 445–451.

120. Kuzu, I., Bicknell, R., Fletcher, C. D., and Gatter, K. C. (1993) Expression of adhesion molecules on the endothelium of normal tissue vessels and vascular tumors. *Lab. Invest.* **69,** 322–328.

121. Wakui, S., Furusato, M., Itoh, T., et al. (1992) Tumor angiogenesis in prostatic carcinoma with and without bone marrow metastases: a morphometric study. *J. Pathol.* **168,** 257–262.

122. Carnochan, P., Briggs, J. C., Westbury, G., and Davies, A. J. (1991) The vascularity of cutaneous melanoma: a quantitative histological study of lesions 0.85–1.25 mm in thickness. *Br. J. Cancer* **64,** 102–107.

123. Svrivastava, A., Laidler, P., Hughes, L., Woodcock, J., and Shedden, E. J. (1986) Neovascularization in human cutaneous melanoma: a quantitative morphological and Doppler ultrasound study. *Eur. J. Cancer Oncol.* **22,** 1205–1209.

124. Vesalainen, S., Lipponen, P., Talja, M., Alhava, E., and Syrjanen, K. (1994) Tumor vascularity and basement membrane structure as prognostic factors in T1-2M0 prostatic adenocarcinoma. *Anticancer Res.* **14,** 709–714.

125. Visscher, D., Smilanetz, S., Drozdowicz, S., and Wykes, S. (1993) Prognostic significance of image morphometric microvessel enumeration in breast carcinoma. *Anal. Quant. Cytol.* **15,** 88–92.

126. Fox, S. B. and Harris, A. (2000) Angiogenesis as a diagnostic and therapeutic target, in *Diseases of the Breast, 2nd edition* (Harris, J., Lippman, M., Morrow, M., Osborn, M., eds.). Lippincott Williams and Wilkins, Philadelphia, PA, pp. 799–809.

127. Vermeulen, P. B., Gasparini, G., Fox, S. B., et al. (2002) Second international consensus on the methodology and criteria of evaluation of angiogenesis quantification in solid human tumors. *Eur. J. Cancer* **38,** 1564–1579.

128. Engels, K., Fox, S. B., Whitehouse, R. M., Gatter, K. C., and Harris, A. L. (1997) Distinct angiogenic patterns are associated with high-grade *in situ* ductal carcinomas of the breast. *J. Pathol.* **181,** 207–212.

129. Weidner, N., Folkman, J., Pozza, F., et al. (1992) Tumor angiogenesis: a new significant and independent prognostic indicator in early-stage breast carcinoma. *J. Natl. Cancer Inst.* **84,** 1875–1887.

130. Barnhill, R. L., Fandrey, K., Levy, M. A., Mihm, M. J., and Hyman, B. (1992) Angiogenesis and tumor progression of melanoma. Quantification of vascularity in melanocytic nevi and cutaneous malignant melanoma. *Lab. Invest.* **67,** 331–337.

131. Sahin, A., Sneige, N., Singletary, E., and Ayala, A. (1992) Tumor angiogenesis detected by Factor-VIII immunostaining in node-negative breast carcinoma (NNBC): a possible predictor of distant metastasis. *Mod. Pathol.* **5,** 17A (abstract).

132. Kumar, S., Ghellal, A., Li, C., et al. (1999) Breast carcinoma: vascular density determined using CD105 antibody correlates with tumor prognosis. *Cancer Res.,* **59,** 856–861.

133. Heimann, R., Ferguson, D., Powers, C., et al. (1996) Angiogenesis as a predictor of long-term survival for patients with node-negative breast cancer. *J. Natl Cancer Inst.* **88,** 1764–1769.

134. Ahlgren, J., Risberg, B., Villman, K., and Bergh, J. (2002) Angiogenesis in invasive breast carcinoma—a prospective study of tumor heterogeneity. *Eur. J. Cancer* **38,** 64–69.

135. Martin, L., Holcombe, C., Green, B., Leinster, S. J., and Winstanley, J. (1997) Is a histological section representative of whole tumor vascularity in breast cancer? *Br. J. Cancer* **76,** 40–43.

136. de Jong, J. S., van Diest, P. J., and Baak, J. P. (1995) Heterogeneity and reproducibility of microvessel counts in breast cancer. *Lab. Invest.* **73,** 922–926.

137. Horak, E. R., Leek, R., Klenk, N., et al. (1992) Angiogenesis, assessed by platelet/endothelial cell adhesion molecule antibodies, as indicator of node metastases and survival in breast cancer. *Lancet* **340,** 1120–1124.

138. Fox, S. B., Leek, R. D., Weekes, M. P., Whitehouse, R. M., Gatter, K. C., and Harris, A. L. (1995) Quantitation and prognostic value of breast cancer angiogenesis: comparison of microvessel density, Chalkley count, and computer image analysis. *J. Pathol.* **177,** 275–283.

139. Axelsson, K., Ljung, B. M., Moore II, D. H., et al. (1995) Tumor angiogenesis as a prognostic assay for invasive ductal breast carcinoma. *J. Natl. Cancer Inst.* **87,** 997–1008.

140. Hansen, S., Grabau, D. A., Rose, C., Bak, M., and Sorensen, F. B. (1998) Angiogenesis in breast cancer: a comparative study of the observer variability of methods for determining microvessel density. *Lab. Invest.* **78,** 1563–1573.

141. Fox, S. B., Leek, R. D., Smith, K., Hollyer, J., Greenall, M., and Harris, A. L. (1994) Tumor angiogenesis in node-negative breast carcinomas—relationship with epidermal growth factor receptor, estrogen receptor, and survival. *Br. Cancer Res. Treat.* **29,** 109–116.

142. Hansen, S., Grabau, D. A., Sorensen, F. B., Bak, M., Vach, W., and Rose, C. (2000) The prognostic value of angiogenesis by Chalkley counting in a confirmatory study design on 836 breast cancer patients. *Clin. Cancer Res.* **6,** 139–146.

143. Dickinson, A. J., Fox, S. B., Persad, R. A., Hollyer, J., Sibley, G. N., and Harris, A. L. (1994) Quantification of angiogenesis as an independent predictor of prognosis in invasive bladder carcinomas. *Br. J. Urol.* **74,** 762–766.

144. Gasparini, G., Toi, M., Verderio, P., et al. (1998) Prognostic significance of p53, angiogenesis, and other conventional features in operable breast cancer: subanalysis in node-positive and node-negative patients. *Int. J. Oncol.* **12,** 1117–1125.

145. Bosari, S., Lee, A. K., DeLellis, R. A., Wiley, B. D., Heatley, G. J., and Silverman, M. L. (1992) Microvessel quantitation and prognosis in invasive breast carcinoma. *Hum. Pathol.* **23,** 755–761.

146. Fox, S. B., Leek, R. D., Bliss, J., et al. (1997) Association of tumor angiogenesis with bone marrow micrometastases in breast cancer patients. *J. Natl. Cancer Inst.* **89,** 1044–1049.

147. Hansen, S., Grabau, D. A., Sorensen, F. B., Bak, M., Vach, W., and Rose, C. (2000) Vascular grading of angiogenesis: prognostic significance in breast cancer. *Br. J. Cancer* **82,** 339–347.

148. Burrows, F. J. and Thorpe, P. E. (1994) Vascular targeting—a new approach to the therapy of solid tumors. *Pharmacol. Ther.* **64**, 155–174.

149. Huang, X., Molema, G., King, S., Watkins, L., Edgington, T. S., and Thorpe, P. E. (1997) Tumor infarction in mice by antibody-directed targeting of tissue factor to tumor vasculature. *Science* **275**, 547–550.

150. Smolle, J., Soyer, H. P., Hofmann-Wellenhof, Smolle-Juettner, F. M., and Kerl, H. (1989) Vascular archictecture of melanocytic skin tumors. *Path. Res. Pract.* **185**, 740–745.

151. Cockerell, C. J., Sonnier, G., Kelly, L., and Patel, S. (1994) Comparative analysis of neovascularization in primary cutaneous melanoma and Spitz nevus. *Am. J. Dermatopathol.* **16**, 9–13.

152. Folberg, R., Rummelt, V., Ginderdeuren, R-V., et al. (1993) The prognostic value of tumor blood vessel morphology in primary uveal melanoma. *Ophthalmology* **100**, 1389–1398.

153. Pezzella, F. (2000) Evidence for novel non-angiogenic pathway in breast-cancer metastasis. Breast Cancer Progression Working Party. *Lancet* **355**, 1787–1788.

154. Pezzella, F., Dibacco, A., Andreola, S., Nicholson, A. G., Pastorino, U., and Harris, A. L. (1996) Angiogenesis in primary lung-cancer and lung secondaries. *Eur. J. Cancer* **32**, 2494–2500.

155. Simpson, J., Ahn, C., Battifora, H., and Esteban, J. (1994) Vascular surface area as a prognostic indicator in invasive breast carcinoma. *Lab. Invest.* **70**, 22.

156. Charpin, C., Devictor, B., Bergeret, D., et al. (1995) CD31 quantitative immunocytochemical assays in breast carcinomas. Correlation with current prognostic factors. *Am. J. Clin. Pathol.* **103**, 443–448.

157. Belien, J. A., Somi, S., de Jong, J. S., van Diest, P. J., and Baak, J. P. (1999) Fully automated microvessel counting and hot spot selection by image processing of whole tumor sections in invasive breast cancer. *J. Clin. Pathol.* **52**, 184–192.

158. Arora, R., Joshi, K., Nijhawan, R., Radotra, B. D., and Sharma, S. C. (2002) Angiogenesis as an independent prognostic indicator in node-negative breast cancer. *Anal. Quant. Cytol. Histol.* **24**, 228–233.

III

ANALYSIS OF TUMOR-DERIVED PROTEINS AND ANTIGENS

15

Immunohistochemistry

Cheryl E. Gillett

Summary

Immunohistochemistry allows specific proteins to be visualized while retaining cellular or tissue structure. Sensitivity of the technique has improved over the years from a single layer of labeled antibody to amplified, labeled polymer-based systems, which enable low levels of antigen to be detected in different types of tissue preparation. However, alongside selecting the most appropriate methods of antigen recovery and enhanced signal amplification is the need to show specificity. As described in this chapter, pertinent and reliable control material must be used to both optimize and monitor performance of novel breast-associated antibodies.

Key Words: Immunohistochemistry; antigen; antibody; breast cancer; methodology; cell pellet; evaluation.

1. Introduction

Immunohistochemistry (IHC) has been used as an important diagnostic, predictive, and research tool in breast cancer since the early 1980s. The ability to identify and locate specific proteins within the tissue structure adds a new dimension to the technique compared with immunoassay/enzyme-linked immunosorbent assay, which uses a very similar methodological approach but on tissue homogenates for example, as described in Chapter 19.

IHC can be carried out on different types of cell and tissue preparation including routine formalin-fixed, paraffin wax-embedded material frozen sections and cytological preparations. The advantage of the former being that antigen expression can be seen in archival material, always a useful way of determining site and level of expression in particular types of breast cancers and relating this to clinicopathological data and patient outcome.

Another advantage of IHC is that by using some chromogen/substrates, the results are permanent, so slides can always be reviewed. As with any cytological or tissue section method, it is important that the samples are interpreted by

From: *Methods in Molecular Medicine, Vol. 120: Breast Cancer Research Protocols*
Edited by: S. A. Brooks and A. L. Harris © Humana Press Inc., Totowa, NJ

someone experienced in breast histopathology. Microscopic examination by an experienced person will elicit far more information and negate errors associated with inaccurate morphological observation.

1.1. Principle of Immunohistochemistry

The basic principle of IHC is the binding of a specific antibody to the target immunogen, followed by the amplification and visualization of that antigen–antibody link *(1)*. The target immunogen may be physically "hidden" from the antibody because of protein folding caused during fixation. A pretreatment or antigen-retrieval step, where enzymes or heat are used to remodel the protein structure and make the antigen accessible, may be required to visualize some antigens *(2,3)*. In the method given in this chapter, heat-mediated antigen retrieval using a pressure cooker is described. Other heat-mediated antigen-retrieval methods are popular, including those using a domestic microwave oven, an approach described in the immunohistochemical method for measurement of estrogen receptor given in Chapter 12. Enzymes, including trypsin and proteases, are also often used to reveal antigenic sites. Trypsinization is described in one of the protocols given in Chapter 16.

The method of detecting the antigen–antibody complex has evolved over the years, consistently aiming to increase the sensitivity, so that very low levels of antigen can be visualized without increasing the nonspecific staining. Other features, which need to be considered in this technical evolution, are the speed and ease of method, consistency in reagent quality, and application to automated staining systems.

1.2. Evolution of IHC Method

1.2.1. Direct

It is now rare for an antibody to be directly conjugated to an enzyme for substrate/chromogen visualization. Not only is this expensive, but there is no amplification of the signal, so the antigen–antibody reaction appears very weak.

1.2.2. Indirect (Two Layers)

The successor to this direct method of detection was the indirect technique, when the unlabeled primary antibody was detected by a second antibody against the species in which the primary antibody was raised. This second antibody had an enzyme conjugated to it for visualization. For example, if a mouse monoclonal antibody was used, the second layer could be a rabbit antimouse or goat antimouse polyclonal antibody. As multiple secondary antibodies attach themselves to the primary antibody, the antigen–antibody signal would be amplified. However, the two-step indirect method only allowed limited amplification, so a third, or tertiary layer, was added to increase the sensitivity.

1.2.3. Indirect (Three Layers)

The most commonly used of these early three-step methods was a soluble-enzyme immune complex. The secondary antibody was unlabeled, and to this was added an anti-enzyme antibody to which the enzyme had complexed. The peroxidase–antiperoxidase and the alkaline phosphatase–antialkaline phosphatase are the most commonly used (*4*).

A more complex arrangement of antibodies and molecules is now used to detect antigenicity, which has been designed to give the greatest sensitivity without compromising the specificity of the assay. The use of biotin and (strept)avidin in these amplifying layers has become the mainstay of IHC methodology, with the majority of laboratories using the standard streptavidin–biotin method, either as a conjugate or a complex (*5*). However, more recently, sensitivity has been further improved by the advent of a peroxidase-labeled polymer to detect antibody binding, such as the Envision™ system by DakoCytomation ([Ely, UK] employed in the protocol for assessing metastases in sentinel lymph nodes in Chapter 11) or the Super Sensitive™ system by Biogenex (San Ramon, CA). These systems fulfill many of the requirements of an IHC method for breast research. The increased sensitivity of the method has a number of advantages:

1. Antigens present at low levels can be detected.
2. Antibodies can be used at greater dilution.
3. As a two-step method, it is quick and easy to use.
4. Reagents are received in a standardized kit.
5. Reagents can be used in an automated stainer.
6. Both mouse and rabbit primary antibodies can be detected with the same kit (*see* **Note 1**).

However, all this comes at a price, and this type of detection system is more expensive than a traditional streptavidin biotin method, particularly when optimizing the technique for each individual antigen.

1.3. Enzyme Detection

The most commonly used conjugated enzymes are peroxidase and alkaline phosphatase (*6*). For peroxidase, the chromogen diaminobenzidine (DAB) is most often used, producing a brown end product. This can be dehydrated and mounted in the usual way and does not fade, making it ideal for long-term storage. Improvements in the production of DAB now mean that when combined with hydrogen peroxide, the product is far more stable. Fast Red used to be the chromogen of choice for alkaline phosphatase, but it is soluble in alcohol and could not, therefore, be dehydrated and mounted in the usual way. New Fuchsin also gives a red end product, but it is not soluble in alcohol, making it a better choice of chromogen. Today, many of the companies producing IHC reagents have detection kits for both peroxidase and alkaline phosphatase that are stable, easy to use, and give enhanced performance.

1.4. Controls

It is paramount to use controls as part of the IHC procedure.

1.4.1. Method Control

A known positive control, i.e., cells/tissues that express the antigen of interest, should always be included as part of the IHC run. With novel antigens, it is usually best to use a characterized cell line, which can be used as a cytospin preparation for cytological/frozen tissue test samples, or can be processed into a paraffin wax block.

1.4.2. Tissue Control

An internal control, i.e., when the antigen is known to be expressed in a particular cell type, is always a bonus. The effects of suboptimal tissue preservation or IHC methodology can be seen if these internal controls are weaker than expected. A negative control should also be carried out on a corresponding test section where the primary antibody is replaced by either Tris-buffered saline or a nonimmune serum. This will demonstrate any staining not associated with binding of the antibody.

1.4.3. Batch Control

By using the same control material from one batch to another, the consistency of the technique can be monitored.

1.5. Research Protocol

When using IHC for breast cancer research, one of the first things to consider is what type of tissue preparation needs to be used. Obviously, when testing out a new antibody, it is vital that the material being used is known to express the protein of interest. Whether this is used in a cytological, frozen, or fixed, paraffin wax format is dependant on the type of test material available. For most research, the ability to detect antigens in conventional paraffin-processed material is the ideal—not only does this give far greater scope to relate expression to morphology, but it also allows specific types of lesion to be assessed. If, ultimately, protein expression is to be assessed in aspirates or cell lines, then the antibody should naturally be assessed using cytological material.

The first IHC run using a new antibody should be as simple as possible; it is always easier to add steps that may improve staining rather than trying to investigate several steps if the technique is not working effectively. If the material definitely expresses the antigen, the only variables that need to be taken

Table 1
Plan of Initial Immunohistochemistry Run With a Novel Antibody

Dilution pretreatment	1:25	1:50	1:100	1:200	1:400	Negative
None	1	2	3	4	5	6
Protease/proteinase K	7	8	9	10	11	12
Pressure cooker	13	14	15	16	17	18

into account with the technique are the need for antigen retrieval and the optimal antibody concentration (*see* **Note 2**). A general starting point is shown in **Table 1**.

Once "staining" is detected in one or more of the 15 test slides, a second run can be done that refines the optimal conditions. However, to maintain consistency of staining, always repeat one of the conditions from the previous batch.

Once an antibody is working on the control material, then the method needs to be transferred to the test material. Do not immediately stain all the cases of interest, particularly if these are diagnostic cases that have been fixed and paraffin wax-processed in slightly different ways (something that occurs with all diagnostic material). Test the antibody again on two to three test cases that either have an internal control or are likely to express the protein of interest (*see* **Note 3**).

1.6. The Scope of This Chapter

This chapter gives a basic protocol for IHC using an autostainer. It can be readily adapted for use in laboratories that do not have this piece of equipment—sections should simply be incubated with the various reagents in a suitable humid, lidded chamber (most simply, a plastic sandwich box lined with damp tissue paper, or commercially available IHC incubation chambers) and washed thoroughly in several changes of buffer between steps. There are many variations on this basic protocol, and the reader is encouraged to experiment. Other approaches may be found in Chapter 16, which gives a range of similar protocols used specifically for detecting altered glycosylation by IHC and an adaptation of the technique lectin histochemistry. Chapters 11 and 12 illustrate the utility of IHC in assessment of metastatic involvement of axillary sentinel lymph node and for measuring estrogen receptor status, respectively.

2. Materials
2.1. Vectabond™ Treatment of Slides

1. Acetone.
2. Vectabond (Vector Laboratories, Peterborough, UK)/acetone solution: 350 mL acetone to one bottle of Vectabond.
3. Distilled water.

2.2. Production of a Cell Pellet

1. Cells suspended in tissue culture medium or formol saline.
2. Formol saline or preferred fixative.
3. 4% electrophoresis grade agarose (Gibco, UK) in distilled water.

2.3. Antigen Retrieval

1. Biogenex protease type XXIV (follow manufacturer's instructions).
2. DakoCytomation proteinase K with diluent (follow manufacturer's instructions).
3. Citrate buffer: 0.01 *M* citric acid, pH 6.0 (6.3 g sodium citrate in 3 L distilled water). Use *N* NaOH to adjust the pH.

2.4. IHC

1. PAP pen (DakoCytomation).
2. Buffer, such as phosphate buffered saline, pH 7.6.

Below is a list of reagents supplied by DakoCytomation for the detection of bound antibody. However, other manufacturers (including Biogenex) also produce sensitive detection methods.

3. Antibody diluent.
4. Peroxidase blocking solution.
5. Envision/horseradish peroxidase.
6. DAB plus chromogen.
7. Substrate buffer.

2.5. Counterstain/Cover Slip

1. Hematoxylin solution.
2. 1% Acid alcohol.
3. 70% Ethanol.
4. Absolute ethanol.
5. Xylene or equivalent clearing agent.
6. Resinous mounting medium, e.g., Depex or Pertex.

3. Methods

3.1. Vectabond Treatment of Slides (Following the Manufacturer's Guidelines)

An alternative protocol using 3-(triethoxysilyl)propylamine (silane) instead of the proprietary brand Vectabond is given in Chapter 16.

1. Place racked slides in acetone to clean them (5 min).
2. Place in Vectabond/acetone solution (350 mL acetone to one bottle of Vectabond, 5 min; this is sufficient for 500 slides).
3. Wash in distilled water for 3 min; change water every 100 slides.
4. Air-dry and store in a clean, dust-free box.

3.2. Production of Cell Pellet

For cells received in media, start at **step 1**; for those received in formalin, go to **step 4**. An alternative protocol is given in Chapter 16.

1. Place cells and solution into a 15- or 50-mL centrifuge tube (depending on the volume of media) and spin at low speed for 2 min at room temperature (RT).
2. Discard the supernatant, leaving the cell pellet.
3. Add 5–10 mL of formol saline (or preferred fixative). Agitate the tube to ensure the cell pellet is disaggregated and fix for 1 h at RT.
4. For cells received in formol saline, proceed from here. Heat 4% agarose in distilled water to 90°C while stirring.
5. When agarose has melted, transfer to a 65°C water bath.
6. Centrifuge cells in formol saline for 2 min (low speed, RT). Remove supernatant, leaving approx 500 µL of formol saline in tube.
7. Disaggregate the pellet and transfer to a 1.5-mL Eppendorf tube. Rinse the old tube with a further 500 µL formol saline to ensure all cells are transferred.
8. Allow cells to settle in Eppendorf tube for 10 min.
9. Centrifuge at low speed for 1 min and remove supernatant, leaving a small amount (approx 200–400 µL) of formol saline in the tube.
10. Warm tube in 65°C water bath for 2 min, making sure pellet does not become dry. Agitate to release cells stuck to side of tube.
11. Add 200–400 µL of agarose solution to the tube (obtaining a final agarose solution of 2%).
12. Cool agarose and pellet for 30 min at RT.
13. Carefully cut down tube to free gel pellet.
14. If required, slice gel into 5-mm slices and wrap in lens tissue paper.
15. Place in processing cassette and process to paraffin wax as normal.

3.3. Tissue Preparation

An alternative protocol is given in Chapter 16.

1. Cut 3-µm sections from the paraffin blocks, float out on warm water, and pick up on Vectabond-treated, clean glass slides.
2. Allow the water to drain from the section and place the slide into a rack and then in a 37°C oven at least overnight. On the day before staining, sections should be baked onto the slide by placing them in a 58°C oven overnight (*see* **Note 4**).

With each batch of test sections, *always* include a positive control section known to contain the antigen of interest. A "negative" control section should also be included for each test case, where the primary antibody is replaced by antibody diluent alone.

3. Dewax the sections by placing the rack of slides in xylene (twice, for 2 min each time).

4. Remove the xylene by placing the rack in absolute alcohol (twice, for 2 min each time), followed by 70% alcohol (once, for 1 min).
5. Place slides into running tap water (at least 5 min).

3.4. Antigen-Recovery Step

Heat-mediated retrieval using a pressure cooker:

1. Fill a 5-L pressure cooker (stainless steel) with 3 L of citrate buffer, place the lid loosely on top, and heat on an electric boiling ring. When the buffer is boiling, place the racks carefully into the pressure cooker.
2. Put the lid on and lock it.
3. Follow the manufacturer's guidelines to set the cooker to increase pressure.
4. Once the cooker has reached sufficient pressure to seal the valves (103 kPa/ 15 psi), "boil" the sections for 2 min. Timing should start immediately once full pressure is reached.
5. After 2 min, release the pressure and remove the pressure cooker from the heat source.
6. Once the pressure has dropped, slide the top and bottom handles apart. Place the cooker in a sink and flush out the buffer with running tap water for at least 5 min (*see* **Note 5**).

3.5. Immunohistochemistry

1. Using a PAP pen, draw a line on the glass slide on either side of the section. Transfer the slides to the autostainer (or a humidity chamber if doing a manual procedure) and cover with buffer (twice, for 3 min each time). A squeezy bottle is ideal for this.
2. Program and run the autostainer in the following sequence, with wash steps between each stage (*see* **Note 6**):
   a. Primary antibody/antibody diluent (negative control), 30 min.
   b. Peroxidase blocking solution, 10 min.
   c. Envision/horseradish peroxidase, 25 min.
   d. DAB plus chromogen, 5 min.
3. If a manual staining procedure is being used, then follow **steps 1** and **2**, with a buffer rinse (twice, for 3 min each time) between each step. Allow approx 100–150 µL per slide (*see* **Note 7**).
4. Wash with buffer, then put slides into a rack and place in running tap water (5 min).

3.6. Counterstain/Cover Slip

1. Lightly stain the nuclei with hematoxylin (1 min).
2. Rinse in tap water to remove excess hematoxylin. Place rack of sections in 1% acid alcohol (5 s) to differentiate, then return immediately to tap water. Leave sections in warm tap water (at least 2 min) so that the nuclei turn blue.
3. Dehydrate through 70% (1 min) then 2X absolute alcohol (1 min each), clear in xylene, and place a cover slip on the section using a resinous mountant.

Sites of antigenicity stain brown, with the nuclei staining blue.

3.7. Evaluation/Assessment

1. Always scan the whole section before higher-power examination, so that any areas of heterogeneic staining are seen.
2. Make a note of the site of antigen localization, including the type of cell, whether it is nuclear, cytoplasmic, or membranous. Always compare localization in normal tissue with that in benign, *in situ*, and invasive lesions.
3. Scoring the level of staining can be difficult. Use a simple method of scoring initially, such as estimating the proportion or intensity of cells labeling for the antigen. A complex scoring regime is not reproducible and can easily be affected by suboptimal fixation and the small variations that occur during the IHC procedure. Automated methods of assessment may well provide a more objective assessment.
4. Make certain to check the negative control as it has been carried out.

4. Notes

1. Remember to check that the detection system will detect the animal in which the primary antibody was raised. The ChemMate™ Envision (DakoCytomation) system detects both mouse and rabbit but is unsuitable for other species. On these occasions, choose either a different pan secondary layer or a specific one.
2. If inexperienced, always run a well-established antibody with the test antibody. These should have exactly the same pretreatment and detection procedures and will highlight any errors with the basic method.
3. Control material, particularly from cell lines, is well and uniformly fixed. Test sections of breast cancer are more variable, with central areas being less well fixed than the edge.
4. To increase the likelihood of the section adhering to the slide, dry the section at 37°C overnight before placing it in a 58°C oven overnight.
5. A reduction in antigen–antibody binding occurs if sections are left in water following the pressure cooker step. To avoid this, continue with the IHC within 30 min.
6. The technique is temperature-sensitive, and a reduction in staining occurs if the lab is too hot or too cold. Ideally, the IHC should be carried out at normal RT (22–25°C). Care should be taken not to place an autostainer or manually carry out the technique under an air conditioning unit or in direct sunlight.
7. Allow sufficient reagent to cover the entire section, ensuring that the edges are covered and that the surface tension does not draw back the solution from the edge. This problem is alleviated by using detergent in the buffer.

References

1. Coons, A. H. and Kaplan M. H. (1950) Localisation of antigen in tissue cells. *J. Exp. Med.* **91**, 1–13.
2. Cattoretti, G., Pileri, S., Parravicini, C., et al. (1993) Antigen unmasking on formalin fixed, paraffin-embedded tissue sections. *J. Pathol.* **171**, 83–98.

3. Norton, A. J., Jordan, S., and Yeomans, P. (1994) Brief, high temperature heat denaturation (pressure cooking): a simple and effective method of antigen retrieval for routinely processed tissue. *J. Pathol.* **173,** 371–379.

4. Sternberger, L. A. (1979) The unlabeled (PAP) method, introduction. *J. Histochem. Cytochem.* **27,** 1657.

5. Hsu, S. M., Raine, L., and Fanger, H. (1981) Use of avidin-biotin-peroxidase complex (ABC) in immunoperoxidase techniques: a comparison between ABC and unlabeled antibody (PAP) procedures. *J. Histochem. Cytochem.* **29,** 577–580.

6. Mason, D. Y. and Sammons, R. E. (1978) Alkaline phosphatase and peroxidase for double immunoenzymic labeling of cellular constituents. *J. Clin. Pathol.* **33,** 454–462.

16

Detection of Aberrant Glycosylation in Breast Cancer Using Lectin Histochemistry

Tracey M. Carter and Susan A. Brooks

Summary

Lectins are naturally occurring, carbohydrate-binding molecules that can be isolated from diverse biological sources and used in the laboratory to investigate the presence of carbohydrate structures in or on cells, in much the same way as antibodies can be used to probe cells and tissues for the presence of specific antigens. As it is becoming increasingly apparent that subtle alterations in the glycosylation of cancer cells can profoundly influence their biological behavior (with consequent implications for patient outcome and prognosis), lectin histochemistry is a potentially useful modification of the more widely used technique of immunohistochemistry. This chapter provides an introductory background to lectins and their use in breast cancer research, and provides basic protocols for lectin histochemistry that highlight the important technical differences between this approach and immunohistochemistry. The methods given here are broadly applicable and can be modified to investigate virtually any glycosylation change of potential interest in breast cancer research.

Key Words: Glycosylation; oligosaccharides; prognostic markers; histochemistry; immunohistochemistry.

1. Introduction

Lectins are a heterogeneous group of naturally occurring proteins and glycoproteins that are able to bind selectively to carbohydrates, rather analogous to monoclonal antibodies binding selectively to their antigens. However, lectins are *not* derived from the immune system and are present in organisms ranging from bacteria and plants to invertebrates as well as mammals. Owing to their ability to precipitate polysaccharides, glycolipids and glycoproteins, and agglutinate cells, lectins were originally known as "agglutinins" before the introduction of the term "lectin" by Boyd and Shapleigh in 1954. The agglutinating property of lectins indicates that they are multivalent and therefore contain two or more carbohydrate-binding sites *(1,2)*.

From: *Methods in Molecular Medicine, Vol. 120: Breast Cancer Research Protocols*
Edited by: S. A. Brooks and A. L. Harris © Humana Press Inc., Totowa, NJ

Lectins are commonly classified according to the monosaccharide that best inhibits their binding—for example, a lectin may be described as being mannose-specific or galactose-specific. However, the actual carbohydrate-combining site of a lectin is believed usually to recognize complex structures composed of between two and six monosaccharide residues, often distinguishing among different anomers, conformations, and linkages. The natural binding partners of most lectins are incompletely defined. The practical consequence of this is that two lectins (e.g., *Helix pomatia* agglutinin [HPA] and *Dolichos biflorus* agglutinin [DBA]) with apparently identical binding preferences (e.g., *N*-acetylgalactosamine [GalNAc]) may actually recognize very different complex carbohydrate structures *(1,2)*. This is an important consideration in lectin histochemistry, because the different lectins may exhibit very different labeling patterns and give different results in clinical samples *(3)*.

Numerous lectins have been isolated and purified from plant and invertebrate sources and are often named according to their source. This is most often the species' Latin binomial, although some lectins are referred to in the literature by their common names *(1,2)*. For example, the lectin derived from *Glycine max* is more usually referred to as "soybean agglutinin," abbreviated to SBA. The lectin from elderberry, conversely, is known as "*Sambucus nigra* agglutinin," abbreviated to SNA. Sometimes more than one lectin has been isolated from the same species and is therefore given a numerical suffix; for example, several lectins have been isolated from *Griffonia (Bandeiraea) simplicifolia* including isolectins-I and -II, abbreviated to GSA-I and GSA-II, respectively, and isolectins from the same source often have differing carbohydrate-binding specificities. In this example, GSA-I has a nominal binding specificity for α-D-galactose, whereas GSA-II recognizes α- and β-D-GlcNAc.

Lectins are useful tools in cancer research because of their property of binding specifically to carbohydrate structures on glycoconjugates of cells and tissues. This allows investigators to identify cellular glycosylation patterns and changes in glycosylation that occur during growth, development, differentiation, and changes that occur during disease states, such as in breast cancer *(1,3)*.

In malignancy, cancer cells synthesize aberrant carbohydrate structures on cell surface glycoconjugates that may be associated with tumor progression or metastatic competence. The most commonly documented glycosylation changes in cancer are as follows:

1. Increased branching of *N*-glycans.
2. Alterations in sialylation.
3. Incomplete biosynthesis resulting in truncated glycans.
4. Increased Lewis antigen synthesis.
5. The re-emergence of fetal antigens (oncofetal antigens).

6. Changes in ABH blood group antigen synthesis.
7. "Neosynthesis" of cancer associated antigens.

A glycosylation change that has been documented in breast and other (*see* **ref. 4** for review) cancers is an increase in oligosaccharide structures recognized by the lectin derived from the Roman snail *H. pomatia* and this may be detected by lectin histochemistry. HPA has a nominal binding specificity for terminal GalNAc, a monosaccharide most commonly located at subterminal positions in oligosaccharide structures of glycoproteins in normal cells. In cancer, owing to failure in the mechanism of normal glycan synthesis, this residue is often exposed. Increased labeling with HPA has been repeatedly described as being associated with metastases in local lymph nodes and distant sites, and hence, poor patient survival. It has also been reported to be a prognostic marker in other tumors including thyroid, gastric, and colorectal carcinomas.

Changes in sialylation in breast cancers have also been documented in the literature (*5,6*). Sialic acid is commonly located at the terminal position of oligosaccharides at the cell surface. They are located at prime positions to mediate essential biological functions involved in cell adhesion, cell motility, and immunogenicity. The lectin derived from the cellar slug *Limax flavus* (*L. flavus* agglutinin) recognizes terminal sialic acid regardless of linkage to underlying subterminal monosaccharides. Linkage-specific sialic acid-binding lectins are also available. For example, the lectin *S. nigra* agglutinin, from elderberry, recognizes terminal sialic acid in α2-6 linkage, and the lectin from *Maackia amurensis* recognizes terminal sialic acid in α2-3 linkage. These lectins may be useful tools for investigating sialylation changes in cellular glycosylation in cancer.

Numerous lectins have been isolated, with wide-ranging carbohydrate-binding specificities, and can be purchased from various companies including Sigma, DakoCytomation, and EY Laboratories, with nominal binding specificities documented in the manufacturers' catalogs. **Table 1** lists some commonly used lectins and their reported nominal binding specificities, but a very wide range of other lectins is readily available. Purified lectins are generally purchased in lyophilized form and are available as the native lectin or, commonly, labeled with biotin, or an enzyme (for example, horseradish peroxidase) or fluorescent (for example, fluorescein isothiocyanate [FITC]) reporter molecule. The type of lectin preparation required (i.e., native or labeled) will depend on the lectin histochemical approach employed. There are many techniques used to visualize lectin binding in cells and tissues and these are largely analogous—with minor technical modifications—to the techniques employed in immunocytochemistry/histochemistry (*see* Chapter 15), but here, lectin takes the place of the primary antisera. In this chapter, two methods are described, a

Table 1
Summary of Carbohydrate-Binding
Characteristics of Some Commonly Used Lectins

Latin binomial name	Common name	Abbreviation	Inhibitory carbohydrate
Arachis hypogae	Peanut	PNA	β-D-Gal(1→3)-D-GalNAc
Canavalia ensiformis	Jack bean	Con A	α-Man
Dolichos biflorus	Horse gram	DBA	α-D-GalNAc
Glycine max	Soybean	SBA	α-D-GalNAc, Gal
Helix pomati	Roman snail	HPA	α-D-GalNAc > α-D-GlcNAc
Limax flavus	Cellar slug	LFA	SA
Phytolacca american	Pokeweed	PWM	α-GlcNAc oligomers
Pisum sativum	Pea	PSA	α-D-Man, α-D-Glc
Triticum vulgaris	Wheat	WGA	β-D-GlcNAc, SA
Ulex europeaeus	Gorse	UEA-I	α-L-Fuc
Wisteria floribund	Wisteria	WFA	D-GalNAc

direct fluorescent and simple, avidin–biotin lectin histochemical method. For an outline of the other main techniques for visualization of lectin binding in cells and tissues, the reader is referred to **ref. 2**.

Direct lectin histochemistry employs a lectin conjugated directly to a fluorescent or enzyme reporter molecule. This method is illustrated in **Fig. 1**. This has the advantage of being simple and quick to perform and is especially appropriate for visualization of lectin binding to cultured cells either in suspension, e.g., for flow cytometry or cultured on cover slips as described in this chapter. The lectin binds to specific cell-bound carbohydrates, and binding is visualized by either fluorescence microscopy in the case of fluorescent labels or light microscopy for the enzyme label. A protocol is given here for visualization of lectin binding in cultured breast cells utilizing FITC-conjugated lectins, but can be readily adapted for use with lectins conjugated to other reporter molecules.

The simple avidin–biotin method, which is illustrated in **Fig. 2**, employs the use of biotinylated lectin. The high affinity between avidin and biotin is exploited in this method whereby lectin binding is detected using an avidin–enzyme conjugate, such as (strept)avidin-horseradish peroxidase. The inclusion of diaminobenzidine as a chromogen with the substrate hydrogen peroxide results in the formation of a brown, insoluble precipitate, readily visible by light microscopy. A protocol is given here for visualization of lectin binding to paraffin wax-embedded breast cancer specimens and cultured breast cell lines. Many other variations on these basic techniques are possible (*see* **ref. 2**).

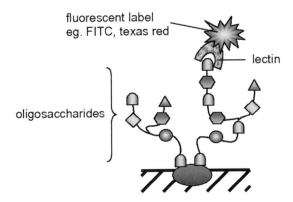

Fig. 1. The direct method. Lectin directly conjugated to a reporter molecule—in this example, a fluorescent label—binds to and labels cell- or tissue-bound oligosaccharides.

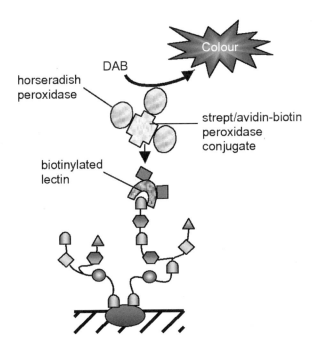

Fig. 2. A simple avidin–biotin indirect method. Biotinylated lectin binds to cell- or tissue-bound oligosaccharides. Labeling is achieved by subsequent layering with avidin or streptavidin, conjugated to a reporter molecule—in this example, the enzyme horseradish peroxidase, which reacts with diaminobenzidine (DAB) to give a brown-colored product visible by light microscopy.

2. Materials

2.1. 3-(Triethoxysilyl)propylamine Treatment of Microscope Slides (see *Notes 1 and 2*)

1. Acetone.
2. Acetone/silane solution: mix 7 mL of 3-(triethoxysilyl)propylamine (silane) with 400 mL of acetone.
3. Distilled water.
4. Microscope slide-carrying racks.
5. 400-mL Glass dishes.

2.2. Preparation of Cultured Breast Cancer Cells for Processing to Paraffin Wax

1. Cells should be cultured under standard culture conditions to 60–70% confluence. Cells should also be grown for 48 h in normal growth media without fetal calf serum (FCS) to 65–70% confluence in T25 flasks (*see* **Note 3**).
2. Phosphate buffered saline (PBS): dissolve 8 g of NaCl, 0.2 g of KCl, 1.44 g of Na_2HPO_4, and 0.24 g of KH_2PO_4 in 800 mL of distilled water. Adjust pH to 7.2, and then make up to 1000 mL with distilled water or commercially available Hank's balanced salts solution (HBSS) without phenol red (*see* **Note 4**).
3. Cell scraper or rubber policeman.
4. 4% (v/v) formol saline, pH 7.2–7.6: dissolve 0.9 g of NaCl in 80 mL of distilled water. Add 10 mL of formaldehyde solution and stir. Adjust pH to 7.2–7.6 using concentrated NaOH solution. Top off with distilled water to bring to a total volume of 100 mL. Filter. This solution can be kept at room temperature and can be stored for up to 2 wk.
5. Lectin buffer, pH 7.6 (*see* **Note 5**): 60.57 g of Tris-HCl, 87 g of NaCl, 2.03 g of $MgCl_2$, and 1.11 g of $CaCl_2$ (*see* **Note 8**). Dissolve in 900 mL of distilled water. Adjust the pH to 7.6 using concentrated hydrochloric acid. Top up with distilled water to 1 L. Check pH again. Then bring volume to a total of 10 L with distilled water.
6. 4% (w/v) low-gelling-temperature agarose: suspend 0.4 g of agarose in 10 mL of lectin buffer. Warm gradually in a water bath or microwave oven with regular stirring. The agarose will dissolve at a temperature of 60°C. Cool to 37–40°C before use.

2.3. Preparation of Formalin-Fixed, Paraffin Wax-Embedded Tissue Sections

1. Formalin-fixed, paraffin wax-embedded clinical breast cancer samples or breast cancer cell lines (prepared according to **Subheading 3.2.**; *see* **Note 6**).
2. Microtome.
3. 20% (v/v) ethanol or industrial methylated spirits (IMS) in distilled water.
4. Crushed ice.
5. Glass tile.

6. Small soft paintbrush.
7. Forceps.
8. Silane-treated microscope slides (*see* **Subheading 2.1.**).
9. Water bath heated to 40°C (*see* **Note 7**).
10. Hot plate heated to 45°C (*see* **Note 7**).

2.4. Direct Lectin Cytochemistry of Cultured Breast Cancer Cell Lines, Using FITC-Labeled Lectins

1. Cells should be cultured under standard culture conditions.
2. Normal growth media, with and without FCS (*see* **Note 3**).
3. Alcohol-sterilized glass cover slips (13-mm diameter, thickness 0 or 1; *see* **Note 8**).
4. 24-well culture plates.
5. PBS or HBSS (*see* **Subheading 2.2.** and **Note 4**).
6. 4% (v/v) formol saline (*see* **Subheading 2.2.**).
7. 50 mM of ammonium chloride in PBS or HBSS. Dissolve 1.337 g of ammonium chloride in PBS or HBSS. Store at 4°C (make fresh weekly). Allow to warm to room temperature before use.
8. Lectin buffer (*see* **Subheading 2.2.**).
9. 0.1% (v/v) Triton X-100 or saponin in lectin buffer (*see* **Note 9**).
10. Humid chamber. A Petri dish or sandwich box lined with Parafilm may be used, with damp blotting paper lining the edges of the dish. The Parafilm provides a nonslip surface for glass cover slips, and the damp blotting paper provides the humid conditions (*see* **Note 10**).
11. Blocking buffer: 3–5% (w/v) bovine serum albumin (Sigma, Dorset, UK) in lectin buffer (*see* **Note 11**).
12. Optimal concentration of FITC-conjugated lectin in blocking buffer (*see* **Note 12**).
13. Ribonuclease A solution (*see* **Notes 13** and **14**): 100 µg/mL ribonuclease type I-A from bovine pancreas (RNAse A, Sigma) in autoclave-sterilized lectin buffer (*see* **Subheading 2.2.**). Make freshly on day needed and store in small (e.g., 5-mL) aliquots at –20°C. Defrost and warm to 37°C immediately before use.
14. 500 nM of propidium iodide (PI) in lectin buffer (*see* **Subheading 2.2.** and **Note 15**).
15. Clean silane-coated glass microscope slides (*see* **Subheading 2.1.**).
16. Citifluor antifade mountant (*see* **Note 16**).
17. Aluminum foil.
18. Clear nail polish.

2.5. Simple Avidin–Biotin Lectin Histochemistry of Paraffin Wax-Embedded Clinical Breast Cancer Samples or Paraffin Wax-Embedded Cultured Breast Cancer Cells

1. Xylene.
2. Absolute ethanol or IMS.
3. 70% (v/v) ethanol or IMS in distilled water.
4. Distilled water.
5. 3% (v/v) hydrogen peroxide in methanol. Make fresh and use within 2 d.

6. Trypsin solution (*see* **Note 17**): dissolve 1 mg/mL of $CaCl_2$ and 1 mg/mL of trypsin (crude, type II from porcine pancreas; Sigma) in lectin buffer (*see* **Subheading 2.2.**). Make solution freshly before use and use immediately. All solutions and glassware should be prewarmed to 37°C.
7. Set incubator to 37°C.
8. Humid chamber. This can simply be a plastic tray or sandwich box lined with damp blotting paper with either plastic wrap or aluminum foil as a lid, or custom-made (usually Perspex) incubation trays are available commercially.
9. Lectin buffer (*see* **Subheading 2.2.**).
10. Blocking buffer (*see* **Subheading 2.4.**).
11. Optimal concentration of biotinylated lectin in blocking buffer (*see* **Note 12**).
12. (Strept)avidin-peroxidase solution. Optimal concentration of (strept)avidin peroxidase in blocking buffer (*see* **Notes 17** and **18**).
13. Diaminobenzidine tetrahydrochloride (DAB) solution: 0.5 mg/mL of DAB and 0.03% (v/v) hydrogen peroxide in lectin buffer (*see* **Subheading 2.2.** and **Notes 19** and **20**).
14. Mayer's hematoxylin solution.
15. Xylene-based mounting medium, e.g., Depex.
16. Glass cover slips.

3. Methods

3.1. Silane Treatment of Microscope Slides

1. Insert glass microscope slides in slide-carrying racks. Lower the racks gently into a glass dish containing acetone and leave submerged for 5 min, with no agitation (to prevent bubbles shielding the solution from evenly bathing the glass surface).
2. Gently transfer the racks to the acetone/silane solution for 5 min, with no agitation, and then transfer through two changes of distilled water for 5 min each. The distilled water must be replaced after every four racks of slides have passed through.
3. Drain racks on paper tissues, then leave the slides to completely dry in dust-free conditions at room temperature or in an incubator or oven overnight.
4. Return the microscope slides to labeled microscope boxes and store at room temperature until required.

3.2. Preparation of Cultured Breast Cancer Cells for Processing to Paraffin Wax

1. Aspirate and discard normal growth media from cells grown in T25 flasks to 65–70% confluence in the presence or absence of FCS (*see* **Note 3**).
2. Wash cells three to fives times, for 4 min each wash, with PBS or HBSS.
3. Add 4 mL of PBS or HBSS and use a rubber policeman to scrape the cells from the culture flasks. Pipet cells up and down gently a few times to disaggregate clumps of cells. The cells should then be transferred to a 15-mL centrifuge tube and pelleted by centrifugation ($1100g$, 4 min).

4. To fix the cells, resuspend them in 4 mL of 4% (v/v) formol saline and pellet by centrifugation (1100*g*, 4 min). Resuspend cells once more in 4 mL of fresh 4% (v/v) formol saline and incubate at room temperature for 30 min. Occasionally invert the tube during the 30-min incubation to mix cells.

5. Pellet the cells by centrifugation (1100*g*, 4 min) and resuspend in 4 mL of PBS or HBSS to wash (*see* **Note 20**). Centrifuge cells and repeat the washes twice. Then, resuspend in 2 mL of lectin buffer. Transfer resuspended cells into two 1.5-mL Eppendorf tubes. Pellet by gentle centrifugation (1100*g*, 4 min) in an Eppendorf centrifuge and aspirate and discard lectin buffer.

6. Resuspend pelleted cells in a few drops of heated (37–40°C) 4% (w/v) low-temperature-gelling agarose and leave to set at room temperature for 30 min (*see* **Note 21**).

7. Process agarose-embedded cell pellets to paraffin wax, using standard protocols.

3.3. Preparation of Formalin-Fixed, Paraffin Wax-Embedded Tissue Sections

1. Place the wax blocks on ice for 15 min before sectioning (*see* **Note 22**).

2. Cut 4–7-μm-thick sections by microtome (*see* **Note 23**).

3. Remove carefully the tissue sections from the microtome knife, using the paintbrush and forceps, taking care not to tear or damage the tissue. Float sections on a few drops of 20% (v/v) ethanol or IMS on a glass tile.

4. Remove carefully creases and folds by manipulating with a soft paintbrush and separate individual sections, using forceps, taking care not to damage the tissue itself. Gently float the sections out into the preheated water bath. Separate the sections further, using the forceps, and collect individual tissue sections onto clean, silane-treated, labeled microscope slides.

5. Drain slides upended on absorbent paper for 5 min to blot excess water.

6. Dry sections on a hotplate for 20 min (*see* **Note 7**) or in a 37°C incubator overnight. Cool to room temperature.

7. Store cut sections at room temperature in labeled boxes or stacked in dust-free conditions until required.

3.4. Direct Lectin Cytochemistry of Cultured Breast Cancer Cell Lines, Using FITC-Labeled Lectins

1. Place dry, sterile glass cover slips into the wells of a 24-well culture plate (*see* **Note 8**).

2. Seed cells at an appropriate density in each well so that they reach 65–70% confluence after 48 h culture (with or without FCS in the normal growth media; *see* **Note 3**).

3. Aspirate and discard the growth media.

4. Wash cells with PBS or HBSS three to five times, for 4 min each wash.

5. Fix cells by incubating with 4% (v/v) formol saline for 30 min at room temperature. Complete all subsequent washes and incubations at room temperature.

6. Wash cells with PBS or HBSS three to five times, for 4 min each wash.

7. Quench free-aldehyde groups by incubating the cells with 50 m*M* ammonium chloride in PBS or HBSS for 10 min.

8. Wash cells with lectin buffer three to five times, for 4 min each wash. All subsequent washes throughout the procedure should be completed in this way unless stated otherwise.

9. Remove carefully the cover slips from each well, using a fine needle slightly bent at the tip and fine forceps (*see* **Note 26**), and transfer to the labeled Parafilm support within the humid chamber.

10. Permeabilize cells with 0.1% (v/v) Triton X-100 in lectin buffer for 10 min (*see* **Note 9**).

11. Wash cells as instructed in **step 8**.

12. Incubate cells with the blocking buffer for 30 min.

13. Drain cells of excess blocking buffer (no need to wash at this stage) and incubate with the FITC-lectin solution for 1 h in the dark (*see* **Note 27**). The remaining incubations and washes should be completed in the dark.

14. Wash cells as instructed in **step 8**.

15. Incubate cells with ribonuclease-A solution for 20 min at 37°C (*see* **Notes 13** and **14**).

16. Wash cells as instructed in **step 8**.

17. To counterstain nuclei, incubate with PI for 30 s to 1 min (*see* **Note 15**).

18. Wash cells as instructed in **step 8**.

19. Mount cover slips, cells face down, onto labeled microscope slides with an antifade aqueous mountant (*see* **Note 28**).

20. Seal the edges of the cover slip with clear nail polish and assess by fluorescent microscopy (*see* **Note 29**).

3.5. Simple Avidin–Biotin Lectin Histochemistry of Paraffin Wax-Embedded Clinical Breast Cancer Samples or Paraffin Wax-Embedded Cultured Breast Cancer Cells

1. Place cut paraffin wax-embedded sections in a metal slide-carrying rack and immerse in xylene for 15–20 min to dissolve wax.

2. To rehydrate tissue sections, transfer the slides through two changes of absolute ethanol or IMS for 1 to 2 min, with agitation at each stage. The slides should then be transferred to 70% (v/v) ethanol or IMS in distilled water for 1–2 min, with agitation. Finally, transfer the sections to distilled water for 1–2 min, with agitation.

3. To quench endogenous peroxidases (*see* **Note 30**), the tissue sections should be transferred to 3% (v/v) hydrogen peroxide in methanol for 20 min. The sections should then be washed in running tap water for 5 min.

4. For carbohydrate retrieval, trypsinization can be carried out (*see* **Note 14**). The sections should be incubated with the prewarmed trypsin solution (37°C) for 20 min in an incubator set to 37°C. The sections should then be washed in running tap water for 5 min.

5. Blot around each of the sections with a soft tissue (*see* **Note 31**) to remove excess buffer and place face up in a humid chamber. Incubate with lectin solution at optimal concentration for 1 h at room temperature (*see* **Note 12**).

6. Remove slides from the humid chamber and wash in several changes of lectin buffer for 1 to 2 min each wash, with agitation. Repeat twice.
7. Drain off excess buffer, blot around each of the sections with a soft tissue (*see* **Note 31**) to remove excess buffer and place face up in a humid chamber.
8. Incubate sections with (strept)avidin peroxidase solution at room temperature for 30 min.
9. Wash sections in lectin buffer as instructed in **steps 6** and **7**.
10. Incubate sections with the DAB solution for 10 min (see **Notes 19** and **32**).
11. Wash sections under running tap water for 5 min.
12. Lightly counterstain nuclei by incubating sections in Mayer's hematoxylin solution for 2 min.
13. "Blue" in running tap water for 5 min (*see* **Note 33**).
14. Dehydrate the tissue sections by transferring to 70% (v/v) ethanol or IMS for 2 min, with slight agitation. Then, transfer through two changes of absolute ethanol or IMS, with agitation (*see* **Note 34**).
15. Clear in xylene and mount with a xylene-based mountant and cover slips. Leave to dry and view by light microscopy.

3.6. Controls for Lectin Histochemistry/Cytochemistry

1. Positive controls. A suitable positive control is a section of a tissue or cell type that has been determined by previous experiments to be positive for particular lectin labeling. Kidney (animal or human) is a good general positive control, as this tissue type has a complex glycosylation profile, and most lectins will give positive labeling of at least some structures. A positive control is essential so that experimental weak or negative labeling for a particular lectin is confirmed to result from absence of the lectin-binding carbohydrates rather than from technical error.
2. Negative controls. These can simply be cells or tissues taken through the lectin-labeling procedures minus the lectin-incubation step. Replace the cells or tissues with blocking buffer for the incubation time. These controls are essential to determine that labeling observed is lectin labeling and not from another part of the protocol.
3. Specificity of binding. The specificity of lectin labeling can be determined by including inhibitory monosaccharides within the lectin solution at a concentration of 0.1–0.2 *M*. It is also advisable to include an additional incubation step with the inhibitory monosaccharide within blocking buffer for 30 min before lectin labeling. When assessing results, total, or at least significant depletion of, lectin labeling should be observed.

4. Notes

1. The acetone–silane solution must be made freshly before use and will be adequate for the treatment of up to 1000 slides. It is convenient to treat large batches of slides and then store them until they are needed.
2. Silane is used to alter the charge on the surface of the microscope slides, so that the tissue sections adhere much more firmly. This is essential, as the washes

throughout the lectin histochemistry procedure are often aggressive and may dislodge the section from the slide.

3. Formalin-fixed, wax-embedded breast cancer samples provide the researcher with an archival source of material for study. These blocks are stored at room temperature and may be kept indefinitely.

4. Phenol red is often added to tissue culture media and buffers such as HBSS in order to detect pH changes. This constituent may contribute to background fluorescence if fluorescent markers are used in lectin histochemistry.

5. Lectin buffer is Tris-HCl buffer with the additional ingredients of $CaCl_2$ and $MgCl_2$. Lectins often require metal ions, such as magnesium and calcium, to bind to carbohydrates effectively. Do not use the buffer PBS as the phosphate ions bind and sequester the metal ions.

6. Ensure that both the hotplate and water bath are at the correct temperature. Too high a temperature may affect lectin binding by damaging the carbohydrate structures. Moreover, if the water bath temperature is too hot, the wax may begin to melt and dissipate. If the water is too cold, the creases and folds may remain in the section.

7. Cells are grown in the presence or absence of FCS. FCS contains a heterogeneous mix of proteins and glycoproteins that may be incorporated in the cells or fixed during fixation, thus causing false-positive results. Therefore, cells are grown without FCS for 48 h. However, this may stress the cells and cause changes in glycosylation profiles. When using cells grown in the presence of FCS, wash thoroughly before fixation.

8. Triton X-100 and saponin are detergents used to permeabilize cells before cytochemical labeling procedures. The liquids are viscous, so it is advisable to cut off the tip from the end of a yellow pipet tip and pipet the detergent slowly. Add 50 µL–50 mL lectin buffer in a 50-mL centrifuge tube. Pipet carefully up and down a few times to expel the viscous detergent from the yellow tip. Mix the solution thoroughly by inverting the tube. Store at 4°C and make freshly weekly. Allow to warm to room temperature before use.

9. Working with cells on cover slips requires considerable manual dexterity. Once the cover slips are placed on the Parafilm, cells face up, solutions can be added or removed, limiting damage to the cells. Add or remove solutions gently from the edge of cover slips, using a micropipet filler fitted with a yellow tip. Approximately 50–200 µL solution will be required to cover the cells adequately. As before, take care that cells do not dry out at any stage of the staining procedure, or this will cause background staining to occur. Furthermore, pipet solutions up and down very gently from the edge of the cover slips to ensure even coverage of solutions over the cells.

10. Bovine serum albumin is used as the blocking solution to block nonspecific sites in lectin histochemistry. Most importantly, it is a nonglycosylated protein that will not interfere with lectin binding. Do not use milk powder or normal serum, both of which are commonly used as blocking solutions in immunocytochemistry/histochemistry, as the glycosylated molecules present may inhibit binding to cells and tissues.

11. Lectins are usually purchased as a lyophilized powder. Upon purchase, add 1 mL of lectin buffer per 1 mg of lectin and dissolve. This is the stock lectin concentration. It is convenient to freeze small aliquots of this, and once thawed, store at 4°C for use. Stock solutions of biotinylated or native lectins can be stored for a few months at 4°C. It is not advisable to repeatedly freeze and thaw the stock solution. For FITC-labeled lectins, use immediately once thawed; do not store at 4°C. The optimal working concentration of the lectin should be determined empirically. Assess labeling of a control tissue, such as animal or human kidney (*see* **Subheading 3.6.**), with lectin solutions of 1.25, 2.5, 5, 10, 20, and 40 mg/mL lectin. Determine the concentration that gives clean (with no background), strong labeling for the method employed. Make all working lectin solutions freshly on the day of lectin labeling.

12. Ribonuclease A is utilized to digest RNA present within the cells, as the nuclear counterstain PI would also bind RNA as well as DNA. This would be evident as background red fluorescent labeling. In the cytoplasm, this treatment is required if cells have been fixed with paraformaldehyde-, formaldehyde-, or glutaraldehyde-based fixatives. The treatment may not be necessary if cells had been fixed with methanol/acetic acid or acetone.

13. It is important that the RNase solution is maintained DNase-free. To ensure this, autoclave the lectin buffer before making stock solutions. Autoclave pipet tips before use. Use a fresh pipet tip for every cover slip of cells. Wear gloves throughout the procedure.

14. PI can be purchased in powder form from Molecular Probes (Eugene, OR). Add distilled water to make a stock concentration of 1 mg/mL and store in the dark at 4°C. A dilution of 1:3000 should be made for a working concentration in lectin buffer. Make freshly before use and cover the tube with aluminum foil. **Caution:** PI is a mutagen; suitable gloves should be worn and solutions should be poured over activated charcoal before disposal. For further information, consult material safety data sheets.

15. Citifluor or other antifade mountants can be purchased commercially. These aqueous-based mountants are used in undiluted form.

16. Trypsin is used for carbohydrate antigen retrieval. The action of the enzyme is thought to break down some of the crosslinking bonds of the formaldehyde-based fixatives, thereby revealing carbohydrate structures.

17. Avidin is a glycoprotein with four binding sites for the small vitamin biotin. Avidin is therefore conjugated with the enzyme label and will bind with high affinity to the biotin of biotinylated lectins. There is a possibility that the glycans of the avidin molecule may bind to lectins within the tissue and cause nonspecific background labeling. Therefore, streptavidin maybe used, a protein (not a glycoprotein) with similar structure to avidin that has been isolated from *Streptomyces avidinii*, a species of bacteria.

18. As with optimizing lectin concentrations, the secondary step of (strept)avidin-peroxidase must also be optimized to produce clean, specific staining. (Strept)avidin-peroxidase is normally purchased lyophilized. Dissolve in lectin buffer at 1 mg/mL and store at 4°C. This is the stock solution. In our laboratory,

we have found that 2.5 µg/mL is a good concentration to work with. Adjust concentration accordingly to optimize.

19. **Caution:** DAB is a potentially carcinogenic substance. Wear gloves, handle, and dispose of DAB according to material safety data instructions. DAB can be purchased from Sigma in powder form. To minimize aerosols produced when weighing powders, purchase 1 g of DAB and dissolve in 200 mL of distilled water in a fume cupboard. Aliquot (1 mL) rapidly (DAB oxidizes at room temperature) into appropriate vials with tight-fitting lids. Freeze at –20°C. These 1-mL stock solution aliquots can then be thawed and can make up to a total of 10 mL of solution at working concentration when required. Alternatively, safer DAB dropper kits are available commercially but tend to be more expensive. Spillages may be swabbed with diluted household bleach. Disposable plasticware must be soaked in diluted household bleach overnight before normal waste disposal.

20. To prepare the working solution, thaw a 1-mL aliquot of DAB and add to 9 mL of lectin buffer containing 10 µL of 30% hydrogen peroxide. Use immediately and always prepare freshly before use.

21. Paraffin wax sections cut more successfully when the blocks are chilled. During cutting process, place an ice cube on the wax block in pauses between taking sections.

22. Cutting sections is quite an art. Better sections will be cut with practice. Always ensure that the microtome blade is sharp; change approximately every three blocks or if it becomes blunt or damaged. Do not touch the blade with the forceps when removing cut sections (use the paintbrush), as this will damage the blade and cause "tramlines" to appear in subsequent sections. When using the same wax block on a different day, make sure that sections are cut in the same orientation as previously to minimize wasting tissue during trimming.

23. Tris-HCl-based buffers (e.g., lectin buffer) should not be used immediately before or after fixation with formaldehyde based fixatives. The amine groups from Tris-HCl are crosslinked by this type of fixative.

24. Warm glass Pasteur pipets in 37°C incubator. Transfer approx 0.5 mL of warmed low-temperature-gelling agarose into Eppendorf tubes containing pelleted cells and stir twice with edge of Pasteur pipet, taking care not to suck cells/agarose back up the pipet. Swirls of cells should be seen within the agarose. Alternatively, tap the Eppendorf tube sharply a couple of times to suspend cells in the agarose. Once set, carefully ease the agarose pellet out of the tube, using a needle, taking care not to tear or damage the cell/agarose pellet.

25. It is essential to keep cell culture materials sterile. Soak forceps in 70% (v/v) ethanol or IMS. Use the sterile forceps to dip individual cover slips in 70% (v/v) ethanol or IMS (for approx 15–30 s), then air-dry.

26. Leave cover slips in buffer at this point. The cells must not dry out at any stage of the staining procedure. Carefully lever the cover slip upward using a needle slightly bent at the end. Once levered slightly, the cover slip can be transferred to the Parafilm support within the humid chamber using the forceps. At this point, it is essential to minimize cellular damage; therefore, the very edge of the cover slip should be picked up with the forceps. When assessing results after lectin

cytochemistry, do not assess potentially damaged cells at the very edges of the cover slips.

27. Fluorescent labels are not permanent and will fade with time. They are photosensitive, and therefore, all solutions and incubations with solutions should be kept dark. Aluminum foil may be used to exclude light from the contents of tubes and plasticware containing solutions. Solutions from frozen stock should be made fresh before use. Results must be assessed as soon as possible (as fluorescence deteriorates) and photographed for permanent record. Until assessment, slides can be stored in the dark at 4°C. Do not stack microscope slides directly on top of one another, as cover slips will slide and the samples will be damaged.

28. Antifade mountant (for example, Citifluor) is an aqueous-based mountant. The mountant does not dry hard like the xylene-based mountants; therefore, the excess should be blotted very carefully and the cover slip sealed in place with clear nail polish. To prevent background fluorescence, the cells should not dry out at any time.

29. Epifluorescent or confocal laser scanning microscopes with suitable light sources and filters are required to visualize lectin binding in tissues labeled with fluorescent markers. FITC emits fluorescent green at 495 nm excitation wavelength. The rhodamine-based fluorescent markers, such as Texas Red and TRITC, emit red fluorescence at an excitation wavelength of 530 nm. To distinguish lectin labeling, red fluorescent markers should not be used in conjunction with a nuclei counterstain, such as PI. Alternative nuclear counterstains include 4',6-diamidino-2-phenylindole.

30. This step is only necessary when using horseradish peroxidase to visualize lectin binding; therefore, it is not required when using fluorescent labels or methods utilizing other enzymes, such as alkaline phosphatase. Endogenous peroxidases within peroxisomes of tissues cause additional labeling. The endogenous peroxidases are therefore quenched in an excess of the hydrogen peroxide substrate.

31. Blot excess buffer very carefully without touching the tissue preparation. Ensure that the tissue section does not dry out at anytime, as this will cause background labeling.

32. Mayer's hematoxylin is a progressive nuclear stain that is deep red in color. The color changes to blue in the presence of slightly alkaline tap water. Alternatively, dip briefly in an alkaline solution, such as dilute NaOH solution.

33. The tissue sections must be thoroughly dehydrated before mounting with xylene-based mountants. The sections are therefore taken through graded alcohols before being cleared in xylene.

References

1. Brooks, S. A., Dwek, M. V., and Schumacher, U. (2002) Carbohydrate binding proteins (lectins) in *Functional and Molecular Glycobiology*. BIOS Scientific, Oxford, UK, pp. 227–247.
2. Brooks, S. A., Leathem, A. J. C., and Schumacher, U. (1997) An introduction to the field, in *Lectin Histochemistry—A Concise Practical Handbook*. BIOS Scientific, Oxford, UK, pp. 1–17.

3. Brooks, S. A. and Carter, T. M. (2001) *N*-acetylgalactosamine, *N*-acetyl-glucosmine and sialic acid expression by primary breast cancers. *Histochem. J.* **103,** 37–51.

4. Brooks, S. A. (2000) The involvement of *Helix pomatia* lectin (HPA) binding *N*-acetylgalactosamine glycans in cancer progression. *Histol. Histopathol.* **15,** 143–158.

5. Julien, S., Krzewinski-Recchi, M. A., Harduin-Lepers, A., et al. (2001) Expression of sialyl-Tn antigen in breast cancer cells transfected with the human CMP-Neu5Ac:GalNAc α2,6-sialyltransferase (ST6GalNAc I) cDNA. *Glycoconjugate J.* **18,** 883–893.

6. Burchell, J., Poulsom, R., Hanby, A., et al. (1999) An α2,3 sialyltransferase (ST3Gal I) is elevated in primary breast carcinomas. *Glycobiology* **9,** 1307–1311.

17

SDS-PAGE and Western Blotting to Detect Proteins and Glycoproteins of Interest in Breast Cancer Research

Chloe Osborne and Susan A. Brooks

Summary

Sodium dodecyl sulfate-polyacrylamide gel electrophoresis (SDS-PAGE) and Western blotting to detect proteins and glycoproteins is one of the most widely used and broadly useful techniques in cancer research, allowing the proteins in a complex sample—such as a blood sample, aspirate, or solid tumor homogenate—to be separated according to molecular weight and visualized within a gel matrix and/or, once separated, transferred onto a supporting membrane, where they may be probed for the binding of antibodies or lectins. In this chapter, the theory and principles of SDS-PAGE and Western blotting are briefly outlined, and basic methods are given that can be applied to investigate virtually any (glyco)protein of interest in breast cancer research.

Key Words: SDS-PAGE; Western blotting; electroblotting; protein analysis; glycoprotein, analysis.

1. Introduction

1.1. Applications of the Technique

Sodium dodecyl sulfate-polyacrylamide gel electrophoresis (SDS-PAGE) *(1)* and electrotransfer of proteins to a solid supporting membrane (Western electroblotting) *(2,3)* are among the most commonly used and versatile laboratory techniques. SDS-PAGE relies on the migration of charged molecules in a gel matrix in response to an electrical field. By this technique, it is possible to separate a complex mixture of proteins, ranging in molecular weight from about 10–200 kDa. Following electrophoretic separation, protein (Western) electroblotting is used to transfer the separated protein bands onto a support membrane, commonly nitrocellulose, where they may be probed, for example, for identification by binding of a particular antibody, or by lectins to map glycosylation. SDS-PAGE and Western blotting enable useful information on

From: *Methods in Molecular Medicine, Vol. 120: Breast Cancer Research Protocols*
Edited by: S. A. Brooks and A. L. Harris © Humana Press Inc., Totowa, NJ

proteins to be obtained, including evidence of their presence and proportion within a complex heterogeneous mixture, such as a serum sample or tissue homogenate, and estimation of molecular weight.

There are countless published studies that have reported analysis of breast cancer-derived proteins using SDS-PAGE and Western blotting techniques. An example is the analysis of different forms of MUC-1 mucin derived from normal and malignant breast epithelium, which has resulted in the generation of monoclonal antibodies that have proved of great interest in breast cancer research and in the clinical setting *(4)*. Our group has used SDS-PAGE and Western blotting to resolve and characterize a profile of shared *Helix pomatia* agglutinin-binding glycoproteins in breast cell lines and clinical tumor samples *(5)*. Characterization of these molecules was of interest, as *H. pomatia* agglutinin is a marker of poor prognosis and metastatic competence in breast cancer (*see* **ref. 6** for review). These studies illustrate the utility of SDS-PAGE and Western blotting techniques, alone or allied with other approaches, for gaining both qualitative and quantitative information.

A variety of sample types, including serum samples, samples of body fluids such as ascites and pleural effusions, and lysates of clinical tissue samples or of cultured cells can be readily analyzed by SDS-PAGE and Western blotting. Generic methods for preparing cell or tissue lysates and for treating serum and other body fluids for analysis by SDS-PAGE and Western blotting are given in this chapter. Generic preparation techniques for tumor homogenates are also given in Chapter 5.

1.2. Principles Underlying SDS-PAGE

SDS-PAGE relies on the migration of charged molecules in a gel matrix in response to an electrical field. This technique facilitates the separation and resolution of a mixture of proteins according to molecular weight. There are two main apparatus types employed for this sort of electrophoresis: the minigel apparatus, which is commonly used for the identification and characterization of proteins; and the large-format gel apparatus sometimes used for preparative work. This chapter will describe generic methods applied to the minigel apparatus, and these can simply be scaled up for large-format gels.

SDS-PAGE can be carried out under reducing or nonreducing conditions. Under reducing conditions, SDS-PAGE involves the linearization of proteins by the dissociation of inter- and intrachain disulfide bonds. This is achieved by heating the protein sample briefly in a boiling water bath in the presence of a reducing agent. The proteins are also coated with a negative charge in the presence of the anionic detergent SDS. They are then separated and resolved as discrete bands as they migrate in an electric field through the "sieving" action of the acrylamide gel matrix.

The polyacrylamide gel slab is cast in two layers, the upper stacking gel and the main separating gel. The stacking gel is a loose meshwork incorporating a low percentage (usually 3% [w/v]) acrylamide through which proteins of all sizes readily migrate in the electric field. The purpose of the stacking gel is to enable all the proteins within the sample to "stack" into a concentrated layer before entering the separating gel. Different percentages of acrylamide incorporated in the separating gel are appropriate to resolve proteins of different molecular-weight ranges. Gels prepared with a lower percentage of acrylamide (for example, 5–7.5% [w/v]) have a larger pore size for the proteins to pass through and will optimally resolve large-molecular-weight proteins. Gels with a higher percentage of acrylamide (for example, 12.5–15% [w/v]) have a smaller pore size and optimally resolve proteins in the lower-molecular-weight range.

It is conventional to separate a standard protein ladder mixture in parallel with test samples. In addition to confirming successful protein separation, measurement of the migration distances of a series of proteins of known molecular weights in the acrylamide gel matrix facilitates molecular-weight determination of sample proteins. Standard protein ladder mixtures of different molecular-weight ranges are widely available commercially and can be purchased as native proteins, labeled with biotin or enzyme labels, radiolabeled, or prestained.

1.3. Principles of Western Electroblotting

Western blotting is the transfer of proteins from the SDS-PAGE gel to a solid supporting membrane. There are three different supports commonly in use: nitrocellulose, nylon, and polyvinylidene fluoride. The choice of membrane depends on the protein being transferred, as different proteins may bind more efficiently to one membrane in comparison with another. Testing of each membrane type is recommended for optimized results. This chapter includes generic techniques for protein transfer to nitrocellulose; the methods are readily adapted for transfer to other membrane types.

There are two types of blotting apparatus used to transfer proteins to solid supports; these facilitate either wet transfer (tank blotting) and semidry transfer. Both give good results, and the choice of technique is mostly a question of personal preference, but semidry blotting is probably more popular, perhaps because it is slightly quicker and easier *(7)*.

Once (glyco)proteins are immobilized on the blotting membrane, they can be probed for the binding of antibodies or lectins. The techniques are largely analogous to those used for immunochemistry and lectin histochemistry (described in Chapters 15 and 16, respectively), with some minor technical modifications. The simplest involves the use of an antibody or lectin directly conjugated to a fluorescent, enzyme, or radiolabel. The principle of this method is straightforward, as it involves direct detection of the antibody or lectin visualized by the label attached to them. The most obvious advantage of direct labeling is it is quick and easy to carry out. It however, is less sensitive than other multistep indirect methods and large, for example, enzyme-label molecules, can alter the binding characteristics of the lectin or antibody *(8)*. One of the most versatile indirect methods of detection involves incubation of the blot with biotinylated primary antibody or lectin. This is followed by incubation with avidin or streptavidin linked to a fluorescent, enzyme, or radioactive reporter molecule. This method is more sensitive than the direct method and does not suffer from the potential steric hindrance from the label affecting the binding site of the antibody or lectin. The use of horseradish peroxidase as a reporter molecule is versatile, as it can be used in conjunction with either a chromogenic substrate (commonly diaminobenzidine and hydrogen peroxide, described here, to give deep-brown-colored bands against a white background) or, for low-level protein expression, it can be used in conjunction with enhanced chemoluminescence for much increased sensitivity. Generic methods are given here, and can be adapted for any individual application.

1.4. Summary

The process of SDS-PAGE and Western blotting includes six main steps:

1. The isolation of the proteins to be analyzed.
2. Separation of the protein using SDS-PAGE and their visualization within the gel.
3. Transfer of the separated proteins to a membrane support.
4. Blocking of nonspecific binding sites on the membrane support.
5. Probing of the proteins.
6. Detection using antibodies or lectins.

This chapter provides a basic protocol that can be adapted to facilitate investigation of virtually any protein/glycoprotein(s) derived from cultured breast cancer cells and clinical tumor samples.

2. Materials

2.1. Release of Proteins From Cell and Tissue Samples by Cell Lysis

1. Triple detergent lysis buffer: make up a solution of 50 mM Tris-HCl, 150 mM NaCl in deionized water, then add 0.02% (w/v) of sodium azide, 0.1% (w/v) SDS, 100 μL/mL phenylmethylsulfonyl fluoride (PMSF) *(see* **Note 1**), 1 μg/mL aprotinin *(see* **Note 2**), 1 μg/mL peptatin A, 1 μg/mL leupeptin, 1% (v/v) Nonident P-40 (NP-40), and 0.5% (w/v) sodium deoxycholate. Adjust pH to 8.0 using HCl.
2. Single-detergent lysis buffer: make up a solution of 50 mM Tris-HCl and 150 mM NaCl in deionized water. Then add 0.02% (w/v) sodium azide, 100 μL/mL PMSF *(see* **Note 1**), 1 μg/mL aprotinin *(see* **Note 2**), 1 μg/mL

peptatin A, 1 µg/mL leupeptin, and 1% (v/v) Triton X-100 or 1% (v/v) NP-40. Adjust pH to 8.0 using HCl.

3. High-salt lysis buffer: make up a solution of 50 m*M* N-2-hydroxyethylpiperazine-*N'*-2-ethansulfonicacid (500 m*M* NaCl) in deionized water, then add 1% (v/v) NP-40, 100 µL/mL PMSF (*see* **Note 1**), 1 µg/mL aprotinin (*see* **Note 2**), 1 µg/mL peptatin A, and 1 µg/mL leupeptin. Adjust pH to 7.0.

4. No-salt lysis buffer: make up a solution of 50mM hydroxyethylpiperazine-*N'*-2-ethansulfonicacid in deionized water, then add 1% NP-40, 100 µL/mL PMSF (*see* **Note 1**), 1 µg/mL aprotinin (*see* **Note 2**), 1 µg/mL peptatin A, and 1 µg/mL leupeptin.

2.2. Removal of Albumin From Tissue and Serum Samples

1. Affigel blue affinity beads (Bio-Rad, Hercules, CA).
2. Deionized water.

2.3. Methanol/Chloroform Precipitation of Proteins Released From Cells and Tissues

1. Chloroform.
2. Methanol.

2.4. Preparation of Polyacrylamide Gels

1. Deionized water.
2. Separating gel buffer: make up a solution of 1.5 *M* Tris-HCl in deionized water and add 0.4% (w/v) SDS. Adjust pH to 8.8 using HCl.
3. Stacking gel buffer: make up a solution of 1.0 *M* Tris-HCl in deionized water and add 0.4% (w/v) SDS. Adjust pH to 6.8 using HCl.
4. Bis/acrylamide stock solution: 29% (w/v) acrylamide and 1% (w/v) *N-N'*-methylenebisacrylamide in deionized water. Check that pH is 7.0 or less and correct as necessary using HCl. Store in a dark bottle at room temperature (*see* **Note 3**).
5. *N,N,N',N'*-tetramethylethylenediamine (TEMED).
6. 10% (w/v) ammonium persulfate solution in deionized water. Make freshly on day of use.

2.5. Sample Preparation

1. Reducing sample buffer: prepare 100 m*M* Tris-HCl with either 200 m*M* dithiothreitol (DTT) or 100 m*M* of β-mercaptoethanol in deionized water. Add 4% (w/v) SDS (electrophoresis grade), 0.2% (w/v) bromophenol blue, 20% (v/v) glycerol. Adjust pH to 6.8 using HCl (*see* **Note 4**).
2. Nonreducing sample buffer as reducing sample buffer, but omit the DTT/mercaptoethanol.

2.6. Running a Gel

1. Running buffer. 25 m*M* Tris, 250 m*M* glycine (electrophoresis grade) dissolved in deionized water. Add 0.1% (w/v) SDS. Adjust pH to 8.3 using HCl.
2. Protein standard ladder made up according to manufacturer's instructions.

2.7. Coomassie Brilliant Blue Total Protein Stain

1. Staining solution: 0.025% (w/v) Coomassie brilliant blue 250, 40% (v/v) methanol, and 10% (v/v) glacial acetic acid in deionized water.
2. Gel destaining solution: 10% (v/v) isopropyl alcohol, 10% (v/v) glacial acetic acid, and 80% (v/v) deionized water.

2.8. Western Electroblotting

1. Whatman 3MM filter paper.
2. Nitrocellulose blotting membrane.
3. Deionized water.
4. Transfer buffer: 25 mM Tris, 190 mM of glycine, and 15% (v/v) methanol in deionized water. Store at 4°C.

2.9. Ponceau Red-S Stain to Assess Transfer Efficiency

1. Ponceau red staining solution: 0.1% (w/v) Ponceau red-S, 5% (v/v) glacial acetic acid in deionized water.
2. Deionized water.

2.10. Antibody and Lectin Probing of Western Blots

1. Lectin buffer: 25 mM Tris base, 150 mM NaCl, 2 mM MgCl$_2$, and 2 mM CaCl$_2$ in deionized water. Adjust pH to 7.6 using HCl (*see* **Note 5**).
2. Phosphate buffered saline (PBS): 137 mM NaCl, 2.7 mM KCl, 10 mM Na$_2$HPO$_3$, and 2 mM KH$_2$PO$_4$ in deionized water. Adjust pH to 7.4 using HCl (*see* **Note 5**).
3. Either:
   a. Nonfat dried milk powder blocking buffer: 5% (w/v) non-fat dried milk powder (e.g. Marvel) and 0.05% (v/v) Tween-20 in PBS.
   or
   b. Albumin blocking buffer: 4% (w/v) bovine serum albumin and 0.05% (v/v) Tween-20 in lectin buffer (*see* **Note 6**).
4. Washing buffer: 0.2% (v/v) Tween-20 in PBS or lectin buffer (*see* **Note 5**).
5. Biotinylated or horseradish peroxidase-conjugated primary antisera or lectin solution made up in PBS-based washing buffer (antibodies) or lectin buffer based washing buffer (lectins) (*see* **Note 5**) at optimum working dilutions. The optimum working dilutions should be determined empirically. As a guide: a concentration of 1–10 µg/mL for lectins is usual.
6. Avidin or streptavidin peroxidase solution: 2.5–5 µg/mL in PBS-based washing buffer (for antibody labeling) or lectin buffer based washing buffer (for lectins) (*see* **Note 5**).
7. Diaminobenzidine hydrochloride (DAB) solution: 0.5 mg/mL DAB in PBS (for antibody labeling) or lectin buffer (for lectins) (*see* **Note 5**). Add hydrogen peroxide immediately before use to give a final concentration of 0.03% (v/v) (*see* **Note 7**).
8. DAB solution (as prepared in **step 7**) can be replaced by an enhanced chemoluminescence kit (Amersham Life Sciences).

3. Methods

3.1. Release of Proteins From Cell and Tissue Samples by Cell Lysis

The most commonly employed lysis buffers used to extract proteins from cultured mammalian cells are given in **Subheading 2.1.** We recommend that triple-detergent lysis buffer/single-detergent lysis buffer be used if little information regarding the target protein is known. Samples should be kept cold and steps performed at 4°C or on ice wherever possible.

1. Chop finely a small sample of fresh, unfixed tissue, using a sharp scalpel.
2. Homogenize chopped tissue in a minimum volume of lysis buffer, i.e., lysis buffer using electric tissue homogenizer and then disrupt cells using a sonicator on ice in 5-s repeated bursts.
3. Check cells are disrupted efficiently by light microscopy.
4. Centrifuge sample for 15 min at 10,000g to pellet solid debris.
5. Aspirate supernatant (containing solubilized proteins) and discard pellet (intact cells/cell debris).

3.2. Removal of Albumin From Tissue and Serum Samples

When resolving proteins from serum, tissue lysates, and other biological samples by SDS-PAGE, the presence of high serum albumin concentrations can cause distortion of the bands. Albumin can be selectively removed using an affinity matrix, which adsorbs albumin from solution (*see* **Note 8**).

1. Pack a small chromatography column with Affigel blue.
2. Wash and equilibrate column with several volumes of deionized water.
3. Load the sample onto the column.
4. Collect eluate.
5. Flush through any additional unbound material using a small volume of deionized water and add to original eluate.

Alternatively, if only a small volume of sample is to be treated, affinity adsorption may be performed in a small tube, rather than a gel column. This is achieved as follows:

1. Place 0.5 mL of Affigel blue in a 1.5-mL Eppendorf tube.
2. Add sample.
3. Mix for approx 30 min, using an end-over-end mixer at room temperature.
4. Centrifuge at 2000g for 2 min to pellet beads.
5. Aspirate supernatant.

3.3. Methanol/Chloroform Precipitation of Proteins Released From Cells and Tissues

This method, based on that given in **ref. 9**, concentrates protein from dilute solution, such as cell or tissue lysates or eluate from an Affigel blue column,

Table 1
Recipes for Separating Gels

Percentage acrylamide in final gel	5%	6%	7.5%	10%	12.5%	15%
Separating gel buffer (mL)	2.5	2.5	2.5	2.5	2.5	2.5
Bis/acrylamide stock (mL)	1.65	2.0	2.5	3.35	4.2	5.0
Distilled water (mL)	5.85	5.5	5.0	4.15	3.3	2.5
APS (µL)	60	60	60	60	60	60
TEMED (µL)	5	5	5	5	5	5

APS, ammonium persulfate solution; TEMED, N,N,N',N'-tetramethylethylenediamine.

and also removes detergents, salts, and other small contaminating molecules that can distort resolution on SDS-PAGE gels.

1. Mix protein sample with methanol and chloroform in a ratio of four parts sample:four parts methanol:one part chloroform.
2. Vortex for 1 min to mix.
3. Centrifuge for 2 min at 10,000*g* (*see* **Note 9**).
4. Aspirate upper layer (methanol/aqueous layer), using a Pasteur pipet and discard.
5. Aspirate lower layer (chloroform/lipid layer), using a Pasteur pipet and discard (*see* **Note 10**).
6. Add a small volume of methanol to rinse precipitated protein.
7. Vortex for 1 min.
8. Centrifuge for 2 min at 10,000*g* to pellet protein.
9. Aspirate supernatant (methanol) to leave behind solid protein pellet.
10. Air-dry protein pellet for 30 min at room temperature in a fume hood.

3.4. Preparation of Polyacrylamide Gels

1. Ensure glass plates are clean (*see* **Note 11**). Assemble plates according to manufacturer's instructions.
2. Prepare separating gel by mixing together reagents listed in **Table 1**, except ammonium persulfate and TEMED (*see* **Note 12**).
3. Add ammonium persulfate and TEMED last and swirl quickly to mix well.
4. Pipet quickly between glass plates (*see* **Note 12**).
5. Pipet a thin layer of deionized water onto the top of the gel (*see* **Note 13**).
6. Allow gel to polymerize for at least 30 min.
7. Remove deionized water from top of gel (*see* **Note 14**).
8. Prepare stacking gel by mixing reagents listed in **Table 2**, except ammonium persulfate and TEMED (*see* **Note 12**).
9. Add ammonium persulfate and TEMED and swirl quickly to mix well.
10. Pipet onto separating gel, leaving a small space to allow for insertion of sample comb (*see* **Note 12**).
11. Insert sample comb and allow to polymerize for at least 30 min (*see* **Notes 15** and **16**).

Table 2
Recipe for Stacking Gel

Stacking gel buffer	1.25 mL
Bis/acrylamide stock	0.5 mL
Distilled water	3.25 mL
APS	30 μL
TEMED	10 μL

APS, ammonium persulfate solution; TEMED, *N,N,N',N'*-tetramethylethylenediamine.

3.5. Sample Preparation (see Note 17)

1. Mix protein sample (e.g., cell or tissue lysate, serum, or ascites sample) in a 1:1 ratio, with reducing or nonreducing sample buffer.
2. If using reducing conditions, heat in boiling water bath for 1–2 min (*see* **Note 18**) and allow to cool.

3.6. Running a Gel

1. Assemble gel apparatus according to manufacturer's instructions.
2. Fill electrophoresis tank with running buffer.
3. Remove gently the sample comb (*see* **Note 19**), ensuring gel is fully submerged in running buffer.
4. Load 10–15-μL sample (depending on size of gel) in each lane, using a Hamilton syringe or micropipet fitted with a fine gel-loading tip.
5. Start the electrophoretic separation at 50–100 V for approx 30 min (or until sample has moved into separating gel) (*see* **Note 20**).
6. Increase voltage to approx 180 V and run until sample has reached end of gel (*see* **Note 20**).
7. Reduce voltage to 0. Turn off power and disconnect.
8. Remove gel from electrophoresis chamber and release gel from between glass plates by levering the plates gently apart using a spatula (*see* **Note 21**).

3.7. Coomassie Brilliant Blue Total Protein Stain

Coomassie blue is a good general protein stain. It is used to visualize all protein bands and should not be used if Western blotting is intended (*see* **Notes 22** and **23**). All steps should be carried out at room temperature, with gentle agitation on a rocking table.

1. Incubate gel in Coomassie brilliant blue staining solution for 4 h.
2. Destain the gel in destaining solution for 4–6 h, with regular changes of destaining solution throughout this period until protein bands appear deep blue against a colorless background.

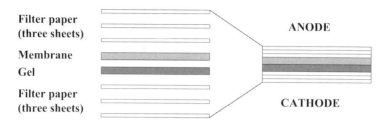

Fig. 1. Schematic representation of blotting sandwich used in both wet and semidry blotting techniques.

3. Wash in deionized water and either photograph and dry, or store in deionized water for future analysis.

3.8. Western Electroblotting

3.8.1. Wet (Tank) Electroblotting

1. Cut six sheets of filter paper (Whatman 3MM) and one sheet of blotting membrane to the same size as the gel.
2. Soak filter papers in transfer buffer. Soak nitrocellulose in deionized water.
3. Assemble the blotting sandwich as follows: three sheets of filter paper then the gel, then the nitrocellulose membrane, and then the remaining three sheets of filter paper (*see* **Note 24**). This is illustrated in **Fig. 1**.
4. Secure the blotting sandwich in the blotting cassette according to manufacturer's instructions.
5. Position the cassette in the blotting tank (membrane facing anode).
6. Run blotting equipment as per manufacturer's instructions. For an average minigel, run for approx 1 h at 0.25 A.

3.8.2. Semidry Electroblotting

1. Cut filter paper and membrane as per wet transfer method.
2. Soak all six sheets of filter paper in transfer buffer.
3. Soak nitrocellulose membrane in deionized water.
4. Assemble blotting sandwich as follows: three sheets of filter paper in the center of the anode, then the nitrocellulose membrane, then the gel, and then the remaining three sheets of filter paper. The blotting sandwich is illustrated in **Fig. 1**. Eliminate any trapped air bubbles (*see* **Note 24**).
5. Position cathode in place.
6. Connect power supply as per manufacturer's instructions. For an average minigel, run for approx 30 min at 0.25 A, according to manufacturer's instructions.

3.9. Ponceau Red-S Stain to Assess Transfer Efficiency

Following transfer of proteins to blotting membrane, blots can be temporarily stained with Ponceau red to assess the efficiency of the transfer. A photographic record can be taken at this stage before destaining the blot completely in preparation for probing the proteins for binding with antibodies/lectins.

1. Immerse blotted membrane in Ponceau red-S solution for 1 min.
2. Wash membrane well in several changes of deionized water until pink/red bands are seen against a white background.
3. After efficiency of transfer has been checked by visual inspection and (if required) photographic record has been made, the membrane can be completely destained by washing in several changes of deionized water.

3.10. Antibody and Lectin Probing of Western Blots

All steps should be carried out with gentle agitation, for example, on a rocking platform.

1. Incubate blot in blocking buffer for 30 min at room temperature.
2. Incubate blot with either horseradish peroxidase-conjugated or biotinylated antibody solution, or lectin solution for 1–2 h at room temperature or overnight at 4°C.
3. Wash blot in washing buffer a minimum of four times (for 10 min each time).
4. For labeling with biotinylated antibody or lectin, incubate with avidin or streptavidin peroxidase solution for 30 min–1 h at room temperature. Wash blot in washing buffer a minimum of four times (for 10 min each time). For labeling with horseradish peroxidase-conjugated antibody or lectin, proceed to **step 5**.
5. Wash blot in PBS (antibodies) or lectin buffer (lectins), both without Tween-20.
6. If using the chromogenic substrate DAB, incubate with DAB solution until dark-brown bands appear against a white background (typically, 5 min–1 h). Wash blot in several changes of tap water and blot dry. If using enhanced chemoluminescence, proceed according to manufacturer's kit instructions.

4. Notes

1. PMSF becomes inactivated in aqueous solutions. Solutions should be made freshly when needed and are safe to discard by flushing to waste with copious amounts of tap water after use.
2. Store aprotinin stock solution in small aliquots at –20°C, as it aggregates upon repetitive thawing and freezing.
3. **Caution:** Acrylamide monomer is a neurotoxin and should therefore be handled and disposed of with the appropriate safety procedures. Once polymerized, polyacrylamide gel is not hazardous. The gel, nonetheless, should still be handled with care, as traces of unpolymerized acrylamide may remain. Bis/acrylamide solution is available commercially, and it may be preferable to purchasing bis and acrylamide in powder form because of the aerosol hazards associated with the latter.
4. Both DTT and β-mercaptoethanol are equally effective. DTT may be preferable, as it is less hazardous than β-mercaptoethanol.

5. Antibody labeling is most usually performed in PBS. PBS is generally not appropriate for lectin labeling, as many lectins require the presence of calcium and magnesium ions. We therefore recommend a general "lectin buffer," which is Tris-HCl-buffered saline with added salts. This buffer, with or without the addition of the calcium and magnesium chloride, may be used for antibody labeling in place of PBS.

6. Nonfat milk powder blocking buffer is commonly used for antibody-labeling experiments. It is not appropriate for lectin labeling, as the glycoconjugates in milk may competitively inhibit lectin binding. The blocking buffer containing (nonglycosylated) bovine serum albumin is preferable. Albumin blocking buffer can also be used in antibody-labeling experiments.

7. **Caution:** DAB is potentially carcinogenic; appropriate handling and disposal procedures should therefore be carried out.

8. Sometimes several cycles of dealbuminization may be necessary before a clean sample is obtained.

9. Centrifugation of the sample:methanol:chloroform mixture results in an upper methanol/aqueous layer and a lower chloroform/lipid layer; the precipitated protein is located at the interface between the two layers and can usually be seen as an opaque disc.

10. Care should be taken during removal of lower chloroform layer to avoid unnecessary disruption of the protein disc.

11. Clean glass plates well after use with a solution of mild detergent in warm water, rinse in distilled water, dry well, and store in a dust-free environment.

12. During gel preparation, the addition of TEMED and ammonium persulfate results in rapid polymerization of the gel. These reagents should be added last, swirled quickly to mix, and the gel cast between the glass plates as swiftly as possible.

13. Layering a little distilled water to the top of the separating gel before it polymerizes ensures a flat interface between the separating and stacking gels.

14. To avoid damaging the gel when removing distilled water, simply invert gel onto some tissue paper and allow water to drain away.

15. When inserting the sample comb, be sure not to capture bubbles. To achieve this, insert the comb at a slanted angle and then lower gently.

16. Gels can be prepared in advance, wrapped in plastic wrap or cling film, and stored for up to 1 wk at 4°C.

17. In order to optimize protein-loading of SDS-PAGE gels, it is a good idea to determine the concentration of each protein in a sample before SDS-PAGE. This is most commonly achieved using a standard colormetric protein quantification assay, kits for which are widely available. With respect to the amount of protein to load into each well, approx 10 µg per well is a good starting point; however, it may be necessary to optimize this to suit the particular experiment.

18. Pierce cap of the tube to prevent pressure build up and consequent explosion during heating.

19. When removing the comb, be sure to avoid bubbles forming in the wells; if bubbles do form, they can be gently removed using a fine pipet tip.

20. Bromophenol blue in the sample buffer runs ahead of the smallest proteins, thus marking the progress of the run.
21. To ensure correct orientation of gel upon analysis, nick off one corner. For example, always nick the bottom left-hand corner.
22. Following Coomassie blue staining, silver staining may be carried out. This is a more sensitive method of detecting proteins in the gel. Silver staining kits are available, for example, from Bio-Rad, which contain all the necessary reagents and full instructions.
23. Sometimes it is helpful to run gels in duplicate and Coomassie blue or silver stain one for total protein, then blot and probe the second to investigate particular (glyco)protein species.
24. Gel, papers, and membrane must be exactly the same size, as the sandwich must be perfectly aligned. If, for example, the filter papers overhang the gel, the electric current will preferentially pass through the papers only, thus bypassing the gel, and the transfer will be compromised. Avoid air bubbles occurring in the layering of the sandwich by rolling over the sandwich using a small roller or the flat edge of a ruler.

References

1. Laemmli, E. K. (1970) Cleavage of structural proteins during the assembly of the head of bacteriophage T4. *Nature* **227,** 680–685.
2. Towbin, H., Staehelin, T., and Gordon, J. (1979) Electrophoretic transfer of proteins from polyacrylamide gels to nitrocellulose sheets: procedure and some applications. *Proc. Natl. Acad. Sci. USA* **76,** 4350–4354.
3. Burnette, W. N. (1981) "Western Blotting": electrophoretic transfer of proteins from sodium dodecylsulfate-polyacrylamide gels to unmodified nitrocellulose and radiographic detection with antibody and radioiodinated protein A. *Anal. Biochem.* **112,** 195–203.
4. Griffiths, A. B., Burchell, J., Gendler, S., et al. (1987) Immunological analysis of mucin molecules expressed by normal and malignant mammary epithelial cells. *Int. J. Cancer* **40,** 319–327.
5. Brooks, S. A., Hall, D. M., and Buley, I. (2001) *N*-acetyl galactosamine glycoprotein expression by breast cell line, primary breast cancer and normal breast epithelial membrane. *BJC* **85,** 1014–1022.
6. Brooks, S. A. (2000) The involvement of *Helix pomatia* lectin (HPA) binding *N*-acetylgalactosamine glycans in cancer progression. *Histol. Histopathol.* **15,** 143–158.
7. Department of Microbiology, University of Capetown, Rondebosch. http://www.mcb.uct.ac.za/manual/SDS-PAGE.htm. Last accessed June 10, 2005.
8. Brooks, S. A., Lymboura, M., Schumacher, U., and Leathem, A. J. (1996) Histochemistry to detect *Helix pomatia* lectin binding in breast cancer: methodology makes a difference. *J. Histochem. Cytochem.* **44,** 519–524.
9. Wessel, D. and Flugge, U. I. (1984) A method for the quantitative recovery of protein in dilute solution in the presence of detergents and lipids. *Anal. Biochem.* **138,** 141–143.

18

Breast Cancer Proteomics Using Two-Dimensional Electrophoresis

Studying the Breast Cancer Proteome

Miriam V. Dwek and Sarah L. Rawlings

Summary

Proteomics has emerged as a powerful approach for studying disease-associated changes in protein levels. The most commonly used method in proteomics studies remains two-dimensional gel electrophoresis, but the methodology, standardization, and interpretation of the results obtained require considerable expertise.

In this chapter, we describe the approaches we have taken to studying the breast cancer proteome, using cells grown in vitro and cancer specimens as the starting materials.

Key Words: Proteome; SDS-PAGE; Western blotting; molecular weight; protein; post-translational modification.

1. Introduction

Proteomics is the study of all the proteins encoded by the genome *(1)*. It has been estimated that a human tissue sample contains at least 10,000 different proteins *(2)*, and in breast cancer, it is likely that even more proteins exist, mainly as a result of inappropriate protein expression because of mutations, mismatching/splicing of genes, and changes in the normal posttranslational modification of proteins. Proteome studies enable changes in a multitude of cellular proteins—perhaps because of a stimulus or treatment regimen—to be identified. In addition, comparisons can be made in the protein expression levels of normal healthy cells or tissues and diseased cells or tissues, often with different clinical behaviors. For example, a number of studies have compared the protein expression levels of normal breast tissue with breast cancer tissue *(3–6)*.

From: *Methods in Molecular Medicine, Vol. 120: Breast Cancer Research Protocols*
Edited by: S. A. Brooks and A. L. Harris © Humana Press Inc., Totowa, NJ

In practical terms, it is still not possible to map the entire tissue or cellular proteome in a single experiment, because the amino acids that make up proteins and their posttranslational modifications mean that no single solubilization protocol is appropriate for all proteins, and no individual separation technique is of sufficiently good resolution.

In recent years, the availability of reliable, commercially available materials for the separation of proteins, first according to their isoelectric point and second, by size, has led to increased use of two-dimensional electrophoresis (2DE) for proteome studies. This technique enables the study of over 1000 proteins from a cell or tissue extract in a single experiment. The recent availability of narrow range immobilized pH gradient (IPG) strips means that literally thousands of proteins can be mapped in a series of experiments with the zoom gel system *(7)*.

In conjunction with newer techniques for protein detection, image analysis, data handling, and protein identification (primarily mass spectrometry), 2DE is a powerful, as yet unsurpassed, technique for proteomics studies *(8)*.

2. Materials

2.1. Sample Preparation

1. Liquid nitrogen.
2. Lysis buffer: 9.5 M urea, 2% (w/v) 3-[(3-cholamidopropyl)dimethylammonio]-1-propanesulfonic acid (CHAPS), 0.8% (v/v) Pharmalyte (Amersham Biosciences, UK) (pH 3.0–10.0 NL), and 1% (w/v) dithiothreitol.
3. Phosphate-buffered saline (PBS): 10X PBS stock is 80 g NaCl, 2.0 g KCl, 14.4 g Na_2PO_4, and 2.4 g KH_2PO_4 in 800 mL of distilled H_2O. Adjust pH to 7.4 with hydrochloric acid (HCl) and adjust volume to 1 L with additional distilled H_2O.
4. 0.35 M Sucrose solution.
5. Cell scraper (rubber policeman).
6. Handheld homogenizer.
7. Bio-Rad (Hercules, CA) protein assay reagent.
8. Distilled or deionized water.
9. Absolute methanol.
10. Absolute chloroform.
11. Rehydration buffer: 8 M of urea, 2% (w/v) 3-[(3-cholamidopropyl)dimethylammonio]-1-propanesulfonic acid, 0.1% (w/v) bromophenol blue.

2.2. Protein Quantification

1. Bio-Rad dye concentrate.
2. Bovine serum albumin (BSA) standard. 5 mg/mL of BSA dissolved in lysis buffer.
3. HCl.

4. Spectrophotometer.
5. Plastic cuvets.

2.3. Isoelectric Focusing

1. IPG Strips (pH 3.0–10.0 NL).
2. Silicone oil.
3. IPG strip reswelling tray.
4. IPG strip aligner tray.
5. Isoelectric focusing (IEF) electrophoresis unit (e.g., Multiphor II, Amersham).
6. Thermostatic circulator set to 20°C (e.g., Multitemp III, Amersham).
7. Tray and electrode holder.
8. IEF electrode strips

2.4. IPG Strip Equilibration

1. Equilibration buffer 1: 50 mM Tris-HCl (pH 8.8), 6 M urea, 30% (v/v) glycerol, 2% (w/v) sodium dodecyl sulfate (SDS), 0.1% (w/v) bromophenol blue, and 10 mg/mL dithiothreitol.
2. Equilibration buffer 2: 50 mM Tris-HCl (pH 8.8), 6 M urea, 30% (v/v) glycerol, 2% (w/v) SDS, 0.1% (w/v) bromophenol blue, and 48 mg/mL iodoacetamide.
3. Tank buffer: 14.4 g glycine, 3.0 g Tris base, and 1.0 g SDS. Make up to 1 L with distilled water.

2.5. SDS-Polyacrylamide Gel Electrophoresis

1. Gel kits (e.g., Miniprotean III for minigels [Bio-Rad] and Hoefer DALT sysytem [Amersham], including gel caster, for large-format gels).
2. Resolving gel buffer: 36.34 g of Tris base, 4.0 mL of a 10% SDS solution. Adjust pH to 8.8 with HCl, and make up to a final volume of 100 mL.
3. 30% Acrylamide solution (it is advisable to purchase this ready-made because of the hazardous, neurotoxic nature of acrylamide).
4. Ammonium persulphate (APS).
5. N,N,N',N'-tetramethylethylenediamine (TEMED).
6. Water-saturated isobutanol.
7. Solidified molecular-weight marker. The marker is made by adding a spatula of agarose to 200 mL of liquid marker and then heating in a beaker of boiling water for a few minutes. This solution is allowed to solidify and then stored at −20°C until use where a small chunk is taken, using a spatula, for each gel.
8. Agarose.
9. Displacing solution: 50 mL resolving gel buffer, 100 mL glycerol, 50 mL distilled water, and 2 mg bromophenol blue.
10. Gel caster.
11. Separator sheets and Perspex filler blocks.
12. Hoefer DALT electrophoresis unit (Amersham).
13. Thermostatic circulator (e.g., Multitemp III, Amersham, set to 10°C).

2.6. Detecting Proteins Separated by 2DE

1. Containers for silver staining (we find that plastic sandwich boxes are ideal). Approximately 100 mL of each of the following solution is required per gel.
2. Fixative: 50% (v/v) methanol and 5% (v/v) acetic acid in distilled water.
3. Distilled or deionized water.
4. Sensitizing solution: 0.02% (v/v) sodium thiosulfate in distilled water.
5. Silver solution: 0.1% (v/v) silver nitrate in distilled water.
6. Developer: 0.04% (v/v) formalin, 35% (v/v) formaldehyde, and 2% (w/v) sodium carbonate in distilled water.
7. After-staining fixative: 5% (v/v) acetic acid in distilled water.

3. Methods

3.1. Sample Preparation

The sample source and preparation need careful consideration in any proteomic study. For cancer studies, there are conflicting opinions regarding the use of whole-tumor samples, cell lines, and microdissected tumor samples. For a more comprehensive discussion of these issues, we refer readers to **refs. 9** and *11*.

We routinely use whole-tumor samples and cell lysate for our breast cancer proteome studies (*see* **Note 1**). It is methods relating to these samples that we discuss here. Sample preparation techniques are also given in Chapter 5.

For tumor tissues:

1. Wrap in foil and crush tissues snap frozen in liquid nitrogen between two heavy metal blocks (*see* **Note 2**).
2. Transfer minced tissue to a porcelain mortar precooled with liquid nitrogen and homogenize with a porcelain pestle to a fine powder. Scrape the powder into an Eppendorf tube containing 1 mL/100 mg tissue of lysis buffer and store on ice.

For cells:

1. Aspirate medium from cells. Wash with 5 mL of cold PBS three times, followed by one wash with cold 0.35 *M* sucrose solution, and aspirate dry.
2. Add 1 mL of lysis buffer, ensuring that the buffer bathes all the cells. Scrape cells into an Eppendorf tube and store on ice (*see* **Note 3**).
3. Homogenize samples on ice using a handheld Ultra-Turrax T8 (IKA-Labortechnik, Staufen, Germany) homogenizer for 5 min.
4. Microcentrifuge samples at 11,000g for 1 h at room temperature and retain supernatant. Determine the protein concentration of each of the samples using a Bio-Rad Bradford protein assay according to the manufacturer's instructions.
5. Remove excess lipid from the samples with a methanol/chloroform extraction *(12)*. Take 1 vol of sample and add 3 vol of distilled water and 4 vol of methanol. Mix well with a vortex mixer and centrifuge at 11,000g for 2 min. Add 2 vol of chloroform and vortex, then centrifuge at 11,000g for 2 min. Remove the upper and lower phases carefully with a syringe, retain the interphase material, and air-dry.
6. Resuspend interphase material in rehydration buffer ready for IEF.

3.2. Protein Quantification

The amount of protein required depends on the size of the IPG strips, the loading capacity of the gel, the defection method, and whether an analytical or preparative run is being performed. Typically, analytical gels in the large format are used with up to 1 mg of protein loading, whereas minigels are used with an order-of-magnitude-lower protein loading. For preparative runs, the loading capacity depends upon the abundance of the spot of interest.

Irrespective of the size of the IPG strip, an accurate comparison of proteins resolved by 2DE requires exact amounts of proteins to be loaded onto each of the IPG strips. There are a number of different protein quantification methods that can be used. One of the most important considerations is that many of the components of the IEF lysis buffer (e.g., urea, nonionic detergents) can interfere with the protein assay (*see* **Note 4**). The following method details the protein assay (a Bradford assay) that we regularly carry out using Bio-Rad dye concentrate.

1. Prepare a 5-mg/mL solution of BSA in IEF lysis buffer. Vortex until dissolved, and then centrifuge at $11,000g$ for 2 min to clear the solution. Simultaneously, centrifuge the samples to be assayed.
2. Prepare a solution of 0.1 M of HCl and make a 1:4 dilution of the dye concentrate with distilled water. **Table 1** details the recipe for the BSA standards.
3. The standard solutions are made up in plastic cuvets and mixed before the absorbance is read at 595 nm. To analyze samples, we usually mix together 10 μL of sample with 10 μL of 0.1 M HCl, 80 μL of distilled water, and 3.5 mL of dye solution. All standards and sample are duplicated and an average absorbance value taken.
4. Graph a standard curve and determine the protein concentration by interpolation.

3.3. Isoelectric Focusing

This method is for Amersham pH 3.0–10.0 NL IPG strips (both 7- and 18-cm size). For details regarding other IPG strips, please refer to **refs. 7 and 13**.

1. Remove IPG strips from freezer, peel off protective plastic backing, and allow the strips to defrost at room temperature for approx 10 min.
2. Pipet 30 μg of protein in 175 μL of rehydration buffer for the 7-cm IPG strips, and 100 μg of protein in 450 μL of rehydration buffer for the 18-cm IPG strips into a reswelling tray. Place the defrosted IPG strips gel side down onto the sample and ensure the IPG strips are not stuck to the bottom of the reswelling tray (*see* **Note 5**).
3. Cover the IPG strips with 2 mL of silicone oil per sample and leave to rehydrate at room temperature overnight.
4. The following day, precool IEF electrophoresis unit to 20°C (we use a Multitemp III thermostatic circulator). Remove strips from reswelling tray and place gel-side up onto a DryStrip (Amersham) aligner tray. Place DryStrip aligner tray into

Table 1
Recipe for Bovine Serum Albumin Standards

Protein concentration (μg)	0	5	10	20	40	50
BSA standard (μL)	0	1	2	4	8	10
Isoelectric focusing lysis buffer (μL)	10	9	8	6	2	0
0.1 *M* Hydrochloric acid (μL)	10	10	10	10	10	10
Distilled water (μL)	80	80	80	80	80	80
Dye solution (mL)	3.5	3.5	3.5	3.5	3.5	3.5

BSA, bovine serum albumin.

Table 2
Running Conditions
for Focus-Immobilized pH Gradient
Strips, Using an Appropriate Power Pack

7-cm IPG strips	18-cm IPG strips
0.05 mA per strip	0.05 mA per strip
3000 V	3000 V
11.5 kVh	60 kVh

IPG, immobilized pH gradient.

a tray and electrode holder and place onto the ceramic cooling block (held in place by first pouring a little silicone oil onto the ceramic block).

5. Soak IEF electrode strips (enough to cover the anode and cathode ends of the IPG strips) in distilled water and place one at the anode and one at the cathode end of the IPG strips. Place anode and cathode electrodes over IEF electrode strips and attach tray and electrode holder electrodes to IEF electrophoresis unit. Fill tray and electrode holder with silicone oil.

6. Focus IPG strips using appropriate power pack (e.g., EPS 3501, Amersham) using the running conditions listed in **Table 2** (*see* **Note 6**).

7. After focusing, place the IPG strips into plastic bags and freeze overnight at –80°C (*see* **Note 7**).

3.4. IPG Strip Equilibration

1. Before SDS-polyacrylamide gel electrophoresis (PAGE), the strips must equilibrated in order to saturate the strip with the SDS buffer system required for the second dimension.

2. Defrost IPG strips at room temperature. Place strips gel side up in DryStrip aligner tray and incubate in equilibration buffer 1 (2 mL per strip) for 15 min.

3. While strips are rehydrating, prepare a 1% (w/v) agarose solution for sealing the IPG strip onto the SDS-PAGE gels by dissolving 0.5 g of agarose in 50 mL of

Table 3
Recipe for Enough Resolving Gel
Solution to Make Two Minigels

Distilled water	5.25 mL
Resolving gel buffer	3.75 mL
30% Acrylamide	6.0 mL
APS	100 µL
TEMED	50 µL

APS, ammonium persulfate solution; TEMED, N,N,N',N'-tetramethylethylenediamine.

tank buffer on a heating magnetic stirrer. Add a little bromophenol to the solution. Keep agarose molten for use later.

4. Aspirate equilibration buffer 1 from DryStrip aligner tray and incubate in equilibration buffer 2 (2 mL per strip) for a further 15 min.
5. After incubation is complete aspirate off equilibration buffer 2 and wash the IPG strips in a little distilled water.

3.5. SDS-PAGE

1. If using 7-cm IPG strips, it is possible, while the strips are incubating in equilibration buffer 2, to prepare the SDS-PAGE gels. If 18-cm IPG strips are being used, SDS-PAGE gel preparation takes considerably longer, and the gels need to be prepared in advance (at least 24 h). The following methods are for 12% acrylamide gels, either 7- × 9-cm gels (for use with 7-cm IPG strips) cast in Bio-Rad Miniprotean III kits or 20- × 25-cm gels (for use with 18-cm IPG strips) cast using a Hoefer DALT system.

3.5.1. Minigels

1. Thoroughly clean glass plates with methanol, air-dry, and assemble. The recipe contained in **Table 3** is enough resolving gel solution to make two minigels.
2. Pour gel solution into assembled glass plates (leaving enough room at the top of the gel for the IPG strip) and overlay with water-saturated isobutanol (*see* **Note 8**). Leave gels to set.
3. Once the gels have set, tip off the saturated isobutanol and pipet some distilled water onto the top of the gel.
4. Gently pick up the IPG strip, using forceps, by grabbing the plastic backing at the cathode (pH 10.0) end of the strip. Place the pointed (pH 3.0) end of the strip towards the left-hand side of the gel. Let the IPG strip float gently down until it touches the top of the gel, and, if necessary, use a spatula to ensure contact with the top of the gel is complete.
5. Pour off the excess water and add a chunk of solidified molecular-weight marker at the pH 3.0 end of the IPG strip.

Table 4
Recipe for Acrylamide Stock Solution

Distilled water	750 mL
Resolving gel buffer	525 mL
30% Acrylamide solution	840 mL
10% SDS solution	21 mL
APS	10 mL
TEMED	301 μL

SDS, sodium dodecyl sulfate; APS, ammonium persulfate solution; TEMED, *N,N,N',N'*-tetramethylethylenediamine.

6. Seal the IPG strip onto the top of the minigel by adding (from the cathode end to the anode end of the strip) the previously prepared and molten 1% agarose (*see* **Note 9**).
7. Electrophorese gels for approx 2 h (or until dye front has reached the bottom of the gels) at 130 V.

3.5.2. Large-Format Gels

This procedure is for the preparation of 10 large gels.

1. Thoroughly clean hinged glass plates with methanol and air-dry.
2. Prepare 200 mL of displacing solution and make up the acrylamide stock solution (without SDS, APS, or TEMED) using the reagents listed in **Table 4**.
3. Degas the acrylamide stock solution for 2 h before use.
4. Load the gel caster with glass plates (hinged end placed vertically opposite the feeding tube), separator sheets and, if not using all the plates, filler blocks.
5. Add the SDS, APS, and TEMED to the acrylamide stock solution (*see* **Note 10**) and slowly pour the solution into the casting chamber using the feeding tube. Be careful not to add any air bubbles to the solution. Once pouring is complete, add displacing solution until it fills the V-well and sloped trough at the bottom of the caster (*see* **Note 11**).
6. Immediately add 750 μL of water-saturated isobutanol to the top of each gel and cover the gel caster with moist tissue and cling film.
7. Leave the gels to set overnight at 4°C.
8. The following day, prepare the tank buffer directly in an Hoefer DALT electrophoresis unit by adding 288 g of glycine, 60.5 g of Tris-HCl base, and 20 g of SDS to 20 L of distilled water in the central chamber. The pump attached to the electrophoresis unit can be turned on and should blow bubbles through the circulating flutes at the base of the tank (*see* **Note 12**). This will mix the buffer mixture.
9. After approx 2 h (or whenever the buffer components have dissolved), use a screwdriver to loosen the white plastic retaining screws on the exterior of the Hoefer DALT tank that hold the barrier combs in place. Raise or remove the two

barrier combs and mix the total Hoefer DALT water contents with the dissolved buffer components of the central chamber.

10. When the buffer is distributed in all chambers, replace the barrier combs to accommodate all of the gels (10 can be run at once). Set the temperature of the tank to 10°C, using a thermostatic circulator.

11. Tip off the saturated isobutanol from the top of the set gels and open the gel caster (*see* **Note 13**). Separate the gels and wipe the excess acrylamide from the surface of each gel, using a damp tissue. Pipet some distilled water onto the top of the gel.

12. Follow **steps 3–6** as for minigels.

13. Once the sealing agarose has completely set, the gels can be placed in the electrophoresis tank by taking one plate at a time (at the unhinged end) and dipping it into the tank buffer. The gels are placed between the grooves on the barrier combs with the IPG strip end of the gel placed towards the cathode.

14. Attach the electrodes of the DALT tank to a power pack and run the gels using the following conditions of 20 mA per gel and at a maximum 3000 V. The gel is run until the dye front is approx 1 cm from the bottom of the gel, which will take about 18 h.

3.6. Detecting Proteins Separated by 2DE

There are essentially two approaches to detect the proteins that have been separated by 2DE. The protein mixture can be either coupled to a tag, such as a fluorescent dye or radioactive tracer before the 2DE steps, or, alternatively, the protein can be detected in-gel after the sample has been separated by 2DE. We use post-2DE protein detection, but the method chosen is ultimately influenced by the image-capture facilities available and the level of sensitivity required. For post-2DE labeling of proteins, two main dye systems are most widely used, Coomassie brilliant blue and silver nitrate staining.

We routinely use silver staining, as kits for this procedure are available from various suppliers and the sensitivity of the detection (1–10 ng of protein) is greater than Coomassie staining (100 ng of protein). There has been some controversy regarding whether silver staining is compatible with mass spectrometry (MS) analysis, because this method requires the proteins to be treated with a strong oxidizing agent, which may lead to chemical modification. Another disadvantage with this method is that sensitizing pretreatments include the use of such reagents as glutaraldehyde, which may result in covalent modifications of the proteins. The latter problem can be overcome by omitting glutaraldehyde from the staining procedure. However, recent publications have detected no problems in analyzing proteins by MS after silver staining and with glutaraldehyde use *(14)*.

The following protocol is based on a number of well-established protocols *(15,16)* and glutaraldehyde is not used (50 mL of each solution is used per minigel, and 200 mL of each solution is used per large-format gel):

1. Fix gel in 50% methanol and 5% acetic acid in distilled water for 20 min at room temperature.
2. Pour off fixing solution and wash gel in distilled water for 10 min.
3. Pour off distilled water and add the sensitizing solution (0.02% sodium thiosulfate in distilled water). Incubate for 1 min.
4. Wash the gel in distilled water (two washes of 1 min each).
5. Pour off distilled water and add 0.1% silver nitrate and incubate for 20 min at 4°C.
6. Wash gel in distilled water (two washes of 1 min each).
7. Develop silver stain by incubating gel in 35 μL of 0.04% formalin, 35% formaldehyde, and 2% sodium carbonate in distilled water. Replace developer as it yellows with fresh developing solution.
8. When proteins are fully developed (*see* **Note 14** and **Fig. 1**), wash the gel in 5% acetic acid in distilled water for 1 min. The gel can be stored in 1% acetic acid for up to 6 mo.

3.7. Data Analysis/Protein Identification

The 2DE-separated proteins are detected by scanning densitometry and manipulated in an image analysis system. Proteins are identified as "landmarks" in each of the gels, and a set of gels produced during a given series of experiments is compared with one another in a match set. Various suppliers produce 2DE analysis systems, and these are indispensable in determining which proteins are altered in the tissue/cellular specimen of interest.

Proteins are detected after separation by 2DE using, most commonly, the technique of MS (*see* **Note 15**). Two main MS methods are used, either matrix-assisted laser desorption/ionization time-of-flight MS or electrospray ionization tandem MS. The reader is referred to **refs. *17*** and ***18*** for further details on this specialist analytical tool.

4. Notes

1. For analysis of a tissue proteome, it is essential that the cells of interest be contained within the tissue. We routinely cut cryostat sections from each of our tissue samples and assess the cells in the specimen before we prepare any samples for separation by 2DE.
2. It is advisable to encase the tissue specimen in two layers of foil, in case the outer layer shatters during the crushing process.
3. We prefer to scrape the cells from the tissue culture flask rather than trypsinize the cells, as the proteolysis may lead to degradation of cell surface glycoproteins.
4. It is advisable to carry out the protein assay at room temperature to prevent the carbamylation of proteins because of the high concentrations of urea in the lysis buffer.
5. A protein sample can be applied to the strip either via the rehydration buffer (as described here) or a sample cup. The method of protein loading depends on the

pH 3.0   ——————————————————————→   pH 10.0

High Mr

Low Mr

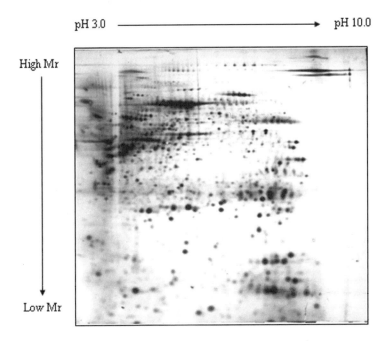

Fig. 1. A large-format (20 × 25 cm) sodium dodecyl sulfate-polyacrylamide gel electrophoresis gel of two-dimensional electrophoresis separated proteins from a breast cancer sample. These proteins were detected with a silver stain.

type of IPG strips used. For example, for pH 6.0–11.0 IPG strips, it is recommended that the protein sample be loaded onto the strip using a sample cup. However, for pH 3.0–10.0 NL IPG strips, protein loading via the rehydration step is considered preferable, as more dilute samples can be loaded, it is technically simpler, and because there is no discrete application point the formation of precipitates at this point is minimized.

6. It is advisable to increase gradually the voltage to ensure that the milliamperes do not exceed the recommended maximum of 0.05 mA per strip. IEF is conducted at very high voltages and very low currents because of the ionic strength within the IPG strips. A low initial voltage will minimize protein aggregation.

7. Typically, proteins that have been separated by IEF can be stored at –80°C for up to 1 mo and then used for the second-dimensional SDS-PAGE analysis.

8. Overlaying the SDS-PAGE with water-saturated isobutanol will ensure that an even surface at the top of the gel is produced. This is particularly important for 2DE gels where a stacking gel is not generally used.

9. Molten agarose is applied from the cathode to anode end of the strip (or the end away from the molecular-weight marker to the molecular-weight marker) to ensure that the molecular-weight marker is not spread across the top of the whole gel. This would ultimately interfere with sample protein detection.

10. After the addition of the APS and TEMED, there is approx 10 min before the gel sets, in which to pour the acrylamide solution into the gel caster. Therefore, the gel caster must be prepared in advance.

11. As the gels polymerize, they will contract, and the acrylamide solution present between the V-well and the bottom of the glass plates will be sucked up into the glass plates.

12. If the pump does not "catch," then there is an air lock within the pump. Quickly turn the pump off and wait for the air bubble to come out through the bypass tubing. Restart the pump. This may have to be done a few times.

13. The gel caster must be opened near a sink to make sure that the displacing solution does not run everywhere.

14. It is up to the researcher to decide when proteins stained using silver nitrate are fully developed; this will often depend on the protein samples used. We have found that protein development will usually take between 5 and 10 min. It is important not to overstain the proteins (resulting in a high background) and when analyzing more than one gel in any given experiment, to develop all gels for the same amount of time.

15. MS is a very sensitive method and as such, the most important consideration for any 2DE study is cleanliness. The importance of this cannot be underestimated. This is to avoid any contaminating proteins, the most common of which is human keratin from hair, skin cells, etc. It is advisable when carrying out any of the methods described in this chapter to wear the appropriate protective clothing, e.g., a nonshedding lab coat, hair net, and powder-free gloves.

References

1. Wilkins, M. R., Sanchez, J. C., Gooley, A. A., et al. (1996) Progress with proteome projects: why all proteins expressed by a genome should be identified and how to do it. *Biotechnol. Genet.c Eng. Rev.* **13**, 19–50.

2. Zuo, X., Echan, L., Hembach, P., et al. (2001) Towards global analysis of mammalian proteomes using sample prefractionation prior to narrow pH range two-dimensional gels and using one-dimensional gels for insoluble and large proteins. *Electrophoresis* **22**, 1603–1615.

3. Czerwenka, K. F., Manavi, M., Hosmann, J., et al. (2001) Comparative analysis of two-dimensional protein patterns in malignant and normal human breast tissue. *Cancer Detect. Prev.* **25**, 268–279.

4. Pucci-Minafra, I., Fontana, S., Cancemi, P., Basirico, L., Caricato, S., and Minafra, S. (2002) A contribution to breast cancer cell proteomics: detection of new sequences. *Proteomics* **2**, 919–927.

5. Bini, L., Magi, B., Marzocchi, B., et al. (1997) Protein expression profiles in human breast ductal carcinoma and histologically normal tissue. *Electrophoresis* **18**, 2832–2841.

6. Williams, K., Chubb, C., Huberman, E., and Giometti, C. S. (1998) Analysis of differential protein expression in normal and neoplastic human breast epithelial cell lines. *Electrophoresis* **19**, 333–343.

7. Gorg, A., Obermaier, C., Boguth, G., et al. (2000) The current state of two-dimensional electrophoresis with immobilised pH gradients. *Electrophoresis* **21,** 1037–1053.

8. Dwek, M. V. and Rawlings, S. L. (2002) Current perspectives in cancer proteomics. *Mol. Biotechnol.* **22,** 139–152.

9. Franzen, B., Linder, S., Okuzawa, K., Kato, H., and Auer, G. (1993) Nonenzymatic extraction of cells from clinical tumour material for analysis of gene expression by two-dimensional polyacrylamide gel electrophoresis. *Electrophoresis* **14,** 1045–1053.

10. Herbert, B. (1999) Advances in protein solubilisation for two-dimensional electrophoresis. *Electrophoresis* **20,** 660–663.

11. Banks, R. E., Dunn, M. J., Forbes, M. A., et al. (1999) The potential use of laser capture microdissection to selectively obtain distinct populations of cells for proteomic analysis: preliminary findings. *Electrophoresis* **20,** 689–700.

12. Wessel, D. and Flugge, U. I. (1984) A method for the quantitative recovery of proteins in dilute solution in the presence of detergents and lipids. *Anal. Biochem.* **138,** 141–143.

13. Hoving, S., Gerrits, B., Voshol, H., Muller, D., Roberts, R. C., and van Oostrum, J. (2002) Preparative two-dimensional gel elctrophoresis at alkaline pH using narrow-range immobilised pH gradients. *Proteomics* **2,** 127–134.

14. Schevchenko, A., Wilm, M., Vorm, O., and Mann, M. (1996) Mass spectrometric sequencing of proteins from silver stained polyacrylamide gels. *Anal. Biochem.* **68,** 850–858.

15. Rabilloud, T., Carpentier, G., and Tarroux P. (1988) Improvement and simplification of low background silver staining of proteins by using sodium dithionate. *Electrophoresis* **9,** 288–291.

16. Swain, M. and Ross, N. W. (1995) A silver stain protocol for proteins yielding high resolution and transparent background in sodium dodecyl sulfate polyacrylamide gels. *Electrophoresis* **16,** 948–951.

17. Gygi, S. P. and Aebersold, R. (2000) Mass spectrometry and proteomics. *Curr. Opin. Chem. Biol.* **4,** 489–494.

18. Aebersold, R. and Goodlett, D. R. (2001) Mass spectrometry in proteomics. *Chem. Rev.* **101,** 269–295.

19

Procedures for the Quantitative Protein Determination of Urokinase and Its Inhibitor, PAI-1, in Human Breast Cancer Tissue Extracts by ELISA

Manfred Schmitt, Alexandra S. Sturmheit, Anita Welk, Christel Schnelldorfer, and Nadia Harbeck

Summary

The determination of the protein content of urokinase-type plasminogen activator (uPA) and its inhibitor, PAI-1, in breast cancer tissue extracts is used clinically to identify patients at risk to experience disease recurrence (metastasis) or early death. The serine protease uPA, in concert with its inhibitor PAI-1, promotes tumor cell adhesion, migration, and proliferation, as well as extracellular matrix degradation and, thus, facilitates tumor cell invasion and metastasis. The various technical steps to recover uPA and PAI-1 protein from archived breast cancer tissues and to quantitatively determine uPA and PAI-1 protein content in tumor tissue extracts by enzyme-linked immunosorbent assay (ELISA) are described in detail. The technical steps involved require fresh-frozen breast cancer tissue, a dismembrator machine (ball mill) to pulverize the tissue in the frozen state, detergent (Triton X-100) containing Tris-buffered saline to extract uPA and PAI-1 from the pulverized breast cancer tissue, an ultracentrifuge to separate the detergent fraction from cellular debris, uPA and PAI-1 ELISA kits, protein determination reagents, and a 96-well spectrophotometer (ELISA reader) to assess uPA, PAI-1, and total protein in the detergent extract. The uPA/PAI-1 ELISAs and the protein determination format described are robust and highly sensitive. In addition to the macromethod of tissue disintegration, we present a simple but sensitive micro-extraction procedure using cryostat sections or core biopsies as the source of breast cancer tissue. Such a technique allows rapid and quantitative determination of uPA and PAI-1, even in small breast cancer specimens.

Key Words: Urokinase; uPA; PAI-1; breast cancer; tissue extract; ELISA; prognosis.

1. Introduction

Tumor cell migration into the extracellular matrix surrounding the primary tumor tissue, as well as intra- and extravasation of malignant cells into and from blood and/or lymph vessels, are multistep processes involved in tumor

From: *Methods in Molecular Medicine, Vol. 120: Breast Cancer Research Protocols*
Edited by: S. A. Brooks and A. L. Harris © Humana Press Inc., Totowa, NJ

cell dissemination and metastasis *(1,2)*. Local proteolysis is a distinctive feature in tumor cell spread and is regulated by complex interactions between various extra- and intracellular proteases and their inhibitors. Key players in the proteolytic scenario are cathepsins, matrix metalloproteinases, and serine proteases of the plasminogen activation system *(1–5)*. The serine proteases plasmin and urokinase-type plasminogen activator (uPA), the uPA receptor (CD87), and the plasminogen activator inhibitor (PAI) type-1 are part of the plasminogen-activation system involved in cancer cell adherence to the extracellular matrix, tumor cell migration, and proliferation *(1,6)*.

Jänicke et al. first demonstrated that determination of the protein content of uPA and PAI-1 in primary breast cancer tumor tissue extracts by enzyme-labeled immunosorbent assay (ELISA) yields strong prognostic information regarding disease-free and overall survival *(7–10)*. In tumors, uPA is produced in its precursor form, pro-uPA, by various normal and cancer cells and is activated by proteases, such as cathepsin B and L, plasmin, kallikreins, or tryptase, to yield enzymatically active uPA *(1,4,5,11)*. In turn, uPA converts the zymogen plasminogen to the active serine protease plasmin, thus facilitating extracellular matrix degradation *(1,5,12)*.

The majority of clinically relevant results on uPA and PAI-1 relating to breast cancer prognosis and response to therapy have been obtained through ELISA *(5,13,14)* for both node-negative and node-positive breast cancer patients *(10,15–21)*. Determination of uPA and PAI-1 in breast cancer tissue extracts allows identification of low-risk, node-negative breast cancer patients who might be spared the burden of adjuvant systemic therapy *(13)*. In addition to their prognostic impact, uPA and PAI-1 are also of predictive value concerning response to adjuvant systemic therapy *(14,22,23)*.

High levels of uPA and/or PAI-1 have been found to be statistically significant indicators of poor patient prognosis, not only in breast cancer, but also in most other solid malignant tumors, such as gastric cancer *(24–26)*, colorectal cancer *(27–29)*, adenocarcinoma of the esophagus *(30)*, ovarian carcinoma *(31,32)*, carcinoma of the cervix uteri *(33)*, renal cell carcinoma *(34)*, prostate cancer *(35)*, and lung cancer *(36,37)*.

The uPA/PAI-1 system has evolved as an important target for cancer therapy *(1,5,38)*. In experimental cancer cell-bearing animals, cell invasion and metastasis is reduced by the action of a synthetic protease inhibitor (e.g., WX-UK1; Wilex AG, Munich, Germany) directed to the proteolytic activity of uPA and plasmin *(1,39–42)*. These results demonstrate the usefulness of synthetic inhibitors as a novel type of cancer therapeutics. A phase II clinical trial involving patients with advanced cancer and receiving this novel drug has been initiated *(43)*.

The various technical steps to recover uPA and PAI-1 protein from archived fresh-frozen breast cancer tissues and to quantitatively determine uPA and PAI-1 protein content in tumor tissue extracts by ELISA are described in detail in this chapter. The technical steps involved require the following:

1. 100–300 mg of frozen breast cancer tissue.
2. A dismembrator machine (ball mill) to pulverize the tissue in the frozen state.
3. Detergent (Triton X-100) containing Tris-HCl-buffered saline to extract uPA and PAI-1 from the pulverized breast cancer tissue.
4. An ultracentrifuge to separate the detergent fraction from cellular debris.
5. uPA and PAI-1 ELISA kits.
6. Protein-determination reagents.
7. 96-Well spectrophotometer (ELISA reader) to assess uPA and PAI-1.

uPA and PAI-1 content is expressed as nanogram of analyte per milligram of protein. The uPA/PAI-1 ELISA (American Diagnostica, Stamford, CT) and the bicinchoninic acid (BCA) protein determination format (Pierce, Rockville, IL) are very robust, highly sensitive, and the results obtained are highly reproducible. In addition, we present a simple but sensitive microextraction procedure using cryostat sections or core biopsies as the source of breast cancer tissue. Such a technique allows rapid and reproducible quantitative determination of uPA and PAI-1, even in small breast cancer specimens. Chapter 29 describes several techniques by which the effects of the urokinase system on adhesion, proliferation, migration, and signal transduction events can be analyzed.

2. Materials
2.1. Freezing and Storing Breast Cancer Tissue Specimens

1. Fresh breast cancer tissue specimen(s).
2. Liquid nitrogen.
3. 1-mL Cryovials (Nunc, Wiesbaden, Germany; **Fig. 1**).
4. Liquid nitrogen tank or –80°C freezer with storage system (**Fig. 2**).
5. Forceps.
6. Scalpel.
7. Latex or plastic gloves.
8. Protective eyewear.
9. Safety gloves to handle devices containing liquid nitrogen.

2.2. Pulverization and Extraction of Deep-Frozen Breast Cancer Tissue Specimens (Macromethod)

1. Deep-frozen breast cancer tissue specimen(s) (100–300 mg each).
2. Microscale.

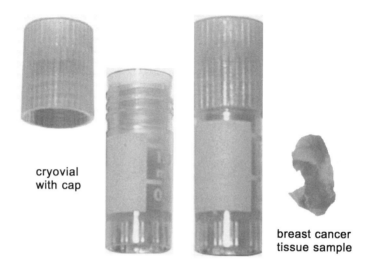

cryovial
with cap

breast cancer
tissue sample

Fig. 1. 1-mL Cryovial plus cap with silicon ring (inside the cap). The breast cancer sample is placed into this vial, closed, and then snap-frozen in liquid nitrogen.

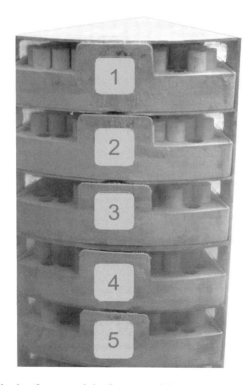

Fig. 2. Storage device for cryovials. Storage of the cryovials in holders and drawers placed into a liquid nitrogen tank is highly recommended. Alternatively, snap-frozen cryovials can be stored at –80°C in a deep freezer.

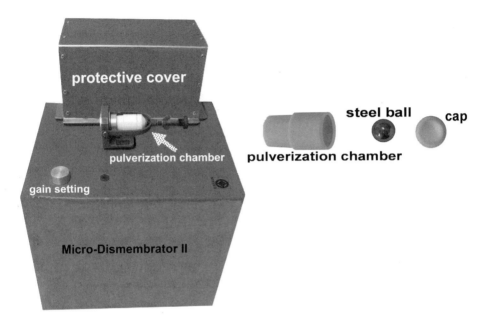

Fig. 3. Microdismembrator plus sample flask to be used for the macromethod of tissue disintegration method. The microdismembrator (ball mill), left, holds a pre-cooled Teflon® sample flask (pulverization chamber) into which the deep-frozen breast cancer tissue is placed and crushed by use of a grinding steel ball. The sample flask is placed and fastened into the holder of the ball mill and then the holder is set in motion (maximum speed, 30 s). As a result, a tissue powder is formed which is taken out of the sample flask by use of a spatula.

3. Spatula.
4. Forceps.
5. Microdismembrator machine, consisting of a ball mill with sample flask (pulverization device) made of Teflon® plus a grinding steel ball (B. Braun Melsungen, Melsungen, Germany; **Fig. 3**).
6. Tris-buffered saline (TBS), containing 0.1 M Tris base and 0.125 M NaCl, adjusted to pH 8.5 with HCl.
7. Tissue extraction buffer: 1% Triton X-100 (Sigma-Aldrich, Munich, Germany) in TBS.
8. Pipets and tips.
9. 2-mL Test tubes.
10. Rocking table to gently rotate the test tubes containing the breast cancer tissue suspended in TBS–1% Triton X-100.
11. Refrigerator or cold room.
12. Ultracentrifuge plus rotor.
13. Ultracentrifuge tubes.

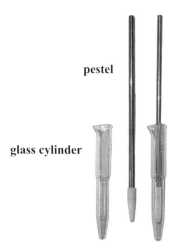

pestel

glass cylinder

Fig. 4. Potter-Elvehjem tissue homogenizer consisting of a glass cylinder with Teflon® pestle to be used for the microtissue disintegration method. TBS-Triton X-100 buffer containing the breast cancer tissue pieces is placed into the glass cylinder and then the pestle is inserted into the cylinder. Several strokes up and down will crush the tissue pieces between the wall of the glass cylinder and the Teflon pestle. Subsequent incubation (2 h at 4°C) will release urokinase-type plasminogen activator and plasminogen activator inhibitor type-1 protein into the buffer fluid.

14. 1-mL Cryovials (Nunc).
15. Liquid nitrogen.
16. Liquid nitrogen tank or –80°C freezer with storage system.
17. Latex or plastic gloves.
18. Protective eyewear.
19. Safety gloves to handle devices containing liquid nitrogen.

2.3. Extraction of Fresh or Deep-Frozen Breast Cancer Tissue Specimens (Micromethod)

1. Fresh or thawed breast cancer tissue specimen(s) (<100 mg each) or 5–10 90-µm-thick cryosections cut from frozen breast cancer tissue specimen(s) or one to three core biopsies (fresh or thawed).
2. Microscale.
3. Spatula.
4. Forceps.
5. Disintegration device (Potter-Elvehjem tissue homogenizer consisting of glass cylinder with Teflon pestle [plunger], Bellco Glass,Vineland, NJ; **Fig. 4**).
6. Ice bath.
7. TBS, containing 0.1 M Tris base and 0.125 M NaCl, adjusted to pH 8.5 with HCl.
8. Tissue extraction buffer: 1% Triton X-100 (Sigma-Aldrich) in TBS.

9. Pipets and tips.
10. 1-mL Test tubes.
11. Rocking table to gently rotate the test tubes containing the breast cancer tissue suspended in TBS–1% Triton X-100.
12. Refrigerator or cold room.
13. Ultracentrifuge plus rotor.
14. Ultracentrifuge tubes.
15. 1-mL Cryovials (Nunc).
16. Liquid nitrogen.
17. Liquid nitrogen tank or –80°C freezer with storage system.
18. Latex or plastic gloves.
19. Protective eyewear.
20. Safety gloves to handle liquid nitrogen-containing devices.

2.4. Determination of uPA Protein in Breast Cancer Tissue Extracts by ELISA

1. ELISA kit. Imubind uPA ELISA kit no. 894 (American Diagnostica), containing:
   a. 12 × 8-Well precoated microtest strips (with catching antibody to uPA).
   b. Strip holder and lid.
   c. Six vials of uPA standards (0, 0.1, 0.25, 0.5, 0.75, and 1.0 ng of pro-uPA), lyophilized.
   d. Two vials of biotinylated detection antibody to uPA (lyophilized).
   e. One vial of streptavidin-horseradish peroxidase (SHP) conjugate.
   f. One vial of SHP diluent (lyophilized).
   g. One vial of peroxidase substrate containing perborate/3,3',5,5'-tetramethyl-benzidine (TMB).
   h. One vial nonionic detergent Triton X-100 (25%) to be added to phosphate-buffered saline (PBS) to prepare wash buffer.
   i. Two packets PBS, pH 7.4.
2. Breast cancer tissue extracts.
3. Control samples (tissue extracts with previously determined amount of uPA protein).
4. Distilled H_2O.
5. 0.5 N H_2SO_4.
6. TBS–1% bovine serum albumin (BSA) solution.
7. TBS, containing 0.1 M Tris base and 0.125 M NaCl, adjusted to pH 8.5 with HCl.
8. Pipets with tips.
9. 96-Well microtiter plate reader with filter set to 450 nm.
10. Computer for data storage and data analysis.
11. Latex or plastic gloves.

2.5. Determination of PAI-1 Protein in Breast Cancer Tissue Extracts by ELISA

1. ELISA kit. Imubind PAI-1 ELISA kit (no. 821, American Diagnostica), containing:
   a. 12 × 8-Well precoated microtest strips (with catching antibody to PAI-1).
   b. Strip holder and lid.

   c. Six vials of PAI-1 standards (0, 1.0, 2.5, 5.0, 7.5, and 10.0 ng of PAI-1), lyophilized.

   d. Two vials of biotinylated detection antibody to PAI-1 (lyophilized).

   e. One vial of SHP conjugate.

   f. One vial of SHP diluent (lyophilized).

   g. One vial of peroxidase substrate containing perborate/TMB.

   h. One vial of nonionic detergent Triton X-100 (25%) to be added to PBS to prepare wash buffer.

   i. Two packets of PBS, pH 7.4.

2. Breast cancer tissue extracts.
3. Control samples (tissue extracts with previously determined amount of PAI-1 protein).
4. Distilled H_2O.
5. 0.5 N H_2SO_4.
6. TBS–1% BSA solution.
7. TBS, containing 0.1 M Tris base and 0.125 M of NaCl, adjusted to pH 8.5 with HCl.
8. Pipets with tips.
9. 96-Well microtiter plate reader with filter set to 450 nm.
10. Computer for data storage and data analysis.
11. Latex or plastic gloves.

2.6. Determination of Protein Content in Breast Cancer Tissue Extracts by the BCA-Microtiter Plate Format

1. Breast cancer tissue extracts.
2. Control samples (tissue extracts with previously determined amount of protein, BSA control samples).
3. TBS (pH 8.5) plus 0.1% Triton X-100 and 0.05% Tween-20 for dilution of samples, controls, and standards.
4. Polystyrene 96-well microtiter plate (Nunc).
5. Pipets with tips.
6. 96-Well microtiter plate reader with filter set to 540 nm.
7. Computer for data storage and data analysis.
8. Latex or plastic gloves.
9. BCA protein assay reagent kit (no. 23225, Pierce) containing:.

   a. BCA reagent A (containing sodium carbonate, sodium bicarbonate, BCA, and sodium tartrate, in 0.1 M sodium hydroxide).

   b. BCA reagent B (containing 4% cupric acid).

   c. Albumin standard ampules (containing 2 mg/mL of BSA in 0.9% saline plus 0.05% sodium azide).

3. Methods

3.1. Tissue Disintegration and Extraction (Macromethod)

1. Provide 100–300 mg of deep frozen tissue (e.g., from liquid nitrogen tank).
2. Transfer the still-frozen tissue block into a precooled (in liquid nitrogen) Teflon sample flask containing a grinding steel ball.
3. Place the still-cool Teflon device into the microdismembrator (ball mill).
4. Set to maximum speed for 30 s to pulverize the still-frozen tissue block.
5. Transfer the still-frozen powder into a test tube.
6. Add 2 mL of cold (4°C) TBS containing 1% Triton X-100.
7. Gently suspend the powder and then rotate the tube for approx 16 h at 4°C.
8. Transfer tissue suspension into an ultracentrifuge tube.
9. Centrifuge at 100,000g for 1 h at 4°C to separate soluble fraction from debris.
10. Recover clear supernatant, discard any lipid layer (at the top), and keep debris for other analyses.
11. Place 50-µL aliquots of supernatant into 1-mL cryovials and store in liquid nitrogen until required.

3.2. Tissue Disintegration and Extraction (Micromethod)

1. Provide one to three breast tissue core biopsies or 5–10 90-µm-thick cryosections of a frozen breast cancer tissue block (how many depends on the size of the tissue block), or less than 100 mg fresh or thawed breast cancer tissue. Keep sections below and above these sections for hematoxylin and eosin staining (in case of cryostat sections).
2. Transfer tissue, sections, or core biopsies into 1-mL Potter-Elvehjem glass cylinder device.
3. Suspend in 200 µL of cold (4°C) TBS containing 1% Triton X-100.
4. By use of this hand-held homogenizer, crush the sample between the cylinder wall and the pestle using about 10 strokes while moving the pestle up and down.
5. Transfer tissue suspension to 1-mL test tube.
6. Gently rotate the tube for about 2 h at 4°C.
7. Transfer suspension to ultracentrifuge tube and centrifuge at 100,000g for 1 h at 4°C to separate soluble fraction from tissue debris.
8. Recover the clear supernatant, discard any lipid layer (at the top), and keep debris for other analyses.
9. Place 10-µL aliquots of supernatant into 1-mL cryovials and store in liquid nitrogen until use.

3.3. Determination of uPA/PAI-1 Protein in Breast Cancer Tissue Extracts by ELISA

Both the uPA and the PAI-1 ELISA kit employ unconjugated antibodies against human uPA and PAI-1, respectively, as the capture antibodies. These antibodies are attached by adsorption to the inner walls of a 96-well microtiter plate, followed by lyophilization. Twelve 8-well strips (96 wells) and a mount-

Std = **Standard provided with the kit to construct standard curve (uPA / PAI-1 / protein)**

Ctr = **Control sample to assure performance of the kit (not provided)**

BE = **breast cancer tissue extract (patient sample)**

Blanks: A1 – H1
Standards: A2 – F2, A3 – F3
Controls: G2 – H3
Breast cancer tissue extracts: A4 – H12

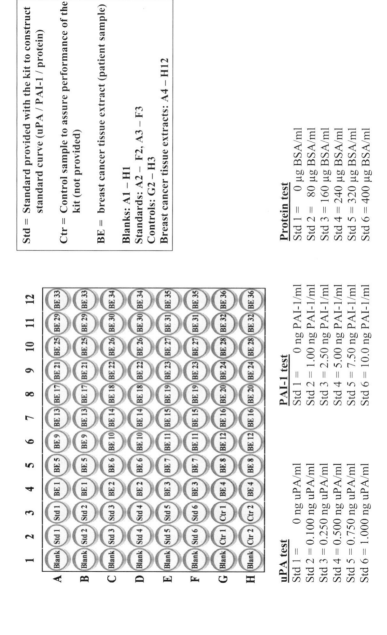

uPA test
Std 1 =   0 ng uPA/ml
Std 2 = 0.100 ng uPA/ml
Std 3 = 0.250 ng uPA/ml
Std 4 = 0.500 ng uPA/ml
Std 5 = 0.750 ng uPA/ml
Std 6 = 1.000 ng uPA/ml

PAI-1 test
Std 1 =   0 ng PAI-1/ml
Std 2 = 1.00 ng PAI-1/ml
Std 3 = 2.50 ng PAI-1/ml
Std 4 = 5.00 ng PAI-1/ml
Std 5 = 7.50 ng PAI-1/ml
Std 6 = 10.0 ng PAI-1/ml

Protein test
Std 1 =   0 µg BSA/ml
Std 2 =   80 µg BSA/ml
Std 3 = 160 µg BSA/ml
Std 4 = 240 µg BSA/ml
Std 5 = 320 µg BSA/ml
Std 6 = 400 µg BSA/ml

Fig. 5. Suggested distribution of blanks, standards, controls, and samples using all 96 wells of a microtiter plate. **Note:** Row 1 is filled with blanks (no standard, control, or sample but dilution buffer added instead). Perform measurements in duplicate.

254

ing frame (holder) are supplied with each kit. Incubate samples, controls, and standards, respectively, in the precoated microtiter plate wells and bound uPA/ PAI-1 is detected by a biotinylated second antibody to either uPA or PAI-1. Addition of horseradish peroxidase (HRP)-conjugated streptavidin to the wells completes the formation of the antibody–enzyme detection complex. Addition of perborate/TMB substrate solution to this antibody–enzyme complex creates a blue color as a measure of HRP activity. The reaction is stopped by addition of sulfuric acid. With the addition of the acid, the color changes from blue to yellow. Solution absorbances are measured at 450 nm in a 96-well microtiter plate spectrophotometer (ELISA reader). The absorption values are compared with those of the uPA and PAI-1 standard curve, respectively (*see* **Fig. 6**).

3.3.1. uPA ELISA

1. Preparation of uPA standard solutions. Add 1 mL of distilled H_2O to each of the 0.1-, 0.25-, 0.5-, 0.75-, and 1-ng uPA standard vials provided with the kit. Agitate gently for 3 min but do not shake.
2. Preparation of biotinylated uPA-detection antibody solution. Add 5.5 mL of distilled H_2O to the antibody-containing vial provided with the kit. Agitate gently for 3 min but do not shake.
3. Preparation of SHP conjugate solution. Add 20 mL distilled H_2O to enzyme diluent vial provided with the kit. Remove 12 mL and mix with 12 µL SHP conjugate provided with the kit.
4. Preparation of sample dilution buffer. Add 200 mg of BSA (not provided) to 20 mL of PBS-0.1% Triton X-100 to yield a 1% BSA solution.
5. Preparation of wash buffer. Add 1 mL of Triton X-100 to 1 L of PBS to yield PBS–0.1% Triton X-100.
6. Preparation of substrate solution. Premixed perborate/TMB solution is provided with the kit.
7. Preparation of enzyme reaction stop solution: 0.5 N H_2SO_4.

3.3.2. PAI-1 ELISA

1. Preparation of PAI-1 standard solutions. Add 1 mL of distilled H_2O to each of the 1-, 2.5-, 5-, 7.5-, and 10-ng PAI-1 standard vials provided with the kit. Agitate gently for 3 min but do not shake.
2. Preparation of PAI-1 detection antibody solution. Add 5.5 mL of distilled H_2O to the biotinylated antibody-containing vial provided with the kit. Agitate gently for 3 min but do not shake.
3. Preparation of SHP conjugate solution. Add 20 mL of distilled H_2O to enzyme diluent vial provided with the kit. Remove 12 mL and mix with 12 µL SHP conjugate provided with the kit.
4. Preparation of sample dilution buffer. Add 200 g of BSA (not provided) to 20 mL of PBS–0.1% Triton X-100 to yield a 1% BSA solution.

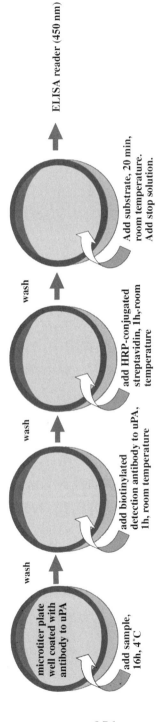

Fig. 6. Outline of the various steps of the urokinase-type plasminogen activator enzyme-labeled immunosorbent assay (ELISA). The same procedure applies to the plasminogen activator inhibitor type-1 ELISA.

microtiter plate well coated with antibody to uPA

add sample, 16h, 4°C

wash

add biotinylated detection antibody to uPA, 1h, room temperature

wash

add HRP-conjugated streptavidin, 1h, room temperature

wash

Add substrate, 20 min, room temperature. Add stop solution.

ELISA reader (450 nm)

5. Preparation of wash buffer. Add 1 mL Triton X-100 to 1 Lr of PBS to yield PBS–0.1% Triton X-100.
6. Preparation of substrate solution. Premixed perborate/TMB solution is provided with the kit.
7. Preparation of enzyme reaction stop solution: 0.5 N H_2SO_4.

3.3.3. Assay Procedure (uPA and PAI-1 ELISA) (*Figs. 5* and *6*)

1. Add 100 µL of standard, control, or sample (diluted in PBS-1% BSA) to microtiter plate well.
2. All samples should be set up in duplicate.
3. Cover plate with lid and incubate overnight at 4°C in a humid chamber.
4. Wash wells four times with wash buffer.
5. Add 100 µL of biotinylated detection antibody to each well.
6. Cover plate with lid and incubate for 1 h at room temperature.
7. Wash wells four times with wash buffer.
8. Add 12 µL of SHP conjugate to 12 mL of enzyme conjugate diluent (provided with the kit).
9. Add 100 µL of this solution to each well.
10. Cover plate with lid and incubate for 1 h at room temperature.
11. Wash wells four times with wash buffer.
12. Add 100 µL of wash solution to each well.
13. Cover plate with lid and place it in the dark.
14. Incubate for 20 min at room temperature; a blue color will develop.
15. Stop the HRP reaction by adding 50 µL of 0.5 N H_2SO_4.
16. The blue solution color will turn yellow.
17. Read absorbances within 30 min on a microtiter plate reader at a wavelength of 450 nm.
18. Deduct the background average of the blanks from the standards and sample readings.
19. Construct standard curve by plotting the mean absorbance value calculated for each uPA/PAI-1 standard vs the corresponding uPA/PAI-1 concentration (**Fig. 7**).
20. Calculate the uPA/PAI-1 concentrations in the test samples by use of this standard curve.
21. Multiply result by dilution factor (e.g., if diluted 1:20, multiply by 20).

3.4. Determination of Protein Content in Breast Cancer Tissue Extracts by the BCA Protein Kit

The Pierce BCA protein assay is a detergent compatible formulation based on BCA for the determination and quantification of protein. This method combines the reduction of Cu^{2+} to Cu^+ by protein in an alkaline medium, with the highly sensitive and selective colorimetric detection of the cuprous cation using a unique reagent containing BCA. A purple color will develop.

1. Mix 20 mL of reagent A with 400 µL of reagent B to generate reagent mix AB.
2. Add 200 µL of reagent mix AB to each well of a 96-well microtiter plate.

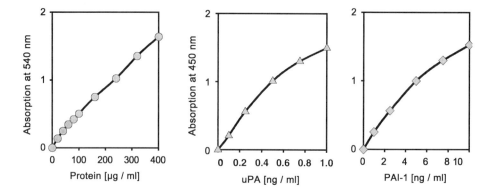

Fig. 7. Determination of protein, urokinase-type plasminogen activator (uPA), and plasminogen activator inhibitor type-1 (PAI-1). Typical standard curves are shown to demonstrate the sensitivity range and performance of 96-well microtiter plate assays for uPA, PAI-1, and protein. Commercially available, quality-assured enzyme-labeled immunosorbent assay test kits for uPA and PAI-1 (Imubind no. 894 and Imubind no. 821; American Diagnostica, Stamford, CT), and the bicinchoninic acid protein assay (Pierce, Rockville, IL) were employed.

3. Add 50 µL of standard (0–400 µg of BSA/mL), control sample, or test sample to each well (*see* **Fig. 5**).
4. Dilute samples with TBS (pH 8.5) plus 0.1% Triton X-100 and 0.05% Tween-20.
5. All samples should be set up in duplicates (*see* **Fig. 5**).
6. Cover plate with lid and incubate it overnight at room temperature, alternatively for 30 min at 37°C.
7. A purple color will develop.
8. Measure absorbance at 540 nm in a 96-well microtiter plate reader.
9. Deduct the background average of the blanks from the standards and sample readings.
10. Construct standard curve by plotting the mean absorbance value calculated for each protein standard vs the corresponding protein concentration (*see* **Fig. 7**).
11. Calculate the protein concentrations in the test samples by use of this standard curve.
12. Multiply result by dilution factor (e.g., if diluted 1:20, multiply by 20).

4. Notes

1. Macromethod needs a deep-frozen tissue block.
2. The micromethod can be performed using small pieces of fresh or thawed tissue blocks, cryostat sections, or core biopsies. Assessment of tumor cell content in parallel hematoxylin- and eosin-stained sections of the piece of tumor investigated is recommended. Because of more efficient, early detection of small breast tumors, there is an ever-increasing demand to measure uPA and PAI-1 in small

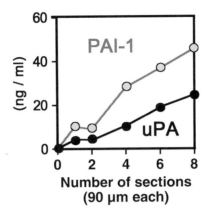

Fig. 8. Determination of urokinase-type plasminogen activator (uPA), plasminogen activator inhibitor type-1 (PAI-1), and protein in primary breast cancer cryostat sections. Up to eight 90-μm-thick cryostat sections were cut and then extracted by the micromethod described using the Potter-Elvehjem tissue homogenizer device (*see* **Fig. 4**). For this, subsequent sections of increasing number (1, 2, 4, 6, and 8) were cut, pooled in five different vials, extracted, and then subjected to uPA, PAI-1, and protein determination as described. Content of nanograms of uPA/PAI-1 per milliliter as a function of increasing number of cryostat sections extracted is shown. Approximately 3 ng of uPA per mg of protein and approx 10 ng of PAI-1 per mg of protein were determined for this breast cancer tissue sample employing uPA ELISA kit no. 894 and PAI-1 ELISA kit no. 821 (both from American Diagnostica, Stamford, CT) and the bicinchoninic acid protein assay (Pierce, Rockville, IL).

pieces of breast cancer tumor specimens, including fine-needle aspirates, core biopsies, and cryostat sections. To meet these demands, a few 90-μm-thick cryostat sections or one to two core biopsies are sufficient to reliably assess uPA and PAI-1 in the resulting tumor tissue extract, using the microdisintegration technique and standard ELISA protein-determination technique *(44)* (**Fig. 8**).

3. 1–5 μL Tissue extract is needed per each measurement of protein, uPA, or PAI-1.
4. Extraction procedures are not possible from formalin-fixed paraffin section.
5. After disintegration (pulverization) of the frozen tissue block by use of the dismembrator machine, addition of TBS (pH 8.5, without the detergent Triton X-100) to the tissue powder, followed by ultracentrifugation, yields the so-called cytosol fraction. A large fraction of uPA and most of all PAI-1 is contained in this cytosol fraction. Addition of 1% of the nonionic detergent Triton X-100 will free additional, membrane-bound uPA and uPA from intracellular stores; additional PAI-1 is not released by this technique. Jänicke et al. *(10)* determined uPA and PAI-1 antigen content in breast cancer tissue extracts by ELISA, in the presence and absence of the nonionic detergent Triton X-100, respectively. For PAI-1, no difference in antigen yield or prognostic impact was found. For uPA,

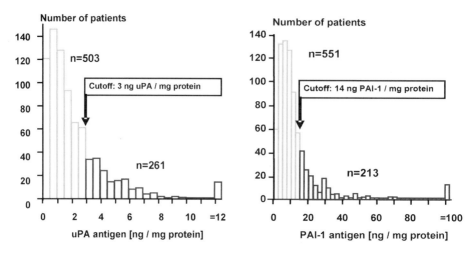

Fig. 9. Histogram of the distribution of urokinase-type plasminogen activator (uPA) and plasminogen activator inhibitor type-1 (PAI-1) protein in tumor tissue extracts of primary breast cancer patients ($n = 764$). Protein levels of the analytes are expressed in nanograms per mg of tumor tissue extract protein. uPA: range, 0.04–66.0; mean, 3.1; median, 2.06. PAI-1: range, 0.06–247.2; mean, 14.7; median, 9.1. Arrows indicate the previously optimized and re-evaluated cutoff values employed to group patients into low- or high- uPA/PAI-1 groups.

however, the detergent-containing extract yielded about twice as much uPA antigen and provided a considerably better assessment of disease-free survival than uPA measured in the detergent-free cytosol fraction.

6. The use of acidic buffers to extract uPA and PAI-1 protein from breast cancer tissues is not recommended. Low pH buffers favor the activation of proforms of cysteine-type proteases cathepsin B and L, with enzyme activity optimal between pH 3.0 and 5.0. At this pH, cathepsins B and L efficiently degrade extracellular matrix proteins but as important, target and degrade/activate other proteins as well. A prime example is pro-uPA, which is activated by the proteolytic action of cathepsins B and L. In addition, activated uPA activates plasminogen to plasmin and may bind to inhibitors PAI-1 and PAI-2 in tissue extracts, thereby constructing complexes between uPA and the inhibitors.

7. In principle, determination of protein, uPA, and PAI-1 can be done in blood serum or plasma. For this, no special extraction is necessary. For breast cancer patients, however, it has been shown that uPA/PAI-1 content in blood is of no prognostic relevance, most probably because of the fact that phagocytic cells (uPA), platelets, and endothelial cells (PAI-1) are also a rich source of these proteolytic factors. Secretion of blood cell uPA/PAI-1 into the blood stream may therefore obscure peripheral blood uPA/PAI-1 protein derived from the tumor tissue.

8. Within various multicenter studies, detailed results regarding performance of ELISA kits to measure uPA and PAI-1 protein in human breast cancer tissue

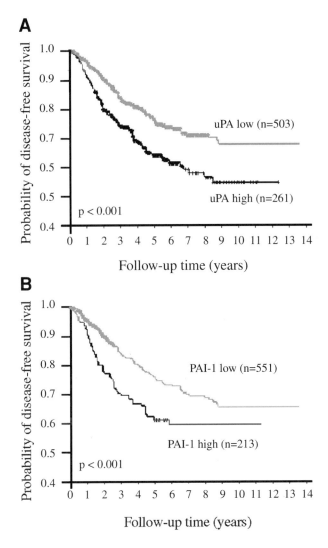

Fig. 10. Increase in urokinase-type plasminogen activator (uPA) or plasminogen activator inhibitor type-1 (PAI-1) in breast cancer tissue is an indicator of poor prognosis. Patients with high-tumor tissue protein content of either factor experience a significantly shorter disease-free survival than patients with low levels of these analytes. Low uPA ($n = 503$, with 106 relapses) vs high uPA ($n = 261$, with 85 relapses). Low PAI-1 ($n = 551$, with 125 relapses) vs high PAI-1 ($n = 213$, with 66 relapses). Cutoffs: uPA, 3 ng/mg protein; PAI-1, 14 ng/mg protein.

extracts were collected. Several commercially available and in-house uPA and PAI-1 ELISA formats were compared and found to be quite comparable and satisfactory for clinical diagnosis (*45,46*). However, the most frequently used uPA and PAI-1 ELISA kits cited in the scientific literature are from American Diagnostica. Therefore, guidelines on how to use these ELISA kits are given in this protocol. An external uPA and PAI-1 control (reference) preparation can be obtained from Prof. Dr. F. Sweep at the University of Nijmegen, The Netherlands (f.sweep@ace.umcn.nl).

9. The statistical approaches to identify and validate cutoff values for uPA and PAI-1 relevant for breast cancer patient prognosis and how to calculate the probability of disease-free survival (Kaplan–Meier plot) have been described by various authors and groups *(2,10,13,15–19,21)*. In **Fig. 9**, an example is given for the distribution of uPA and PAI-1 in tumors of a collective of 764 breast cancer patients. Based on the tumor tissue uPA and PAI-1 values determined, breast cancer patients can be grouped into low- and high-risk groups. Patients with uPA or PAI-1 values exceeding the threshold level of 3 ng of uPA/mg protein or 14 ng of PAI-1/mg protein may experience a higher risk of developing disease recurrence (**Fig. 10**).

10. Visit the website www.piercenet.com to learn about compatible substance concentrations allowed in the BCA protein assay. Technical assistance is available by e-mailing ta@piercenet.com.

11. Visit website www.americandiagnostica.com to get information about the uPA and PAI-1 ELISA assays and to learn about the performance of the kits, including publications on breast cancer prognosis and therapy response. Technical support is available by e-mailing services@amdiag.com.

12. **Caution:** When working with liquid nitrogen, always wear protective eyewear and use special gloves designed for this purpose.

13. When working with breast cancer material, always wear latex or plastic gloves.

References

1. Schmitt, M., Wilhelm, O. G., Reuning, U., et al. (2000) The urokinase plasminogen activator system as a novel target for tumour therapy. *Fibrinol. Proteol.* **14,** 114–132.

2. Andreasen., P. A., Kjöller, L., Christensen, L., and Duffy, M. J. (1997) The urokinase-type plasminogen activator system in cancer metastasis: a review. *Int. J. Cancer* **72,** 1–22.

3. Duffy, M. J. (1996) Proteases as prognostic markers in cancer. *Clin. Cancer Res.* **2,** 613–618.

4. Schmitt, M., Jänicke, F., and Graeff, H. (1992) Tumor-associated proteases. *Fibrinolysis* **6,** 3–26.

5. Schmitt, M., Harbeck, N., Thomssen, C., et al. (1997) Clinical impact of the plasminogen activation system in tumor invasion and metastasis: prognostic relevance and target for therapy. *Thromb. Haemost.* **78,** 285–296.

6. Reuning, U., Magdolen, V., Wilhelm, O., et al. (1998) Multifunctional potential of the plasminogen activation system in tumor invasion and metastasis. *Int. J. Oncology* **13,** 893–906.

7. Jänicke, F., Schmitt, M., Ulm, K., Gössner, W., and Graeff, H. (1989) Urokinase-type plasminogen activator antigen and early relapse in breast cancer. *Lancet* **2,** 1049.

8. Jänicke, F., Schmitt, M., Hafter, R., et al. (1990) The urokinase-type plasminogen activator (u-PA) is a potent predictor of early relapse in breast cancer. *Fibrinolysis* **4,** 69–78.
9. Jänicke, F., Schmitt, M., and Graeff, H. (1991) Clinical relevance of the urokinase-type and tissue-type plasminogen activators and of their type 1 inhibitor in breast cancer. *Sem. Thromb. Hemost.* **17,** 303–312.
10. Jänicke, F., Pache, L., Schmitt, M., et al. (1994) Both the cytosols and detergent extracts of breast cancer tissues are suited to evaluate the prognostic impact of the urokinase-type plasminogen activator and its inhibitor, plasminogen activator inhibitor type 1. *Cancer Res.* **54,** 2527–2530.
11. Stack, M. S. and Johnson, D., A. (1994) Human mast cell tryptase activates single-chain urinary-type plasminogen activator (pro-urokinase). *J. Biol. Chem.* **269,** 9416–9419.
12. Dano, K., Andreasen, P. A., Grondahl-Hansen, J., Kristensen, P., Nielsen, L.S., and Skriver, L. (1985) Plasminogen activators, tissue degradation, and cancer. Adv. Cancer Res. **44,** 139–266.
13. Jänicke, F., Prechtl, A., Thomssen, C., et al. (2001) Randomized adjuvant chemotherapy trial in high-risk, lymph node-negative breast cancer patients identified by urokinase-type plasminogen activator and plasminogen activator inhibitor type 1. *J. Natl. Cancer Inst.* **93,** 913–920.
14. Harbeck, N., Kates, R. E., Look, M. P., et al. (2002) Enhanced benefit from adjuvant chemotherapy in breast cancer patients classified high-risk according to urokinase-type plasminogen activator (uPA) and plasminogen activator inhibitor type 1 (n = 3424). *Cancer Res.* **62,** 4617–4622.
15. Grøndahl-Hansen, J., Christensen, I. J., Rosenquist, C., et al. (1993) High levels of urokinase-type plasminogen activator and its inhibitor PAI-1 in cytosolic extracts of breast carcinomas are associated with poor prognosis. *Cancer Res.* **53,** 2513–2521.
16. Foekens, J. A., Schmitt, M., van Putten, W. L. J., et al. (1994) Plasminogen activator inhibitor-1 and prognosis in primary breast cancer. *J. Clin. Oncol.* **12,** 1648–1658.
17. Fernö, M., Bendahl, P. O., Borg, Å., et al. (1996) Urokinase plasminogen activator, a strong independent prognostic factor in breast cancer, analysed in steroid receptor cytosols with a luminometric immunoassay. *Eur. J. Cancer* **32A,** 793–801.
18. Harbeck, N., Dettmar, P., Thomssen, C., et al. (1999) Risk-group discrimination in node-negative breast cancer using invasion and proliferation markers: six-year median follow-up. *Br. J. Cancer* **80,** 419–426.
19. Harbeck, N., Thomssen, C., Berger, U., et al. (1999) Invasion marker PAI-1 remains a strong prognostic factor after long-term follow-up both for primary breast cancer and following first relapse. *Breast Cancer Res. Treat.* **54,** 147–157.
20. Duffy, M. J., O'Grady, P., Devaney, D., O'Sioran, L., Fennelly, J. J., Lijnen, H. (1988) Urokinase-plasminogen activator, a marker for aggressive breast carcinomas. *Cancer* **62,** 531–533.
21. Bouchet, C, Hacene, K., Martin, P. M., et al. (1999) Dissemination risk index based on plasminogen activator system components in primary breast cancer. *J. Clin. Oncol.* **17,** 3048–3057.

22. Jänicke, F., Thomssen, C., Pache, L., Schmitt, M., and Graeff, H. (1994) Urokinase (uPA) and PAI-1 as selection criteria for adjuvant chemotherapy in axillary node-negative breast cancer patients, in *Prospects in Diagnosis and Treatment of Cancer* (Schmitt, M., Graeff, H., Jänicke, F., eds.). Elsevier Science, Amsterdam,, pp. 207–218.

23. Foekens, J. A., Look, M. P., Peters, H. A., van Putten, W. L. J., Portengen, H., and Klijn, J. G. M. (1995) Urokinase-type plasminogen activator and its inhibitor PAI-1: Predictors of poor response to tamoxifen therapy in recurrent breast cancer. *J. Natl. Cancer Inst.* **87,** 751–756.

24. Nekarda, H., Schmitt, M., Ulm, K., et al. (1994) Prognostic impact of urokinase-type plasminogen activator and its inhibitor PAI-1 in completely resected gastric cancer. *Cancer Res.* **54,** 2900–2907.

25. Heiss, M. M., Babic, R., Allgayer, H., et al. (1995) Tumor-associated proteolysis and prognosis, new functional risk factors in gastric cancer defined by the urokinase-type plasminogen activator system. *J. Clin. Oncol.* **8,** 2084–2093.

26. Ganesh, S., Sier, C. F. M., Griffioen, G., et al. (1994) Prognostic relevance of plasminogen activators and their inhibitors in colorectal cancer. *Cancer Res.* **54,** 4065–4071.

27. Sato, T., Nishimura, G., Yonemura, Y., et al. (1995) Association of immunohistochemical detection of urokinase-type plasminogen activator with metastasis and prognosis in colorectal cancer. *Oncology* **52,** 347–352.

28. Ganesh, S., Sier, C. F. M., Heerding, M. M., et al. (1996) Prognostic value of the plasminogen activation system in patients with gastric carcinoma. *Cancer* **77,** 1035–1043.

29. Verspaget, H. W., Sier, C. F., Ganesh, S., Griffioen, G., and Lamers, C. B. (1995) Prognostic value of plasminogen activators and their inhibitors in colorectal cancer. *Eur. J. Cancer* **31A,** 1105–1109.

30. Nekarda, H., Schlegel, P., Schmitt, M., et al. (1998) Strong prognostic impact of tumor-associated urokinase-type plasminogen activator in completely resected adenocarcinoma of the esophagus. *Clin. Cancer Res.* **4,** 1755–1763.

31. Kuhn, W., Pache, L., Schmalfeldt, B., et al. (1994) Urokinase (uPA) and PAI-1 predict survival in advanced ovarian cancer patients (FIGO III) after radical surgery and platinum-based chemotherapy. *Gynecol. Oncol.* **55,** 401–409.

32. Kuhn, W., Schmalfeldt, B., Reuning, U., et al. (1999) Prognostic significance of urokinase (uPA) and its inhibitor PAI-1 for survival in advanced ovarian carcinoma stage FIGO IIIc. *Br. J. Cancer.* **79,** 1746–1751.

33. Kobayashi, H., Fujishiro, S., and Terao, T. (1994) Impact of urokinase-type plasminogen activator and its inhibitor type 1 on prognosis in cervical cancer of the uterus. *Cancer Res.* **54,** 6539–6548.

34. Hofmann, R., Lehmer, A., Buresch, M., Hartung, R., and Ulm, K. (1996) Clinical relevance of urokinase plasminogen activator, its receptor, and its inhibitor in patients with renal cell carcinoma. *Cancer* **78,** 487–492.

35. Miyake, H., Hara, I., Yamanaka, K., Arakawa, S., and Kamidono, S. (1999) Elevation of urokinase-type plasminogen activator and its receptor densities as

new predictors of disease progression and prognosis in men with prostate cancer. *Int. J. Oncol.* **14,** 535–541.

36. Pedersen, H., Brünner, N., Francis, D., et al. (1994) Prognostic impact of urokinase, urokinase receptor and type 1 plasminogen activator inhibitor in squamous and large cell lung cancer tissue. *Cancer Res.* **54,** 4671–4675.

37. Pedersen, H., Grøhndahl-Hansen, J., Francis, D., et al. (1994) Urokinase and plasminogen activator inhibitor type 1 in pulmonary adenocarcinoma. *Cancer Res.* **54,** 120–123.

38. Rosenberg, S. (2000) Modulators of the urokinase-type plasminogen activation system for cancer. *Exp. Opin. Ther. Patents* **10,** 1843–1852.

39. Bürgle, M., Kessler, H., Stürzebecher, J., Magdolen, V., Wilhelm, O., and Schmitt, M. (2002) The urokinase-type plasminogen activator system—a new target for tumor therapy, in *Proteinase, Peptidase Inhibition: Recent Potential Targets for Drug Development* (Smith H. J., Simons, C., eds.). Harwood Academic, New York, pp. 231–248.

40. Mühlenweg, B., Sperl, S., Magdolen, V., Schmitt, M. and Harbeck N. (2001) Interference with the urokinase plasminogen activator system: a promising therapy concept for solid tumors. *Exp. Opin. Pharmacother.* **1,** 683–691.

41. Magdolen, U., Krol, J., Sumito, S., et al. (2002) Natural inhibitors of tumor-associated proteases. *Radiol. Oncol.* **36,** 131–143.

42. Setyono-Han, B., Stürzebacher, J., Schmalix, W. A., et al. (2005) Suppression of rat breast cancer metastasis and reduction of primary tumor growth by the small synthetic urokinase inhibitor WX-UK1. *Thromb. Haemost.* **93,** 779–786.

43. http://www.medicalnewstoday.com/index.php?newsid=8684.

44. Schmitt, M., Lienert, S., Prechtel, D., et al. (2002) The urokinase protease system as a target for breast cancer prognosis and therapy: technical considerations. *J. Clin. Ligand Assay* **25,** 43–52.

45. Benraad, T. J., Geurts-Moespot, J., Grøndahl-Hansen, J., et al. (1996) Immunoassays (ELISA) of urokinase-type plasminogen activator (uPA): Report of an EORTC/BIOMED-1 workshop. *Eur. J. Cancer* **32A,** 1371–1381.

46. Sweep, C. G. J., Geurts-Moespot, J., Grebenschikov, N., et al. (1998) External quality assessment of trans-European multicentre antigen determinations (ELISA) of urokinase-type plasminogen activator (uPA) and its type-1 inhibitor (PAI-1) in human breast cancer tissue extracts. *Br. J. Cancer* **78,** 1434–1441.

IV

ANALYSIS OF GENES AND GENE EXPRESSION IN TUMOR SPECIMENS

20

Fluorescence *In Situ* Hybridization and Comparative Genomic Hybridization

Patricia Gorman and Rebecca Roylance

Summary

This chapter discusses the complementary methodologies of fluorescence *in situ* hybridization and comparative genomic hybridization. Fluorescence *in situ* hybridization uses fluorescently labeled DNA probes (whole chromosomes, centromere, or locus-specific sequences) to visualize complementary DNA sequences in the target DNA (metaphase chromosomes or interphase nuclei). Comparative genomic hybridization is essentially a modified *in situ* hybridization, whereby the whole genome can be screened for gains and losses in a single experiment. Tumor and normal DNA are differentially fluorescently labeled and competitively co-hybridized to normal metaphase spreads. Both techniques require multiple steps in their preparation. These can be divided into preparation of the target, preparation of the probes, hybridization, post-hybridization washes, and image acquisition and analysis, each of which will be described in detail. Success of each experiment is dependent on all of these steps, but where steps are of critical importance to particular techniques, they will be highlighted, together with notes on how to optimize the process.

Key Words: Comparative genomic hybridization; fluorescence *in situ* hybridization; DNA probes; fluorescence; tumor.

1. Introduction

Fluorescence *in situ* hybridization (FISH) and comparative genomic hybridization (CGH) are molecular cytogenetic techniques that have been widely used in the study of breast and other cancer types. FISH is used to detect structural and numerical chromosomal aberrations, i.e., simple copy-number alterations and the presence of DNA amplification, present either as double minutes or homogeneously staining regions (HSRs), whereas CGH detects only numerical aberrations. The techniques can be used either in isolation or in conjunction to provide complementary information.

From: *Methods in Molecular Medicine, Vol. 120: Breast Cancer Research Protocols*
Edited by: S. A. Brooks and A. L. Harris © Humana Press Inc., Totowa, NJ

FISH uses fluorescently labeled DNA probes to visualize complementary DNA sequences in the target DNA. Suitable DNA probes for FISH include whole chromosome, centromere, or locus-specific sequences, whereas the target DNA can be either metaphase chromosomes or interphase nuclei. Metaphase chromosomes can be obtained from normal individuals, cell lines, or tumors. "Normal" metaphase spreads would be used for FISH when mapping the position of a probe and will not be discussed further in this chapter. Obtaining metaphase spreads from solid tumors is notoriously difficult and often, complex changes are often found. This is particularly true of breast cancers, with many rearrangements, marker chromosomes, and DNA amplifications seen. Interphase nuclei can be obtained from a range of clinical materials, including touch preparations, fine-needle aspirates, bone marrow smears, and importantly, archival (formalin-fixed, paraffin wax-embedded) material. For the study of breast tumors and, thus, the purposes of this chapter, we will limit our discussion to the use of archival material.

Whereas a review of the entire FISH literature in breast cancer is not within the remit of this chapter, the specific example of amplification of the *HER2/ERBB2* gene is worth mentioning because of its important clinical implications *(1)* and is discussed in Chapter 22. FISH assessment of c-*myc* gene amplification is also described in detail in Chapter 21 (which also reviews the FISH technique, and the reader is referred to this material as well).

Using conventional FISH, several different probes can be used in a single experiment if they are labeled differently. However, a specific variant of FISH, multicolor FISH (M-FISH) or spectral karyotyping (SKY) *(2,3)*, has been introduced, which uses a combination of fluorochromes to simultaneously label all chromosomes in different colors, therefore enabling visualization of every chromosome in a single experiment. This permits cryptic rearrangements, marker chromosomes, and double minutes to be easily identified, although small deletions and intrachromosomal rearrangements will still go undetected. However, these techniques have limited usefulness for the analysis of breast tumors because of the difficulty of obtaining chromosome preparations, as discussed above. Thus, realistically, the utility of M-FISH/SKY for breast cancer research lies in the analysis of breast cancer cell lines. Only M-FISH will be discussed specifically here, as it is the more adaptable method. It is essentially simply a modification of normal FISH protocols and uses the same type of microscope, but with modifications.

The ability to perform FISH on tissue sections is particularly useful for assessing the amount of genetic heterogeneity within tumors and for establishing genotype–phenotype correlations. However, in order to study multiple different genetic regions, multiple experiments need to be set up, which is clearly very time-consuming. One way of overcoming this obstacle is the use of tissue arrays *(4)*, described in Chapter 4. Many tumor sample cores (up to 1000) are arrayed in a "new" paraffin block, and then multiple sections of the array provide targets for parallel *in situ* detection of DNA, RNA, and protein in each specimen (*see* Chapter 23 for the methodology for RNA and protein detection). The advantages of this technique are that multiple samples can be analyzed very rapidly, the significance of novel genes can be confirmed, and it is possible to correlate genetic findings with clinical information. At present, the use of FISH on tissue arrays is predominantly confined to assessing increased copy number or amplification.

CGH is essentially a modified *in situ* hybridization, which is capable of screening the entire genome for gains and losses of genetic material in a single experiment *(5)*. Two differentially labeled DNA probes are used: the test/tumor sample (green) and the reference or normal DNA sample (red) are competitively co-hybridized to the target DNA; normal metaphase spreads. Differences in the copy number between test and reference DNA are seen as differences in the ratio of green-to-red fluorescence intensity. Images of the metaphases are captured and quantification of the fluorescence ratios performed using a digital image analysis system. Regions of chromosomal gain are seen as an increased fluorescence ratio, whereas regions of loss are seen as a decrease in the fluorescence ratio. Losses are detectable when the region affected exceeds 10 Mb *(6)*; smaller regions of gain are detected if there is high-level amplification; for example, a 2-Mb region that is amplified five times will be visualized *(7)*. For each tumor, 5–10 metaphases are analyzed and an average fluorescence ratio for each chromosome obtained. Once regions of gain or loss have been identified, these regions can be defined further using FISH or molecular genetic techniques. There are now many established examples of the utility of CGH in identifying genetic regions worthy of further investigation. With specific reference to breast cancer, positional cloning of amplified regions has lead to the identification of *STK15 (8)* and *AIB-1 (9)*, both on the long arm of chromosome 20, and *PS6K* on the long arm of chromosome 17 *(10)*.

One of the major limitations to the use of CGH, as already discussed, is the resolution of the target DNA. This has been overcome with the recent introduction of array-based CGH, where the target DNA is replaced by arrays of genomic bacterial artificial chromosomes (BACs), bacteriophage P1, cosmids, or complementary (c)DNA clones, which results in resolution in the order of approx 1.4 Mb *(11)*. Even-higher resolution arrays of regions of interest are possible by the use of overlapping clones; resolution here can be down to less than the clone length (<50 kb). Furthermore, the use of arrays also permits more accurate relative copy-number estimation. Approaches to gene analysis using cDNA microarrays are described in Chapters 27 and 28.

FISH and CGH depend on the same basic principles, and many of the steps involved are identical, so it is logical that the techniques are discussed together. However, there are important differences that need to be highlighted. The setting up of both experiments depends on multiple steps, all of which are important for a successful result. These steps are as follows.

1.1. Preparation of the Target

1.1.1. Preparation of Metaphase Spreads

These can be prepared from blood, cell lines, or tumors. To obtain metaphase spreads from breast cancers is difficult for the reasons outlined above and will not be discussed further in this chapter. It is important to note that for CGH, the target must be normal metaphases that are typically prepared using blood from a healthy volunteer. The basic method for preparation of metaphase spreads is the same for both blood and established breast cancer cell lines. Following a period in culture, the cells are harvested. Breast cell lines are grown in culture until they are growing exponentially. Blood is typically cultured for 72 h and in the presence of a mitogen (e.g., phytohemagglutinin [PHA]), which specifically stimulates cell division of the T-lymphocytes. Just before harvesting, cell division is arrested in metaphase by the addition of colcemid. The cells are treated with hypotonic solution to make them swell, and then fixed using methanol/acetic acid. The metaphase "spreads" are prepared by dropping the fixed cells onto cleaned microscope slides.

1.1.2. Preparation of Interphase Nuclei

The preparation of interphase nuclei depends on the source material from which they are derived. The most common source of interphase nuclei for FISH will be archival (formalin-fixed, paraffin wax-embedded) material. For confirmatory studies, i.e., when FISH is being done to confirm CGH findings, the sections used are ideally adjacent to the material from which the DNA has been extracted to perform CGH. If tissue arrays are being used, the preparation is the same as for single sections.

Before use, it is necessary to dewax the samples.

1.2. Preparation of Probes: DNA Extraction and Labeling

DNA is extracted from source material using standard methods. For FISH probes, source material refers to P1-derived bacterial artificial chromosomes (PACs), BACs, and cosmids, whereas for CGH, this refers to tumor material and normal tissue, ideally from the same subject. Probes for both FISH and CGH are labeled by nick translation, but there are important methodological differences, depending on whether FISH or CGH is being set up.

FISH probes are labeled either directly or indirectly by nick translation to achieve an ideal probe fragment size of between 200 and 500 bp. Direct labeling uses fluorescently labeled nucleotides, which are incorporated directly into the DNA, whereas for indirect labeling, the probe is labeled with either biotin or digoxigenin, and the signal is detected later with the use of fluorescent antibodies. The number of probes that can be detected in a single experiment depends on a number of factors, including the method of labeling used (direct vs indirect), and the type of filter equipment fitted to the microscope (filter set or filter wheel). Direct labeling permits visualization of more probes than indirect, because there are an increased variety of fluorescently labeled nucleotides that can be used. A microscope equipped with a filter wheel will permit visualization of more fluorochromes than a filter set. A typical number of probes that can be visualized in a single experiment would be in the range of one to three. Specifically, for M-FISH, the probes are commercially available and are already labeled.

For CGH, it is preferable to use direct labeling and providing there is sufficient DNA (at least 1 μg); it is also labeled by nick translation. Two probes must be labeled "the test" and "the reference," and conventionally, these are labeled green and red, respectively. However, if only a small amount of DNA is available, it must first be amplified using degenerate oligonucleotide primed-polymerase chain reaction (DOP-PCR) *(12)*. This uses a degenerate primer and has two stages, initial low-stringency cycles, where the specific bases at the 3' end of the oligonucleotide theoretically primes every 4 kb along the template DNA, and then an increased number of cycles with high stringency, whereby the oligonucleotide "tailed" DNA from the initial cycles is then amplified. DNA amplified in this way can be labeled either by nick translation or by further DOP-PCR, with fluorescent nucleotides incorporated into the PCR reaction. The ideal fragment size is a smear ranging from 500 to 2 kb.

1.3. Hybridization

Labeled probes are precipitated in the presence of an excess of unlabeled human Cot I DNA, resuspended in hybridization mix, denatured, and preannealed before being applied to the denatured metaphase or interphase DNA on the slides. The presence of Cot I DNA and the preannealing step are to suppress hybridization of the interspersed repetitive DNA sequences present in the DNA probes. The length of time the slides are left to hybridize is variable, depending on whether FISH (2–16 h, depending on the size of probe), M-FISH (16 h), or CGH (72 h) is being set up.

1.4. Post-Hybridization Washes

The slides are washed using solutions of differing stringency to remove unbound probe and any nonspecific hybridization. If indirect labeling has been used for FISH a detection step, using fluorescently labeled antibodies, is required.

1.5. Image Acquisition and Analysis

Images are captured using an epifluorescence microscope equipped with appropriate filters and a cooled charge-coupled device camera. The analysis will depend on the type of *in situ* hybridization that has been performed. Most of the analysis is done using specific commercially available software.

2. Materials

2.1. Preparation of Target

2.1.1. Breast Cancer Cell Lines, Harvesting of Cells, and Preparation of Metaphase Spreads for FISH and M-FISH

1. Versene: 0.2 g/L phosphate-buffered saline (PBS) with PBSA.
2. Trysin-versene (0.25% trysin in versene), stored at –20°C.
3. Culture medium: according to published protocols for the cell lines.
4. 10 µg/mL of colcemid solution, stored at 4°C.
5. Hypotonic solution: 0.075 *M* of potassium chloride warmed to 37°C before use.
6. Fixative solution: 3 vol:1 vol methanol:acetic acid (glacial), prepared freshly before use and kept at 4°C.
7. Clean 76 × 26-mm microscope slides stored in 500 mL of 70% ethanol with 0.05% concentrated hydrochloric acid and dried immediately with lint-free tissues (e.g., Kimwipes) before cells are dropped.
8. Series of 70, 95, and 100% ethanol washes.

2.1.2. Blood Cultures, Harvesting of Cells, and Preparation of Metaphase Slides for CGH

1. 50 mg/mL of sodium heparin, stored at 4°C.
2. Lyophilized PHA stored at 4°C. It is made up in sterile water to 9 mg/mL and stored in aliquots at –20°C.
3. Culture medium: RPMI-1640, fetal calf serum (10%), L-glutamine (4 m*M*).
4. Then, the same materials listed as **items 4–8** of **Subheading 2.1.1.**

2.1.3. Preparation of Interphase Nuclei in Formalin-Fixed, Paraffin Wax-Embedded Tissues for FISH

1. 4- to 6-µm sections of formalin-fixed, paraffin wax-embedded tissues, either single tissue block or from tissue arrays.
2. Xylene (low in sulfur).
3. Sterile water.
4. 1 *M* Sodium thiocyanate, prepared freshly before use.
5. PBS.
6. 0.4% Pepsin in 0.1 *M* HCl, prepared freshly before use.
7. 4% Paraformaldehyde, prepared freshly before use.
8. Series of 70, 90, and 100% ethanol washes.

2.2. DNA Extraction

2.2.1. DNA Extraction From BACs, PACs, and Cosmids for FISH

1. Luria-Bertani ([LB] Bacto-tryptone, Bacto-yeast extract, NaCl) agar (LB and agar), stored as solid at room temperature (RT). Before use, LB agar should be melted (e.g., in a microwave) and allowed to cool to 55°C before adding an appropriate antibiotic and pouring into Petri dishes. Once prepared, the dishes can be wrapped in parafilm and stored at 4°C for up to 1 mo.
2. Appropriate antibiotic: ampicillin made up in sterile water (50 µg/mL), kanamycin made up in sterile water (25 µg/mL), or chloromphenicol made up in 100% ethanol (20 µg/mL). Store stocks at –20°C.
3. LB broth.
4. Glycerol, warmed to 37°C before use.
5. Solution 1: 50 m*M* glucose, 10 m*M* ethylenediaminetetraacetic acid ([EDTA] pH 8.0), and 25 m*M* Tris-HCl (pH 8.0).
6. Solution 2: 0.2 *N* NaOH, 1% sodium dodecyl sulfate (SDS).
7. Solution 3: 5 *M* KOAc (pH 5.5).
   Note: Solutions 1–3 are all stored at RT.
8. Phenol:chloroform:isoamyl alcohol (25:24:1), stored at 4°C.
9. Chloroform:isoamyl alcohol (24:1), stored at RT.
10. Isopropanol, stored at RT.
11. 70% Ethanol stored, at –20°C.
12. Tris-HCl/EDTA ([TE] pH 8.0).
13. 10 mg/mL of RNase A solution. Made up in 10 m*M* Tris-HCl (pH 7.5), 15 m*M* NaCl, and heated to 100°C for 15 min, before cooling slowly to RT. Store in aliquots at –20°C.
14. An alternative to preparing FISH probes is to buy them commercially. Many probes, particularly whole-chromosome and centromere probes, are available commercially and are already labeled, and should be used according to the manufacturers' guidelines. As already discussed, M-FISH probes are purchased commercially (Vysis, Downers Grove, IL).

2.2.2. DNA Extraction From Fresh/Frozen Tissue for CGH

1. Digestion buffer: 100 m*M* NaCl, 10 m*M* Tris-HCl (pH 8.3), 25 m*M* EDTA, 0.5% SDS, and 0.1mg/mL proteinase K. The buffer should be prepared freshly before use. All stock solutions, except the proteinase K, should be autoclaved. Stock proteinase K should be 20 mg/mL and stored in aliquots at –20°C.
2. Phenol:chloroform: 50:50 buffered phenol and chloroform, stored at 4°C.
3. Chloroform:isoamyl alcohol (24:1), stored at 4°C.
4. Distilled water.
5. 3 *M* Sodium acetate (pH 5.2): 246.12 g anhydrous sodium acetate dissolved in 800 mL water, and pH adjusted to 5.2 with glacial acetic acid, before making up to a total volume of 1 L. Store in autoclaved aliquots before use.
6. 70 and 100% ethanol.
7. 10 mg/mL of RNase A solution, stored in aliquots at –20°C.

2.2.3. DNA Extraction From Blood for CGH

This is for the reference DNA, although normal tissue adjacent to the tumor can also be used. It is preferable that the reference DNA from the same patient as the tumor DNA, but if necessary, it can be obtained from a healthy volunteer.

1. Ice-cold distilled water.
2. Nuclei lysis buffer: 10 mM Tris-HCl, 400 mM NaCl, and 2 mM EDTA (0.6 g of Tris-HCl, 11.70 g of NaCl, and 0.37 g of Na-EDTA dissolved in 500 mL of water). Autoclave and store at 4°C before use.
3. 0.1% Nonidet P-40 (NP-40).
4. Proteinase K buffer: 2 mM of EDTA and 1% SDS, autoclaved before use and stored at 4°C.
5. Proteinase K solution: 2 mg proteinase K dissolved in 1 mL of proteinase K buffer, and prepared freshly before use.
6. Saturated ammonium acetate: 148 g of NH_4Ac in 100 mL of water.
7. 10% SDS solution.
8. 70 and 100% ethanol.

2.2.4. DNA Extraction From Formalin-Fixed, Paraffin Wax-Embedded Tissue for CGH

1. Xylene (low in sulfur).
2. 30, 60, 80, and 100% ethanol.
3. Digestion buffer: 75 mM of NaCl, 2.5 mM of EDTA, and 100 mM Tris-HCl (pH 8.0), with 0.5% Tween-20 and 0.5 mg/mL of proteinase K.
4. Then, the same materials as listed as **items 2–7** of **Subheading 2.2.2**.

2.3. Labeling of Probes

2.3.1. Nick Translation: Direct Labeling

2.3.1.1. NICK TRANSLATION: DIRECT LABELING FOR FISH

1. DNA solution to be labeled (at least 1 µg is required).
2. 10X Nick translation buffer: 0.2 mM deoxyadenosine 5'-triphosphate (dATP), 0.2 mM deoxycytidine 5'-triphosphate (dCTP), 0.2 mM deoxyguanosine 5'-triphosphate (dGTP), and 0.05 mM of deoxythymidine 5'-triphosphate (dTTP) in 500 mM Tris-HCl (pH 7.8); 50 mM $MgCl_2$; 100 µM of β-mercaptoethanol; and 100 µg/mL of BSA (nuclease free), stored in ready-to-use aliquots at –20°C.
3. Fluorochromes: fluorescein isothiocyanate (FITC)-12-deoxyuridine 5'-triphosphate (dUTP) and Rhodamine-5-dUTP; these are light-sensitive and so should be handled in low-lighting conditions.
4. Nick translation enzyme mix (cat. no. 1745808; Roche, UK).
5. Distilled water.
6. 0.5 M EDTA.

2.3.1.2. NICK TRANSLATION: DIRECT LABELING FOR CGH

1. The same materials listed as **items 1–3** and **5–6 Subheading 2.3.1.1.**
2. 0.5 U/μL of DNA polymerase I/0.4 mU/μL of DNAse I enzyme mix (Gibco–BRL, Paisley, UK).
3. 10 U/μL of DNA polymerase I (Promega, Southampton, UK).

2.3.2. Nick Translation: Indirect Labeling (see **Note 1**)

1. DNA solution to be labeled (at least 1 μg is required).
2. Bio Nick™ Labeling System (Invitrogen, Paisley, UK) for biotin labeling including: 10X dNTP mixture, containing 0.2 mM each of dCTP, dGTP, and dTTP; 0.1 mM dATP; and 0.1 mM biotin-14-dATP.
3. 10X Digoxigenin mix: 0.2 mM each of dCTP, dGTP, and dATP; 0.1 mM dTTP, 0.1 mM dig-dUTP, 500 mM Tris-HCl (pH 7.8), 50 mM MgCl$_2$, 100 μM β-mer-captoethanol, and 100 μg/mL of BSA.
4. 10X Enzyme mixture: 0.5 U/μL DNA polymerase1, 0.007 U/μL of DNase 1.
5. Stop buffer: 0.5 M EDTA (pH 8.0).
6. Distilled water.

2.3.3. DOP-PCR

1. DNA solution (100 pg–100 ng).
2. 10X PCR buffer: 30 mM MgCl$_2$, 500 mM KCl, 100 mM Tris-HCl (pH 8.4), and 1 mg/mL of gelatin. All stock solutions should be autoclaved before preparation of the buffer.
3. Nucleotides for primary reaction: 2.5 mM each of dATP, dGTP, dCTP, and dTTP, made up in sterile distilled water.
4. Nucleotides for labeling reaction: 2.5 mM dATP, dGTP, and dCTP and 1.25 mM of dTTP, made up in sterile distilled water.
5. 6-MW primer: 50 μm 5'CCG ACT CGA GNN NNN NAT GTG G3', where N = A, C, G, or T in roughly equal proportions.
   Note: Items 2–5 should be stored in ready-to-use aliquots at –20°C.
6. Distilled water.
7. *Taq* polymerase (5 U/μL).

2.4. Mixing, Precipitating, and Denaturing of Probes

1. Labeled DNA.
2. 1 mg/mL Human Cot 1 DNA (Roche).
3. 3 M Sodium acetate (pH 5.2).
4. 100% Ethanol stored at –20°C.
5. 20X Saline sodium citrate (SSC): 175.3 g of NaCl and 88.2 g of sodium citrate dissolved in 800 mL of water, pH adjusted to 7.0 with a few drops of a 10 N solution of NaOH before adjusting volume to 1 L. Store in autoclaved aliquots.
6. Hybridization buffer: 10% dextran sulfate, 50% deionized formamide (molecular biology grade), 2X SSC (pH 7.0), stored at –20°C in ready-to-use aliquots.

2.5. Denaturing of Target DNA

2.5.1. Denaturing of Metaphase/Interphase DNA on Slides for FISH and CGH

1. Denaturation solution for slides: 70% formamide (deionized, as in **step 6**, **Subheading 2.4.**), 2X SSC, pH 7.0.
2. 22 × 50-mm cover slips.
3. Series of 70 (ice-cold), 95, and 100% ethanol washes.

2.5.2. Denaturing of Metaphase/Interphase DNA on Slides for M-FISH

1. Denaturation solution as detailed in **step 1**, **Subheading 2.5.1.**, but must be in a Coplin jar and heated to 72°C before use.
2. 10 mg/mL of RNase A, diluted to working concentration of 100 µg/mL in 2X SSC.
3. SSC solution: 2X SSC (pH 7.0).
4. 100 mg/mL of pepsin solution, stored in 35-µL aliquots at –20°C. Just before use, thaw an aliquot and dissolve in 69.3 mL of distilled water and 0.7 mL of 0.1 *M* HCl that has been prewarmed to 37°C in a Coplin jar.
5. PBS with BSA.
6. Formaldehyde solution: 1.89 mL of 37% formaldehyde, 57.6 mL of distilled water, 3.5 mL of 1 *M* MgCl$_2$, and 7 mL of 10X PBS; make just before use and place in a Coplin jar.
7. Then, the same materials listed as **items 2** and **3**, **Subheading 2.5.1.**

2.6. Hybridization

1. 22 × 22-mm or 22 × 50-mm cover slips.
2. Rubber sealant.
3. Moist chamber, e.g., plastic slide box with a lid and a layer of moistened paper in the bottom. The slides can then be placed horizontally in the boxes resting on the side "ledges" above the moistened paper. Boxes should be sealed with tape.

2.7. Post-Hybridization Washes

2.7.1. Post-Hybridization Washes for Directly Labeled Probes for FISH and CGH

1. Formamide solution: 50% formamide and 2X SSC (pH 7.0). **Note:** The formamide used here does not need to be deionized.
2. 2X SSC solution (pH 7.0).
   Note: Solutions 1 and 2 should both be prepared freshly before use and then warmed to 42°C. It is important to check they are at the correct temperature before use.
3. SSC/Tween-20 (SSCT): 4X SSC and 0.05% Tween-20, pH 7.0.
4. Series of 70, 95, and 100% ethanol washes.
5. 4,6-diamidino-2-phenylindole (DAPI), which is a counterstain, made up in Citifluor, a mounting medium containing Antifade, (0.15 µg/mL), stored at 4°C.

2.7.2. Post-Hybridization Washes for M-FISH

1. 0.4X SSC/0.3% NP-40, warmed to 72°C before use.
2. 2X SSC/0.1% NP-40.
3. DAPI III, a more-dilute DAPI than used for other *in situ* hybridizations, is necessary, and it is provided with the probes.

2.7.3. Post-Hybridization Washes and Detection of Signal for Indirectly Labeled Probes

1. Same materials listed as **items 1–5** of **Subheading 2.7.1.**
2. SSCT plus Marvel nonfat dried milk powder (5%).
3. Avidin-FITC/Texas Red (Vector Labs, Peterborough, UK): 1 in 300 dilution in SSCT plus Marvel, made up immediately before use.
4. Antidigoxigenin-Rhodamine/FITC (200 µg/mL): 1 in 100 dilution in SSCT plus Marvel, made up immediately before use.

2.8. Image Acquisition and Analysis

1. Epifluorescence microscope equipped with a filter wheel with specific filters in combination with a cooled charge-coupled device camera and suitable computer hardware. The number of filters will determine which fluorochromes it is possible to detect. The minimum number of filters required for detection of FISH (using two different fluorochromes) and for CGH is three: a Spectrum Green filter that will detect Spectrum Green and FITC, a Spectrum Orange filter to detect Rhodamine, and a DAPI filter. For M-FISH, a filter wheel containing filters for spectrums Red, Green, Aqua, Far Red, Gold, and DAPI are all required.
2. Software for capturing and analysis of FISH, M-FISH, and CGH images is all commercially available (e.g., Smart capture for capturing FISH and CGH, QUIPS XL SpectraVision™ for capturing and analysis of M-FISH, and QUIPS™ CGH analysis for CGH analysis, is all from Applied Imaging, UK).

3. Methods

3.1. Preparation of Target

3.1.1. Culture of Cell Lines, Harvesting of Cells, and Preparation of Metaphase Spreads (see Note 2)

Obviously, care needs to be taken when working with biological material. A laboratory coat and gloves should be worn, and all steps should be carried out in a tissue culture hood, until the cells are fixed. Tubes containing blood should be disposed of carefully before incineration. The supernatant from all steps up to the fixative steps should be disposed of into Vercon.

1. Add 50–100 µL of colcemid (*see* **Note 3**) to a 75-cm² cell culture flask containing 15 mL of culture medium, for 1 h (cells are ideally harvested when growing exponentially, so 24 h before harvesting, they should have either been subcultured or have had their medium changed, depending on their rate of growth).

2. Remove the 15 mL of culture medium, discarding 10 mL and retaining 5 mL in a 15-mL Falcon tube.

3. Add 5 mL of versene to the flask to wash the cells, swirl, and then remove it and add to the retained 5 mL culture medium from **step 2**.

4. Adherent cells are removed from the flask by addition of 3–4 mL trypsin/versene and incubation at 37°C, for approx 5–10 min, until the cells become detached.

5. The 10 mL of retained medium (from **steps 2** and **3**) is then added to inactivate the trypsin, and the contents of the flask are all transferred to the original 15-mL Falcon tube.

6. Centrifuge at 500*g* for 5 min.

7. Remove all of the supernatant with a pipet and resuspend the pellet in the very small amount of remaining medium by flicking the tube gently.

8. Add 10 mL of prewarmed hypotonic KCl. The first few drops should be added carefully, flicking the tube gently the entire time. Make up to 10 mL and incubate at 37°C for 15–20 min.

9. Add 0.6 mL of ice-cold fixative solution (as a top layer to the hypotonic solution), close the lid, and gently invert the tube twice to mix the solutions.

10. Centrifuge at 500*g* for 5 min.

11. Remove the supernatant with a pipet and resuspend the pellet completely by flicking the tube gently.

12. Add a few drops of fixative solution *very carefully* while gently flicking the tube (*see* **Note 4**), and then make up to 10 mL, gently agitating the tube the entire time.

13. Centrifuge at 500*g* for 5 min.

14. Remove the supernatant with a pipet.

15. Resuspend the pellet by flicking the tube gently, and again, add carefully 10 mL of fixative solution, agitating the tube the entire time.

16. Repeat **steps 13–15** twice. After the second fixative step, the tubes should be left on ice for 30 min. Thereafter, fixative solution does not need to be added slowly.

17. Repeat **steps 13** and **14**, and then resuspend the pellet in 0.5–1 mL of fixative solution.

18. Using a siliconized glass pipet, drop from a distance of about 40 cm one drop of fixed material onto each end of a clean microscope slide (*see* **Subheading 2.1.1.**, **item 7** and **Note 5**), which has been moistened by breathing on it (the slide should still be moist when the fixed material hits the slide). **Note:** Two separate drops on each slide means two hybridizations can be done on the same slide.

19. Using a pipet, the slides should be "washed" with fixative (before they dry) and then placed in a warm, humid environment to dry (e.g., over a water bath set at 55–60°C; *see* **Note 6**).

20. Slides should be examined using a microscope to ensure there are sufficient metaphases (*see* **Note 7**). If there are too many, then more fixative can be added to the pellet; if there are too few, then spin again and resuspend the pellet in less fixative. The amount of cytoplasm should also be noted (*see* **Note 8**). Even if the slides look satisfactory when examined under phase contrast microscopy, they

may not hybridize well for CGH and so need to be tested before hybridization (*see* **Note 9**).

21. Once the slides have dried, they should be dehydrated in an ethanol series of 70, 95, and 100% for 3 min each, and then left at RT overnight before storage.

22. Slides being prepared for M-FISH should be used fresh, i.e., within 2–3 d of preparation. Slides for other uses should be stored at –20°C, in a box containing a desiccant, e.g., a small amount of silica gel wrapped in a piece of perforated parafilm, until use.

23. Fixed material can be stored temporarily (days) at 4°C, or for longer periods (months) at –20°C.

3.1.2. Blood Cultures, Harvesting of Cells, and Preparation of Metaphase Spreads

1. Take 4 mL of blood from a volunteer and place immediately into a tube containing 40 µL of sodium heparin (10 µL of heparin/1 mL of blood), then agitate the tube gently to ensure thorough mixing. (The amount of blood taken is arbitrary— 4 mL gives eight tubes, which can be reasonably harvested by one person and can yield approx 160 slides, if good metaphases are obtained from each tube).

2. In separate universal tubes, add 0.5 mL of heparinized blood to 9.5 mL culture medium and 0.1 mL PHA solution and mix.

3. Incubate the tubes at 37°C with 5% CO_2 for 72 h, with the lids left loose. Agitate gently the tubes each day.

4. Before harvesting, add 100 µL of colcemid (final concentration 0.1 µg/mL) and incubate for 15–20 min at 37°C (*see* **Note 3**).

5. Transfer blood to 15-mL Falcon tubes and centrifuge at 500*g* for 5 min.

6. Then, go to **steps 7–18** of **Subheading 3.1.1. Note:** the only difference is that the fixed blood cells should be washed more rigorously, so **step 16** of **Subheading 3.1.1.** should read "repeat **steps 13–15** up to five times."
   Note: Prepared slides with metaphase spreads, specifically for CGH, are available commercially.

3.1.3. Preparation of Interphase Nuclei

Paraffin wax-embedded material needs to be dewaxed before use.

1. Dewaxing the slides: take 4-µm sections which are not hematoxylin and eosin (H&E)-stained and place in xylene twice for 10 min each, then 10 min in 100% alcohol, and 5 min each in 80, 60, and 30% ethanol, taking care not to let the slides dry out at all between steps.

2. After dewaxing and rehydration, permeabilize by incubating in sodium thiocyanate for 10 min at 80°C.

3. Wash in PBS twice for 5 min each wash, at RT.

4. Digest in pepsin for between 5 and 30 min at 37°C.

5. Repeat **step 3**.

6. Fix in paraformaldehyde for 2 min.

7. Dehydrate through a 70, 90, and 100% ethanol series.

3.2. DNA Extraction

Phenol/chloroform should be used in a fume hood and disposed of appropriately.

3.2.1. DNA Extraction From BACs, PACs, and Cosmids for FISH

Perform **steps 1–4** near a naked Bunsen burner flame.

1. Streak bacteria containing the plasmid onto LB agar plates supplemented with the appropriate antibiotic. Incubate inverted overnight at 37°C.
2. Inoculate a single bacterial colony into 7 mL of LB broth plus antibiotic in a 15-mL Falcon tube and shake overnight in an orbital shaker at 200 rpm at 37°C.
3. Streaked plates can be stored inverted and wrapped in parafilm at 4°C for up to 1 mo. If it is necessary to repick a colony, this can be done, but it should be noted that care must be taken, as contaminant growth is likely to occur during prolonged storage.
4. Mix 0.5 mL of the culture from **step 2** with 0.5 mL of prewarmed glycerol for long-term storage at –70°C. When preparing further DNA from this sample, the glycerol stock should be partially thawed and the bacteria streaked as described in **step 1**.
5. Centrifuge the remaining 6.5 mL at 1500g for 10 min.
6. Discard supernatant and dry pellet by inverting the tube carefully onto a paper tissue.
7. Resuspend the pellet in 300 μL of solution 1 by vortexing and transfer to a 1.5-mL Eppendorf tube (the volume of solution 1 used is dependent on the size of the pellet and can be varied, but then, solutions 2 and 3 must be scaled accordingly).
8. Add 300 μL of solution 2 and invert the tube gently. Leave at RT for 5 min; the contents of the tube will become transparent.
9. Add 300 μL of solution 3, invert gently, and place on ice for 5 min; a white precipitate will form.
10. Spin in a minifuge at 15,000g for 10 min at 4°C.
11. Place tubes on ice. Carefully remove the supernatant and add it to an equal volume of phenol:chloroform:isoamyl alcohol. The white precipitate can be discarded.
12. Mix by inverting and spin in a minifuge at 15,000g for 5 min at 4°C.
13. Remove the top layer, place in a clean tube, and add an equal volume of chloroform:isoamyl alcohol.
14. Repeat **step 12**.
15. Remove the top layer, place in a clean tube, and add 800 μL of ice-cold isopropanol.
16. Mix by inverting and place on ice for 5 min.
17. Spin in a minifuge at 15,000g for 15 min at 4°C; a white pellet should be visible.
18. Remove supernatant and discard. Add 500 μL of cold 70% ethanol to the pellet and invert several times to wash the pellet.
19. Spin in a minifuge at 15,000g for 5 min at 4°C.
20. Remove the supernatant and air-dry the pellet.

21. Resuspend in 40 μL TE.
22. Add 100 μg/mL RNaseA to the resuspended DNA and leave for 30 min at 37°C.
23. Incubate at 70°C for 5 min to inactivate the RNaseA.
24. Measure the amount of DNA using a spectrophotometer (OD 260 and 280).
25. DNA can be stored until use at −20°C.

3.2.2. DNA Extraction From Frozen/Fresh Tissue for CGH

It is very important that the tissue samples are examined first by a pathologist to confirm that there is at least 70% of tumor present in the samples for CGH. The presence of contaminating normal tissue means that genetic changes are much more difficult to detect reliably *(7)*. For the following methods, the volumes used will depend on the amount of tissue available and should therefore be adjusted accordingly. Tissue-handling steps should be carried out in a laminar flow cabinet.

1. Tissue chunks should be minced in a Petri dish using a scalpel, and then placed in approx 1 mL of extraction buffer. Tissue should be scraped from slides using a drawn-out sterile glass capillary tube, and then placed into a small Eppendorf tube with 50–300 μL of digestion buffer (depending on size of sections).
2. Leave in buffer at 37°C for 1 h if very small, or overnight for bigger samples.
3. Add an equal volume of phenol/chloroform, mix by inverting the tube, and spin at 20,000g at 4°C for 15 min.
4. Remove the top layer and place in fresh tube, carefully avoiding the white interface and discarding the bottom layer.
5. Repeat **steps 3** and **4**.
6. Add an equal volume of chloroform/isoamyl alcohol, mix by inverting the tube several times, and spin at 20,000g at 4°C for 15 min.
7. Remove the top layer and put in a fresh tube, again avoiding the interface and discarding the bottom layer.
8. Add 0.1 volume of 3 M of sodium acetate (pH 5.2) and add 2–3 volumes of ice-cold 100% ethanol.
9. Gently invert the tube. If there is a large amount of DNA, it should now be visible as a precipitate, which can be hooped out using a sealed glass Pasteur pipet. Wash briefly in 70% ethanol, and allow to dry, before resuspending in distilled water and proceeding to **step 12**.
10. If, however, no DNA is visible (and very small amounts of DNA may not be), the tube should be put at −70°C for 2 h or up to overnight, and then spun at 20,000g at 4°C for 15–30 min. A pellet should now be visible.
11. Remove as much as possible of the supernatant, wash with 70% ethanol, and spin again at 20,000g at 4°C for 15 min. Remove the ethanol and air-dry the pellet at RT before resuspending in distilled water.
12. Add 100 μg/mL RNaseA, and then leave at 37°C for 30 min–1 h. Then, incubate at 70°C for 5 min to inactivate the RNaseA.

13. Determine the quantity of DNA spectrophotometrically and the quality by running on a 1% agarose gel.
14. DNA should be stored at 4°C short term, but at –20°C for the longer term. **Note:** Alternatively, a kit for extracting DNA from tissue can be used, which also gives good results (cat no. 51304; Qiagen, Valencia, CA).

3.2.3. DNA Extraction From Blood for CGH

1. Take 50-mL Falcon tubes and add 5–10 mL blood (it can be fresh or frozen; if frozen, allow to thaw first) into each tube.
2. Add ice-cold water to each tube to make a final volume of 50 mL, then invert tubes to mix well and lyse the red blood cells.
3. Spin for 20 min at 4°C and 1300*g*.
4. Discard supernatant by pouring off into Vircon, and then carefully invert over a paper towel to remove the remaining lysed red blood cells, leaving a white nuclear pellet.
5. Add 25 mL of 0.1% NP-40 to the nuclear pellet and spin at 4°C and 1300*g*.
6. Discard the supernatant and invert carefully over a paper towel to remove remaining liquid, then add 3 mL of nuclei lysis buffer and vortex to resuspend the pellet completely.
7. Add 200 µL of 10% SDS and 600 µL of proteinase K solution, mix by inversion, and incubate at 60°C for 1.5–2 h (or overnight at 37°C).
8. Add 1 mL of saturated ammonium acetate and shake vigorously for 15 s. Allow to stand at RT for 10–15 min, and then spin for 20 min at 1300*g*.
9. Pour the supernatant into a separate tube. Precipitate the DNA by adding 2 volumes of cold 100% ethanol to the supernatant and mix gently by inversion. The DNA should become visible as a precipitate and can be hooped out on the tip of a sealed glass Pasteur pipet.
10. Wash in 70% ethanol, and then resuspend in distilled water.
11. Proceed to **step 12** of **Subheading 3.2.2.**

3.2.4. DNA Extraction From Formalin-Fixed, Paraffin Wax-Embedded Tissue for CGH

This method is for tissue sections on slides, but it can be easily adapted to tissue sections in Eppendorf tubes. Five 10-µm sections should yield sufficient DNA to nick translate, but obviously, it depends on the area of the sections; generally, 1 cm^2 should give a reasonable yield.

1. Dewaxing the slides: take five 10-µm sections that are not H&E-stained (*see* **Note 12**); however, one H&E slide is needed for reference. Place slides in xylene for 15 min; then 10 min in 100% alcohol; and 1 min each in 80, 60, and 30% ethanol, taking care not to let the slides dry out at all between steps. Slides can be left at this stage in sterile water, but if they are to be left for a few weeks, they should be stored at 4°C and the water changed regularly.

2. By comparing the slides to the H&E slide, scrape off the regions of tumor, using a drawn-out sterile glass capillary tube and place into an Eppendorf tube containing 300 μL of digestion buffer.
3. Leave at 55°C overnight, add more proteinase K to a final concentration of 1 mg/mL, and then leave at 55°C for at least 3 d.
4. Proceed to **step 3**, **Subheading 3.2.2**. (**Note:** the Qiagen kit can also be used for formalin-fixed, paraffin wax-embedded tissue.)

3.3. Probe Labeling

3.3.1. Direct Labeling by Nick Translation

The main difference in the labeling conditions for FISH and CGH is due to the optimum size of probe required for each method; hence, the differences in the concentration of enzymes and incubation times. For FISH, a variable number of probes can be labeled, but for CGH, two probes must be labeled. Remember that once the fluorochromes are added, all the steps should be done in low-lighting conditions.

3.3.1.1. FOR FISH

1. Combine 5 μL of nick translation buffer, 1 μL of fluorochrome-conjugated dUTP, 1 μg of DNA, and 10 μL of enzyme mix and distilled water to make a total volume of 50 μL. **Note:** the enzymes should be added last and the tubes kept on ice.
2. Incubate at 15°C for 1–2 h, then leave on ice while 5 μL is run on a 1% agarose gel.
3. Probe fragments should form a smear ranging in size between 200 and 500 bp (*see* **Note 10**).
4. If the fragments are the correct size, the reaction should be stopped by adding 2 μL of EDTA and heating to 70°C for 5 min to denature the enzymes.
5. Probes can be stored until use at –20°C.

3.3.1.2. FOR CGH

1. Combine 5 μL of nick translation buffer, 1 μL of FITC-12-dUTP to label the test DNA or 1 μL of Rhodamine-5-dUTP to label the reference DNA (*see* **Note 11**), 1 μg DNA, 10 μL DNA polymerase I/DNase mix, 1 μL DNA polymerase I, and distilled water to make a total volume of 50 μL.
2. Proceed to **step 2**, **Subheading 3.3.1.1**. The important exception being **step 3**, where the probe fragments should form a smear ranging in size between 500 and 2000 bp. This is particularly important (*see* **Note 10**).

3.3.2. Indirect Labeling by Nick Translation

1. Combine 5 μL of dNTP mix (either BioNick™ [Gibco–BRL] mix or digoxigenin mix), 1 μg of DNA, and 5 μL of enzyme mix for biotin and make up to a total volume of 50 μL with distilled water.

2. Proceed to **step 2**, **Subheading 3.3.1.1. Note:** there is a stop buffer provided in the BioNick kit.

3.3.3. DOP-PCR Labeling (see *Notes 11* and *12*)

Small amounts of DNA cannot be labeled by nick translation. The DNA is amplified using DOP-PCR, and as little as 100 pg has been reported to give reproducible amplification *(13)*. If sufficient DNA is produced, some label the products using nick translation (*see* **Note 10**). However, in our experience, a satisfactory-sized probe, particularly from formalin-fixed, paraffin wax-embedded tissue, is not achieved in this way, so the DNA should be labeled also by DOP-PCR.

3.3.3.1. PRIMARY REACTION

1. Mix 5 µL of 10X of PCR buffer, 5 µL of primary dNTPs, 2 µL of 6 MW, 100 pg– 100 ng DNA (optimum 20–100ng), 0.5 µL of *Taq* polymerase, and distilled water to make a total of 50 µL. DNA should be added last. **Note:** it is very important to have a negative control in each experiment, i.e., a tube containing all the above but with no DNA.
2. Primary reaction conditions: 96°C for 10 min; then nine cycles of 94°C for 1 min, 30°C for 1.5 min, 72°C for 3 min with ramp to 72°C; 1°C for 4.2 s; then 35 cycles of 94°C for 1 min, 62°C for 1 min, and 72°C for 3 min; and then 72°C for a further 10 min.
3. Run 10 µL on 1% agarose gel. The PCR product varies in size, particularly if the source of DNA is formalin-fixed, paraffin wax-embedded tissue, when the fragments may be in the range of 50–1000 bp. The negative control should not contain a smear; if it does, then the products should be discarded and not used (*see* **Note 12**). Unused product should be stored at –20°C.

3.3.3.2. LABELING REACTION

1. Mix 1–5 µL of (depending on concentration as determined by gel) DNA from the primary reaction, 5 µL of PCR buffer, 4.4 µL of labeling nucleotides, 2 µL of 6 MW, 1 µL FITC-12-dUTP (for the test) or 1 µL Rhodamine-5-dUTP (for the reference), 1 µL of *Taq* polymerase, and distilled water to make a total of 50 µL. Again, set up a negative control.
2. Labeling reaction conditions: 96°C for 10 min; then 40 cycles of 94°C for 1 min, 55°C for 1 min, and 72°C for 3 min; and then 72°C for 10 min.
3. Run 10 µL on 1% agarose gel. If not used immediately, products should be stored at –20°C.

3.4. Mixing, Precipitating, and Denaturing of Probes

3.4.1. For FISH

1. Mix 100–200ng of labeled probe (*see* **Note 13**), 5 µL of human Cot 1 DNA, and 0.1 volume of 3 *M* sodium acetate and 2 volumes of cold absolute ethanol. These

amounts are for a single area on a slide. If, for example, there is a large tissue section, then amounts would need to be doubled.
2. Place on dry ice for 30 min or leave at –20°C overnight.
3. Spin at 15,000*g* at 4°C for 15min.
4. Aspirate supernatant carefully and leave pellet to air-dry, taking care not to overdry the pellet; otherwise, it will be very difficult to resuspend.
5. Resuspend pellet in 10 μL of hybridization mix; leave at 37°C for 15 min, with intermittent vortexing.
6. If probes are being prepared for use on paraffin sections, go straight to **Subheading 3.5.3.** and do not proceed further here; otherwise, proceed to **step 7**.
7. Denature at 75°C for 5 min.
8. Preanneal at 37°C for 30 min (while the probes are preannealing, the slides can be prepared (*see* **Subheading 3.5.** and **Note 14**).
9. Place the 10 μL of the denatured probe onto the denatured slide that has been placed on a hotplate at 37°C. Cover the probe with a 22 × 22-mm cover slip, taking care to ensure there are no air bubbles.
10. Seal cover slip with rubber sealant and leave on the hotplate until the rubber sealant dries.
11. Leave to hybridize in a humid chamber for 2 h for a repetitive centromere probe, to overnight (i.e., 16 h) for a single-copy, locus-specific probe.

Commercially available probes will have specific instructions that may vary from the instructions above, and of course, should be followed.

3.4.2. For M-FISH

1. Denature 10 μL of labeled probe should be at 72°C for 5 min.
2. Place denatured probe onto denatured slide, cover with a 22 × 22-mm cover slip, taking care to ensure there are no air bubbles.
3. Seal cover slip with rubber sealant and leave to hybridize in a humid chamber for 16 h.

3.4.3. For CGH

1. Mix 1 μg of test and reference labeled DNA (*see* **Note 15**), 50 μL of human Cot 1 DNA (*see* **Note 14**), 0.1 volume of 3 *M* sodium acetate, and 2 volumes of cold absolute ethanol.
2. Proceed to **step 2**, **Subheading 3.4.1.**, with three distinctions:
   a. **Step 8**. Preannealing can be up to 1 hour (*see* **Note 14**).
   b. **Step 11**. Hybridization should be for 72 h.
   c. Also **note step 9**. If there are suitable metaphases, both halves of the slide can be used, so 10 μL of denatured probe can be placed on each half and covered with a 22 × 22-mm cover slip.

3.5. Denaturation of Target DNA

This is a particularly crucial step for both M-FISH and CGH. For M-FISH, a particularly important factor is that the slides must have been prepared freshly. For CGH, each batch of slides must have the optimal denaturation conditions determined, and to do this, test slides must be denatured for different times (e.g., range of 2–5 min), stained with DAPI, and then examined using a microscope (*see* **Note 9**). For FISH, the denaturation steps are less critical.

3.5.1. Denaturation of Metaphase DNA for FISH/CGH

1. Remove slides from storage just before use and mark the areas of interest with a diamond pen (this may or may not apply).
2. Denature slide on a hot plate at 73°C for 2 min for FISH or for the predetermined optimum denaturation time (depending on slide batch as discussed in **Subheading 3.5.**) for CGH with denaturation solution under a 22 × 50-mm cover slip.
3. Place immediately into ice-cold 70% ethanol for 3 min, and then dehydrate through an ethanol series for 3 min each.
4. Air-dry the slides. They are then ready for use.
5. Just before use, place slides on a hot plate at 37°C.

3.5.2. Denaturation of Metaphase DNA for M-FISH

For M-FISH, slides need to be pretreated.

1. Place 100 μL RNaseA onto slide.
2. Cover with 22 × 50-mm cover slip and leave for 30 min at 37°C in a humid chamber.
3. Wash twice, for 5 min each wash, in 2X SSC at RT in a Coplin jar.
4. Place slides in a Coplin jar containing pepsin solution for 5 min at 37°C.
5. Wash twice, for 5 min each wash, PBS at RT.
6. Fix in formaldehyde for 2 min at RT.
7. Repeat **step 5**.
8. Dehydrate through ethanol series of 3 min each.
9. Air-dry the slides.
10. Slides should now be placed in a Coplin jar containing denaturation solution at 72°C for 1–3 min. No more than four slides should be placed in a jar at any one time, as this will cause too great a drop in the temperature of the denaturation solution.
11. Proceed to **steps 3** and **4** of **Subheading 3.5.1**.

3.5.3. Denaturation of Interphase Nuclei From Deparaffinized Samples for FISH

1. Take 10 μL of resuspended probe (from **step 6** of **Subheading 3.4.1.**) and place directly onto the deparaffinized slide. (**Note:** for a tissue array or large tissue section, this will be 20 μL of probe.)
2. Cover each probe with a 22 × 22-mm cover slip (22 × 50-mm cover slip if a larger area is to be covered), taking care to ensure there are no air bubbles.
3. Seal cover slip with rubber sealant.
4. Denature on hotplate at 72°C for 5 min.
5. Proceed to **step 11** of **Subheading 3.4.1.**

3.6. Post-Hybridization Washes

All the steps for directly labeled probes should be done in low lighting conditions.

3.6.1. Post-Hybridization Washes for Directly Labeled Probes *(see **Note 16**)*

Formamide waste should be carefully disposed of.

1. The rubber cement should be removed gently and the slide shaken to flick off the cover slips; if they do not come off, then they can be made to come off by putting the slide in the Coplin jar containing formamide solution.
2. Three 5-min washes in formamide solution in a water bath.
3. Three 5-min washes in SSC solution in a water bath.
4. One 5-min wash in SSCT at RT. **Note:** during **steps 2–4**, the slides should never become completely dry.
5. Dehydrate slides in an ethanol series for 2 min each and air-dry in dark.
6. Mount in DAPI solution, approx 30 µL per slide, and cover with a 22 × 50-mm cover slip.
7. Store slides in a cardboard folder at 4°C, but capture images as soon as possible.

3.6.2. Post-Hybridization Washes for M-FISH

1. The rubber cement should be removed gently and the slide shaken to flick off the cover slips.
2. Wash in 0.4X SSC/0.3% NP-40, shaking for 1–3 s, and then leave for up to 2 min.
3. Wash in 2X SSC/0.1% NP-40, shake for 1–3 s, and then leave for 5 s–1min.
4. Air-dry, then mount in DAPI III solution and cover with a 22 × 50-mm cover slip.
5. Store slides at 4°C, but capture images as soon as possible; this is particularly important for M-FISH.

3.6.3. Post-Hybridization Washes for Indirectly Labeled Probes

1. This should proceed as for **steps 1–4, Subheading 3.6.1.**, except that these steps do not need to be done in low-lighting conditions.
2. Remove slides from Coplin jar and add 100 µL of SSCT plus Marvel solution to block nonspecific hybridization. Cover with 22 × 50-mm cover slip.
3. Place slides in a humid chamber and leave at 37°C for 30 min.
4. Remove cover slip and wash in SSCT at RT for 1min.
5. Add 100 µL of avidin-FITC/SSCT plus Marvel solution to slide *or* 100 µL of antidigoxigenin-FITC/SSCT plus Marvel, depending on how the probe was labeled. Cover with 22 × 50-mm cover slip. If two probes have been used together, then to detect the two colors, combine avidin-FITC/antidigoxigenin-Rhodamine to make a total of 100 µL in SSCT plus Marvel.
6. Place slides in a humid chamber for 30 min at 37°C.
7. Three 3-min washes in SSCT at RT.
8. Proceed to **step 5** of **Subheading 3.6.1.**

3.7. Image Acquisition and Analysis

3.7.1. FISH

The number of images it is necessary to capture will depend on the question under investigation. When assessing copy-number changes from cell lines, the number of metaphase spreads it is necessary to examine will depend on the heterogeneity seen—the greater the degree of variability, the greater the number of spreads it will be necessary to examine. However, a conventional number would be 20. For assessing changes in interphase nuclei, it would be necessary to examine 100 nuclei. It is important to check that the probes map to the correct position, and this is done by the acquisition of a digitally inverted DAPI image that gives a banding pattern resembling classical G banding. When using probes on interphase nuclei, it is sensible to check the probe maps to the correct position before use.

3.7.2. M-FISH

It is very important to follow the instructions for the appropriate software for successful capture and analysis. For analysis of each cell line, at least 20 metaphases should be captured. Some of the fluorochromes fade very easily, so care must be taken when scanning; the slide should be scanned using a low-power objective and the Gold filter. Metaphases should be captured in the order recommended by the manufacturers, namely, Spectrum Gold, Spectrum Far Red, Spectrum Aqua, and then Spectrum Red and Spectrum Green in any order, and finally, the DAPI image. Metaphases should be captured immediately and saved in an appropriate format. When all metaphases have been captured, they can be processed using the semiautomated software. The chromosomes have to be separated, and this is best done using the chromosome segmentation software, which can separate touching and overlapping chromosomes. The software can also assign axes and the *p*-telomere. Chromosomes are then arranged in a karyotype based on their color profiles, using the color classifier. It is then very important to check each chromosome has been assigned correctly and to correct manually any errors. Care should be taken when attempting to assign breakpoints based on the color profiles, as there is invariably some blending of color profiles at the breakpoint.

3.7.3. CGH

For analysis of each sample, images of 5–10 metaphases should be captured and the raw data saved. Metaphases should be captured using the ×63 or ×100 objective, with the field diaphragm closed down to the edge of the image acquisition area (this increases the contrast within the image). It is most important that the bulb is well focused and that there is homogeneous illumination of the optical field to avoid variations of the fluorescence ratio. Metaphases should have smooth intense color that is not granular in appearance, and heterochromatin regions should not be brightly stained (*see* **Notes 2–6, 8–10**, and **14**).

Semiautomated karyotyping and CGH analysis is done using commercially available software. First, a digitally inverted DAPI image is generated that gives a banding pattern resembling classical G banding and is used for karyotyping. The software has tools to divide touching and crossed-over chromosomes (alternatively, crossovers can be excluded). The position of axes and centromeres for each chromosome are checked. An automated karyotype is then generated, but the accuracy does need to be confirmed, and any corrections made. Once the karyotype is acceptable, the software generates CGH profiles for each chromosome by calculating the green-to-red ratio, pixel by pixel, along the length of each chromosomal axis. After each metaphase has been analyzed separately, a collection of 5–10 metaphases is combined and an average ratio for each chromosome obtained. Conventionally, gains are considered significant when the ratio of test to reference DNA is 1.2:1 or greater, and losses considered significant when the ratio is 0.8:1 or less, although other limits are used, e.g., 1.15 and 0.85. For an improved interpretation of the CGH ratio profiles, the analysis software can be extended to calculate statistical confidence intervals. There is generally no concordance regarding the limits used for high-level amplification; some will consider it when the ratio exceeds a certain threshold, the minimum value used being 1.4, whereas others will infer high-level amplification when by visual inspection there are areas of discrete intense green signal noted, with a corresponding profile suggesting gain.

4. Notes

1. Although some would use indirect labeling for CGH, we would not recommend this as in our hands it does not give as good results.
2. The quality of the metaphase-spread preparation is probably the single most important factor in determining the success of a CGH experiment *(14)*, and it is also critical to the success of M-FISH experiments. Whereas the quality of the preparation is much less important for FISH, **Notes 3–6** and **8** pertain to the preparation of metaphase spreads for all *in situ* work.
3. The chromosome size and quantity of metaphases is variable. Colcemid times longer than 20 min will give more metaphase spreads, but they will be more condensed. Therefore, a balance needs to be achieved between chromosome length and number. Some breast cancer cell lines may be slow growing and require long colcemid times to ensure sufficient metaphases at the expense of their quality.
4. It is most important to add the first fix slowly, as if it is added too quickly, it will result in the pellet clumping and poor fixation. Proper fixation ensures crisp, well-spread chromosomes. Placing the cells on ice also helps facilitate fixation.

The more times the pellets are washed with fixative, the cleaner the final preparation will be, with less cytoplasm.

5. Spreading of the metaphase chromosomes is variable. Ideally, metaphases should be well spread with not too many overlapping chromosomes. Metaphases spread well when they are well fixed (*see* **Note 4**) and when the microscope slides are clean, hence, the importance of storing them in ethanol with a small amount of hydrochloric acid and drying them, just before dropping the spreads, with lint-free tissue. The other important factor is the atmospheric conditions (*see* **Note 6**).

6. Slide-making conditions are important. However, conditions can vary considerably (temperature and humidity), and so if the metaphase spreads do not look optimal on one day, store the fixed material and try again another day. The conditions noted here work well in our laboratory, but they are subject to great variability. If the conditions are too cold/dry, the metaphases will not spread. Conversely, if the conditions are too hot/humid, the metaphases overspread and indeed in extreme cases appear as a "chromosome soup."

7. It should be noted that interphase nuclei will be present among the metaphase spreads. If interphase nuclei are required for study (and this only applies to FISH) the cells should ideally all be in G_0, but when cells have been pretreated with colcemid, the nuclei will reflect cells at different stages in the cell cycle; therefore, any copy number estimates must be interpreted with caution.

8. The amount of cytoplasm is critical. If the metaphases appear to be embedded in too much cytoplasm, then washing the pellet and/or the slides with more fixative may be tried. The amount of cytoplasm is critical, as too much prevents both optimal denaturation and probe penetration, with a resulting poor hybridization. However, a small amount of cytoplasm may allow the chromosomes to withstand the necessary denaturation. Some authors pretreat slides for CGH with proteinase K or pepsin to remove excess cytoplasm, but we find that if the slides are of sufficient quality, pretreatment is not necessary. However, pretreatment with pepsin is necessary for M-FISH. If a batch of slides has a large amount of cytoplasm, they will not be useful for CGH and so should be discarded. Although it is time-consuming to prepare a new batch, it is ultimately worthwhile compared with setting up many CGH experiments that yield doubtful results. If a new batch has to be prepared, a longer hypotonic stage may be helpful.

9. It is necessary to test the quality of each batch of slides for CGH, before use; again, if they are of poor quality, then they should be discarded. Slides are quality-tested by denaturing them (using a range of denaturation times, e.g., 2–5 min), staining with DAPI, and then examining them using a microscope. This is necessary, as slides that look satisfactory by microscopy may not necessarily withstand denaturation well. Optimal metaphase spreads are ones that tolerate enough denaturation to achieve uniform hybridization along each chromosome but do not lose their structure and morphology. By implication from this, slides that are underdenatured will not hybridize, and if overdenatured, the chromosomes appear fat, without normal morphology. Once an optimal denaturation time has been defined, the slides should have a test hybridization with normal male and female

DNA; all autosomes should have a ratio between 0.9 and 1.1, and the X chromosome should have a ratio of less than 0.6.

10. The size and quality of the probe is an important step in determining the quality of both FISH and CGH. If the probe fragments are too large, then the incubation time should be increased or more enzyme (DNase/polymerase mix) added; if the fragment size is too small, then repeat with a shorter incubation time or by adding less enzyme. If the probes are too large, then the resulting hybridization will be poor with typically a spotty or speckled appearance. DNA contaminated with protein will label inefficiently and give a similar hybridization appearance. A large amount of contaminating protein and the probe will fail to label, and in this situation, the DNA needs to be repurified. If it is desirable to attempt nick translation of DOP-PCR'd DNA, then less enzyme and shorter incubation times are needed.

11. As method of quality control, controls can be set up, for example, with normal male (green) and normal female DNA (red). The fluorescence ratios, particularly of the X chromosome, should be as in **Note 9**. If using DOP-PCR to label DNA, a useful internal control for an experiment is to pair tumor DNA with DNA from a normal sample taken from an individual of the opposite sex. The profile of the X chromosome will be a guide to the quality of the experiment, i.e., a ratio that is less than expected will suggest a poor-quality experiment. It is also important if using a DOP-PCR'd probe to ensure that the reference probe has been prepared in the same manner. So, for example, if the test probe is derived from paraffin wax-embedded material, then the reference probe should also use normal DNA extracted from paraffin wax-embedded.

12. DOP-PCR is a difficult technique. It is often not very reproducible and is prone to contamination. Separate pipets should be used for PCR only. If possible, it should be done in a dedicated room or area with surfaces, pipets, and tubes subjected to ultraviolet irradiation. If contamination occurs, this should be dealt with by preparing fresh stock solutions and cleaning the pipets used and taking the usual precautionary methods for any PCR. DNA that has been extracted from H&E sections will not PCR. Although such DNA run on a gel will look satisfactory, it is only when it is amplified that the problem will become known. Similarly, if only small amounts of frozen tissue are available that need to be amplified, problems arise if the tissue has been placed in optimum cutting temperature (OCT) compound. In this situation, in our experience, the DNA does PCR, and reasonable smears are obtained, but it results in very poor quality hybridization. In addition, *see* **ref. 15** with regard to trying to optimize DOP-PCR.

13. The amount of labeled probe used for FISH depends on the size of the probe. The bigger the probe, then the greater the amount required, e.g., 100 ng for cosmids and 200 ng for PACs. Any combination of commercial and homemade probes may be used, so long as they are labeled with different fluorochromes, and the microscope has the necessary filters for capturing. Similarly, if using indirect labeling, different combination of fluorescent antibodies must be used.

14. The amount of Cot I and preannealing times are important for both FISH and CGH. If there is insufficient suppression of the repetitive sequences in a CGH

experiment, this will result in strong labeling of the heterochromatin regions of chromosomes 1, 9, 16, and 19 and high intensity of nonspecific fluorescence at chromosomal regions that have a high content of repetitive sequences. Neither change can be corrected for during image analysis and make it difficult to detect small copy-number alterations in the heterochromatin regions and inaccuracies in the fluorescence ratio in regions of repetitive sequences.

15. Some use less than 1 μg of nick-translated-labeled probe for CGH; however, in our experience, this amount gives a strong, uniform hybridization. Nonetheless, if using DOP-PCR-labeled products, it may be necessary to use less probe.

16. Post-hybridization washes are probably subject to the most variability among different methods. Those outlined here give good results, with a very good signal-to-noise ratios.

Acknowledgment

We would like to thank to Andrew Rowan for helpful comments on this manuscript.

References

1. Slamon, D. J., Clark, G. M., Wong, S. G., Levin, W. J., Ullrich, A., and McGuire, W. L. (1987) Human breast cancer: correlation of relapse and survival with amplification of the *HER-2/neu* oncogene. *Science* **235,** 177–182.

2. Schrock. E., du Manoir, S., Veldman, T., et al. (1996) Multicolor spectral karyo-typing of human chromosomes. *Science* **273,** 494–497.

3. Speicher, M. R., Gwyn Ballard, S., and Ward, D. C. (1996) Karyotyping human chromosomes by combinatorial multi-fluor FISH. *Nat. Genet.* **12,** 368–375.

4. Kononen, J., Bubendorf, L., Kallioniemi, A., et al. (1998) Tissue microarrays for high-throughput molecular profiling of tumor specimens. *Nat. Med.* **4,** 844–847.

5. Kallioniemi, A., Kallioniemi, O-P., Sudar, D., et al. (1992) Comparative genomic hybridization for molecular cytogenetic analysis of solid tumors. *Science* **258,** 818–821.

6. Bentz, M., Plesch, A., Stilgenbauer, S., Dohner, H., and Lichter, P. (1998) Minimal sizes of deletions detected by comparative genomic hybridization. *Genes Chromosomes Cancer* **21,** 172–175.

7. Kallioniemi, O-P., Kallioniemi, A., Piper, J., et al. (1994) Optimizing comparative genomic hybridization for analysis of DNA sequence copy number changes in solid tumors. *Genes Chromosomes Cancer* **10,** 231–243.

8. Zhou, H. Y., Kuang, J., Zhong, L., et al. (1998) Tumor amplified kinase *STK15/ BTAK* induces centrosome amplification, aneuploidy and transformation. *Nat. Genet.* **20,** 189–193.

9. Anzick, S. L., Kononen, J., Walker, R. L., et al. (1997) *AIB1*, a steroid-receptor coactivator amplified in breast and ovarian cancer. *Science* **277,** 965–968.

10. Couch, F. J., Wang, X. Y., Wu, G. J., Qian, J., Jenkins, R. B., and James, C. D. (1999) Localization of PS6K to chromosomal region 17q23 and determination of its amplification in breast cancer. *Cancer Res.* **59,** 1408–1411.

11. Pinkel, D., Segraves, R., Sudar, D., et al. (1998) High resolution analysis of DNA copy number variation using comparative genomic hybridization to microarrays. *Nat. Genet.* **20,** 207–211.
12. Telenius, H., Carter, N. P., Bebb, C. E., Nordenskjold, M., Ponder, B. A., and Tunnacliffe, A. (1992) Degenerate oligonucleotide-primed PCR: general amplification of target DNA by a single degenerate primer. *Genomics* **13,** 718–725.
13. Speicher, M. R., du, M. S., Schrock, E., et al. (1993) Molecular cytogenetic analysis of formalin-fixed, paraffin-embedded solid tumors by comparative genomic hybridization after universal DNA-amplification. *Hum. Mol. Genet.* **2,** 1907–1914.
14. Karhu, R., Kahkonen, M., Kuukasjarvi, T., Pennanen, S., Tirkkonen, M., and Kallioniemi, O. (1997) Quality control of CGH: impact of metaphase chromosomes and the dynamic range of hybridization. *Cytometry* **28,** 198–205.
15. Kuukasjarvi, T., Tanner, M., Pennanen, S., Karhu, R., Visakorpi, T., and Isola, J. (1997) Optimizing DOP-PCR for universal amplification of small DNA samples in comparative genomic hybridization. *Genes Chromosomes Cancer* **18,** 94–101.

21

Fluorescence *In Situ* Hybridization Assessment of c-*myc* Gene Amplification in Breast Tumor Tissues

Jan K. Blancato, Mary Steele Williams, and Robert B. Dickson

Summary

This chapter details methods used for analysis of DNA copy-number changes in breast tumor tissues through the use of fluorescence *in situ* hybridization. The specific DNA probe described herein is the oncogene c-*myc*, although the tissue fluorescence *in situ* hybridization methodology presented is suitable for dual-color studies of most unique sequence and chromosome specific control probes.

The breast tumor tissue sections are first deparaffinized in a solvent and clearing agent, and then pretreated with a protease to allow the target DNA within the breast tissue cells to be uncovered. This allows the DNA to be available for hybridization with the labeled c-*myc* probe. The tissue sections are then analyzed to assure that appropriate digestion of cellular material has been attained. The tissues are then denatured. The c-*myc* probe and control probe for the centromere of chromosome 8 are commercially available as differentially labeled and are cohybridized to the tissue and sealed beneath a cover slip in a humid chamber. They are incubated for 12–16 h. The cover slip is then removed, and the section is postwashed in 2X saline sodium citrate at 72°C for 5 min and allowed to cool to room temperature in a detergent solution. The slides are then counterstained with 4',6-diamidino-2-phenylindole, and a cover slip is applied. The slides are then viewed with fluorescence microscopy using filters that allow the c-*myc* and chromosome 8 signals to be visualized. If possible, 50 cells are counted, and the data are expressed as number of c-*myc* signals/number of chromosome 8 signals.

Key Words: c-*myc* FISH; tissue FISH; gene amplification; probe; chromosome 8.

1. Introduction

In the past decade, the cytogenetics lab has seen a major advance in diagnostic and prognostic capabilities, with the use of molecular cytogenetics. The development of a combination of cytogenetics and molecular biology, the technique of fluorescence *in situ* hybridization (FISH) has increased the resolution and application of cytogenetics (*1*). The availability of quality-controlled DNA probes from commercial sources has expedited the research and clinical uses

From: *Methods in Molecular Medicine, Vol. 120: Breast Cancer Research Protocols*
Edited by: S. A. Brooks and A. L. Harris © Humana Press Inc., Totowa, NJ

of this technique and the acceptance of these tests. FISH is a technique that allows a DNA sequence to be detected on a metaphase chromosome or in interphase nuclei within a tissue section. This technique uses a DNA probe that can be made to entire chromosomes or single, unique sequence genes and serves as a powerful adjunct to tumor marker tests. Generic methods for this technique are given in Chapter 20.

The steps of a FISH protocol are similar to those of Southern blot hybridization, but in the *in situ* experiment, the DNA is not extracted and run in a gel, but studied in its original place in fixed cells or on the chromosomes. The DNA and surrounding material is fixed in a non-nucleic acid-precipitating fixative. The specimen is then treated with heat and formamide to denature the double-stranded DNA to render it single stranded. The target DNA is made available for binding to a DNA probe with a complementary sequence that is similarly denatured and single stranded. The probe and target DNA then hybridize or anneal to each other in a duplex, based on complementary base pairing. The probe DNA is commonly directly labeled with a fluorescent dye. Fluorescence microscopy then allows the visualization of the hybridized probe on target material.

In situ hybridization with radionuclide labeled probes has been used by a select number of laboratories for more than 25 yr *(2)*, and an example of this approach is given in Chapter 23. Fluorescence nucleic acid-labeling systems have the advantage of providing dual- or triple-target detection using different fluorescent dyes in the same experiment. The signal intensity with fluorescence is greater than with *in situ* hybridization performed with immunochemical labels using enzymes, such as horseradish peroxidase. Versatile labeling systems, streamlined protocols, and vastly improved fluorescence microscopes have enabled most cytogenetics laboratories, and some pathology laboratories, to perform FISH tests as a part of their repertoire.

There are three major categories of DNA sequences used for probes in FISH studies. They are α-satellite or centromeric DNA probes, whole-chromosome probes (WCPs), and unique-sequence probes. Satellite sequences are repetitive DNA sequences in the genome, which do not code for a gene product, and are polymorphic. Different individuals have variation in their number of copies of these DNA. The α satellite DNA is a 171--bp pair DNA monomer, which is repeated n number of times as a tandem repeat. That block of tandem-repeated DNA is copied n number of times, in a higher order repeat, at the centromere of each chromosome *(3,4)*. The majority of this DNA is identical in all of the human chromosomes, but 2–3% of the DNA is variable, to the degree that centromeres of each individual chromosome can be distinguished, and probes to those chromosomes can be produced *(5)*. The exception is the shared homology between chromosomes 13 and 21 and 14 and 22, which are not distinguishable through centromeric FISH studies.

Repeat-sequence probes are useful for counting specific chromosomes, as in aneuploidy determinations; they can be used on both interphase and metaphase cell preparations. Simultaneous visualization can be accomplished with up to three different satellite probes, using different-colored labels or label mixing. These probes are robust, because the targets are large and repeated many times. This allows the hybridization to take place rapidly, allowing for a very large signal.

WCPs are composed of numerous unique and repetitive sequences from an entire chromosome *(6)*. They can be produced through somatic cell hybrids, flow sorting of the specific chromosome, or microdissection of specific chromosomes with PCR amplification of the DNA *(7,8)*. WCPs are also called paint probes, because of the painted appearance of the metaphase chromosomes when hybridized. These probes are designed for use on metaphase chromosome preparations. Their use in interphase results in a splotchy, undefined fluorescence because the interphase chromatin, to which they hybridize, is decondensed, as opposed to the compact, condensed state of metaphase.

For the best results, tissues fixed in formalin or paraformaldehyde are appropriate for FISH analysis. The first step in addressing paraffin wax-embedded tissues is the thickness of the section. The 4-μ section is optimal for FISH studies. Some laboratories have had success with thicker sections and with the use of confocal microscopy to visualize FISH results in these sections. It is best to cut the sections and float them onto a microscope slide coated with silane to avoid sample loss through the many experimental steps. Most investigators air-dry these preparations and bake them overnight at 65°C before storage.

The paraffin is removed from the tissue section with successive washes in xylene or nonorganic clearing agents. Dehydration of the tissue is accomplished in a wash of 100% ethanol. Most tissues will require pretreatment with a proteinase K, pepsin, and/or a chaotropic solution before denaturation of the DNA for FISH. The concentration and duration of the treatment is dependent on the tissue type. Some tissues, such as placenta, kidney, and adrenal gland, are more resistant to digestion than others, such as lung tissue. These conditions must be determined for each specimen block and may vary for similar specimens. Conditions, such as duration and temperature of fixation and age of specimen, affect these variables and require careful monitoring of the pretreatment conditions. It is also commonly noted that tumor cells require less rigorous digestion than normal cells within the same tissue. When evaluating digestion, one must focus on the cell type and the area of the slide of most

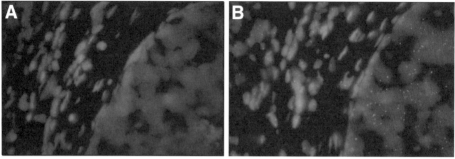

Under-digestion of tissue   **Effective digestion of tissue**

Fig. 1. Fluorescence *in situ* hybridization results after effective pretreatment and digestion of breast tumor tissues. (**A**) Under-digestion of tissue. Breast tumor tissue was hybridized with a fluorescein labeled centromeric probe and counterstained with propidium iodide. (**B**) Effective digestion of tissue. The same sample after further digestion and hybridization with the same probe.

interest. **Figure 1** shows photographs of a breast tumor tissue FISH experiment with different pretreatment regimens after the hybridization experiment is undertaken.

Control probes and control cell specimens should be used when performing FISH studies. Control probes can be run to assure that successful hybridization is accomplished. Control specimens provide essential information about the success of the experiment. For interphase studies, a control probe such as an alpha satellite labeled in a fluorochrome with a different color than the test unique-sequence probe can be hybridized, and both the control and test probe can be counted on 100 or more cells. **Figure 2** shows an example of a c-*myc* FISH study with dual-label hybridization. The number of cells one needs to score for a particular experiment depends on the sensitivity and specificity one would like for the test. These statistical measures quantify how well the test works in determining true positives and true negatives relative to another test. These numbers can be derived from a pilot study, which should include hybridization efficiency, percentage of cells discarded, and normal cut-offs derived from results from normal specimens. A consultation with a statistician may be helpful in these cases.

Reporting results of FISH studies should include the numbers of test and control cells scored and the number of signals of the test and control probe. A narrative analysis of the result should accompany the appropriate International System for Human Cytogenetic Nomenclature 1995 nomenclature (*9*). Specific information about the probe, such as manufacturer and lot number, may also be useful in reports.

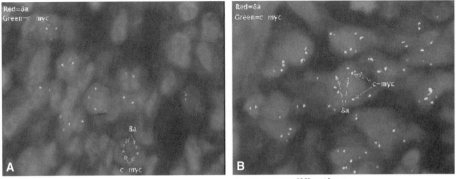

Normal results   **c-*myc* amplification**

Fig. 2. Fluorescence *in situ* hybridization assessment of c-*myc* gene amplification in human breast tumor tissues using a Spectrum Orange labeled c-*myc* and a Spectrum Green chromosome 8 control probe. (**A**) Normal results. (**B**) c-*myc* amplification.

FISH analysis for unique sequence probes is targeted at genes that, when amplified, provide information on the diagnosis and prognosis of specific cancers. These genes include *HER-2/neu*, *p53*, N-*myc*, and c-*myc*. The amplification of *HER-2/neu* is a prognostic indicator in node-negative breast cancer, and its investigation using this technique is the subject of Chapter 22. The *p53* gene may be deleted in B-cell lymphocytic leukemia in a subset of patients *(10)*. The N-*myc* gene is amplified in neuroblastoma, and c-*myc* is commonly amplified in breast carcinoma *(11)*. For the most part, these probes are used on interphase cells in touch-print preparations or paraffin wax-embedded tissues. FISH in these cases is used to enhance the information from other biological marker studies.

An optimally functioning fluorescence microscope is required for FISH analysis, whereas such sensitive instrumentation many not be required for other techniques, such as monoclonal antibody analysis using fluorescence. There are two types of available fluorescence microscopes, which differ in the way the light contacts the specimen. Transmitted light microscopes reflect light from above onto the specimen. Of the two types, incident illumination is better for FISH analysis. The 100-W bulb is preferable for use with unique-sequence probes and situations in which smaller signals are expected. Microscope bulb age and alignment can also affect the apparent strength of the signal. If the microscope is not properly aligned, or if the bulb has been used for greater than 100 h, the nuclei may appear dark and the signal may appear weak.

Objectives that are manufactured specifically for fluorescence microscopy are also optimal, because they are made of low-fluorescing glass and have few lens corrections. Many fluorescence microscopes are equipped with an automatic camera device or image capture software. The optimal camera settings will depend on the type of microscope and should be determined empirically.

When film is exposed for long periods—as with FISH—the sensitivity gradually becomes lower than the labeled value, and a longer exposure time than indicated is necessary. Many fluorescence microscopes are equipped with an automatic camera device. The optimal camera settings will depend on the type of microscope and should be determined empirically.

2. Materials

1. c-*myc* FISH probes directly labeled with a red fluorochrome are the preferable DNA probe for these studies. They are commercially available from Appligene (Strasbourg, France) and from Visis/Abbott (Chicago, IL).
2. 4-μm-thick, paraffin wax-embedded breast tissue specimens on silanized or other adhesive-coated slides are obtained from a tissue bank or pathologist. At least three serial sections must be requested for the studies, as one will be stained for examination by light microscopy.
3. Proteinase K: prepare 25 mg/mL stock solution in distilled water. Add 400 mL of stock solution to 40 mL of distilled water to make protein digestion solution. Store the remaining solution in aliquots of 400 μL at –20°C.
4. 20X saline–sodium citrate (SSC) may be stored at room temperature (18–25°C) until the expiration date on the bottle. Before use, verify that the pH of the solution is 7.0 and adjust with HCL and NaOH, if necessary.
5. 2X SSC/0.5% Nonidet P-40 solution: prepare 1 L and store at room temperature. It is stable for 1 yr.
6. Epifluorescence microscope, equipped with a 100-W Mercury arc lamp and DAPI, red, green, and double- or triple-band pass filters.
7. Glass Coplin jars (50 mL) and plastic Coplin jars for steps that do not require heating.
8. Glass cover slips (22 × 50 mm, 25 × 25, 22 × 22, or 18 × 18).
9. Silanized, frosted-glass microscope slides.
10. Ethanol series: prepare 500 mL (v/v) solutions of 70, 80, 95, and 100% ethanol in distilled water. Store tightly capped at room temperature. Solutions can be kept for 1 mo if exposure to ambient air is limited.
11. Staining solutions hematoxylin and eosin Y Signature Series stains and clarifier reagent (Richard Allen Scientific, Kalamazoo, MI).
12. Xylene.
13. CitriSolv (Fisher Scientific): store in a vented cabinet at room temperature.
14. Humidified chamber for incubation: line empty plastic pipet box or similar container with Whatman filter paper and dampen until moist with distilled water.
15. Incubator or lab oven with thermostat set at 37°C.
16. Micropipetors for P2–P200 mL and tips.
17. Small water baths with thermostat set at 37°C and 70–74°C.
18. Slide warmer with surface thermometer or PCR machine with accommodations for microscope slides.

19. Sodium borohydride.
20. A solution of 2.5 μg/mL propidium iodide in an antifade-containing mounting media can be purchased or made in the lab.
21. Microcentrifuge tubes.
22. Rubber cement for sealing cover slips.
23. 1 *N* HCl for adjusting pH.
24. Concentrated NaOH solution for adjusting pH.

3. Methods

3.1. Slide Preparation (see Note 1)

Paraffin-embedded tissues should be fixed with 10% neutral buffered formalin or paraformaldehyde. Certain fixatives, such as alcohols, can cause nucleic acid precipitation and are thus best avoided. At least five serial sections from each case should be cut, as one will be stained for light microscopic analysis of the sample characteristics including the location of blood vessels, tumor cells, and connective tissue. This slide will be used for orientation in the final scoring of the adjacent FISH treated slide to ensure that the appropriate cell types are scored. Additional slides may also be necessary if a section does not contain the required number of tumor cells or is otherwise inadequate for analysis.

1. Cut formalin-fixed, paraffin wax-embedded tissue sections into 4-μm-thick sections and apply to silanized slides by floating the section in warmed distilled water, then scooping the silanized slide under the tissue section and lifting the slide with the attached tissue section up and out of the water.
2. Include blocks of normal breast tissue for use as a negative control.
3. Allow to air-dry and bake slide at 65°C for 8–16 h.
4. Slides can be stored indefinitely at room temperature, but long-term storage may change the pretreatment conditions.

3.2. Deparaffinating Slides

The following steps should be performed in a fume hood. Solutions can be placed in individual Coplin jars or in a Histotek apparatus specifically designed for sequential slide treatments.

1. Place up to four slides in a Coplin jar containing 40 mL of fresh CitriSolv and incubate slides for 10 min at room temperature. Repeat in a fresh container of CitriSolv for an additional 10 min.
2. Remove the slides and place in a 100% ethanol solution and allow to soak for 5 min.
3. Repeat for an additional 5 min.
4. Remove the slides from the ethanol and allow to air-dry at room temperature. It is best to process the slides for FISH as soon as possible after this step.

3.3. Hematoxylin and Eosin Staining for Section Orientation

1. Rinse slides with deionized water at room temperature for 2 min.
2. Immerse slide in hematoxylin 1 solution for 5 min at room temperature.
3. Rinse slide in running tap water until no more blue strain runs off the slide.
4. Immerse slide in clarifier reagent for 30–60 s.
5. Rinse slide in running tap water 30 s.
6. "Blue" slide in running tap water 1 min.
7. Rinse slide in 95% ethanol.
8. Immerse slide in the eosin Y for 2 min.
9. Dehydrate slide in 100% ethanol for 1-min intervals, three times.
10. Immerse slide in three successive xylene baths for 1-min intervals.
11. Apply cover slip to slide.

3.4. Slide Pretreatment

Pretreatment solutions should be prepared fresh on the day of use.

1. Dissolve 10 g of sodium bisulfite in 30 mL of 2X SSC in a 50-mL tube at 45°C for 5–10 min and transfer to 10 mL of 2X SSC in a Coplin jar within in a water bath heated to 45°C. Incubate specimens in solution for 15 min.
2. Prepare digestion solution of 0.25 mg/mL proteinase K in 2X SSC in a Coplin jar, at 43°C, and incubate slide for 10 min. It is best to monitor the digestion step carefully, as no signal will be revealed if the tissue is underdigested, and the tumor DNA will be degraded if overdigestion occurs. Protein digestion is variable with different specimens, and somewhat dependent on the original fixation times and the nature of the specimen. An assessment can be made before going on to hybridization and additional digestion time can be added.
3. Following the initial 10-min digestion, place 20 µL of the propidium iodide solution on the specimen and cover slip with a glass cover slip. Propidium iodide is water-soluble and will wash out of the specimen easily, following digestion evaluation.
4. Examine using the green filter of the fluorescence microscope. An appropriately digested sample will demonstrate clear borders, and individual nuclei can be discerned and show little background fluorescence. An underdigested sample will show persistent green autofluorescence and poor propidium iodide staining. The amount of additional protein digestion that will be required may be tested in 5-min intervals and depend on the particular sample. Breast tissue samples may have considerable connective tissue and digestion may be difficult. Sometimes, one of the serial sections may be more suitable for the FISH analysis than others.
5. An overdigested sample may show loss of nuclear borders, and the nuclei may appear lost or indistinct. Overdigestion may also result in the loss of the tissue from the slide. If this is the case, start with a new slide with a shorter, 10-min protein digestion, and then evaluate the sample with propidium iodide staining and fluorescence observation.
6. When suitably digested, process slides through a graded ethanol series of 70, 80, and 95% ethanol, for 2 min each, in Coplin jars, at room temperature.
7. Allow slides to air-dry at room temperature.

3.5. Probe Preparation

1. c-*myc* probes directly labeled with Spectrum Orange are available for purchase from Vysis/Abbott and Appligene. A directly labeled control probe for the centromere of chromosome 8, labeled in Spectrum Green or another green fluorophore, can be obtained from Vysis/Abbott, Appligene, or Cytocell (UK), and must be included in the hybridization for analysis.
2. Dilute the concentration of DNA of the control chromosome probe to one half of what is indicated in package insert when mixing with hybridization solution so that the signal does not cross-hybridize when postwashed at a stringency appropriate for the c-*myc* unique-sequence probe.

3.6. FISH Hybridization

1. Prepare a humid chamber for hybridization and prewarm at 37° C, 30 min before hybridization. Codenaturation of the DNA probe and DNA target sequence in the tissue section is accomplished by incubation on a heat block or slide warmer at 85°C for 10 min (*see* **Note 2**).
2. Preheat the surface and place prepared slide on the surface.
3. Denature probe in a 75°C water bath for 5 min and place on ice until ready to hybridize.
4. Apply 10 μL of probe to section and cover slip with a 22 × 22-mm glass cover slip.
5. Seal cover slip edges with rubber cement delivered in a plastic disposable syringe without a needle.
6. Place slides in prewarmed humid chamber and allow to hybridize overnight in a 37°C oven or incubator for 16 h.

3.7. Posthybridization Wash

1. Postwash slides in a Coplin jar preheated to 72°C in a water bath. Be sure to measure the temperature of the wash solution with a calibrated thermometer within the Coplin jar itself. Place slides in the solution for 5 min. This step is critical, and attention to the temperature and time will insure scorable results.
2. Remove slides and place in a Coplin jar containing 4X SSC, with 0.05% Tween-20, at room temperature for 5 min.
3. Rinse once in distilled water at room temperature to remove excess salts and detergents.
4. Allow slide to dry at room temperature, shielded from light.
5. Apply 20 μL of DAPI counterstain diluted in an antifade solution (*see* **Note 3**).
6. Place a 22 × 22-mm glass cover slip over the section.
7. Store slides in a dark slide box at –20°C. Slides can be stored for up to 1 yr, but are best viewed within 2 d of hybridization.

3.8. Microscopy and Scoring

Analyze cells with the use of fluorescence microscopy (*see* **Note 4**). To assure scoring of the appropriate regions of the tissue section, refer to hematoxylin and eosin-stained serial section for orientation and place FISH slide at similar coordinates.

1. In the most robust hybridizations, the DAPI counterstain, red c-*myc* signal, and green, chromosome 8 control signal may be visualized with a triple-band pass filter. The red and green fluorochromes can be distinguished with use of a double-band pass filter and, usually, nuclear definition can be ascertained using this scheme. It may be necessary to view the red and green signals with the individual filters, as these will be the most sensitive for the individual fluorochromes. Results may be variable within the section, and some areas may demonstrate better results than others, so it is worthwhile to scan the hybridized region for the best outcome.

2. Score cells in areas of tissue section that demonstrate unambiguous clear signals and distinct nuclear borders. Score only cells that have both red and green signals. Score distinct signals using ×63 or ×100 objectives by focusing up and down and record the number of red and green signals within 100 clearly defined nuclei.

3. Score a control breast slide at the same time.

3.9. Data Analysis

1. Score data as a ratio of number of c-*myc* signals/number of chromosome 8 signals for each slide. The normal ratio is 1.0.

2. We use the ratio of 1.6 as the low-end cutoff for c-*myc* gene amplification, which is a smaller number than some other amplicons, such as *HER-2/neu.*

4. Notes

1. The most critical considerations in the success of tissue FISH are related to the fixation and processing of the tissue. Breast tissue can be particularly tricky to study, as much connective tissue is present, which may cause autofluorescence and difficulty in scoring the hybridization. It may be necessary to examine multiple slides for scoring. It is practical to realize that hybridization conditions on the experimental slide can vary greatly, with certain parts demonstrating perfect results, and others showing lack of probe penetration and excess autofluorescence.

2. It is also important to be certain that the probe and target are fully denatured. It may be of assistance to denature the DNA probe solution in a 72–75°C water bath before placing it on the tissue. This will assure adequate probe denaturation, and it is unlikely that the probes will become overdenatured.

3. One problem that is simple to avoid with multiple fluorescence stains is a higher-than-necessary concentration of the counterstain. A very bright counterstain can overpower the test and control probe signals so they are not visible.

4. Photography of results can be thorny when the signals are on different planes. The number of signals that are counted through focusing through the planes of the tissue section may not always be simply represented; therefore, confocal microscopy with reconstruction may be helpful in special cases such as a formal publication or grant application.

   This method has been successfully used in a recent study correlation c-*myc* gene amplification expression of its mRNA and protein in high-grade human breast cancer *(12)*.

References

1. Pinkel, D., Gray, J., Trask, B., van den Engh, G., Fuscoe, J., and van Dekken, H. (1986) Cytogenetic analysis by in situ hybridization with fluorescently labeled nucleic acid probes. *Cold Spring Harbor Symp. Quant. Biol.* **51,** 151–157.
2. Pardue, M. L. (1969) Molecular hybridization of radioactive DNA to the DNA of cytological preparations. *Proc. Natl. Acad. Sci. USA* **63,** 378
3. Jabs, E. W., Wolf, S. F., and Migeon, B. R. (1984) Characterization of a cloned DNA sequence that is present at centromeres of all human autosomes and the X chromosome and shows polymorphic variation. *Proc. Natl. Acad. Sci. USA* **81,** 4882–4888.
4. Waye, J. S. and Willard, H. F. (1985) Chromosome-specific alpha satellite DNA: nucleotide sequence analysis of the 2.0 kilobase repeat from the human X chromosome. *Nucleic. Acids Res.* **12,** 2731–2734.
5. Aleixandre, C., Miller, D., Mitchell, A., et al. (1987) p82H identifies sequences at every human centromere. *Hum. Genet.* **77,** 46–50.
6. Lengauer, C., Reithman, H., and Cremer, T. (1990) Painting of human chromosomes generated from hybrid cell lines by PCR with Alu and P1 primers. *Hum. Genet.* **86,** 1–6.
7. Lichter, P., Ledbetter, S. A., Ledbetter, D. H., and Ward, D. C. (1990) Fluorescence *in situ* hybridization with ALU and L1 polymerase chain reaction probes for rapid characterization of human chromosomes in hybrid cell lines. *Proc. Natl. Acad. Sci. USA* **85,** 9138–9142.
8. Guan, X. Y., Meltzer, P., and Trent, J. (1994) Rapid generation of whole chromosome painting probes (WCPs) by chromosome micro-dissection. *Genomics* **22,** 101–107.
9. International System for Human Cytogenetic Nomenclature (1995), in *An International System for Human Cytogenetics Nomenclature* (Mitelman, F., ed.). S. Karger, Farmington, CT, pp. 94–98.
10. Hoff, E. R., Tubbs, R. R., Myles, J. L., and Procop, G. W. (2002) *HER2/neu* amplificaton in breast cancer: stratification by tumor type and grade. *Am. J. Clin. Pathol.* **117,** 916–921.
11. Aulmann, S., Bentz, M., and Sinn, H. P. (2002) c-*myc* oncogene amplification in ductal carcinoma *in situ* of the breast. *Breast Cancer Res. Treat* **74,** 25–31.
12. Blancato, J. A., Singh, B., Liu, A., Liao, D. J., and Dickson, R. B. (2004) Correlation of amplification and over-expression of c-*myc* oncogene in high-grade breast cancer: FISH, *in situ* hybridization, and immunohistochemical analyses. *Br. J. Cancer* **90,** 1612–1619.

22

Detection of *HER2* Gene Amplification by Fluorescence *In Situ* Hybridization in Breast Cancer

John M. S. Bartlett and Amanda Forsyth

Summary

Fluorescence *in situ* hybridization (FISH) is increasingly recognized as the most accurate and predictive test for both *HER2* gene amplification or expression and response to Herceptin™ therapy in breast cancer. Diagnostic procedures for FISH require rigorous quality control, as with all diagnostic procedures, which rely on standardized methodologies. We describe the use of FISH for *HER2* in our own laboratory, based on more than 4000 diagnostic assays, and the optimal approaches to scoring *HER2* gene amplification in breast cancer.

Key Words: Fluorescence *in situ* hybridization; breast cancer; *Her-2*; *neu*; *c-erbB-2*; gene amplification.

1. Introduction

The assessment of *HER2/c-erbB-2/neu* (hereafter *HER2*) gene amplification and protein expression has become one of the central debating points in current breast cancer diagnosis and biology (*see* **refs.** *1* and *2*). The debate around whom to test, when testing should be offered, and most importantly, which method to use, is represented at most current conferences where breast cancer pathology is under discussion.

Overexpression of the p185[HER2] protein product of *HER2/neu* is closely related to gene amplification in breast cancer *(3–8)*. Slamon et al. first described the biological importance of HER2 in breast cancer in 1987 *(9)* and many subsequent publications *(10)* confirm the prognostic significance of HER2 amplification and overexpression in breast cancer *(11–14)*. There has been controversy regarding node-negative carcinomas *(12–14)*, but some of the reported differences may be methodological *(15–17)*. HER2 is one of four homologous receptors that, together, make up the HER (or type I or erbB) family of transmembrane-receptor tyrosine kinases. These receptors form

From: *Methods in Molecular Medicine, Vol. 120: Breast Cancer Research Protocols*
Edited by: S. A. Brooks and A. L. Harris © Humana Press Inc., Totowa, NJ

homo- or heterodimers, following ligand binding to their external domains and activate a complete series of intracellular signaling pathways via autophospho- rylation of tyrosines on their intracellular domains.

Recent clinical trials implicating HER2 in modified responses to antiestrogens and anthracyclins *(11,18–25)* has stimulated interest in accurate and reliable identification of patients with carcinomas driven by HER2 ampli- fication and overexpression *(19)*. Most critically, the recent FDA approval for the first anti-HER2 therapy, Herceptin™, and the wide licensing of this agent throughout the world, coupled with the likelihood of further targeted therapies, has thrown the need for HER2 testing into sharp relief and has intensified the debate.

Fluorescence *in situ* hybridization (FISH) is a technique used to study gene and chromosome copy number *in situ*. It has found clinical application in the assessment of gene rearrangements in leukemia and lymphoma *(26)*, and, recently, forms part of the routine diagnostic assessment of amplification of the gene *HER2/neu* in breast cancer *(27–30)*. There are now a number of dif- ferent commercially available fluorescent and chromogenic *in situ* hybridiza- tion systems, and their use is reviewed elsewhere *(1,2)*. Generic methods for FISH are given in Chapter 20. Recent studies using chromogenic *in situ* hybridization *(1,2,31)* show a high concordance with FISH only when selected cases are also assessed for chromosome 17 copy number. There remains a debate as to how such cases may be prospectively identified in clinical diag- nostic laboratories. The current UK guidelines *(30,32)* therefore recommend the use of systems where chromosome 17 is used as a control for the high level of aneusomy observed in breast cancers *(29,33)*.

2. Materials
2.1. Slide Pretreatment
2.1.1. Manual Protocol

Many of the reagents required for this protocols form part of the Abbott/ Vysis (UK) Paraffin Pretreatment Reagent Kit (cat. no. 32-801200); alterna- tively, they can be made up as described here.

1. Silanized microscope slides (*see* **Note 1**).
2. Control sections (*see* **Note 2**), for example, "Probe check" quality-control slides (Abbott).
3. Water baths set at 80 and 37°C.
4. 0.2 N HCl, pH 2.0.
5. Pretreatment reagent: 8% (w/v) sodium thiocyanate in distilled water.
6. Pepsin (Fluka or Sigma, UK): prepare a 10% (w/v) stock solution in 0.2 N HCl, aliquot, and store at –20°C for up to 4 mo (*see* **Note 3**). Dilute to 25 mg/50 mL

with 0.2 *N* HCl immediately before use or use protease from a Vysis (Chicago, IL) slide pretreatment kit (25-mg lyophilized aliquot in 50 mL 0.2 *N* HCl).

7. Two staining dishes with 100% xylene.
8. Two staining dishes with 100% methanol.
9. Wash buffer: 2X saline–sodium citrate (SSC), pH 7.0: dissolve 175.3 g NaCl and 88.2 g sodium citrate in 800 mL distilled water, pH to 7.0 with 10 *M* NaOH. Make up to 1 L with distilled water and autoclave. Dilute 1:10 with distilled water for 2X SSC).
10. Staining dish with 70% methanol.
11. Staining dish with 85% methanol.
12. 4,6-Diamidino-2-phenylindole-2-hydrochloride ([DAPI] Sigma, UK) in Vecta-shield (Vectorlabs, UK):Vectashield with 200 ng/mL DAPI added.
13. 100-W Epifluorescence microscope with appropriate filters (*see* **Note 4**).

2.1.2. Automated Slide Pretreatment

Where large numbers of FISH samples are being analyzed, we have found that the use of the VP2000 tissue processor (Vysis) produces significant advantages in both tissue-processing time and consistency of results.

1. VP2000 Tissue-processing robot.
2. 2X SSC, pH 7.0: dissolve 175.3 g NaCl and 88.2 g sodium citrate in 800 mL distilled water, and adjust pH to 7.0 with 10 *M* NaOH. Make up to 1 L with distilled water and autoclave. Dilute 1:10 with distilled water for 2X SSC.
3. Silanized microscope slides (*see* **Note 1**).
4. Control sections (*see* **Note 2**), for example, "Probe check" quality-control slides (Abbott).
5. Xylene.
6. 95% Ethanol.
7. Distilled water.
8. 0.2 *N* HCl, pH 2.0.
9. Pretreatment reagent: 8% (w/v) sodium thiocyanate in distilled water.
10. Pepsin (*see* **Note 3**): 250 mg in 500 mL 0.2 *N* HCl (Vysis protease buffer).
11. 10% Neutral buffered formalin.
12. 70% Ethanol.
13. 85% Ethanol.
14. 100-W Epifluorescence microscope with appropriate filters (*see* **Note 4**).

2.2. Denaturation and Probe Hybridization

1. Omnislide hybridization platform (Thermo-Hybaid, UK) with dark, plastic lid.
2. 2X SSC, pH 5.3: dissolve 175.3 g NaCl and 88.2 g sodium citrate in 800 mL distilled water and adjust pH to 5.3 with 10 *M* HCl. Make up to 1 L with distilled water and autoclave. Dilute 1:10 with distilled water for 2X SSC (pH 5.3). Alternatively, take 66 g of 20X SSC salts (provided with PathVysion™ kit [Vysis]) and dissolve in 200 mL distilled water, and then adjust pH to 5.3 with 10 *M* HCl.

Make up to a final volume of 250 mL with distilled water.

3. Denaturing solution, pH 7.0–8.0: 49 mL ultrapure formamide (Fluka, UK), 7 mL 2X SSC (pH 5.3) and 14 mL distilled water. Check pH is between pH 7.0 and 8.0 before each use (*see* **Note 5**).
4. Temporary "cover slips": cut Parafilm into temporary cover slips (*see* **Note 6**).
5. Staining dish with 70% alcohol.
6. Staining dish with 85% alcohol.
7. Staining dish with 100% alcohol.
8. HER2/chromosome 17 probe mixture (from PathVysion kit).
9. Rubber cement (*see* **Note 7**).

3. Methods
3.1. Manual Pretreatment of Slides

Note: This method has been adapted from the PathVysion pretreatment protocol, Abbott Diagnostics, and Vysis.

1. Cut 5-μm tissue sections onto silanized slides (*see* **Note 1**) and bake at 56°C overnight. Store at room temperature until required (*see* **Note 8**).
2. Prepare two water baths, one at 85°C and one at 37°C; place one Coplin jar per five slides to be treated in each water bath. Fill those at 80°C with 8% sodium thiocyanate solution, and those at 37°C with 0.2 N HCl for protease digestion (do not add protease at this time).
3. Immerse slides to be analyzed in xylene for 10 min to remove wax (*see* **Note 9**).
4. Repeat **step 3** with a fresh xylene bath.
5. Transfer slides into 100% methanol for 5 min.
6. Repeat **step 5**.
7. Place slides in 0.2 N HCl for 20 min (*see* **Note 10**) at room temperature.
8. Wash slides in distilled water for 3 min at room temperature.
9. Wash in wash buffer for 3 min at room temperature.
10. Place slides in 8% sodium thiocyanate in distilled water at 80°C for 30 min (*see* **Note 11**).
11. Wash in distilled water for 1 min at room temperature.
12. Wash in wash buffer for 5 min at room temperature.
13. Repeat **step 12** with fresh wash buffer and remove excess fluid before proceeding (*see* **Note 12**).
14. Place in protease buffer at 37°C for 22 min (*see* **Note 13**).
15. Immerse slides in 2X SSC buffer for 5 min at room temperature.
16. Repeat **step 15** with fresh wash buffer.
17. Place slides in 70% alcohol for 1 min at room temperature.
18. Place slides in 85% alcohol for 1 min at room temperature.
19. Place slides in 100% alcohol for 1 min at room temperature.
20. Allow slides to air-dry.
21. Apply DAPI in mountant and apply cover slips.

22. Assess the extent of tissue digestion with a 100-W epifluorescence microscope that incorporates a filter block specific for the excitation and emission wavelengths of DAPI (*see* **Note 14**). If digestion is optimal, then proceed to **step 23**. If sections are underdigested, then proceed to **step 23** and replace sections in protease buffer (**step 14**) for 2–20 min, depending on the extent of underdigestion. Repeat **steps 15–21** and reassess digestion. If sections are overdigested, discard and repeat with new section, reducing the incubation time in protease (**step 14**).

23. Place slides in 2X SSC (pH 7.0) buffer until the cover slips fall off, then dry in an oven at 45°C before proceeding with *in situ* hybridization.

3.2. Automated Pretreatment of Slides

The VP2000 is an automated tissue-processing station with a robotic arm that moves slides (up to 50) among 12 reagent basins, up to three temperature-controlled water baths, a rinse bath (with circulating distilled water), and a drying station. Movement of slides is controlled by a computer with steps programmable for position and duration in each wash. The temperature-controlled baths can also be agitated. The protocol below describes the use of the system for pretreatment of batches of breast tumors.

1. Switch on the VP2000 and computer control station (*see* **Note 15**). Lift the protective plastic covering from each side of the VP2000 processor and remove any metal lids covering solutions. Check the levels of each solution in basins 4–15. The plastic containers have a fine groove; approx 700-mL containers should be topped up to this line with the appropriate solution every time the machine is run.

2. Basins 1–3 are the temperature-controlled water baths. Basin 1 contains the pretreatment solution and basin 3, the protease buffer. The pretreatment solution should be topped up to 500 mL before each use with distilled water (*see* **Note 16**).

3. If required, top up the protease buffer in basin 1 to 500 mL with fresh protease buffer (*see* **Note 17**); do not add protease at this time.

4. Allow the water bath to fill with distilled water from the reservoir.

5. Place slides (up to 50) into the slide holder and mount on the robotic arm.

6. Allow the water baths to reach target temperatures (80 and 37°C). Add protease to protease buffer and select a program. For HER2 FISH pretreatment, we use the following:

    a. Xylene (basin 4) for 5 min at room temperature.

    b. Xylene (basin 5) for 5 min at room temperature.

    c. Xylene (basin 6) for 5 min at room temperature.

    d. 95% Ethanol (basin 7) for 1 min at room temperature.

    e. 95% Ethanol (basin 8) for 1 min at room temperature.

    f. 0.2 *N* HCl (basin 9) for 20 min at room temperature.

    g. Water rinse (water bath set to recirculate) for 3 min at room temperature.

    h. Pretreatment reagent (basin 1) for 30 min at 80°C.

    i. Water rinse (water bath set to recirculate) for 3 min at room temperature.

    j. Protease digestion (basin 3) for 18 min (*see* **Note 18**) at 37°C.

k. Water rinse (water bath set to recirculate) for 3 min at room temperature.

l. Fix in 10% neutral buffered formalin (basin 11) for 10 min at room temperature.

m. Water rinse (water bath set to recirculate) for 3 min at room temperature.

n. 70% Ethanol (basin 12) for 1 min at room temperature.

o. 85% Ethanol (basin 13) for 1 min at room temperature.

p. 95% Ethanol (basin 14) for 1 min at room temperature.

q. Air-dry (drying station) at 28°C for 3 min.

7. At this point, digestion should be checked using **steps o–q** (*see* **Note 14**) of the manual pretreatment protocol above before proceeding to denaturation and probe hybridization (**Subheading 3.3.**).

3.3. Denaturation and Probe Hybridization

1. Ensure pretreated slides prepared as directed in **Subheadings 3.1.** or **3.2.** are dry.

2. Check pH of denaturing solution and apply 100 μL to each slide in a fume hood (*see* **Note 5**). Cover with a temporary cover slip (*see* **Note 6**). Place slides on Omnislide in rack, with light shielding.

3. Denature slides for 5 min at 72°C, using Omnislide.

4. Remove slide rack from Omnislide and remove temporary cover slips in fume hood.

5. Place in 70% alcohol in fume hood for 1 min at room temperature.

6. Place in 85% alcohol for 1 min at room temperature.

7. Place in 100% alcohol for 1 min at room temperature.

8. Remove slides, remove excess ethanol, and allow to air-dry.

9. Apply 10 μL of HER2/chromosome 17 probe mixture to a 22 × 26-mm cover slip. Invert the slide and lower gently onto cover slip.

10. Seal the slide with rubber cement.

11. Repeat for each slide to be analyzed and place on Omnislide.

12. Hybridize slides overnight at 37°C on the Omnislide, shielded from light (*see* **Note 19**).

3.4. Post-Hybridization Wash

1. Place a Coplin jar containing 50 mL of post-hybridization wash buffer into a water bath set at 72°C. Prepare a staining dish with post-hybridization wash buffer at room temperature.

2. Remove slides from Omnislide hybridization station.

3. Using forceps, remove rubber cement from each slide and place in post-hybridization wash buffer at room temperature to allow cover slip to float off.

4. Check temperature of 72°C post-hybridization wash buffer is 72 ± 1°C before proceeding.

5. Remove slides from room temperature wash and carefully remove excess buffer (*see* **Note 12**).

6. Place slides into post-hybridization wash at 72°C for 2 min. Do not add more than five slides per jar (*see* **Note 20**).

7. Allow slides to air-dry shielded from light (*see* **Note 21**).

8. Mount slide in mountant with 0.2 ng/mL DAPI and seal with clear nail polish (*see* **Note 22**).

3.5. Quantitation of Hybridization Signals

The description below relates specifically to the scoring scheme used in our laboratory for scoring of *HER2* gene amplification; alternative systems for scoring chromosome copy, and androgen receptor amplification are described elsewhere *(34)*.

1. Identify regions for analysis by FISH using adjacent hematoxylin and eosin (H&E)-stained sections for each case (*see* **Note 23**).
2. Count signals for HER2 (orange) and chromosome 17 in 60 nonoverlapping tumor cell nuclei in the control and carcinoma sections (*see* **Note 24**). Record the individual results in the sheet shown below (*see* **Appendix A**), noting the case number, coordinates, batch number of probe, date, and observer code. Score 20 nuclei each from separate tumor areas within the slide where possible (*see* **Note 25**).
3. Calculate the total number of HER2 and chromosome 17 signals observed for each area by summing the counts for each cell in the spreadsheet (*see* **Appendix A**).
4. Calculate the HER2/chromosome 17 ratio for each area by entering the individual counts for HER2 and chromosome 17 into the results spreadsheet as shown in **Appendix B**. This spreadsheet can be set up in programs such as Microsoft Excel or Lotus to automatically calculate variation among area scores and among observers (*see* **Note 26**).

4. Notes

1. Silanized slides can be purchased from several suppliers (e.g., Sigma) or prepared as follows:
   a. Immerse slides in acetone for 5 min (400 mL in a glass container).
   b. Transfer to 2% silane in acetone (8 mL 3'-aminopropyl-triethoxysilane in 392 mL acetone).
   c. Wash slides in water for 25 min (under a running tap). Air-dry slides and store dry until use.
2. In performing diagnostic FISH analysis, it is essential to include internal and external quality controls. We routinely include sections from amplified and nonamplified controls within each diagnostic run, as well as a negative control section, omitting the probe cocktail controls for hybridization efficiency, and nonspecific staining. In addition, we currently participate in a local external quality control scheme. The UK National External Quality Assurance Scheme is currently being expanded to include HER2 FISH testing. We would recommend participation in this or another equivalent scheme.
3. Pepsin activity can be highly variable between suppliers and batches, and therefore activity should be tested before the use of a new batch. Pepsin is also highly labile, and activity declines rapidly once diluted. Pepsin should be added to

digestion buffer immediately before starting digestion and fresh pepsin added for each batch of slides to be digested. If more than 30 min is required for digestion, additional pepsin should be added.

4. The use of a 100-W epifluorescence microscope is essential if good results are to be obtained. Filters specific for DAPI, Spectrum Orange, and Spectrum Green are required, along with a triple-band pass filter for all flourophores. We would also recommend the use of a dual-band pass Spectrum Orange/Green filter for the HER2 test. For other flourophores, appropriate filters will need to be purchased. For many applications, a ×40 or ×63 objective is sufficient; however, when scoring FISH, we prefer to use a ×100 objective.

5. The denaturing solution contains formamide, which is toxic and should be handled within a fume cabinet.

6. The use of temporary cover slips in conjunction with a humidified hybridization chamber, such as that present on the Omnislide, provides a convenient alternative to glass cover slips. Temporary cover slips are made by cutting Parafilm to the appropriate size. Following addition of the denaturation solution, the Parafilm is used to cover the slide during the 5-min denaturation period.

7. Routinely, we use rubber cement supplied for cycle puncture repair, as it is provided in easy to use tubes.

8. Unlike some immunohistochemistry procedures, we have not observed any deterioration of slides when stored for prolonged periods (6–24 mo) before FISH analysis. However, we recommend the use of slides within a period of 6 mo of cutting.

9. Xylene should be used with care and within a fume hood. The solvent should be changes periodically to avoid wax buildup in the wash bath. The use of nonorganic solvents such as Hemo-De, where available, may provide a safer alternative to xylene.

10. 0.2 N HCl is thought to act by acid deproteination of tissue, thus increasing probe penetration, possibly because a partial reversion of the fixation process. The use of a pretreatment permeabilization step reduces the requirement for prolonged incubation in proteases and allows preservation of better tissue morphology.

11. Sodium thiocyanate acts as a reducing agent to break the protein–protein disulphide bonds formed by formalin fixation and facilitates subsequent proteolytic digestion.

12. Fluid can be removed by gently touching the slide, edgewise, onto a pad of absorbent tissues.

13. The duration of exposure of the slides to protease is perhaps the most critical step in ensuring adequate pretreatment of formalin fixed tissues before application of DNA probes for FISH. The extent of treatment required varies according to the tissue and to a far lesser extent, to the degree of fixation. We recommend digestion times be evaluated in each laboratory to optimize results. In our laboratory and in many others, the optimal protease digestion time for breast cancer specimens is between 22 and 28 min. This is significantly longer than that described within the PathVysion protocol. In our experience, one of the main reasons for the failure of a laboratory to establish FISH is over-rigid adherence to an inad-

equate digestion period. The importance of ensuring adequate digestion cannot, therefore, be underestimated. When performing FISH for the first time, we would recommend performing a digestion series on representative samples, using the digestion assessment protocol defined in **Note 14**. Selected slides, with optimal morphology, can then be identified for hybridization with probes. The duration of exposure of tissue sections to pepsin required for adequate digestion will vary from tissue type to tissue type and, to a far lesser degree, within tissues. In our experience, tissues such as breast require digestion times of between 18 and 22 min, whereas tissues from bladder cancers require digestion times of 25–30 min. The concentration and activity of pepsin will also influence the duration of this step (*see* **Note 3**), and therefore, digestion times should be reassessed each time the pepsin batch is changed.

14. When assessing the nuclei for extent of digestion, the staining intensity resulting from the intercalation of DAPI with DNA in the nucleus is a good indicator. Nuclei that stain gray to gray-blue are underdigested and, once the cover slip is removed, can be reintroduced to a fresh batch of pepsin/HCl for up to 15 min. Nuclei that stain blue with clearly visible nuclear borders are suitably digested. Where nuclear borders are lost, these sections are overdigested and are discarded. The digestion is repeated with different sections for 30 min. It is important to examine areas from different parts of the slide when dealing with thin sections that have been formalin-fixed and paraffin-processed, as there will inevitably be variations in the fixation effects and therefore, in the effect of pepsin digestion. If the digestion of at least two-thirds of the tumor is acceptable, then these slides will be suitable for hybridizing.

15. The VP2000 should be switched on before the computer to allow the computer to recognize the VP2000.

16. Pretreatment solution contains 8% (w/v) sodium thiocyanate: during each run at 80°C, some water is lost from this solution, and this is replaced by topping up the solution with distilled water. We recommend replacing the solution either every 2 wk or after between 5 and 10 runs.

17. Use protease buffer from the same batch number. The pH of the protease buffer should be checked before use and adjusted, if required, with 0.1 M HCl to pH 2.0 ± 0.1. We recommend replacing the solution either every 2 wk or after between 5 and 10 runs.

18. Digestion times on the VP2000 tend to be slightly shorter than those for manual pretreatment, possibly because of greater circulation of buffer within the digestion chamber. However, similar principles apply and a digestion series (*see* **Note 13**) should be produced before commencing FISH routinely. We have found sections digested using the automatic protocol to be more reproducibly digested and have a greater success rate, with less requirement for redigestion than those treated manually.

19. A minimum hybridization time of 12–14 h is recommended.

20. Addition of slides to the posthybridization wash will lower the temperature. A maximum of five to six slides per Coplin jar should be added, because addition of

further slides may compromise the stringency of the posthybridization wash. If large batches of slides are to be washed simultaneously, either prepare multiple Coplin jars or use larger staining dishes.

21. Simply placing the slides in a cupboard will suffice, although use of light shielded boxes is a useful alternative.

22. Clear nail polish is a useful sealant and can be used to prevent slides from drying out.

23. With experience, it is possible to identify areas for scoring; in most cases, without detailed reference to an adjacent H&E-stained slide. However, because of the high rate of amplification observed in ductal carcinoma *in situ*, which is currently not clinically relevant in regard to HER2-based therapies, confirmation of the tumor morphology by examination of an H&E-stained section by a trained histopathologist should be regarded as central to the diagnosis of HER2 amplification. For samples where dual scoring is to be performed, note the coordinates either on a New England Finder or using the vernier scales on the microscope stage.

24. It is essential that only cells with clear nuclear boundaries are scored. Only nuclei with signals for both chromosome 17 and HER2 signals should be included. Our recent data *(28)* show a high rate of aneusomy for chromosome 17 in breast cancer (>55% cases); therefore, the chromosome 17 copy number should be scored in each case.

25. In a small number of cases (1–2% *[28]*), heterogeneity of amplification may be observed, scoring cells from three separate areas of the tumor markedly increases the likelihood that such heterogeneity will be correctly observed. In cases where only one or two areas are amplified, we recommend scoring additional cells from these areas and reporting the maximum HER2/chromosome 17 ratio with a note to the effect that the tumor was heterogeneous for HER2 amplification.

26. There are a number of principles embodied in the scoring of FISH signals in tissue sections, many of which are detailed within the PathVysion protocol document. Dual-observer scoring is a valuable means of ensuring accurate results are obtained, particularly when new observers are being trained in the interpretation of FISH signals. In our extensive experience, interobserver variation for absolute counts of signals can be routinely controlled below 10% *(35–37)*. Periodic review of scoring by selective sampling of diagnostic results can be a valuable means of ensuring continued quality control.

References

1. Bartlett, J. M. S., Mallon, E. A., and Cooke, T. G. (2003) The clinical evaluation of HER2 status, which test to use? *J. Pathology* **199,** 411–417.
2. Bartlett, J. M. S., Mallon, E. A., and Cooke, T. G. (2003) Molecular diagnostics for determination of HER2 status. *Diag. Pathol.* **9,** 48–55.
3. Slamon, D. J., Clark, G. M., and Wong, S. G. (1987) Human breast cancer: correlation of relapse and survival with amplification of the *HER-2/neu* oncogene. *Science* **235,** 217–227.
4. Coombs, L. M., Pigott, D. A., Sweeney, E., et al. (1991) Amplification and overexpression of c-*erb-B2* in transitional cell carcinoma of the urinary bladder. *Br. J. Cancer* **63,** 601–608.

Appendix A
Scoring Template for HER2 Fluorescence *In Situ* Hybridization

| Case | | Probe Batch No: | | Date | |
| Number | | Protease batch Number | | Observer | |

AREA 1: Ordinates	Green	Orange	AREA 2	Green	Orange	AREA 3	Green	Orange
1			1			1		
2			2			2		
3			3			3		
4			4			4		
5			5			5		
6			6			6		
7			7			7		
8			8			8		
9			9			9		
10			10			10		
11			11			11		
12			12			12		
13			13			13		
14			14			14		
15			15			15		
16			16			16		
17			17			17		
18			18			18		
19			19			19		
20			20			20		
TOTAL			TOTAL			TOTAL		

5. Reles, A., Marx, D., Meden, H., Hammadi, H., Schauer, A., and Friedmann, W. (1991) *c-erb-B2* oncogene expression in ovarian cancers. *Arch. Gynecol. Obstet.* **250,** 183–184.
6. Tyson, F. L., Boyer, C. M., Kaufman, R., et al. (1991) Expression and amplification of the *HER-2/neu* (*c-erB-2*) protooncogene in epithelial ovarian-tumors and cell-lines. *Am. J. Obstet. Gynecol.* **165,** 640–646.
7. Albino, A. P., Jaehne, J., Altorki, N., Blundell, M., Urmacher, C., and Lauwers, G. (1995) Amplification of *HER-2/neu* gene in human gastric adenocarcinomas. *Eur. J. Surg. Oncol.* **21,** 56–60.

Appendix B
Result Spreadsheet for HER2 Amplification (Giving Worked Example)

Pathology Number:			Batch No:	
			Date	

Observer 1		Observer 2	

	Chromosome 17	HER-2	Ratio	Chromosome 17	HER-2	Ratio	Mean Ratio
Area 1	50	190					
Area 2	45	180					
Area 3	48	195					

Score Obs 1	Score Obs2

Inter-Observer variation

Overall c-erbB2 ratio is	

Tumour is   **Amplified**   **Normal**   (circle 1)

8. Underwood, M. A., Bartlett, J., Reeves, J., Gardiner, D. S., Scott, R., Cooke, T. (1994) *C-erbB2* gene amplification as a molecular marker in bladder cancer. *Cancer Res.* **81,** 1822–1822.

9. Slamon, D. J., Godolphin, W., Jones, L. A., et al. (1989) Studies of the *HER-2/neu* proto-oncogene in human breast and ovarian cancer. *Science* **244,** 707–712.

10. Revillion, F., Bonneterre, J., and Peyrat, J. P. (1998) *ERBB2* oncogene in human breast cancer and its clinical significance. *Eur. J. Cancer* **34,** 808.

11. Ross, J. S. and Fletcher, J. A. (1998) The *HER-2/neu* oncogene in breast cancer: prognostic factor, predictive factor, and target for therapy. *Stem Cells* **16,** 413–428.

12. Andrulis, I. L., Bull, S. B., Blackstein, M. E., et al. (1998) *neu/erbB-2* amplification identifies a poor-prognosis group of women with node-negative breast cancer. Toronto Breast Cancer Study Group. *J. Clin. Oncol.* **16,** 1340–1349.

13. Dalifard, I., Daver, A., Goussard, J., et al. (1998) p185 overexpression in 220 samples of breast cancer undergoing primary surgery: comparison with c-*erbB-2* gene amplification. *Bioorg. Med. Chem. Lett.* **1,** 855–861.

14. Press, M. F., Bernstein, L., Thomas, P. A., et al. (1997) *HER-2/neu* gene amplification characterized by fluorescence *in situ* hybridization: Poor prognosis in node-negative breast carcinomas. *J. Clin. Oncol.* **15,** 2894–2904.

15. Piffanelli, A., Dittadi, R., Catozzi, L., et al. (1996) Determination of ErbB2 protein in breast cancer tissues by different methods. Relationships with other biological parameters. *Breast Cancer Res. Treat.* **37,** 267–276.

16. Press, M. F. (1990) Oncogene amplification and expression. Importance of methodologic considerations. *Am. J. Clin. Pathol.* **94,** 240–241.

17. Press, M. F., Hung, G., Godolphin, W., and Slamon, D. J. (1994) Sensitivity of HER-2/neu antibodies in archival tissue samples: Potential source of error in immunohistochemical studies of oncogene expression. *Cancer Res.* **54,** 2771–2777.

18. Goldenberg, M. M. (1999) Trastuzumab, a recombinant DNA-derived humanized monoclonal antibody, a novel agent for the treatment of metastatic breast cancer. *Clin. Therap.* **21,** 309–318.

19. Giai, M., Roagna, R., Ponzone, R., De Bortoli, M., Dati, C., and Sismondi, P. (1994) Prognostic and predictive relevance of c-*erbB-2* and ras expression in node positive and negative breast cancer. *Anticancer Res.* **14,** 1441–1450.

20. Rosen, P. P., Lesser, M. L., Arroyo, C. D., Cranor, M., Borgen, P., and Norton, L. (1995) Immunohistochemical detection of *HER2/neu* in patients with axillary lymph node negative breast carcinoma. A study of epidemiologic risk factors, histologic features, and prognosis. *Cancer* **75,** 1320–1326.

21. Carlomagno, C., Perrone, F., Gallo, C., et al. (1996) c-*erbB2* overexpression decreases the benefit of adjuvant tamoxifen in early-stage breast cancer without axillary lymph node metastases. *J. Clin. Oncol.* **14,** 2702–2708.

22. Muss, H., Berry, D., and Thor, A. (1999) Lack of interaction of tamoxifen (T) use and *ErbB-2/Her-2/Neu* (H) expression in CALGB 8541: a randomized adjuvant trial of three different doses of cyclophosphamide, dooxrubicin and fluorouracil (CAF) in node positive primary breast cancer (BC). *Proc. Am. Soc. Clin. Oncol.* **18,** 68A (abstract).

23. Paik, S., Bryant, J., Park, C., et al. (1998) *erbB-2* and response to doxorubicin in patients with axillary lymph node- positive, hormone receptor-negative breast cancer. *J. Natl. Cancer Inst.* **90,** 1361–1370.

24. Ravdin, P. M., Green, S., Albain, V., et al. (1998) Initial report of the SWOG biological correlative study of c-*erbB-2* expression as a predictor of outcome in a trial comparing adjuvant CAF T with tamoxifen (T) alone. *Proc. Am. Soc. Clin. Oncol.* **17,** 97A (abstract).

25. Thor, A. D., Berry, D. A., Budman, D. R., et al. (1998) *erbB-2, p53,* and efficacy of adjuvant therapy in lymph node-positive breast cancer. *J. Natl. Cancer Inst.* **90,** 1346–1313.

26. Arber, D. A. (2000) Molecular diagnostic approach to non-Hodgkin's lymphoma. *J. Mol. Diag.* **2,** 178–190.

27. Mitchell, M. S. and Press, M. F. (1999) The role of immunohistochemistry and fluorescence *in situ* hybridization for *HER-2/neu* in assessing the prognosis of breast cancer. *Sem. Oncol.* **26,** 108–116.

28. Pauletti, G., Godolphin, W., Press, M. F., and Slamon, D. J. (1996) Detection and quantitation of *HER-2/neu* gene amplification in human breast cancer archival material using fluorescence *in situ* hybridization. *Oncogene* **13,** 63–72.

29. Bartlett, J. M. S., Reeves, J., Stanton, P., et al. (2001) Evaluating *HER2* amplification and overexpression in breast cancer. *J. Pathol.* **195,** 422–428.

30. Ellis, I. O., Dowsett, M., Bartlett, J., et al. (2000) Recommendations for HER2 testing in the UK. *J. Clin. Pathol.* **53,** 890–892.

31. Isola, J., Tanner, M., Forsyth, A., Cooke, T. G., Watters, A. D., and Bartlett, J. M. S. (2004) Interlaboratory comparison of HER2 oncogene amplification as detected by chromogenic and fluorescence *in situ* hybridization. *Clin. Cancer Res.* **10,** 4793–4798.

32. Ellis, I. O., Bartlett, J., Dowsett, M., et al. (2000) Recommendations for HER2 testing in the UK. *J. Clin. Pathol.* **53,** 890–892.

33. Watters, A. D., Going, J. J., Cooke, T. G., and Bartlett, J. M. S. (2003) Chromosome 17 aneusomy is associated with poor prognostic factors in invasive breast carcinoma. *Breast Cancer Res. Treat.* **77,** 109–114.

34. Edwards, J., Krishna, N. S., Mukherjee, R., Watters, A. D., Underwood, M. A., and Bartlett, J. M. S. (2001) Amplification of the androgen receptor may not explain the development of androgen-independent prostate cancer. *Br. J. Urol.* **88,** 633–637.

35. Bartlett, J. M. S., Watters, A. D., Ballantyne, S. A., Going, J. J., Grigor, K. M., and Cooke, T. G. (1998) Is chromosome 9 loss a marker of disease recurrence in transitional cell carcinoma of the urinary bladder? *Br. J. Cancer* **77,** 2193–2198.

36. Bartlett, J. M. S., Adie, L., Watters, A. D., Going, J. J., and Grigor, K. M. (1999) Chromosomal aberrations in transitional cell carcinoma that are predictive of disease outcome are independent of polyploidy. *BJU Int.* **84,** 775-779.

37. Watters, A. D., Ballantyne, S. A., Going, J. J., Grigor, K. M., and Bartlett, J. M. S. (2000) Aneusomy of chromosomes 7 and 17 predicts the recurrence of transitional cell carcinoma of the urinary bladder. *BJU Int.* **85,** 42–47.

23

In Situ Hybridization Combined With Immunohistochemistry to Localize Gene Expression

Rosemary Jeffery, Toby Hunt, and Richard Poulsom

Summary

This chapter describes methods that allow researchers to localize sites of gene expression at both the mRNA and protein levels, within a histological section of a single tissue or tissue microarrays.

Identification of the cells within a tumor specimen that express a specific mRNA (assessed by hybridization *in situ*) or protein (assessed by immunohistochemistry) is a significant step toward understanding tumor behavior that is not possible using methods in which tissues are homogenized before analysis. Combined detection of mRNA and protein may permit effects of subtle regulatory processes such as translational repression to be observed and allow coexpression of genes to be detected. Application of such combined techniques to tissue microarrays of tumor tissues from cohorts of patients with known clinical outcome would allow the predictive value of specific patterns of expression to be tested retrospectively.

Key Words: Microarray; gene expression; screening; *in situ* hybridization; cancer; phenotype; genotype.

1. Introduction

In situ hybridization (ISH) can provide crucial information about where a specific gene is expressed and has been applied successfully to a great variety of breast cancer research projects. The Cancer Research UK *In Situ* Hybridization Service has hybridized more than 51,000 tissue sections. Our preferred method for detecting mRNA in routinely fixed paraffin wax-embedded materials, developed over several years from the method described by Senior and colleagues *(1)*, continues to rely on ^{35}S-labeled riboprobes, despite the high profile in the literature of nonisotopic methods. We consider that ^{35}S provides the best balance of specificity, sensitivity, and cost *(2)*. Most importantly, isotopic, unlike nonisotopic ISH, gives reproducible and easily interpretable results, without the need to adjust the method to individual cell types within

From: *Methods in Molecular Medicine, Vol. 120: Breast Cancer Research Protocols*
Edited by: S. A. Brooks and A. L. Harris © Humana Press Inc., Totowa, NJ

tissue sections *(3)*. Other experienced ISH facilities confirm that isotopic ISH is more sensitive than nonisotopic, even when signal amplification steps are included *(4)*. Fluorescence ISH methods are given in Chapter 20, and the application of this approach is the subject of Chapters 21 and 22.

For many genes, the sites where protein is present, revealed by immunohistochemistry (IHC), do not correspond to the sites of synthesis, revealed by *in situ* hybridization to the mRNA, often because the protein is secreted and taken up elsewhere. ISH and IHC are methods that complement each other, revealing different aspects of the gene's expression. ISH can be applied to look for sites of potential synthesis as soon as a sequence has been cloned, much more quickly than a specific antibody can be produced *(5,6)*; indeed, ISH can sometimes be used to help validate a candidate antibody *(7)*. Immunohistochemistry is the subject of Chapter 15.

Some research projects require comparison of the patterns of expression of mRNA and protein on the same histology section, and we have recently developed protocols that can accomplish this in sections of conventional blocks and tissue microarrays (*see* Chapter 4). Our experience of combined IHC/ISH is relatively limited; we believe that the distributions revealed are not significantly different from those seen using the methods singly, but this should be established for each study.

Our ISH protocol gives good results, allowing localization of moderately abundant mRNA in the vast majority of routine surgical specimens. With the economies of scale, reagent costs are approx $22 per slide.

Comparison of many published ISH protocols reveals that "essential steps" highlighted by one group may not be used by another. Nevertheless, there are common principles and quality control checkpoints that are very useful to observe.

The key stages in a successful ISH study are:

1.1. Probe Design and Synthesis

Riboprobes are single-stranded RNA molecules synthesized by in vitro transcription using a DNA-directed RNA polymerase (SP6, T3, or T7), sufficient nucleoside triphosphates (including ^{35}S UTP), and a suitable DNA template. *Templates* are lengths of double-stranded DNA bearing the sequence for RNA polymerase binding and initiation, followed by a sequence that is specific to the target RNA. A riboprobe capable of binding to an mRNA must be a strand complementary to the target mRNA, i.e., an RNA version of the noncoding strand. Usually, templates are made from *plasmid* DNA that has been linearized with a restriction endonuclease. A convenient way to prepare large amounts of good-quality template is to start from a cloned cDNA fragment in a plasmid vector. Alternatively, specific cDNA fragments can be amplified by reverse transcriptase-polymerase chain reaction using primers containing RNA polymerase sequences, for example *(4)*. Ideal features of a plasmid for making an antisense riboprobe are shown in **Fig. 1** and explained in **Note 1**. Template DNA must be of good quality, as explained in **Note 2** and **Fig. 2**.

1.2. Preparation of Tissues

Results in **Fig. 3** were all obtained using paraffin blocks of tissues fixed with a formalin fixative and processed routinely as if for pathological evaluation. Postmortem specimens should be avoided, but even 35-yr-old blocks of routinely processed clinical specimens may work well if they have intact mRNA (check with a β-actin probe; *see* **Note 3**). Reblocking small fragments of tissue from one wax block to another does not usually cause problems, and tissue arrays (described in **Chapter 4**) made using needle biopsies of suitable donor blocks are a convenient way to survey large numbers of cases for population studies of mRNA expression. Frozen tissues may give good mRNA labeling, but are awkward to store and handle, and above all, give poor morphology. Cell cultures can be studied as cytospins or directly if grown on glass slides.

1.3. Immunohistochemistry

Conventional IHC is used to deposit a stable reaction product at precisely those sites where the primary antibody has bound.

1.4. Permeabilization of Tissues

This step enables the probe to gain access to the target and is standard for routinely processed blocks. Frozen sections and cell cultures do not usually need this step.

1.5. Hybridization

The riboprobe is encouraged to base pair with homologous complementary sequences in conditions designed to speed up the rate of association, yet minimize nonspecific binding to other sequences and proteins.

1.6. Washing

Following hybridization, sections are treated with RNaseA to degrade unhybridized riboprobe and to cleave imperfect hybrids. The resultant fragments are then washed out at higher stringency to reduce background signals.

1.7. Autoradiography

Slides are dipped in sensitive photographic liquid emulsion to form a thin layer, dried, and then kept for 2–70 d to allow a latent image to form. A perma-

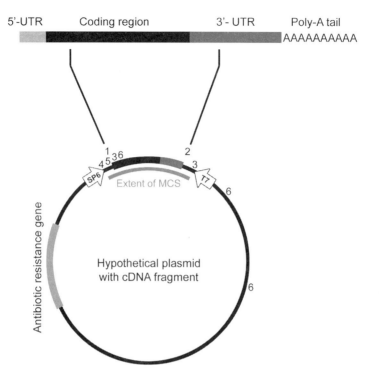

Fig. 1. Designing an ideal plasmid for making a riboprobe. The target mRNA has coding and untranslated regions and a poly (A) tail. Following database searches, the region 1,2 (between 100 and 1.3 kb, being free of repeat elements, areas of strong homology with other mRNA, and its poly [A] tail) was selected and cloned into the plasmid as shown, using conventional restriction cloning or reverse transcriptase-poly-merase chain reaction of the region. The recipient plasmid bears two DNA-directed RNA polymerase-binding sites, one for the T7 polymerase and one for SP6; in this example, the T7 will make antisense riboprobes capable of detecting the mRNA. Mul-tiple cloning sites vary considerably among vectors. For making riboprobes, use a vector with a short multiple cloning site that allows the 3'-end of the cDNA fragment to be close to the RNA polymerase start to minimize undesired probe sequence and irrelevant binding (*see* **Note 1**). Members of the pGEM series (Promega) are preferred to pBluescript (Stratagene), or pCR series vectors (Invitrogen). Clones from the I.M.A.G.E. Consortium *(18)* sets using the vector pT7T3D-pac (modified from the Pharmacia parent) are also preferred. 3,3: Sites cut by a restriction endonuclease that could not make a useful template because one cut occurs between the antisense-pro-ducing polymerase site and the cDNA fragment. 4: A potentially useful restriction site for making template, except that undesired vector sequence is added to the riboprobe (need to cut closer to the insert). 5: A better location for restriction, except that this enzyme leaves a 3' overhang (potentially problematic). 6, 6, 6: Sites cut by the selected restriction enzyme (generating ideally 5' overhangs or blunt ends). The number of cuts is irrelevant, but there must be a fragment containing the template sequence and the RNA polymerase binding site.

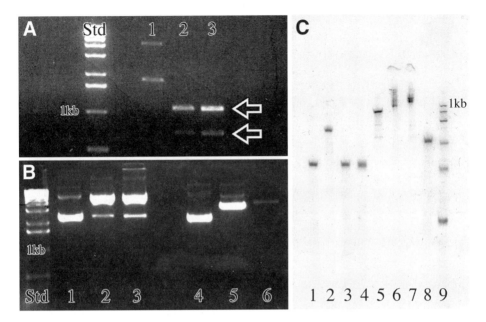

Fig. 2. Quality control by gel analysis (*see* **Note 2**). (**A**) Aliquots of plasmid DNA before restriction (lane 1), after restriction (lane 2), and "final template sample" after clean up (lane 3) reveals that the linearization process is broadly complete (no bands of supercoiled plasmid remain). In this example, a plasmid for the positive control riboprobe to detect human β-actin *(12)* has been digested with *Dra*I, producing two bands (arrows). A standard DNA ladder helps establish that fragment sizes are correct. (**B**) In these two examples, aliquots of plasmid DNA before restriction (lanes 1, 4), after restriction (lanes 2, 5) and after clean up (lanes 3, 6) reveal poor preparation of template: the linearization process is incomplete (bands of supercoiled plasmid remain in lanes 2, 3), and recovery of DNA after clean up was poor (lane 6 very weak band). (**C**) Autoradiographs of approx 10^6 cpm of each riboprobe were separated on a 6% polyacrylamide gel in the presence of 6 *M* urea (cat. no. EC 6865580X; Invitrogen, UK), dried, and exposed to Kodak (UK) X-AR film at room temperature for approx 15 min. Lanes 1–4 and 8 (the human β-actin control probe *[12]*) show good riboprobes, with distinct single bands of radioactivity at the correct size, a very weak tail of shorter fragments, and no bands of "wrap-around" transcripts. Lane 5 shows a good riboprobe (the two additional bands may be because of some secondary structure in the template and are acceptably weak). In contrast, lanes 6 and 7 show poor riboprobes of uncertain size, with evidence of wrap-around transcripts; such probes are unlikely to give good ISH results. Lane 9 contains 10^6 cpm of an RNA transcript size-standard (*see* **Subheading 2.2.9.**).

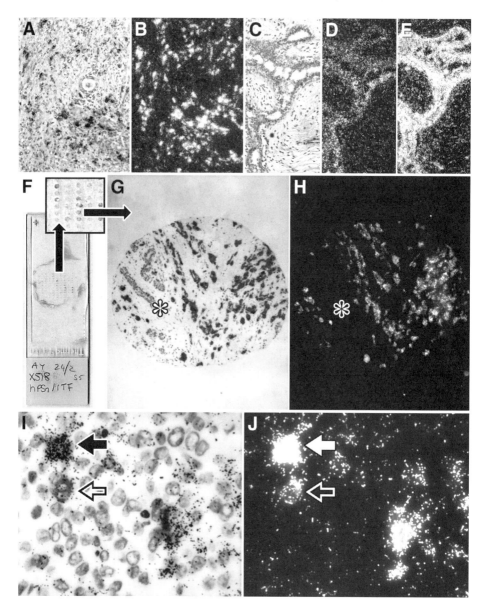

Fig. 3. Micrographs showing localization of mRNA and combined immunohistochemistry/*in situ* hybridization using routine histology blocks. Most bright-field images are accompanied by their reflected-light, dark-field counterpart, obtained simply by switching from conventional illumination to epi-illumination (*see* **Note 7**). **(A,B)** Detection of human stromelysin 3 mRNA in breast cancer using a 467-base probe (plus some vector sequence) and exposing for 13 d. Only the most intense clusters of silver grains can be seen at this magnification (*continued on next page*)

nent image made up of silver grains is then developed, a counterstain used to reveal the tissue architecture, and a glass cover slip applied to protect the completed preparation.

1.8. Interpretation of Results

Dense clusters of black–silver grains, visible with most microscopes at moderate magnification (100–200× overall), are produced with long exposure times. However, if reflected-light, dark-field conditions are used to look at the slides, much shorter exposure times are needed, and clusters of even a few grains can be appreciated at moderate magnification and a true assessment of background graininess can be made.

ISH is an excellent technique for revealing the cell types that express the highest levels of the target, compared to surrounding tissue, and can readily identify just a few cells that express a target at moderate levels, even when a Northern blot is negative (8). Conversely, if a target is expressed widely at moderate levels, for example glyceraldehyde-3-phosphate dehydrogenase, the impression may be simply that of a generally grainy high background, even though a Northern blot of homogenized tissue would be strongly positive.

The entire ISH procedure, from labeling probes and cutting sections through to dipping, takes 4–5 d (**Fig. 4**), plus autoradiographic exposure time (2–3 d for abundant mRNA targets and 10 d for a moderately abundant mRNA target; prolonged exposure times are limited by background grain formation that depends on many variables). For convenience and economy, slides are processed in batches of 100 or 200.

Combining IHC with ISH successfully depends on carrying out conventional IHC in RNase-free conditions and making a reaction product stable to subsequent steps that contrasts well with the ISH grains. We prefer Vector Red precipitate to the brown deposits made by 3,3'-diaminobenzidine.

Fig. 3. (*continued from opposite page*) unless using reflected light imaging (24). (**C,D**) The level of expression of Wnt 5a mRNA in a phyllodes tumor (25) cannot be seen unless reflected-light, dark-field imaging is used: a 385-base probe and exposing for 11 d. (**E**) The positive control section shows that β-actin mRNA was detectable at various signal levels in all regions of this tissue: 11 d exposure. (**F–J**) Combined immunohistochemistry and *in situ* hybridization on a tissue microarray: pS2 (TFF1) protein in red and TFF3 mRNA silver grains. In the samples shown at high magnification, TFF1 peptide is present in most carcinoma cells but not other cell types (asterisk). Most tumor cells express both TFF1 peptide and TFF3 mRNA, although individual cells can be found with just TFF3 mRNA ([**I,J**] solid arrow) and virtually only TFF1 peptide ([**I,J**] open arrow). The TFF3 probe contained 221 bases of specific sequence: 5 d exposure.

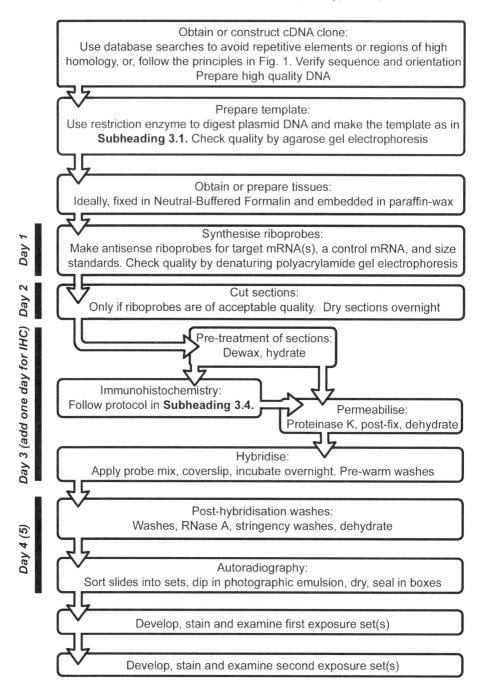

Fig. 4. Flow chart of the principal steps involved.

2. Materials

Be aware of the health and safety requirements involved in working with all reagents, because many require considerable care. We use Milli-Q water for all solutions unless specified, although other high-quality water should be satisfactory.

2.1. Template Preparation

1. Nuclease-free water: water shaken with 0.1% vol. diethylpyrocarbonate (DEPC) then autoclaved.
2. Tris-HCl/ethylenediaminetetraacetic acid (EDTA) (TE) buffer: 10 mM Tris-HCl (pH 8.0) and 1 mM EDTA. Store at room temperature after autoclaving.
3. Phenol/chloroform/isoamyl alcohol (cat. no. 15593-031; Invitrogen, Carlsbad, CA), stored as directed.
4. Chloroform/isoamyl alcohol (cat. no. C-0549; Sigma, Poole, UK) stored at 4°C.
5. 7.5 M Ammonium acetate: 14.44g (cat. no. A 1542, Sigma) made up to 25 mL with water. Store at room temperature after autoclaving.

2.2. Probe Labeling (In Vitro Transcription)

1. 5X Transcription buffer: supplied with RNA polymerases purchased from Promega (Southampton, UK). Store at –20°C.
2. RNase inhibitor: 20 U/µL (cat. no. N2111, Promega), store at –20°C.
3. Dithiothreitol ([DTT] cat. no. D 9779, Sigma): For 1M, dissolve 19.25 g and make up to 125 mL with water. Prepare 100-mM and 10-mM stocks and autoclave. Store single-use aliquots in microfuge tubes at –20°C for up to 1 yr.
4. AGC mix: ATP, GTP, CTP each at 6.25 mM in water. Prepare from Boehringer Ingelheim (Germany) stocks and store 25-µL reusable aliquots in microfuge tubes at –20°C for up to 6 mo.
5. ^{35}S UTP at 40 mCi/mL, 800 Ci/mmol (cat. no. SJ 40383; GE Healthcare, Little Chalfont, UK, or cat. no. NEG 039H; DuPont, Stevenage, UK).
6. DNase I: RNase-free grade from Boehringer Ingelheim or Promega. Store at –20°C.
7. Chromaspin-30 columns: DEPC-equilibrated type from Clontech (UK).
8. Ribosomal RNA: dispense 25 U DEPC-treated water directly into the vial (cat. no. R 5502, Sigma) to achieve a final concentration of 10 mg/mL. The RNA content per unit varies between batches. Store 25-µL aliquots in microfuge tubes at –20°C for up to 1 yr.
9. Control templates: "Perfect RNA marker" templates provide transcripts of 0.1–1.0 kb (cat. no. 69003-3; Novagen Merck KGaA, Darmstadt, Germany).

2.3. Cutting and Preparing Paraffin Sections

1. Microscope slides. These need to be RNase-free and treated to encourage adhesion of the section, for example, "colorfrost" charged slides (cat. no. 9991002; Thermo Shandon, Runcorn, UK).

2. Rehydrating alcohols plus DEPC: used before permeabilization. Prepare 500 mL each of a series of ethanol solutions using high-quality ethanol and DEPC-treated water: 100, 80, 60, and 30% ethanol. Add 0.1% vol of DEPC but *do not* autoclave. Use for only approx 400 slides.

3. Phosphate-buffered saline (PBS): for example, dissolve one PBS tablet (cat. no. P4417, Sigma) in 400 mL water. For PBS+, treat with 0.1% vol. DEPC and then autoclave.

4. Proteinase K: dissolve 200 mg of proteinase K (cat. no. P 4914, Sigma) in 20 mL TE buffer, making a 10-mg/mL stock. Store as 1-mL aliquots in microfuge tubes at –20°C. Just before use, add 1 mL to 500 mL of 37°C TE buffer to make the working solution of 20 µg/mL.

5. Glycine/2X PBS: 0.2% glycine (cat. no. G 4392, Sigma) dissolved in 2X PBS, and then autoclaved.

6. 4% Paraformaldehyde (PFA) in PBS: add 20 g of PFA (cat. no. P 6148, Sigma) to 500 mL of PBS, warm carefully to approx 80°C in a fume hood. If necessary, use a few drops of 1 M NaOH to dissolve resistant solids. Cool on ice to approx 20°C. Make freshly each time.

7. 100 mM Triethanolamine buffer: dissolve 37.5 g of triethanolamine (cat. no. T 1502, Sigma) in DEPC-treated water and make up to 2 L. Autoclave and store for up to 3 mo.

8. Acetylation buffer: within *seconds* before use, add 1.25 mL of acetic anhydride (cat. no. A 6404, Sigma) to 500 mL of 0.1 M triethanolamine buffer.

9. Dehydrating alcohols plus DEPC: used before hybridization. Prepare 500 mL each of a series of ethanol solutions, using high-quality ethanol and DEPC-treated water: 30, 50, 70, 90, and 100% ethanol. Add 0.1% vol DEPC but *do not* autoclave. Use for only approx 400 slides.

2.4. Immunohistochemistry (Optional)

See Chapter 15 for more guidance on immunohistochemistry.

1. Acetic acid solution: 20% vol glacial acetic acid in methanol. Prepare freshly for single use.

2. Serum block: for this example, rabbit serum (cat. no. X0902; DakoCytomation, Ely, UK). Store as directed. Dilute 1:25 with PBS+ just before single use.

3. Primary antibody: for this example, a mouse monoclonal antibody (cat. no. 18-0162; Zymed, Cambridge Bioscience, Cambridge, UK) against the estrogen-inducible peptide pS2 (TFF1). Store as directed. Dilute 1:50 in PBS+ just before single use.

4. Secondary antibody: for this example, to detect a mouse monoclonal with human tissue sections use biotinylated rabbit antimouse (cat. no. E0354, Dako-Cytomation). Store as directed. Dilute 1: 500 in PBS+ just before single use.

5. Detection conjugate: streptavidin–alkaline phosphatase (cat. no. D0396, DakoCytomation).

6. Detection substrate: vector Red (cat. no. SK5100; Vector Labs, Peterborough, UK).

2.5. Hybridization

1. RNase-free cover slips: open a new pack of precleaned cover slips, wrap approx 25 in aluminum foil, and then bake at 180°C in 50-mL beakers covered in aluminum foil.
2. Ribosomal RNA: as described in **Subheading 2.2.**
3. Formamide (deionized): for hybridization buffer only. Take 400 mL of formamide and 20 g of ion exchange resin (501–×8, 20–50 mesh fully regenerated; Bio-Rad, Hemel, Hempstead, Germany). Stir in fume hood cupboard overnight. Filter using a no. 1 filter paper to remove resin. Store at –20°C in small aliquots (approx 1 mL).
4. 10X Salts solution: dissolve 14.2 g Na_2HPO_4 in stages in 100 mL of water and adjust to pH 6.8. Add 176.2 g NaCl, then 100 mL of 1 M Tris-HCl (pH 7.6) and 250 mL of 0.2 M EDTA (pH 7.5) and mix. Make up to final volume of 1 L with water. Do not autoclave or filter. Store at room temperature.
5. Dextran sulfate solution: Dissolve 50 g of dextran sulfate (cat. no. D8906, Sigma) into 100 mL of autoclaved water in a sterile bottle at 80°C (water bath). Store 1-mL aliquots in microfuge tubes at –20°C.
6. Denhardt's and salts solution: add 5 mL of 10X salts solution directly to the vial (cat. no. D-9905, Sigma; store at 0–5°C) containing a powder that is very hard to dissolve. Transfer to a 50-mL plastic tube and dissolve in a total of 25 mL of 10X salts solution. Store 300-μL aliquots in microfuge tubes at –20°C.
7. Hybridization buffer: for 1 mL, combine the following in a microfuge tube in order:
   a. 100 μL Denhardt's and salts solution.
   b. 500 μL Formamide (deionized).
   c. 30 μL rRNA.
   d. 200 μL Dextran sulfate solution (prewarmed to reduce viscosity).
   e. 10 μL 1 M DTT.

Mix well. May be stored at –20°C for a few months.

2.6. Washing

1. Formamide wash buffer: add 250 mL 10X salts solution to 1.25 L of formamide (nondeionized; BDH, Poole, Dorset, UK). Make up to 2.5 L with DEPC-treated water.
2. Tris-HCl/NaCl/EDTA (TNE) buffer: for RNase A digestion. Combine 146 g of NaCl, 50 mL of 1 M Tris-HCl (pH 7.6), 25 mL of 0.2 M EDTA (pH 7.5), and make up to 5 L with water. Adjust to pH 7.2–7.6.
3. Stock RNase A: dissolve 500 mg of ribonuclease A (cat. no. R-5503, Sigma) in 10 mL of 10 mM sodium acetate (pH 5.2). Heat to 100°C for 15 min, cool, and adjust to pH 7.4 with 1 M Tris-HCl. Store 1-mL aliquots in microfuge tubes at –20°C.
4. 20X saline–sodium citrate (SSC): dissolve 175.3 g of NaCl and 88.23 g of sodium-citrate in 750 mL of water. Adjust to pH 7.0 if necessary, and then make up to 1 L. Autoclave and store at room temperature.

5. 5 *M* Ammonium acetate solution: 96.25 g made up to 250 mL with water. Autoclave and store at room temperature.
6. Dehydrating alcohols plus acetate: used before autoradiography. Prepare 500 mL each of a series of ethanol solution, using high-quality ethanol and DEPC-treated water: 30, 50, 70, 90, and 100% ethanol containing 30 mL of 5 *M* ammonium acetate in 500 mL each solution. Use for only approx 400 slides.

2.7. Autoradiography

1. Emulsion (Ilford [Mobberley, UK] K5 in gel form, size A): 50 mL is the preferred pack size. Store at 4°C in original light-proof packing away from any radioactive source. Once opened, use within 3–4 wk. Do not reuse diluted emulsion.
2. D-19 developer: purchased from Kodak (UK), diluted, and stored as described by manufacturer.
3. Stop solution: 1% vol glacial acetic acid in water. Use once only. Store up to 6 mo.
4. Fixer: 30% (w/v) sodium thiosulfate in water. Use once only. Store up to 6 mo.
5. Dilute Giemsa solution (cat. no. 350864X, BDH): Dilute 1:5 with water and then filter. May be reused. Store up to 3 mo or until staining becomes weak.
6. DPX (a mixture of distyrene [a polystyrene], tricresyl phosphate [a plasticizer] and xylene): synthetic mountant DePeX (cat. no. 36125-2B, DBH).

3. Methods

3.1. Template Preparation

1. To a microfuge tube, add 50 µg plasmid DNA (approx 1 mg/mL solution in TE or water), 35 µL of 10X restriction endonuclease buffer appropriate to the chosen restriction enzyme, and nuclease-free water to 340 µL. Mix, and then remove 3.5 µL as a "predigest" sample to be kept at –20°C for later analysis.
2. Add 10 µL of chosen restriction enzyme (10 U/µL), mix, and incubate at the temperature specified by the enzyme supplier for 3–4 h. Mix, and then remove 3.5 µL as a "postdigest" sample to be kept at –20°C for later analysis.
3. Add 350 µL of phenol/chloroform, shake gently to emulsify for 2 min, then centrifuge at 13,000*g* for 5 min in a bench-top microcentrifuge.
4. Transfer the upper (aqueous) phase to a fresh microfuge tube, taking care to avoid the interphase.
5. Repeat **steps 3** and **4**.
6. Add 300 µL of chloroform/isoamyl alcohol, shake gently to emulsify for 2 min, and then centrifuge at 13,000*g* for 5 min.
7. Transfer the upper (aqueous) phase to a fresh microfuge tube, taking care to avoid the interphase.
8. Add 100 µL of 7.5 *M* ammonium acetate, mix, and then add 750 µL of ethanol and mix again.
9. Allow to stand for approx 30 min at room temperature.
10. Pellet the DNA at 13,000*g* for 15 min.
11. Discard the supernatant, and then add 1 mL of 70% ethanol.

12. Pellet the DNA at 13,000*g* for 15 min.
13. Discard all of the supernatant by careful pipeting, and allow the pellet to air-dry (about 15 min).
14. Add 25 µL of 10 m*M* Tris-HCl and 0.1 m*M* EDTA (pH 7.6) and dissolve the template DNA (37°C, 10 min).
15. Remove 1 µL as a "final template sample." The stock template solution may be stored at –20°C for several years.
16. Assess the efficiency of plasmid cleavage production by conventional 1% agarose ethidium bromide gel electrophoresis of the three samples taken.
17. Measure the concentration of the final template solution spectrophotometrically, or estimate by comparing the fluorescence of its band with those in the pre- and postdigestion samples. If necessary, adjust the concentration of the final template solution to approx 1 mg/mL.

3.2. Probe Labeling (In Vitro Transcription)

1. To a microfuge tube at room temperature, add in order:
   a. 2.5 µL of 5X transcription buffer.
   b. 1.0 µL of RNase inhibitor.
   c. 0.7 µL of DTT (100 m*M*).
   d. 2.0 µL of AGC mix.
   e. 2.4 µL of stock template solution/nuclease-free water (to give 1 µg template DNA).
   f. 3.5 µL of ^{35}S UTP.
   g. 0.4 µL (6–8 U) of appropriate RNA polymerase from Promega.
2. Incubate at 37–40°C, 60 min.
3. Destroy template by adding DNase I (1 U, 1 µL) and incubating at 37°C, 15 min. During this time, prepare a Chromaspin-30 column by centrifugation as described by manufacturer.
4. Add DTT (10 m*M*, 25 µL) and carrier Ribosomal RNA (10 mg/mL, 1.5 µL) to reaction mixture tube, and mix well.
5. Remove a 1-µL sample, dilute with 50 µL water, and add 3 mL scintillant to estimate initial ^{35}S present.
6. Add bulk of reaction mixture to top of gel in a Chromaspin-30 column.
7. Centrifuge at 700*g* for 3 min at 15°C, collecting eluate into a new tube containing DTT (100 m*M*, 4 µL) and RNase inhibitor (2 µL).
8. Mix well and remove 1 µL for dilution with 50 µL water and 3 mL scintillant to estimate total ^{35}S incorporated.
9. Assess riboprobe quality by standard 6% polyacrylamide denaturing gel electrophoresis (cat. no. EC 6865580X; Invitrogen, UK) of duplicate aliquots of 10^6 cpm riboprobes (and standard riboprobes) for 55 min, dry gel, and expose to X-ray film for 15 min. Meanwhile, store riboprobes at –20°C until use within a few days.
10. Discard columns and vials as appropriate for ^{35}S waste.

3.3. Cutting and Preparing Paraffin Sections (see Note 3)

1. Wearing gloves, cut sections at 4 μm, using a microtome with disposable blades.
2. Float sections using a clean brush or forceps onto DEPC-treated water (fresh daily), degassed before use if necessary.
3. Collect sections onto treated microscope slides.
4. Dry sections overnight in 40°C oven in racks or card slide trays protected from dust.
5. Dewax in fresh xylene for 8 min (two changes).

   Note: Alcohols and xylene are not autoclaved!

6. Rehydrate by sequential immersion in the rehydrating alcohols plus DEPC, 5 min each.
7. Rinse in PBS+.

3.4. Optional Steps for Immunohistochemistry

1. Block endogenous alkaline phosphatase in the acetic acid solution at room temperature for 5 min.
2. Wash in PBS+, twice, for 5 min each wash.
3. Block nonspecific serum binding by covering entire area of tissue with 200 μL diluted rabbit serum. Incubate in a humid chamber for 15 min.
4. Shake off serum, then cover area of tissue with 200 μL of diluted primary antiserum. Incubate in a humid chamber for 35 min.
5. Wash in PBS+, twice, for 5 min each wash.
6. Shake off PBS+ and apply 200 μL of diluted secondary antiserum. Incubate in a humid chamber for 35 min.
7. Wash in PBS+, twice, for 5 min each wash.
8. Shake off PBS+ and apply 200 μL diluted detection conjugate. Incubate in a humid chamber for 35 min.
9. Wash in PBS+, twice, for 5 min each wash.
10. Prepare Vector Red substrate: add 2 drops of reagent 1 to 5 mL of 200 mM Tris-HCl (pH 8.2), mix well, and then add 2 drops of reagent 2. Mix again and then add 2 drops of reagent 3. Mix and then apply approx 250 μL of this solution to cover the tissue on each slide. Incubate in a humid chamber for 5–15 min as appropriate (examine using microscope).
11. Wash in PBS+. Proceed directly to **Subheading 3.5.**, or, if necessary, dehydrate slides through ascending alcohol series (plus DEPC), air-dry, and then store in dust-free conditions for a few days.

3.5. Permeabilization and Postfixation

1. Permeabilize tissue with proteinase K at 37°C for 10 min.
2. Rinse in glycine/2X PBS for 5 min to block the proteinase.
3. Rinse in PBS+ for 5 min.
4. Postfix in 4% PFA in PBS for 10 min.
5. Rinse in PBS+, three times, for 5 min each rinse.
6. In a fume hood, immerse slides in 500 mL of acetylation buffer for 10 min.

7. Wash in PBS+, three times, for 5 min each wash.
8. Dehydrate by sequential immersion in the dehydrating alcohols plus DEPC, 5 min each.
9. Air-dry. The specimens are now ready for hybridization.

3.6. Hybridization

1. Add riboprobe/water (*see* **Note 4**) to hybridization buffer in a microfuge tube, heat at 80°C for 1 min to "denature" probe, mix well, centrifuge briefly to reduce aerosols, and then chill the mix on ice.
2. Pipet 20 µL onto each section (the mix is viscous, so volumes are approximate).
3. Gently lower an RNase-free glass cover slip onto each slide until it makes contact with the hybridization buffer, and then allow the buffer to spread under the weight of the cover slip.
4. Working in a fume hood, place the slides horizontally in, for example, plastic slide-mailing boxes or Sakura slide racks, and place in lunch boxes humidified with blotting paper saturated with 1X salts and 50% formamide.
5. Seal the lunch boxes with PVC tape and incubate overnight at 55°C.

3.7. Washing

Prewarm all solutions before use.

1. Place the first wash buffers in water baths ready for use the following day: per 25–50 slides, 5 L of TNE buffer at 37°C, and 2 L of formamide wash buffer at 55°C.
2. In a fume hood, open the lunch box containing the slides.
3. Remove the slides, gently remove each cover slip by soaking in buffer if necessary, and place in a slide rack immersed in 500 mL of formamide wash buffer at 55°C on a rocking table, four changes over a total of 3–4 h.
4. Remove all traces of the formamide wash buffer using nine changes of 500 mL of TNE buffer at 37°C, shaking over approx 45 min.
5. During the TNE washes, thaw 1 mL of stock RNase A, and then add to 500 mL of TNE.
6. Incubate the slides with the RNase A solution at 37°C for 1 h in a plastic lunch box. Keep specific containers for this step. Dispose of RNase-contaminated gloves.
8. Wash slides in 2X SSC for 30 min at 65°C with agitation, twice.
9. Wash slides in 0.5X SSC for 30 min at 65°C with agitation (*see* **Note 5**).
10. Pass slides through graded ethanols (30, 50, 70, 90, and 100% ethanol), all containing 0.3 *M* ammonium acetate.
11. Air-dry covered to avoid dust. The specimens are now ready for autoradiography.

3.8. Autoradiography

1. In a darkroom, using a 902 filter and a 15-W bulb, heat a water bath to 42°C.
2. Cool a metal plate on ice.
3. Add 25 mL of water to a cut-down, 100-mL measuring cylinder or beaker in the 45°C bath. Add Ilford K5 emulsion until volume is 40 mL and leave at least

10 min to allow emulsion to melt, and then use a glass rod to stir the solution thoroughly. Leave for 20 min.

4. Stir slowly again. Dip a test slide, wipe the back of it on a paper towel, and then place it on the cooled plate to chill the emulsion layer. Hold the slide up to the safelight; there should be no bubbles (if so, allow emulsion to rest for another 5 min) and the layer of emulsion should be smooth and even with no streakiness (if not, mix again and retest).

5. Dip slides one at a time by dipping vertically into the warm emulsion until the tissue section is immersed. In one smooth movement, lift the slide clear of the emulsion and rest the end on the dipping vessel for approx 10 s to recover the excess. Wipe the end and back of the slide with a paper towel before placing on the cooled plate.

6. Allow slides to dry for about 2.5 h, in total darkness if possible, until the surface of the emulsion is hard when scratched with a fingernail.

7. Place dry slides in a wooden (or plastic but not metal) slide rack/holder/box. Seal into light-proof, black plastic bag.

8. Store in 4°C fridge to expose emulsion (2–70 d as appropriate; *see* **Note 6**).

9. Develop sets of exposed slides in safelight conditions by immersion in preprepared Kodak D-19 developer at approx 18°C for 4 min, agitating each minute (use glass or plastic slide carriers).

10. Immerse in 400 mL of stop solution for 30 s.

11. Immerse in tap water for 30 s.

12. Immerse in 400 mL of sodium thiosulfate fixer, two changes of 4 min each.

13. Wash extensively in many changes of (preferably running) cold tap water over 1 h. Slides may now be exposed to light.

14. Counterstain tissues by immersing racked slides in diluted Giemsa solution for 3–4 min.

15. Wash out excess stain with tap water for 30 s.

16. Air-dry and then mount in DPX under glass cover slips.

17. When the DPX is set, clean the back of the slides with a hard-backed blade, then front and back with 70% ethanol and paper tissue to remove all traces of emulsion and grease.

3.9. Interpretation

If possible, arrange to view the sections using a microscope that allows rapid switching between conventional illumination and reflected light (*see* **Note 7**).

Under conventional illumination with 100× overall magnification and moderate exposure times, only the most intense clusters of black-silver grains can be seen (*see* **Fig. 3A**), unless much higher magnification is used and the field of view was limited to perhaps 100 or 200 cells. In contrast, looking at the same slide in reflected light (*see* **Fig. 3B**), much lower densities of silver grains are seen easily. More importantly, the quality of background obtained can be assessed in moments. Sections that in conventional illumination appear to have no labeling, may, in fact, reveal significant patterns of mRNA expression in reflected light (*see* **Fig. 3C,D**). With Giemsa's counterstain, the nuclei of cells without nearby grains appear greenish-yellow or golden in reflected light, and the threshold for deciding whether a cell or cell type is labeled can be chosen while looking at thousands of cells and associated extracellular matrices.

Switching between conventional illumination and reflected-light, dark-field conditions is an extremely useful way to assess whether there are any significant patterns of silver grains on the section, or if significant "expression" is occurring in specific regions.

If ISH and IHC have been combined (*see* **Fig. 3F–J**), it may be difficult in reflected light to detect silver grains revealing mRNA over intense red reaction product for protein. However, many advantages remain, and it is clear even from moderately low magnification views of a single-tissue microarray core (*see* **Fig. 3G,H**) that some epithelial and vascular structures express neither TFF1 protein or TFF3 mRNA *(8)*, and that the majority of tumor cells express both to varying extents.

Certain cell types have well-deserved reputations for nonspecific binding. Eosinophils frequently show nonspecific binding *(9)* despite the fact that their granules are rich in RNases. Stratified squamous epithelium in the skin can give high background, and melanin can confuse, although in reflected light, melanin is brownish unlike the bright, silver grains.

Routine use of sense strand controls is of dubious value. Sense strand probes made from the same plasmid as the antisense probe contain different domains of vector sequence. These will have a different propensity to bind nonspecifically *(10)*. Careful attention to probe design (*see* **Note 1** and **Fig. 1**) should reduce the likelihood that probes contain promiscuous regions.

Consider whether there may be related mRNA targets that the antisense probe should also recognize *(11)*.

The principal concern should be with the specificity of signals obtained with the antisense probe. Was the stringency high enough to give specific signals? When riboprobes are used as cross-species, with low-stringency washes, it is possible that some signals derive from homologous targets, for example, other members of a multigene family.

Patterns of expression derived from using several riboprobes on near serial sections can be compared and used to establish that specific, differential patterns of labeling occurred. To establish that there was hybridizable mRNA within all cell types within a section, use a probe to β-actin (*see* **Fig. 3E** and **ref. *12***). Signals from β-actin mRNA are usually strongest over vascular smooth muscle cells and the centers of inflammatory cell aggregates, and are variable among other cell types. In contrast, the levels of signal produced by a probe to the "housekeeping gene" glyceraldehyde-3-phosphate dehydrogenase are less variable and thus, difficult to distinguish from a high background.

Sites of expression of an mRNA can conflict with expectations. For example, immunohistochemistry for gelatinase A (MMP-2) in blocks of breast carcinoma indicates that this metalloproteinase is present principally in the tumor epithelium, yet the mRNA is localized principally to stromal cells with low or undetectable levels of gelatinase A mRNA in the tumor epithelium *(13)*.

The density of silver grains over cells can be scored semiquantitatively *(14)*, as is often done for immunohistochemical staining intensity (0, 1+, 2+, 3+).

Riboprobe ISH offers greater specificity and sensitivity than other ISH methods, because more reporting labels can be hybridized specifically to each target. Nonisotopic riboprobe methods may have some advantages, but their value in experiments intended to screen for sites of expression is severely limited by the fact that peak sensitivity is dependent on the cell type and fixation conditions. With such protocols, permeabilization conditions usually need to be "titrated" for individual blocks and even cell types within a block *(3)*. Signal amplification methods, for example, using tyramide deposition to increase the number of signal-forming sites derived from each probe *(4)*, are less satisfactory than isotopic ISH. *In situ* PCR amplification has been used effectively to increase ease of detection *(15)* but is not robust enough for screening purposes and can be prone to PCR errors *(16)*.

4. Notes

1. The sequence selected to make a probe should not contain intron sequences (which will bind to all nuclei and increase background labeling), common repetitive elements such as Alu repeats or poly (A) tracts (which could increase background by labeling all cells weakly), or domains that are highly conserved among members of a family (which will reduce the specificity of the probe).

   Careful selection of probe sequence can allow ISH to reveal patterns of expression of even closely related mRNA *(6,12)*. Attempts to use riboprobes "across" distant species are risky; lowering the stringency enough to get signals may permit detection of homologous targets. Domains from the 3' untranslated region are especially useful for making probes *(12,13)*; they may be less conserved and also label more intensely and give less background because they are generally AT-rich, so fragments remaining after RNase digestion will wash off at lower stringency.

   Carry out a database search to see what the intended probe is homologous to and, if necessary, linearize the template closer to the RNA polymerase binding site, or clone a different region of cDNA. It does not matter if the enzyme cuts several times, as long as the desired island is created. As a rough guide to avoiding crosshybridization, exclude stretches of perfect match longer than 15 bases. Minimize the amount of GC-rich sequence derived from the multiple cloning site of plasmids, as this can increase background *(10)*, or use a control vector-only riboprobe to assess this irrelevant binding *(17)*.

A simple way to find a cDNA for ISH studies is to use the Unigene search engine of the National Center for Biotechnology Information (http://www.ncbi.nlm.nih.gov/). This will reveal listings of clones available from resources such as the I.M.A.G.E clone sets *(18)*, distributed by, for example "MRC geneservice," a division of the UK Medical Research Council's Human Genome Mapping Project Resource Centre (http://www.hgmp.mrc.ac.uk/geneservice/index.shtml). Clones in the vector pT7T3D-pac are well suited to ISH, as this vector contributes little to the riboprobe. Always verify the sequence of any clone intended for ISH use.

2. Traditional alkaline lysis methods give good-quality plasmid DNA. Qiagen and Wizard preparations are acceptable if care is taken afterward to ensure that the DNA is made protein- and RNase-free. Starting with small amounts of plasmid (<20 µg) often results in poor-quality templates. Linearize plasmid DNA with up to fivefold excess of restriction enzyme that produces 5' protruding or blunt ends to make an "island" of DNA bearing the appropriate RNA polymerase site and part or all of the cDNA insert. Do not proceed to make riboprobes if the gel (*see* **Subheading 3.1.15.** and **Fig. 2B**) shows incomplete linearization of plasmid DNA. Intact plasmids yields "wrap-around" transcripts, made very efficiently because of the polymerase repeatedly circling the plasmid (**Fig. 2C**). These will impair the final signal-to-noise ratio. Nonspecific initiation from 3' protruding ends (as created by digestion with restriction endonucleases *Kpn*I, *Pst*I, *Pvu*I, *Sac*I, and *Sph*I) has been reported; if there are no alternative restriction sites, use Klenow to blunt such templates by adding 5 U Klenow DNA polymerase to the transcription reaction *before* adding any nucleosides or RNA polymerases; incubate at 22°C for 15 min and then add the other components.

Use moderate-specific activity ^{35}S UTP (approx 800 Ci/mmol at 40 mCi/mL) to make probes with approximately three out of four U residues labeled; it allows efficient synthesis of long probes at approx $1.3–1.7 \times 10^9$ cpm/µg RNA. Never add cold UTP to the transcription reaction. We prefer ^{35}S UTP, rather than ATP, GTP or CTP, which need higher molarities to label efficiently. Double-label synthesis (^{35}S UTP and ^{35}S CTP together, aiming for high specific activity) is inefficient.

Incorporation of ^{35}S should be more than 40%, but is no indication of probe quality; this should be assessed on a 6% polyacrylamide denaturing gel that removes secondary structure and resolves the RNA species by length. If transcripts are not of the expected length, consider the possibility of incorrect orientation of the insert, relative to the RNA polymerase site used. Good probes (*see* **Fig. 2C**) are characterized by a single band of the anticipated size (size standards in lane 9 were made using Novagen's control templates; *see* **Subheading 2.2.9.**). Secondary structures in individual templates give characteristic fingerprints of less-abundant shorter fragments. Nicked DNA templates from poor plasmid preparations give smears of highly variable sizes. RNase contamination often gives a smear of fragments low down the gel, but less severe contamination gives a complex pattern of fragments, and such probes should be discarded. Further examples are shown in **ref. 2**. When RNase contamination is detected, it is usually best to discard all current labeling reagents and start with new stocks.

[33]P is a more expensive alternative to ^{35}S, with similar spatial resolution *(4)* and a short half-life that makes exposure difficult to control *(19)*. [3]H offers excellent spatial resolution but requires lengthy exposure times.

Inappropriate transcription from other RNA polymerase sites is reportedly possible when exceeding 10 U of RNA polymerase per pmol of template; 1 μg of a 3-kb vector contains approx 0.5 pmol of template and thus needs just 5 U of enzyme.

Hydrolysis of probes is often recommended, but this is wasteful of probe and does not improve the final signal-to-noise ratio. Short riboprobes (80 bp) work, but the best signal-to-noise ratios are obtained with longer probes (0.3–1.0 kb, and even 1.6 kb can work well), nonhydrolyzed, and with permeabilization of sections carried out as described.

Do not use riboprobes that have been made more than a few days earlier (reexamination on a 6% polyacrylamide denaturing gel usually reveals some degradation).

Do not cut sections for an ISH run until confident that the probes are acceptable.

3. Many formalin-based fixatives are well suited to ISH studies, for example, neutral buffered formalin, formal saline, phenol formalin, and formal calcium. Limit fixation time to no longer than one overnight, and then replace the fixative with 70% ethanol. For small pieces of gut, at least 5 h fixation is adequate, and perfusion fixation does not seem to give better results than immersion. Glutaraldehyde-fixed tissues are too resistant to protease digestion. Avoid the coagulating fixatives Carnoy's *(20)* and Methacarn, and citrus oil substitutes for xylene during processing. Tissues fixed in the presence of mercury give autoradiographic artifacts.

Chill paraffin blocks face up on ice as needed, but do not use any block face treatments to assist cutting. Discard the first five sections from the block, even if you have used it recently. Lift sections onto the floating-out bath with a clean brush. Sections of pancreas seem able to leak RNases into the bath, but DEPC-treated water in the bath appears to help.

Label slides with pencil or an engraving slidewriter. Commercial sources of precut tissue sections exist, for example Ambion (http://www.ambion.com/index.html), BD Biosciences (http://www.bdbiosciences.com/), BioCat (http://www.biocat.de/), and academic users may obtain sections of cancer tissue arrays at low cost through the National Cancer Institute's Tissue Array Research Program (http://resresources.nci.nih.gov/tarp/index.cfm). Despite widespread availability of precut sections, we consider that sections are best used for ISH within a week, otherwise, the signal strength is reduced *(2,21)*.

For cell cultures, consider Nunc multiwell slides, as the effects of different culture conditions can be compared on a single slide. Cells on slides should be fixed with 4% PFA in PBS, or in neutral buffered formalin for a few hours, then rinsed in PBS, dehydrated through an ascending alcohol series and air-dried. Use slides fresh if possible, or store slides dry at –70°C for several weeks.

Protease treatment seems unnecessary with frozen sections or cultured cells. Postfixation in 4% PFA in PBS ensures inactivation of the proteinase (and of any RNases). Acetylation is thought to reduce background *(22)*. Sections should be permeabilised, dehydrated, and hybridized on the same day.

For each block of tissue, use a section hybridized to a positive-control-probe, usually β-actin *(12)*, and two sections of each "query" probe to allow two exposure times.

For combined ISH and IHC, we have not explored in detail the use of antisera that require antigen retrieval steps; we have obtained combined results where pepsin digestion has been required (unpublished results). Other combined methods suggest using RPMI tissue culture medium as a diluent for the antibodies *(23)*, but this does not appear to be critical.

4. The volume of hybridization buffer needed is approx 20 µL per section if the tissue is covered completely by a 22 × 42-mm cover slip. For 100 µL of probe mix, use 84 µL of hybridization buffer with 16 µL of probe/water. Use approx 10^6 cpm probe per 20 µL final probe mix. Arrange slides in a fume hood in groups for specific probes on a sheet of paper or purpose-made plastic boxes (Slide Show; BioGenex, UK). Cover slips marked with a permanent marker are easier to see to remove.

   Hybridization is reasonably stringent at 55°C. The combination of a relatively high temperature and a low ion concentration is aimed at reducing the strength of binding between probe and tissue RNA. Bovine ribosomal RNA is used during hybridization to reduce nonspecific binding. Humidification with formamide and salts as used in the hybridization buffer minimizes evaporation and edge effects, but chambers should be filled and emptied in a fume hood.

5. Posthybridization RNase treatment and stringency washes are key steps affecting the signal to noise ratio, and the certainty with which the signal can be considered specific.

   The repeated post-RNase washes are important. Remember that gloves spread RNases by contact. There is no advantage in including mercaptoethanol in the stringency washes that remove remaining short probe segments.

   The use of higher stringency washes (0.1X SSC at 65°C after **step 9, Subheading 3.7.**) may be more reassuring if discrimination among highly homologous targets is needed, but specific signals will be weaker.

6. The dark room must be dark; even indicator lamps on equipment or switched power points may expose emulsion. Test the room by leaving out dipped slides (or X-ray film) partly shielded with aluminum foil for 4 h, develop, and then compare the background graininess. Expose slides away from high-energy radioisotopes.

   Avoid problems by using only high-quality solvents and changing xylene and alcohols frequently.

Forty milliliters of prepared emulsion is enough for 150 slides if a narrow dipping chamber is used. Sections that were mounted away from the frosted end need less emulsion. Lead "doughnuts" (cat. no. L2775, Sigma) help keep the emulsion chambers steady in the water bath. Do not leave the metal plate on ice while dipped slides are drying or condensation will ruin the emulsion.

Anticipate exposure times of 2–5 d for extremely abundant mRNA, 7–10 d for β-actin and other moderately abundant mRNA, and 21–35 d for less abundant mRNA. For a new target with new tissue blocks, develop the positive-control set of slides hybridized for β-actin mRNA and a set of the test riboprobe after 10 d; if the β-actin set have worked well but there are no patterns or background graininess apparent for the test set, try developing the second set after approx 25 d.

Giemsa's stain is good for discriminating many tissue structures and cell types. ISH slides stained with hematoxylin and eosin look "abnormal," because proteinase digestion increases the eosinophilia.

7. Reflected-light, dark-field illumination, as used for metallurgy, can be produced using an epi-illumination lamp and objectives with an outer prism sheath that directs the light down on to the specimen. We use an old Olympus BH-2 with 100-W tungsten epi-illumination lamp housing (BH2-UMA and BH2-HLSH) and 10× and 20× Neo S Plan IC objectives, and a Nikon ME600, again with 100-W epi-illumination).

Several alternative systems are available using epifluorescence microscopes (with or without cross-polarizing filters to obscure most elements of the tissue section). However, condenser block, dark-field systems cannot reveal good results if there are dense clusters of silver grains, because light scattered from the grains illuminates the object as well.

Plastic film cover slips (used by some automated cover slipping machines) produce much poorer dark-field images.

Acknowledgments

This work was supported by Cancer Research UK. We are grateful to those who developed the basis of the method (*1*), to Jan Longcroft and the late Len Rogers, and other colleagues who have helped us carry out the techniques with such care. The tissue microarray used in **Fig. 3** was generously provided by Professor A. M. Hanby.

References

1. Senior, P. V., Critchley, D. R., Beck, F., Walker, R. A., and Varley, J. M. (1988) The localisation of laminin mRNA and protein in the postimplantation embryo and placenta of the mouse: an *in situ* and immunohistochemical study. *Development* **104,** 431–446.
2. Poulsom, R., Longcroft, J. M., Jeffery, R. E., Rogers, L. A., and Steel, J. H. (1998) A robust method for isotopic riboprobe *in situ* hybridisation to localise mRNAs in routine pathology specimens. *Eur. J. Histochem.* **42,** 121–132.

3. Steel, J. H., Jeffery, R. E., Longcroft, J. M., Rogers, L., and Poulsom, R. (1998) Comparison of isotopic and non-isotopic labelling for *in situ* hybridisation of various mRNA targets with cRNA probes. *Eur. J. Histochem.* **42**, 143–150.

4. Frantz, G. D., Pham, T. Q., Peale, F. V., and Hillan K. J. (2001) Detection of novel gene expression in paraffin-embedded tissues by isotopic *in situ* hybridization in tissue microarrays. *J. Pathol.* **195**, 87–96.

5. Burchell, J., Poulsom, R., Hanby, A., et al. (1999) An α2,3 sialyl transferase (ST3 GalI) is elevated in primary breast carcinomas. *Glycobiology* **9**, 1307–1311.

6. Poulsom, R., Hanby, A. M., Lalani, E-N., Hauser, F., Hoffman, W., and Stamp, G. W. H. (1997) Intestinal trefoil factor (TFF3) and pS2 (TFF1), but not spasmolytic polypeptide (TFF2) mRNAs are co-expressed in normal hyperplastic and neoplastic human breast epithelium. *J. Pathol.* **183**, 30–38.

7. Srinivasan, R., Poulsom, R., Hurst, H. C., and Gullick, W. J. (1998) Expression of the c-erbB-4/HER4 protein and mRNA in normal human foetal and adult tissues and in a survey of nine solid tumor types. *J. Pathol.* **185**, 236–245.

8. Chinery, R., Poulsom, R., Rogers, L. A.,et al. (1992) Localisation of intestinal trefoil–factor mRNA in rat stomach and intestine by hybridization *in situ.* *Biochem. J.* **285**, 5–8.

9. Ellis, R. D., Ashwood, P., Powell, J. J., et al. (2002) Selective binding of nucleotide probes by eosinophilic cationic protein during *in situ* hybridisation. *Histochem. J.* **34**, 153–160.

10. Witkiewicz, H., Bolander, M. E., and Edwards, D. R. (1993) Improved design of riboprobes from pBluescript and related vectors for *in situ* hybridisation. *Biotechniques* **14**, 458–463.

11. Moorwood, K., Charles, A. K., Salpekar, A., Wallace, J. I., Brown, K. W., and Malik, K. (1998) Antisense WT1 transcription parallels sense mRNA and protein expression in fetal kidney and can elevate protein levels in vitro. *J. Pathol.* **185**, 352–359.

12. Zandvliet, D. W. J., Hanby, A. M., Austin, C. A., et al. (1996) Analysis of foetal expression sites of human type II DNA topoisomerase α and β mRNAs by *in situ* hybridisation. *Biochim. Biophys. Acta* **1307**, 239–247.

13. Poulsom, R., Hanby, A. M., Pignatelli, M., et al. (1993) Expression of gelatinase A and TIMP-2 mRNAs in desmoplastic fibroblasts in both mammary carcinomas and basal cell carcinomas of the skin. *J. Clin. Pathol.* **46**, 429–436.

14. Dorudi, S., Hanby, A. M., Poulsom, R., Northover, J., and Hart, I. R. (1995) Level of expression of E-cadherin mRNA in colorectal cancer correlates with clinical outcome. *Br. J. Cancer* **71**, 614–616.

15. Mee, A. P., Dixon, J. A., Hoyland, J. A., Davies, M., Selby, P. L., and Mawer, E. B. (1998) Detection of canine distemper virus in 100% of Paget's disease samples by in situ-reverse transcriptase-polymerase chain reaction. *Bone* **23**, 171–175.

16. Steel, J. H., Morgan, D. E., Poulsom, R. (2001) Advantages of *in situ* hybridisation over direct or indirect *in situ* RT-PCR for localisation of galanin mRNA expression in rat small intestine and pituitary. *Histochem. J.* **33**, 201–211.

17. Dunne, J., Hanby, A. M., Poulsom, R., et al. (1995) Molecular cloning and tissue expression of FAT, the human homologue of the *Drosophila* fat gene that is

located on chromosome 4q34-q35 and encodes a putative adhesion molecule. *Genomics* **30,** 207–223.

18. Lennon, G., Auffray, C., Polymeropoulos, M., and Soares, M. B. (1996) The I.M.A.G.E. Consortium: an integrated molecular analysis of genomes and their expression. *Genomics* **33,** 151–152.

19. Longcroft, J. M., Jeffery, R. E., Rogers, L. A., Hanby, A. M., and Poulsom, R. (1994) ^{33}P is a poor alternative to ^{35}S for routine isotopic *in situ* hybridisation. *Cell Vis.* **1,** 90–91.

20. Urieli-Shoval, S., Meek, R. L., Hanson, R. H., Ferguson, M., Gordon, D., and Benditt, E. P. (1992) Preservation of RNA for *in situ* hybridization: Carnoy's versus formaldehyde fixation. *J. Histochem. Cytochem.* **40,** 1879–1885.

21. Lisowski, A. R., English, M. L., Opsahl, A. C., Bunch, R. T., and Blomme, E. A. (2001) Effect of the storage period of paraffin sections on the detection of mRNAs by *in situ* hybridization. *J. Histochem. Cytochem.* **49,** 927–928.

22. Hayashi, S., Gillam, I. C., Delaney, A. D. and Tener, G. M. (1978) Acetylation of chromosome squashes of *Drosophila melanogaster* decrease the background in autoradiographs from hybridization with [^{125}I]-labelled RNA. *J. Histochem. Cytochem.* **26,** 677–679.

23. Spiegel, H., Herbst, H., Niedobitek, G., Foss, H-D., and Stein, H. (1992) Follicular dendritic cells are a major reservoir for human immunodeficiency virus type 1 in lymphoid tissues facilitating infection of CD4+ T-helper cells. *Am. J. Pathol.* **140,** 15–22.

24. Ahmad, A., Hanby, A. M., Poulsom, R., et al. (1998) Stromelysin 3: an independent prognostic factor for relapse-free survival in node-positive breast cancer and demonstration of novel breast carcinoma cell expression. *Am. J. Pathol.* **152,** 721–728.

25. Sawyer, E. J., Hanby, A. M., Rowan, A. J., et al. (2002) The Wnt pathway, epithelial-stromal interactions, and malignant progression in phyllodes tumors. *J. Pathol.* **196,** 437–444.

24

Quantitation of RNA by Ribonuclease Protection Assay

John W. Moore

Summary

A robust ribonuclease protection assay is described here. In brief, total cellular RNA, carrier yeast transfer RNA, and ^{32}P-labeled antisense riboprobes, (one or more designed to detect the RNA species being studied and another to detect a suitable RNA species to act as a loading control) are combined and made 0.5 M with respect to ammonium acetate. Absolute alcohol (2.5 vol) is added, and tubes are incubated at $-20°C$ for 30 min. Precipitated RNA and riboprobes are pelleted by centrifugation and, after removal of the supernatants, dissolved in a small volume of hybridization buffer. After hybridization for 16 h at 55°C, a ribonuclease cocktail is added to digest the unhybridized RNA. This is followed by a proteinase K digestion step that degrades the ribonucleases. Finally, the hybridized complex is precipitated at $-20°C$ using isopropanol:4 M guanidium thiocyanate (2:1), with added glycogen as a coprecipitant, and harvested by centrifugation. The pellet is dissolved in loading buffer, and the sample is electrophoresed in a polyacrylamide gel. The intensities of the bands in the gel representing the protected fragments for the target RNA and the loading control are quantitated by phosphorimager analysis.

Key Words: Ribonuclease protection assay method; RNA quantitation; RNA analysis; riboprobe; quantitation.

1. Introduction

The current interest in gene discovery using microarray analysis has resulted in an explosion of RNA species shown to be regulated under different experimental conditions. Confirmation of array data by other quantitative techniques of RNA analysis such as Northern blotting, reverse transcriptase-polymerase chain reaction (PCR), or ribonuclease protection assay protection analysis are usually required, and each technique has its place in the laboratory. Northern blots are useful in determining molecular size but are less sensitive than protection assays when it comes to assessing up- or downregulation of RNA. Reverse transcriptase-PCR is useful in quantifying expression of RNA species but has quite a narrow linear range. Real-time PCR can be used, but this is very

From: *Methods in Molecular Medicine, Vol. 120: Breast Cancer Research Protocols*
Edited by: S. A. Brooks and A. L. Harris © Humana Press Inc., Totowa, NJ

expensive, requiring specialized equipment and commercially prepared reagents and is more suited to the routine laboratory. In the research environment, ribonuclease protection assay is versatile, capable of high throughput and is the preferred choice of method.

To the uninitiated, setting up a protection assay can be a daunting task, so in this chapter points of detail are emphasized, which, if followed, should help researchers to master this powerful technique.

The method of detecting RNA species by ribonuclease protection analysis depends on the resistance of RNA/RNA hybrids to digestion by ribonucleases. In brief, 5–50 µg of total cellular RNA (the amount required depends on the level of expression of the RNA species being studied) is incubated with a ^{32}P-labeled antisense riboprobe. This is transcribed from template DNA, homologous to the RNA species of interest, which has been cloned into a vector bearing suitable bacterial promoter sequences. The probe is made by incubating ^{32}P-labeled nucleotide triphosphate (in this method, ^{32}P-CTP is used) along with nonradiolabeled nucleotides and a suitable RNA polymerase.

The method used in this chapter is adapted from one previously described *(1)*. Total cellular RNA, carrier yeast transfer RNA, and probes are combined and made 0.5 *M* with respect to ammonium acetate. Absolute alcohol (2.5 vol) is added and tubes are incubated at –20°C for 30 min. Precipitated RNA and riboprobes are pelleted by centrifugation at max. speed in a bench-top centrifuge and, after removal of the supernatants, dissolved in a small volume of hybridization buffer. After hybridization for 16 h at 55°C, a ribonuclease cocktail is added to digest the unhybridized RNA. This is followed by a proteinase K digestion step that degrades the ribonucleases. Finally, the hybridized complex is precipitated at –20°C, using isopropanol:4 *M* guanidium thiocyanate (2:1), with added glycogen as a coprecipitant, and harvested by centrifugation. The pellet is readily dissolved in loading buffer and the sample is electrophoresed on a polyacrylamide gel.

Chapter 7 covers the extraction of RNA from tumor and other cell and tissue samples. Ribonucleases are inactivated during the process, and it is obviously extremely important not to reintroduce these enzymes during the analysis. Gloves should always be worn and changed frequently. Use only disposable plasticware, because it is considered ribonuclease-free if touched only by the gloved hand. Store RNA samples at –80°C, thaw quickly, and keep on ice. To remove a sample for analysis, vortex mix and pulse centrifuge the tube before opening. Refreeze the stock immediately. If the samples are extracted correctly and stored in ribonuclease-free water, freezing and thawing up to 10 times has been shown not to affect the quality of the RNA.

2. Materials

Chemicals, reagents, enzymes, etc, should be the best molecular biology grade and can be purchased from any reputable supplier. Specific suppliers of equipment are named in this chapter because the author uses them in his laboratory, and they are reliable. Other equipment, designed for the job, from reputable suppliers should work just as well, although design and directions for use may be, of course, different.

2.1. Specialized Equipment

1. Sequi-Gen GT polyacrylamide gel electrophoresis systems and a Power Pac 3000 (Bio-Rad Laboratories, UK). The electrophoresis system comes in two sizes (21×50 cm and 38×50 cm) and comprises an integrated plate assembly (IPC) with a bonded inner glass plate and an outer glass plate that, when assembled into the working unit, is clamped to the IPC. The two plates are separated by two machined vinyl spacers, 0.4 mm thick. (*See* the Bio-Rad Laboratories catalog for an exploded diagram.) In addition, plastic well-forming combs, 0.4 mm thick (14 cm, 16 wells for the smaller system and 31 cm, 32 wells for larger one), are required.
2. SG210D Integrated Speed Gel Slab Gel Dryer manufactured by Savant (UK).
3. Autoradiography cassettes with intensifier screens.
4. Fuji Medical X-Ray Film, Super RX (Fuji Medical Systems, UK).
5. Phosphorimager screens, cassettes, scanning equipment (Molecular Dynamics, UK) and imaging software (ImageQuant; Amersham Biosciences, UK).
6. Duck bill gel loading tips 0.2-10 µL (Rainin, Oakland, CA).
7. Safelock 1.5-mL Eppendorf microcentrifuge tubes (Merck Biosciences, UK).
8. Screw-capped, 1.5-mL microtubes (Merck Biosciences).
9. Mini Quick Spin RNA columns (Roche Diagnostics, UK).
10. Saran Wrap 450×300 mm (Dow Chemical Company, UK).

2.2. General Reagents

1. Diethyl pyrocarbonate (DEPC)-treated water: add 1 mL of DEPC (Sigma-Aldrich, UK) to 1 L of Milli-Q water (distilled water that has been further purified by passing through the Milli-Q system [Millipore, UK]) or an equivalent process. Shake to dissolve and leave overnight at room temperature. Autoclave to remove remaining traces of DEPC. **Caution:** DEPC is a suspected carcinogen and can also decompose to form an explosive mixture of ethanol and carbon dioxide. Handle with care in a fume hood.
2. Deionized formamide 99.5% (Sigma-Aldrich). To keep the formamide fully deionized, 1 g of resin AG 501-X8 (D), (Bio-Rad Laboratories) can be added to 50-mL of deionized formamide in a 50 mL-Falcon tube and agitated gently for 30 min. The tube, including the resin, is kept at $-20°C$ and thawed for use.

Initially, the resin is a greenish blue color, but as it becomes exhausted, over several weeks, the color changes to yellow and should be replaced.

2.3. Gel Preparation and Running

1. SequaGel concentrate and SequaGel diluent (cat. nos. EC830 and EC840, respectively, National Diagnostics, UK).
2. 10X Tris-borate–ethylenediaminetetraacetic acid (EDTA) (TBE) buffer: 0.89 M Tris, 0.89 M boric acid, and 0.02 M EDTA in best-quality distilled water.
3. Electrophoresis running buffer: 1X TBE made by diluting 10X TBE in Milli-Q water.
4. Gel loading buffer: 80% deionized formamide, 1 mM EDTA (pH 8.0), 0.1% bromophenol blue, and 0.1% xylene cyanol in DEPC-treated water.
5. 10% Ammonium persulfate (APS).
6. N,N,N',N'-tetramethylethylenediamine ([TEMED] Sigma).

2.4. Template, Probe, and Marker Preparation

1. Mix of four ribonucleoside triphosphates (NTP mix with CTP): 4 mM each of ATP, UTP, GTP, and CTP, prepared from 100 mM NTP solutions (Roche Diagnostics) in DEPC water.
2. Mix of three ribonucleoside triphosphates (NTP mix without CTP): 4 mM each of ATP, UTP, and GTP, prepared from stocks as above. Store NTP mixes at –20°C.
3. RNA polymerases T3, T7, and SP6 and transcription buffer at 10X concentrate (Roche Diagnostics).
4 Placental ribonuclease inhibitor (Pharmacia, UK). Store at –20°C.
5. Dithiothreitol, 200 mM in DEPC-treated water. Store in 0.5-mL aliquots at –70°C.
6. DNASE I, ribonuclease-free (Roche Diagnostics). Store at –20°C.
7. Mini Quick Spin Sephadex G50 RNA columns (Roche Diagnostics). Store at 4°C.
8. *Msp*I digest of pBR322, 1 µg/µL (N3032; New England Biolabs, UK). Store at –20°C.
9. [a-^{32}P]-CTP (specific activity, 370 MBq/mL; Amersham International, UK). Store at –20°C.
10. Phenol/chloroform/isoamyl alcohol (26:24:1, Sigma-Aldrich). Store at 4°C.
11. Absolute alcohol and 70% alcohol.

2.5. Protection Assay

1. 2 M Ammonium acetate in DEPC water. Store at room temperature.
2. 10 mg/mL yeast tRNA in DEPC water, 100,000 U/mL RNase T1, 10 mg/mL RNaseA, and 10 mg/mL proteinase K (all from Sigma-Aldrich). Store at –20°C.
3. Glycogen for molecular biology (20 mg/µL) from Roche Diagnostics. Store at –20°C.
4. 5X Hybridization buffer: 200 mM piperazine-1,4-*bis*(2-ethanesulfonic acid) buffer (pH 6.4), 2 M NaCl, and 5 M EDTA in DEPC water. Aliquot into 1.5-mL vol and store at –20°C. The working solution is prepared by mixing one part of the concentrate with four parts of deionized formamide.
5. Digestion buffer: 10 mM Tris-HCl (pH 7.5), 300 mM NaCl, and 5 mM EDTA. Store at room temperature.

6. Guanidium thiocyanate (GdSCN) solution: Prepare a solution of 4 *M* GdSCN (Merck) and 25 m*M* sodium citrate (pH 7.0) in DEPC-treated water. Store at room temperature in the dark.

3. Methods

3.1. Preparation of the Gel Apparatus

The Sequi-Gen (Bio-Rad Laboratories) inner and outer plates, spacers, and combs should be cleaned scrupulously using detergent and warm water, and then thoroughly rinsed in tap water and distilled water to remove all traces of detergent. Remove the water with paper towels before wiping the glass with another paper towel soaked with few milliliters of 95% ethanol. Dry the glass once more. Transfer the IPC to the fume hood and wipe a few milliliters of dimethyldichlorosilane all over the fixed inner plate with a paper towel and leave for a few seconds for the fumes to evaporate. Dry the spacers and place in position before assembling the apparatus. To facilitate the injection of the "plug" (*see* **Subheading 3.2.**), offset the two glass plates slightly so that the outer plate finishes 2–3 mm above the bottom of the inner plate bonded to IPC. Set the washed comb aside on a clean piece of aluminum foil.

3.2. Preparing the Polyacrylamide Gel

The volumes described are sufficient to prepare enough mix for the smaller (21 × 50-cm) Sequi-Gen gel electrophoresis system. For the larger (38 × 50-cm) apparatus, simply double the quantities.

Caution: unpolymerized polyacrylamide is neurotoxic, so gloves should always be worn, and gels should be prepared on a large containment tray.

Most of the prepared liquid polyacrylamide will be introduced between the glass plates from the top of the apparatus. To prevent the liquid running straight through, however, load approx 10 mL of gel mix between the plates from the bottom of the assembly. Once polymerized this will form a 2- to 3-cm plug.

For a 6% gel, mix in a beaker:

1. 50 mL of SequaGel diluent.
2. 18 mL of SequaGel concentrate.
3. 7.5 mL of 10X TBE.

Remove 15 mL of the above mix into a plastic universal container (setting carefully aside and covering the remaining mix) and add:

1. 75 µL of 10% APS.
2. 30 µL of TEMED.

Mix well and load rapidly into a 20-mL syringe. With the gel apparatus laying perfectly flat, connect a 19- or 21-gage needle to the syringe and evenly inject the mixture between the plates from the bottom of the apparatus, using the ridge made by offsetting the plates. Using these amounts of TEMED and

10% APS, the polyacrylamide should polymerize in about 10–15 min. Once the plug has set, the upper half of the rig can be supported on an empty pipet tip box in preparation for the introduction of the remaining polyacrylamide solution, this time from the top of the apparatus.

To the 60 mL of gel mix remaining in the beaker, add:

1. 250 µL of 10% APS.
2. 30 µL of TEMED.

Load this into a 50-mL syringe (no needle required), tilt the apparatus to about 45°, and allow carefully a steady, controlled trickle of the mix to flow from the syringe to fill the space between the glass plates. When the plates are one quarter filled, stop pouring, put the syringe down, and tilt the rig so that it is upright. Look for bubbles and if any are seen, tilt the fluid between the plates back and forth to remove them. Once done, continue the filling half way. Once again, stop and remove any bubbles that may have been introduced. Do the same again when the gel is three-fourths poured before filling carefully to the top of the smaller glass plate.

Once full, lay the assembly so that it is almost but not completely flat (use something like a screw top from a universal container to support the upper edge of the rig). The final stage is the insertion of the comb. Change gloves at this point to avoid contaminating the comb and slide it between the glass plates to a depth of 1 cm or so. Avoid the use of bulldog clips or other clamps; they are not necessary if the apparatus is laid almost flat as described. Leave for 1–2 h to polymerize.

3.3. Preparation of Template DNA for Riboprobe Synthesis

To prepare a construct suitable for making a riboprobe, the cDNA appropriate to the gene of interest should be cloned into a vector bearing the T3, T7, or SP6 RNA polymerase promoter sequences (e.g., pBluescript from Stratagene or pGEM3Z from Promega). The orientation of the cDNA must be known so that the appropriate promoter can be chosen to allow transcription of the antisense probe. The DNA downstream of the chosen promoter sequence should be linearized with a restriction enzyme, giving a 5' overhang or a blunt end (*see* **Note 1**). Linearizing with an enzyme yielding a 3' overhang should be avoided, because extraneous transcripts may be generated. The restriction site chosen for linearization of the plasmid should ensure that between 100 and 600 nucleotides (nt) of the insert DNA is available for transcription. Riboprobes greater than 600 nt may work, but they are less stable and are not recommended.

3.3.1. Digestion, Purification, and Quantitation of the Template DNA

1. To an Eppendorf tube, add 50 µg of plasmid DNA, 20 µL of 10X concentrated buffer, 2 µL of albumin (100X concentrated), if required, and enough double-distilled water to make the final volume in the tube up to 200 µL (allowing for enzyme addition). Centrifuge and add 20 µL of the chosen restriction enzyme. Vortex mix and incubate at the recommended temperature for 2 h.
2. Add an equal volume of phenol/chloroform/isoamyl alcohol (26:24:1) and vortex vigorously for 15 s.
3. Centrifuge at 13,000g for 30 s and remove the upper aqueous layer into another microtube. To the aqueous phase add an equal volume of fresh phenol/chloroform/isoamyl alcohol (26:24:1), vortex mix as before, recentrifuge, and again remove the upper aqueous layer to a fresh tube. Discard the phenol chloroform fractions according to local rules.
4. Add an equal volume of chloroform to the aqueous phase. Centrifuge and remove the upper, aqueous layer to another tube. Repeat the chloroform extraction to ensure complete removal of traces of phenol from the aqueous phase.
5. Traces of chloroform can be easily seen and removed from under the aqueous layer with a fine pipet. Add 3 M sodium acetate to give a final concentration of 0.3 M. Add 2.5 vol of absolute alcohol and place at –70°C for 30 min.
6. Centrifuge at 13,000g for 15 min to recover the DNA pellet. Remove the supernatant and wash the pellet with 70% ethanol. Recentrifuge and remove excess supernatant completely.
7. Air-dry for 30 min and take up in 30 µL of DEPC water.
8. Dilute the dissolved DNA 1:50 in distilled water and measure the OD_{260}.
9. Calculate the concentration of DNA from the known relationship between OD and DNA concentration (OD_{260} of 1.0 = 50 µg/mL).

3.4. Preparation of ^{32}P-CTP-Labeled Probes (see Note 2)

Usually, a probe to detect the target RNA is made to as high a specific activity as is possible (using only one ^{32}P-labeled nucleotide). This is done by including unlabeled ATP, UTP, and GTP in the mix, along with ^{32}P-CTP, so that every CTP introduced into the riboprobe is radiolabeled.

Loading controls (*see* **Note 3**) such as glyceraldehyde 3-phosphate dehydrogenase, β-actin, or U6 small-nuclear RNA are usually of much higher abundance compared to the target RNA. Therefore, if all probes were made to a high specific activity, the signal from the loading control would be so intense that quantitation on a phosphorimager or other image analyzer would be very difficult. To overcome this, the loading control probe should be made to a much lower activity. This is done by using much less ^{32}P-CTP in the reaction and by diluting the labeled CTP with unlabeled CTP in addition to ATP, UTP, and GTP.

To a 1.5-mL Safelock tube, add the reagents listed in **Table 1**.

Table 1
Reagents for Preparation of ^{32}P-CTP-Labeled Probes

	High-activity probe (μL)	Low-activity probe (μL)
10X transcription buffer (*see* **Note 4**)	1	4
200 m*M* DTT	0.5	2
RNase inhibitor	0.5	2
NTP mix without CTP	1	
NTP mix with CTP		4
Linearized template DNA, 0.3–0.6 μg/μL	1	2
DEPC-treated water	3	23
^{32}P-CTP	2.5	1
Vortex mix and spin briefly then add:		
RNA polymerase (SP6, T7 or T3)	0.5	2
Vortex mix, spin briefly, incubate at 37°C for 15 min, respin, and then add:		
DNase I (RNase-free)	1	4
Final volume (*see* **Note 5**)	11	44
Vortex mix, spin briefly, and incubate at 37°C for 30 min.		

DTT, dithiothreitol; NTP, nucleoside triphosphate; DEPC, diethyl pyrocarbonate.

3.4.1. Purification of the Probe Using Quick Spin Columns

1. Resuspend the Sephadex G50 by tapping gently.
2. Remove the lid of column, using the tool provided, and then snap off spout.
3. Place the column in an Eppendorf tube and spin at 500*g* for 1 min to remove excess buffer without drying out the Sephadex (*see* **Note 6**). Discard the eluate.
4. Carefully add the unpurified probes and place the loaded columns into a screw-capped, 1.5-mL microtube, appropriately labeled. Centrifuge in a microcentrifuge at 2400*g* for 4 min.
5. Discard the column and place the screw cap on to the microtube containing the eluate (*see* **Note 7**).
6. To quantitate the probe, transfer 2 μL to a counting vial and count the cycles per minute by Cherenkov counting in a scintillation counter.
7. To check quickly that the probe has been successfully prepared, transfer 2 μL to an Eppendorf tube and add 8 μL of gel loading buffer.
8. Heat for 3 min at 95°C and load on to a 21 × 50-cm sequencing gel.
9, Run the gel at 50 W for about 30 min.
10. Separate the glass plates and transfer to filter paper (Whatman 3MM; *see* **Note 8**).

11. Cover the gel with Saran Wrap and expose the wet gel to film in a cassette at –80°C for 15 min. Using the wet gel saves time. It may be more convenient, however, to dry the gel as described in **Subheading 3.6.3.**

12. Develop the film and confirm that the labeling of the RNA transcript has worked (*see* **Fig. 1**) and that there is a minimal amount of unincorporated ^{32}P-CTP in the preparation (*see* **Note 9**). The labeled probe should be stored at –20°C and can be used for up to 1 wk after preparation.

3.5. Labeling of Molecular Size Markers

DNA markers, rather than RNA markers, are used, because they are more stable when labeled with ^{32}P and have a useful life of about 2 mo. Although the mobility on polyacrylamide gels is about 10% faster than that of RNA of the same size, DNA markers are quite adequate for assessing the size of bands on a ribonuclease protection gel.

Suitably cut circular DNA such as λ or φX174 can be used. Here, we use an *Msp*I digest of pBR322, which gives size markers between 50 and 600 nt in length. The fragments generated by this endonuclease have a projecting 5' terminus and can therefore be end-labeled with the Klenow fragment of DNA polymerase 1 (*see* **Note 10**).

1. To a 1.5-mL Safelock tube, add the reagents listed in **Table 2**. Incubate at room temperature for 30–60 min and pass through a Sephadex G50 Quick Spin column to remove unincorporated dCTP (*see* **Subheading 2.4.**). Place 2 μL in a scintillation counter.

2. Mix in a screw-capped, 1.5-mL tube, 3×10^5 cpm of labeled, cut pBR322, and make up to 90 μL with formamide loading buffer (*see* **Subheading 2.3.**). Add 10 μL of yeast tRNA solution (10 mg/mL). For use, take about 5 cpm on a handheld monitor (this will be about 0.5 μL when prepared with fresh isotope) and dilute to 10 μL with formamide loading buffer.

3.6. Ribonuclease Protection Assay

3.6.1. Hybridization

1. The concentration of RNA in the sample is determined by measuring the OD_{260} and the quality assessed by the 260/280 nm ratio and by running a gel (*see* Chapter 7). The number of counts needed to provide excess should be determined by experiment. Usually, 2×10^5 cpm of the high-activity probe and 0.6×10^5 cpm of the low-activity probe is sufficient for between 5 and 50 μg of cellular RNA. As shown in the **Fig. 1**, the optimal amount of RNA to be used should also be determined for each probe. For most probes, 20 μg will be enough and is used in the example below.

2. Thaw the RNA samples quickly, vortex mix, pulse spin, and place on ice.

3. Aliquot 20 μg of each test sample into 1.5-mL Safelock tubes. Add DEPC H_2O so that the final volume is the same in all of the tubes. To one tube, which will be

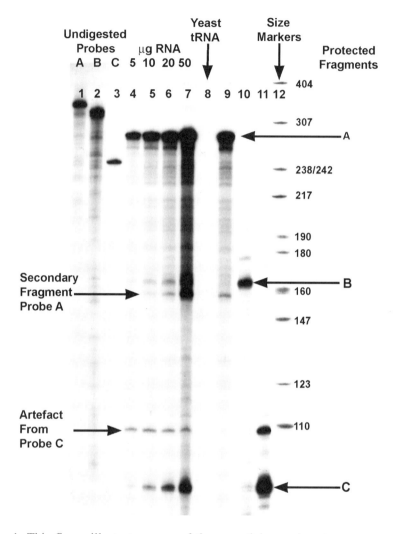

Fig. 1. This figure illustrates some of the essential experiments necessary when setting up ribonuclease protection assays. ^{32}P-CTP-labeled probes A and B were made to high activity and probe C (the loading control probe) to low activity. Lanes 1–3 show the bands from the undigested probes and confirm that the probes were satisfactory as discussed in **Note 9**. Lanes 4–7 show the patterns of labeled fragments, following hybridization and digestion of increasing amounts (5, 10, 20, and 50 μg) of total cellular RNA that were mixed with the three riboprobes (2×10^5 cpm each of probes A and B and 0.6×10^5 cpm of probe C). Lane 8 shows the absence of bands when yeast transfer RNA only was incubated with all three riboprobes and taken through the method. When attempting assays using multiple probes, it is essential to identify clearly which protected fragments are specific for each probe. This can be achieved by running each probe separately. Thus, probes A–C were added separately to aliquots of

Table 2
Reagents for Labeling
of Molecular Size Markers

*Msp*I digest of pBR322	2 µL
^{32}P-dCTP	3 µL
10X Buffer	2 µL
Water	12 µL
Klenow enzyme	1 µL

a background control, add DEPC water only. Because this has no target RNA, any bands observed on the film will represent background and can be ignored.

4. To each tube add the target probe(s) (2×10^5 cpm), the low-activity loading control probe (0.6×10^5 cpm), 2.5 µL yeast tRNA (25 µg), and enough 2 *M* ammonium acetate to achieve a final concentration of 0.5 *M*. Calculate the volumes required for each component, and then make up enough premixed solution for all of the tubes in the batch.

5. Add 2.5 vol of absolute ethanol to each tube. Mix well and place at –20°C for 30 min.

6. Centrifuge at 13,000g in a refrigerated microfuge for 15 min. A good-sized pellet should be visible. Remove the supernatant and confirm, using a handheld monitor, that the overwhelming number of counts is in the pellet.

7. To each tube, add 20 µL of freshly prepared hybridization buffer (one part of 5X hybridization buffer plus four parts deionized formamide). Again, prepare a premixed solution, in excess of the number of tubes in the batch. After addition of the hybridization buffer, vortex each tube vigorously and incubate at 85–90°C for 2–3 min. Vortex mix again, pulse spin, and confirm that the pellets are fully dissolved by aspirating, momentarily, the contents of a small representative number of tubes and checking with a handheld Geiger counter.

Fig. 1. (*continued from opposite page*) RNA and processed as above (lanes 9–11). The first thing to observe is the absence of undigested probe (compare lanes 1, 2, and 3 with 9, 10, and 11), indicating that the conditions for digestion were satisfactory. Lane 9 shows that the highly expressed RNA, complementary to probe A generates a main protected fragment, just below the 307-nucleotide size markers and a clearly visible, though weaker fragment, just below the 160-nucleotide marker. The pattern observed in lane 10 allows the secondary band from probe A to be distinguished from that of probe B in lanes 4–7. For probes A and B, increasing the amounts or cellular RNA as in lanes 4–7 clearly results in a proportionate increases in the intensity of the signal generated and shows that the amount of label used for each target is saturating. Probe C in lane 11 shows two protected fragments. However, it is obvious from lanes 4–7 that only in the lower band is the intensity related to the concentration of target RNA, indicating that this band should be used as the loading control and that the upper band is an artifact and should not be used.

8. Place at 95°C for 4 min to unwind all secondary and tertiary structures in the RNA and transfer the tubes to a 55°C water bath for at least 16 h.

3.6.2. Ribonuclease and Proteinase K Digestion

1. The hybridized solution is cooled briefly on ice and spun at 13,000*g* to spin down any condensed water.
2. Prepare ribonuclease solution: mix 5 µL of ribonuclease T1 (100,000 U/mL) and 20 µL of ribonuclease A (10 mg/mL) in 10 mL digestion buffer.
3. Add 200 µL of ribonuclease solution to each tube. Vortex mix and briefly centrifuge.
4. Incubate at a 22°C in a water bath for 40 min (*see* **Note 11**).
5. Add 35 µL of a premixed solution of 10% *N* lauroylsarcosine:stock proteinase K (25:10) to each tube and incubate for 30 min at 37°C.

3.6.3. Precipitation of Hybridized-Protected Fragment and Gel Loading

1. Prepare enough premixed solution of isopropanol:4 *M* GdSCN (2:1) and 80 mg (4 µL) of glycogen per sample. Add 750 µL to each tube, vortex well, and place at –20°C for 30 min.
2. Centrifuge at full speed for 15 min in a refrigerated microfuge.
3. Remove the supernatant completely (*see* **Note 12**) and dissolve the pellet in 10 µL of loading buffer.
4. Vortex well, warm to 80–90°C for 2–3 min, and vortex again to completely dissolve the pellet. Again, check that counts are predominantly in the loading buffer.
5. The samples are incubated at 95°C for 4 min and then loaded on to the gel using a P20 Gilson pipet and a duck bill tip (*see* **Note 13**).
6. The small-gel apparatus is run at 50 W and the large-gel apparatus is run at 100 W. The resistance should start at 1200–1300 V, rising to about 1800 V as the run nears completion. Run until the lower dye is about 5 cm above bottom edge of the gel (nearly 2 h).
7. The gel is carefully removed on to Whatman 3MM paper (*see* **Note 8**), covered in Saran Wrap, and dried using a gel drier for 40 min at 80°C.
8. After removal of the Saran Wrap, the dried gel is transferred to an autoradiograph cassette and secured with a minimal amount of tape. In a darkroom, the gel is overlaid with X-ray film, and the cassette securely fastened and left overnight at room temperature before developing. Longer periods of exposure or exposure at –70°C may be necessary for weak bands. To quantitate the bands, exposure to a phosphorimager screen is recommended.

3.6.4. Quantitation of the Bands

The bands on exposed X-ray film can be quantitated by densitometry, using suitable equipment. The major drawback with this method of analysis is that quantitation is linear over a narrow range, so bands of low and high intensity cannot be quantified from the same film. Although this can be overcome by taking several images at varying exposure times, the preferred method of measurement is phosphorimagery. This technology relies on the sensitivity of a patented phosphorimagery screen to strong β-emissions. The dried gel is transferred to a specialized cassette and a screen, previously "blanked" on a light box to erase any existing image, and exposed to it for several hours. The image is then scanned into a computer loaded with the appropriate software (e.g., ImageQuant). The image can be intensified electronically if necessary, and the number of pixels in individual bands are counted by using the various tools in the software package.

To correct for variations in loading, the number of pixels in the protected fragment(s) corresponding to the target RNA species (e.g., *see* **Fig. 1**, probes A and B, in lanes 4–7) is divided by the number of pixels in the loading control (*see* **Fig. 1**, probe C in lanes 4–7) and the ratio obtained used to compare the result of one lane to another.

3.7. General Comments

The method described in this chapter is one that we have found to be generally applicable to most of the probes and RNA species that we have studied. It is most important, however, that investigators validate their assays under their conditions, and it is recommended that as a minimum, experiments as outlined in the legend for **Fig. 1** be carried out. Although the method, as described, uses two probes (i.e., those complementary to the loading control and to the target RNA), three or four probes can be incubated at the same time if it is certain that one protected fragment or breakdown bands will not interfere with other targets. Using **Fig. 1** as an example, it would not be advisable to use multiple probes when 50 μg of RNA is used (lane 7), because of the high background from the probe A-protected fragment.

It is important to be consistent at all stages of the procedure. This will make it easier to troubleshoot if things go wrong. It is advisable, initially at least, to carry out assays in triplicate. This will give some idea of the precision of the assay. Another way to inspire confidence in the results is to keep an aliquoted stock of RNA frozen at −70°C, which can be used as a control to assess consistency between batches and provide a point of reference for comparison of results on different gels.

An examination of the short reference list will provide further insight into several of the issues not covered in this article.

4. Notes

1. The restriction site used to linearize the template can be internal to the insert DNA, or it can be located in the multicloning site. It is advisable to run an agarose gel to make sure that the enzyme has cut properly. If uncut vector is present,

repeat the digest with fresh enzyme. Sometimes, if the cDNA is very large, the restriction site chosen may not be unique, and several bands may be seen on an agarose gel. As long as no uncut vector is present and the chosen promoter region is contiguous with the selected stretch of cDNA, transcription should still be satisfactory, and gel purification should not be necessary.

2. When working with isotopes, local rules should be followed meticulously. By adopting the following basic precautions, contamination of gloves, centrifuges, and so on, can be avoided. Solid, perspex Eppendorf tube racks are recommended. Never use light polystyrene racks for anything other than water bath floats. They sit unevenly on the work surface and can easily be upended with obvious consequences. Always use Eppendorf Safelock (or equivalent) microtubes and make sure that the hinged cap locks firmly into place before going on to the next stage of the procedure. When using a vortex mixer, keep one finger of a gloved hand firmly over the cap and after mixing; spin briefly in a microfuge to get the contents of the tube to the bottom. After an incubation step, a "pulse" spin is essential for the removal of the water of condensation, which may have accumulated around the rim of a microtube. If not removed, gloves will become contaminated. Always have the Geiger counter switched on and get into the habit of checking gloves after any manipulation involving isotopes. Monitor working surfaces, centrifuges, racks, and so on, continuously, and deal with any contamination immediately.

3. The loading control is used as a standard against which the gene of interest is to be compared by phosphorimagery or densitometry. It should therefore be stably transcribed and not strongly affected by the conditions of the experiment.

4. Examine the thawed transcription buffer for precipitated salts. Redissolve these by incubating at 37°C for a few min. All reactants in microtubes should be gently vortex mixed and briefly centrifuged before use.

5. By scaling the volume of the mix for the low-activity probe up to 40 µL, a proportionately much lower amount of ^{32}P-CTP can be accurately pipeted (i.e., 1 µL in 40 µL as compared to 0.25 µL in 10 µL for the high-activity probe). These final volumes are within the manufacturer's range for the Quick Spin columns.

6. If a fixed angled rotor is used on the microfuge, the surface of the gel will be sloping after proceeding as in **step 3**, **Subheading 3.6.1.**

7. Pass the tube in front of the monitor. If the synthesis of the probe has been successful, an intense signal will be emitted.

8. This step is probably the most daunting of the whole procedure. The first stage is to separate the outer glass plate from the inner plate on the IPC. This is best done by placing the rig on the bench so that the outer glass plate is face down with the open end of the IPC towards the front. By exerting gentle leverage with, for example, a sturdy ballpoint pen or a P1000 Gilson pipetman, the outer plate can be separated from the bonded plate of the IPC. In theory, the gel should stick to the outer plate, because the plate in the IPC has been rendered "nonstick" by silanizing (*see* **Subheading 3.1.**). If the gel behaves as it should, a controlled lift

and removal of the IPC should leave the gel ready for lifting on to Whatman 3MM paper. Problems can arise if parts of the gel stick to both plates and here, the advice is: do not panic. Take the needed time; allow gravity to work on the gel so that it rolls off on to the outer plate. It may stretch a bit, but that is not a major problem. There may also be the odd crease or air bubble, which is usually best left alone.

After removal of the spacers, the gel is overlaid with an oversized piece of Whatman 3MM paper and gently pressed on to the gel. The paper, with gel attached, is carefully lifted off the glass plate and the gel side of the paper covered with Saran Wrap. Trim the Saran Wrap and the Whatman 3MM paper on all sides to within about 2 cm of the gel and place face up on the gel dryer. There is no need to fix the gel.

9. There should be one major band on the gel representing the full-length riboprobe. If there is more than one significant band it may necessary to design another probe or use a more rigorous purification method (*see* **ref. 2**).

10. The *Escherichia coli* enzyme DNA polymerase I, in addition to its 5'-to-3' polymerase activity, has two intrinsic nuclease activities, one of which digests DNA in a 5'-to-3' direction and the other in the opposite, 3'-to-5' direction. These enzymes are responsible for correcting errors introduced during DNA synthesis in vivo. The Klenow fragment of polymerase I retains only the 3'-to-5' exonuclease activity and lacks 5'-to-3' activity and can therefore be used to fill in DNA with a 5' overhang.

11. Some methods recommend a temperature of 37°C for this step. However, some hybridized fragments can be overdigested at this temperature. If the temperature is too low, unhybridized fragments may not be fully digested. In this author's experience, room temperature (22°C) for 40 min is satisfactory for most probes.

12. It is very important, for the even running of the gel, that the supernatant be removed completely. This will mean recentrifuging and aspirating several times and even removing the final droplet that clings to the pellet.

13. The gel apparatus should be fully assembled with 1X TBE in the bottom trough and the same buffer, prewarmed to 55°C, in the integral plate chamber. Before loading, the well forming comb must be removed. Remember that after heating at 95°C, the labeled fragment is single stranded and therefore susceptible to attack by ribonuclease. Therefore, change gloves before immersing fingers in the buffer and removing the comb. This latter step should be done carefully so as not to disturb the well uprights. Before loading, carefully wash each well twice with buffer using a P1000 Gilson pipet.

14. Time considerations: the synthesis and checking of the probes take about 3 h. Probes can be used immediately or stored at –20°C for several days before use. The prehybridization steps take 2–3 h, depending on the number of samples being processed. The hybridization step can be conveniently done overnight, and the posthybridization steps culminating in the loading of the gel will take 3–4 h. Gel running and drying will take another 3 h.

References

1. Petersen, N. E., Larsen, L. K., Nissen, H., et al. (1995) Improved RNase protection assay for quantifying LDL-receptor RNA: estimation of analytical imprecision and biological variance in peripheral mononuclear cells, *Clin. Chem.* **41,** 1605–1613.
2. Tymms, M. J. (1995) Quantitative measurement of mRNA using RNase protection assay. *Methods Mol. Biol.* **37,** 31–46.

25

Identification of Steroid Hormone-Regulated Genes in Breast Cancer

Bruce R. Westley and Felicity E. B. May

Summary

The measurement of the expression of hormonally regulated genes in breast cancer may provide an indication of its hormone responsiveness. In addition, these genes may provide novel therapeutic targets. This chapter reviews the hormonally responsive genes that have been identified in breast cancer cell lines and tumors, using differential hybridization, differential display, serial analysis of gene expression, and array technology. The biological relevance of the genes identified is discussed.

Key Words: Estrogen; breast cancer, gene expression; SAGE; regulation of gene expression; microarray.

1. Introduction

The search for, and identification of, hormonally regulated genes in breast cancer has been ongoing for more than 20 yr. This research is based on the observation that breast cancer can be hormonally responsive *(1)*, the discovery of the estrogen receptor *(2)*, and the demonstration of the estrogen receptor in a majority of breast tumors *(3)*. The rationale for searching for hormonally regulated genes has been manyfold. First, genes might be identified that could be useful for studying the molecular mechanism of action of steroid hormones. Second, these genes may play important roles in mediating the effects of hormones on cancer cells. Third, the genes identified may be useful diagnostic or prognostic markers or predictive of response to therapy.

Breast cancer is one of a few hormonally responsive cancers where endocrine therapy is an important therapeutic option, and it would be particularly useful to identify the most valuable set of genes for predicting the potential benefit of endocrine therapy. To date, markers can predict the benefit of a particular treatment for a population, but give limited information for an indi-

From: *Methods in Molecular Medicine, Vol. 120: Breast Cancer Research Protocols*
Edited by: S. A. Brooks and A. L. Harris © Humana Press Inc., Totowa, NJ

vidual. The "Holy Grail" is, therefore, to identify one, or a set of, genes whose level of expression would predict the amount of benefit that an individual would receive from hormone therapy and the most appropriate form of endocrine therapy. The ability to predict the response to different endocrine agents is of increasing relevance, with the introduction of pure estrogen antagonists such as Faslodex and potent aromatase inhibitors such as Letrozole and Arimidex. These are likely to supplement or replace the partial estrogen agonist tamoxifen, which has been the mainstay of endocrine therapy for many years.

A landmark discovery was that of the estrogen receptor by Toft and Gorski (2). Initially, this involved the demonstration of preferential uptake of radiolabeled estrogen into estrogen-responsive tissues (4) and was followed by the identification and characterization of a protein that had a high affinity and specificity for estrogens. This was followed by the purification of the receptor protein, the preparation of monoclonal antibodies against the receptor, (5) and the cloning of the estrogen receptor mRNA sequence and gene (6). These early studies spawned extensive work into the identification of the repertoire of genes controlled by estrogens in target tissues and the mechanisms by which the estrogen receptor controls the expression of these genes.

Almost all attempts to identify hormonally regulated genes in breast cancer have used estrogen responsive breast cancer cell lines such as MCF-7, ZR-75, and T47D, because they are tractable model systems in which culture conditions such as exposure to steroid hormones can be controlled with some precision. However, it is important to realize that these cells are grown routinely in culture in the presence of estrogens and other steroid hormones, as most media formulations include fetal calf serum. As well as containing significant levels of a variety of steroids and growth factors, most media also contain phenol red, a pH indicator, which is itself a weak estrogen. Before embarking on an experiment to identify hormone responsive genes it is, therefore, necessary to culture cells in an estrogen-free environment for several days to remove estrogens from the cells and allow the mRNA levels of estrogen-regulated genes to subside to their unstimulated levels.

The focus of this chapter is to describe the methodologies used to identify estrogen-regulated genes in breast cancer cells and the genes that have been identified. This is relevant to breast cancer, because estrogens promote cell proliferation and tumor progression. The identification of the repertoire of estrogen-regulated genes should clarify the proteins involved in these processes and identify potential new therapeutic targets for the treatment of breast cancer.

The reagents required for the techniques described in this chapter are readily available as kits from a number of suppliers. As the protocols for these techniques are varied, change frequently, and are available freely on the websites of the companies providing these technologies (e.g., www.affymetrix.com, www.clontech.com, www.promega.com, and www.stratagene.com), this chapter does not detail precise protocols. Instead, it focuses on the different methods that have been used to identify hormonally regulated genes, reviews the genes that have been identified to date, provides some information on their known and predicted biological functions, and addresses the extent to which the genes identified have fulfilled the original aims of the search. It also reviews recent microarray studies on breast tumors, which have identified genes whose expression is related to that of the estrogen receptor.

2. Strategies for the Identification of Hormonally Regulated Genes in Breast Cancer

2.1. Known Estrogen-Regulated Genes

The expression of the estrogen receptor α is regulated by estrogen. The effect of estrogen varies with the breast cancer cell line. Estrogen receptor α-expression is decreased by estradiol treatment in MCF-7 cells (7) but is increased in three other cell lines, EFM-19, T47D, and ZR-75 (7,8). This differential regulation may result from the repertoire of transcription factors present in the different cells rather than the selective use of the three estrogen receptor α-promoters that are active in breast cancer cell lines (9).

The first hormonally regulated genes to be identified in breast cancer were based on the prior knowledge that their expression was regulated by estrogen in other tissues. The classic example of this is the progesterone receptor (10), which is regulated by estrogen in the uterus. Expression of the progesterone receptor is regulated by estrogen in breast cancer cells (11), and of all the markers of estrogen responsiveness that have been identified to date, the expression of the progesterone receptor is currently the most widely used in clinical practice (12).

Estrogens modulate the responsiveness of estrogen-responsive breast cancer cells to insulin-like growth factors, and this led to a search for components of the insulin-like growth factor signal transduction pathway whose expression is regulated by estrogen. The insulin-like growth factor receptor (13) and insulin receptor substrate-1 (14) are both regulated by estrogens, and the induction of insulin receptor substrate-1 expression may be particularly important for the effects of estradiol on insulin-stimulated growth.

2.2. Protein Gel Electrophoresis

Early studies on breast cancer cell lines used labeling of newly synthesized proteins with radioactive amino acids. An estrogen-induced protein of 24 kDa was identified, using double-isotope labeling by Edwards et al. (15). This was later identified as the heat shock protein Hsp27, which is regulated by protein kinase C (*16*) as well as by estrogen and is thought to be involved in both cell proliferation and differentiation. Westley and Rochefort (*17*) used one- and two-dimensional gel electrophoresis to identify estrogen-induced proteins of 46 and 160 kDa. The 46-kDa protein was identified as cathepsin D, an aspartyl protease (*18*). The same technique was used to identify progesterone-induced proteins in MCF-7 and T47D cells (*19*). The progestin-induced protein of 250 kDa was identified as fatty acid synthetase (*20*).

Studies such as these were an early version of what is now referred to as proteomics, which links the resolution of two-dimensional gel electrophoresis with the power of mass spectrometry (this is the subject of Chapter 18). This is widely used for the identification and characterization of proteins in the postgenomic era. It is, however, somewhat ironic that in 2005, the most commonly used method to resolve complex protein mixtures remains two-dimensional gel electrophoresis with protocols similar to those described by O'Farrell in 1975 (*21*). In contrast to current proteomic techniques, these early studies were characterized by the length of time taken to identify and characterize the regulated proteins. For example, the 46-kDa estrogen-regulated protein was first described in 1979, but was not identified as cathepsin D until 1988.

2.3. Colony Hybridization

Recombinant DNA techniques subsequently became the method of choice for identifying differentially expressed genes. The first technique used colony hybridization in which bacteria carrying cDNA corresponding to individual mRNA sequences are fixed as gridded arrays on membranes, and hybridized with cDNA synthesized from total mRNA extracted from control or hormonally treated cells. All studies have used cell lines, because the procedure required manipulation of the hormonal environment to achieve differences in the mRNA levels of specific responsive genes. A variety of regulated mRNAs was identified (**Table 1**) in this way, including a trefoil factor family (TFF) protein TFF1 (*22,23,24*); the pNR series, which included TFF1 and cathepsin D (*18,24,25,22*); RNA that is differentially regulated by antiestrogens (*26*); pLIV1 (*27*); the pSyd series (*28*); and pMGT1, an RNA whose expression is reduced by estradiol in T47D cells (*29*). Studies to understand the function of proteins encoded by these genes in normal and malignant breast cancer cells continue to this day (*30,31,32,33*).

2.4. Subtraction Hybridization

Subtraction hybridization is a powerful way of removing common sequences from mRNA populations, thereby enriching for mRNAs that differ in abundance. Several methods of subtraction hybridization have been described. The early methods involved multiple rounds of hybridization of cDNA prepared

Table 1
Identification of Estrogen-Regulated Genes by Differential Hybridization

Name of clone	Protein	Cell line	Hormone	Reference
pS2	TFF1	MCF-7	Estradiol	*22*
BCE1	TFF1	MCF-7	Estradiol	*23*
pNR-1	—	MCF-7	Estradiol	*24*
pNR-2	TFF1	MCF-7	Estradiol	*24*
pNR-3	—	MCF-7	Estradiol	*24*
pNR-4	—	MCF-7	Estradiol	*24*
pNR-7	Hsp27	MCF-7	Estradiol	*25*
pNR-8	Aldolase A	MCF-7	Estradiol	*25*
pNR-13	—	MCF-7	Estradiol	*25*
pNR-17	—	MCF-7	Estradiol	*25*
pNR-20	—	MCF-7	Estradiol	*25*
pNR-21	—	MCF-7	Estradiol	*25*
pNR-22	—	MCF-7	Estradiol	*25*
pNR-23	A-tubulin	MCF-7	Estradiol	*25*
pNR-25	—	MCF-7	Estradiol	*25*
pNR-100	Cathepsin D	ZR-75	Estradiol	*18,25*
pNR-101	GAPDH	ZR-75	Estradiol	*25*
pNR-102	Aldolase A	ZR-75	Estradiol	*25*
pNR-105	TFF1	ZR-75	Estradiol	*25*
pLIV-1	LIV1	ZR-75	Estradiol	*27*
pLIV-2	TFF1	ZR-75	Estradiol	*27*
pSyd	—	T47D	Estradiol	*28*
pSyd-1	—	T47D	Estradiol	*28*
pSyd-2	—	T47D	Estradiol	*28*
pSyd-3	—	T47D	Estradiol	*28*
pSyd-4	—	T47D	Estradiol	*28*
pSyd-5	—	T47D	Estradiol	*28*
pSyd-6	—	T47D	Estradiol	*28*
pSyd-7	—	T47D	Estradiol	*28*
pSyd-8	—	T47D	Estradiol	*28*
pMGT1	—	T47D	Estradiol	*29*

from mRNA extracted from treated cells (tester RNA), to an excess of mRNA extracted from untreated cells (driver) followed by physical separation of single-stranded cDNA from the RNA–cDNA duplex and cloning of the single-stranded cDNA that had not hybridized. Recent methods can be performed with as little as 2 µg of mRNA, use a single round of subtractive hybridization, and exploit polymerase chain reaction to selectively amplify differentially expressed genes.

Table 2
Identification of Estrogen-Regulated Genes by Suppression Subtractive Hybridization

Name of clone	Name of protein	Cell line	Hormone	Reference
DEME-2	—	MCF-7	Estradiol	*34*
DEME-12	Neuropeptide peptide Y receptor Y1	MCF-7	Estradiol	*34*
DEME-31	—	MCF-7	Estradiol	*34*
DEME-40	TFF1	MCF-7	Estradiol	*34*
DEME-47	—	MCF-7	Estradiol	*34*
Clones 59, 65, 229	Thrombospondin	MCF-7	Estradiol	*35*
Clones 71, 155, 203	PDZK1	MCF-7	Estradiol	*35*
Clones 76, 239	Ig-like protein	MCF-7	Estradiol	*35*
Clone 223	GREB1	MCF-7	Estradiol	*35*

Subtraction hybridization has been used to identify genes in a variety of contexts such as genes that differ in their levels of expression during malignant progression. It was used by Kuang et al. *(34)* and Ghosh et al. *(35)* to identify estrogen-regulated mRNA in breast cancer cells (**Table 2**). Kuang et al. *(34)* compared gene expression in estrogen receptor-positive MCF-7 and estrogen-receptor negative MDA-MB-231 cells. They identified 29 differentially expressed sequences, five of which (DEME-2, -12, -31, -40, and -47) were shown to be regulated by estrogen, using Northern transfer analysis. DEME-12 was identified as neuropeptide Y receptor Y1 and DEME-40 as TFF1. DEME-6 is regulated by estradiol and was characterized in some detail. Its expression is correlated with estrogen receptor in a panel of breast cancer cell lines, and it is expressed in primary breast cancers but not in normal breast tissue.

Ghosh et al. *(35)* identified 15 sequences, of which 11 were novel, in a cDNA library constructed with mRNA from MCF-7 breast cancer cells using estrogen-treated cells as the tester and cells grown in the absence of estradiol as the driver. Four genes were identified from databases and were commented on in detail (*see* **Table 2**). *PDZK1* contains a PDZ domain. Proteins containing this domain organize proteins at the cell membrane and are involved in linking transmembrane proteins to the actin cytoskeleton, controlling signal transduction, determination of cell polarity, cell differentiation, and ion transport. Thrombospondin is a matrix-bound adhesive glycoprotein expressed in mammary cells and one that colocalizes with transforming growth factor-1 and insulin-like growth factor-1. A novel gene identified by Ghosh et al. *(35)* was termed GREB1 (gene regulated by estrogen in breast cancer). *GREB1* and *GREB2* were derived from this same gene, and *GREB2* matched an expression sequence tag from human brain. The predicted protein is at least 1949 amino

Table 3
Steroid Hormone-Regulated Genes Identified by Differential Display

Name of protein	Cell line	Hormone	Reference
Na⁺/H⁺ exchanger regulatory factor.	MCF-7	Estrogen	*37*
Megakaryocyte CD63	MCF-7 and T47D	Estrogen	*38*
UDP-glucose dehydrogenase	ZR-75	Androgen	*40*
G protein-coupled receptor 30 (GPR30)	MCF-7	Progesterone	*44*
hD1g5	MCF-7, T47D, and ZR-75	Progesterone	*43*
Flavin-containing monooxy-genase 5 (FM05)	T47D	Progesterone	*42*
6-phosphofructo-2-kinase/ fructose-2,6-bisphosphatase	T47D	Progesterone	*41*
CD-9/MRP-1	T47D	Progesterone	*45*
CD-59/protectin	T47D	Progesterone	*45*
TSC-22	T47D	Progesterone	*45*
Desmoplakin	T47D	Progesterone	*45*
FKBP51	T47D	Progesterone	*45*
Na⁺/K⁺ ATPase subunit α-1	T47D	Progesterone	*45*

acids long and is encoded within an 8-kb mRNA containing at least three noncoding 5' exons.

2.5. Differential Display

Differential display was invented in 1992 by Liang and Pardee *(36)* to characterize altered patterns of gene expression. It exploits the polymerase chain reaction to amplify the 3' terminal portion of mRNA, using anchored primers designed to bind to the 5' boundary of the poly (A) tail at the 3' end of mRNA and upstream primers of arbitrary sequence. The polymerase chain reaction products from different mRNA preparations are then displayed by denaturing polyacrylamide gel electrophoresis, and measurement of the relative intensities of bands allows differentially expressed genes to be identified. The amplified sequences are then cloned and sequenced. Although this technique has been used successfully, a major drawback has been the high proportion of false-positive, regulated bands identified.

Differential display has been used to identify estrogen-, androgen-, and progesterone-regulated genes in breast cancer cells (**Table 3**). Ediger et al. *(37)* identified the Na⁺/H⁺ exchanger regulatory factor, a PDZ domain-containing protein that is enriched in polarized epithelia and regulates protein kinase A inhibition of the Na^+/H^+ exchanger and may act a scaffold adaptor protein that contributes to the specificity of signal transduction events. Stephen et al. *(38)* identified an mRNA for human megakaryocyte CD63 antigen, whereas Thompson and Weigel *(39)* cloned a gene, *ICERE-1*, whose expression is inversely correlated with that of estrogen receptor. The study of Lapointe and Labrie *(40)* is one of very few to search for androgen-regulated genes in breast cancer. Androgens inhibit the proliferation of breast cancer cells, and they identified UDP-glucose dehydrogenase an enzyme involved in the control of steroid inactivation.

Several groups have used differential display to identify progesterone-regulated genes. Hamilton et al. *(41)* identified an mRNA-encoding a protein with a high degree of homology with isoforms of the enzyme 6-phophofructo-2-kinase/fructose-2,6-bisphosphatase. Miller et al. *(42)* identified flavin-containing monooxygenase 5 as being regulated specifically by only one form, the B form, of the progesterone receptor. This enzyme is involved in the metabolic activation of drugs and xenobiotic compounds, and the authors speculated that progesterone could enhance the carcinogenicity of drugs such the antiestrogen tamoxifen. The group of Ylikomi *(43,44)* identified two progesterone-regulated mRNAs, including a G protein-coupled receptor (GPR30) and a member of the MAGUK protein family, hDlg5, in MCF-7 cells. This protein plays a role in cell growth control and maintenance of cell adhesion and polarity and has been implicated as a tumor suppressor gene. Kester et al. *(45)* identified a series of progesterone-regulated mRNAs from T47D cells whose growth is inhibited by progestins. Changes in the pattern of expression of these genes, including desmoplakin, CD-9, CD-59, Na^+/K^+-ATPase α-1, and annexin-VI, suggested that estradiol dedifferentiates these cells, whereas progestins have the opposite effect.

2.6. Serial Analysis of Gene Expression

Serial analysis of gene expression (SAGE) is a technique that allows the absolute abundance of thousands of different mRNAs to be measured simultaneously in a comprehensive and unbiased way and hence, the detection of differences in expression among samples. The comprehensive coverage and absence of bias are advantages over other methods described herein, and SAGE has the advantage over gene microarrays where only genes that have been identified previously can be analyzed. SAGE libraries are created by the concatenation of short sequences (called sequence tags) from mRNA. The abundance of mRNA is reflected by the number of times a particular tag is identified by sequencing.

Inadera et al. *(46)* analyzed approx 30,000 sequence tags from control and estrogen-treated MCF-7 cells. In addition to identifying the previously known

Table 4
Estrogen-Regulated Genes Identified by Serial Analysis of Gene Expression

Name of clone	Name of protein	Cell line	Hormone	Reference
E2IG1	—	MCF-7	Estradiol	*47*
E2IG2	—	MCF-7	Estradiol	*47*
E2IG3	—	MCF-7	Estradiol	*47*
E2IG4	—	MCF-7	Estradiol	*47*
	Heat shock 90-kDa protein 1-β	MCF-7	Estradiol	*47*
	Pescadillo (zebrafish) homolog 1	MCF-7	Estradiol	*47*
	Stanniocalcin 2	MCF-7	Estradiol	*47*
	Inhibin-β B	MCF-7	Estradiol	*47*
	Proteasome subunit, β type, 4	MCF-7	Estradiol	*47*
	TFF1	MCF-7	Estradiol	*47*
	Cathepsin D	MCF-7	Estradiol	*46*
	TFF1	MCF-7	Estradiol	*46*
	High mobility group-1 protein	MCF-7	Estradiol	*46*
	Wnt-1-inducible signaling pathway protein 2	MCF-7	Estradiol	*46*
EIT-6	Homologous to rat immediate early SM-20	ZR-75	Estradiol	*48*
TIT-5	—	ZR-75	Estradiol	*48*
DET-2	—	ZR-75	Estradiol	*48*
EIT-10	Cathepsin D	ZR-75	Estradiol	*48*

estrogen-regulated genes cathepsin D, TFF1, and high-mobility group 1 protein, they also identified WISP-2 (*Wnt-1*-inducible signaling pathway protein 2), which belongs to the CCN family of growth factors and is upregulated in mammary epithelial cells transformed by the *Wnt-1* oncogene (**Table 4**). Charpentier et al. *(47)* analyzed 190,000 mRNA transcripts also from control and estrogen-treated MCF-7 cells. The most-induced estrogen-regulated genes identified are shown in **Table 4**. They include heat shock 90-kDa protein 1-β protein, pescodillo 1, TFF1, and stanniocalcin 2. Novel genes, *E2IG1–E2IG5*, standing for E_2-induced genes, were also identified. E2IG1 is a novel member of the family of small heat shock proteins; E2IG4 is a new member of leucine-rich repeat containing proteins. Many other genes, which had not been described previously as being estrogen-regulated, were identified, including genes that the authors classified as being chaperone and cell cycle progression proteins and paracrine or autocrine growth factors; however, the fold induction by estradiol was small. Seth et al. *(48)* analyzed approx 450,000 transcripts from ZR-75 breast cancer cells treated with estradiol or the antiestrogen 4-hydroxytamoxifen, and reported the identification of four regulated genes. *EIT-6* is homologous to rat immediately early gene *SM-20* and is proposed to be involved in transmitting growth-promoting signals initiated by estrogen; *EIT-10* is cathepsin D; and the other two, *TIT-5* and *DET-2*, were not identified (**Table 4**).

2.7. Array Technology

The principle of array technology is, in essence, similar to that of colony hybridization. Known DNA sequences are immobilized instead of DNA from bacteria harboring unknown cDNA sequences. The first arrays to be made available were large nylon or nitrocellulose filters with spots of DNA that were hybridized with radiolabeled cDNA prepared from total or subtracted mRNA populations. Comparison of the intensity of hybridization of radiolabeled cDNA from two mRNA preparations to all the immobilized DNA identified those that give different intensities of signal and are candidate regulated genes. There have been several modifications and improvements to this technique, including the immobilization of DNA at high density on glass slides, the use of fluorescent probes, which allows two probes to be hybridized simultaneously, and the development of lithographic techniques by Affymetrix (Santa Clara, CA), which allow high densities of oligonucleotides to be synthesized directly on silicon wafers. cDNA arrays are the subject of Chapters 27 and 28.

One major advantage of this technique is that the DNA immobilized on the filter is known, and therefore, the regulated gene is identified immediately. In addition, advances in the fluidics systems used for the hybridization enable the detection of rare mRNA. The other major advantage is that many different genes (currently up to 33,000 genes, using the Affymetrix U133 plus 2.0 chips) can be analyzed in a single experiment. The advances in array technology and the statistical techniques for handling the data have resulted in it becoming a major tool in the hunt for genes, or groups of genes, with diagnostic or prognostic value and for potential drug targets in a variety of diseases including breast cancer.

The results from array studies on estrogen-regulated genes are difficult to summarize, because they comprise long lists of genes whose expression varies, and it is difficult to evaluate the relative importance of the genes on the lists. In addition, the statistical analysis used to analyze the data can lead to different conclusions *(49)*. As the first publications in breast cancer were published in 2000, it is too soon to expect follow-up data to have emerged that might lead to a consensus on the most valuable genes. However, the statistical

Table 5
Estrogen-Regulated Genes Identified by Microarray Technology

Name of protein	Cell line	Hormone	Reference
Cytochrome P450-IIB	ZR-75	Estradiol	*52*
Gap junction protein (α-1)	ZR-75	Estradiol	*52*
Insulin-like growth factor binding protein-4	ZR-75	Estradiol	*52*
TFF1	ZR-75	Estradiol	*52*
TFF3	ZR-75	Estradiol	*52*
Cationic amino acid transporter E16	ZR-75	Estradiol	*52*
TFF1	MCF-7	Estradiol	*56*
PDZK1	MCF-7	Estradiol	*56*
IGFBP4	MCF-7	Estradiol	*56*
Solute carrier family 7 member-5	MCF-7	Estradiol	*56*
Tumor protein D-52-like-1	MCF-7	Estradiol	*56*
Estrogen receptor-α	MCF-7	Estradiol	*56*
Stanniocalcin-2	MCF-7	Estradiol	*56*
IGFBP5	MCF-7	Estradiol	*56*
Ras-related and estrogen-regulated growth inhibitor (RERG)	MCF-7	Estradiol	*55*
Stanniocalcin-2	MCF-7	Estradiol	*53*
X-box binding protein-1	MCF-7	Estradiol	*53*
Insulin growth factor-binding protein-4	MCF-7	Estradiol	*53*

analysis of microarray data ranks genes, and this review will discuss the genes reported by the authors as being the most potentially important.

The majority of studies using arrays for breast cancer have focused on the identification of genes whose expression correlates with clinicopathological features or surrogates of clinical outcome. Recently, however, important papers have been published showing that gene signatures are more powerful predictors than standard systems based on clinical and histological criteria *(50,51)*.

Array studies on hormonal responsiveness of breast cancer have focused on two areas. These are the identification of hormonally regulated genes in cell lines and the identification of mRNA whose expression is associated with estrogen receptor status in breast tumors. In the cell line studies (**Table 5**), genes are generally ranked according to the degree of induction, whereas in the tumor studies, they tend to be ranked by their importance in contributing to the estrogen receptor phenotype or other clinical parameters.

2.7.1. Cell Lines

Soulez and Parker *(52)* used the estrogen-responsive ZR-75-1 cell line treated with estradiol, 4-hydroxytamoxifen, Raloxifene, and Faslodex in the presence of cyclohexamide to identify estrogen-regulated genes. Fifty-three genes that were regulated more than 1.5-fold by estrogen were identified. Of the novel estrogen-induced mRNAs, the authors emphasized the induction of the enzyme cytochrome *p450-II b* as the most highly induced estrogen-regulated gene, followed by cationic amino acid transporter E16, gap junction protein, and insulin-like growth factor binding protein-4. However, some known estrogen-regulated proteins were also identified such as TFF1 and TFF3. In a comprehensive study, Bouras et al. *(53)* used microarrays to identify genes regulated by estrogens in the MCF-7 breast cancer cell line and then to correlate the expression of these genes with estrogen receptor status in a panel of breast cancer cell lines and primary tumors. This study identified stanniocalcin 2 as an estrogen-regulated gene. This gene had been identified by Charpentier et al. *(47)* using SAGE analysis. Hoch et al. *(54)* used cDNA arrays to identify estrogen receptor-associated genes in human breast cancer cell lines. The transcription factor GATA-3 was more highly associated with expression of the estrogen receptor than the progesterone receptor in both cell lines, and showed that GATA-3 expression was also associated with estrogen- and progesterone-receptor expression, using immunohistochemistry. It is important to note, however, that expression of GATA 3 has not been reported to be regulated by estradiol. Finlin et al. *(55)* also used MCF-7 cells to identify estrogen-regulated mRNAs by microarray and focused on a novel *ras*-related gene named *RERG* (*ras*-related and estrogen-regulated growth inhibitor). Inoue et al. *(56)* profiled 9000 genes to identify estrogen-regulated mRNA in MCF-7 breast cancer cells. A custom array comprising 138 estrogen-regulated and 10 nonregulated mRNAs was then used to analyze the kinetics of estrogen induction in more detail. The mRNA encoding TFF1 was the most induced, but induced mRNAs identified in other array studies such as stanniocalcin 2 were also identified.

A summary of the estrogen-regulated genes that have been identified most frequently using the various technologies described above is given in **Table 6**. Also included are the estrogen receptor-α and progesterone receptor genes. It is noteworthy that the former has only been identified by recent microarray studies, and the latter has not been identified, despite being very sensitive to estrogen regulation in a number of cell lines *(11)*. The genes identified most frequently are those encoding cathepsin D and TFF1. The association of the estrogen-regulated gene products with estrogen receptor α protein expression in breast tumors is shown. TFF1, TFF3, pLIV1, and Hsp27 are associated with estrogen receptor protein expression, whereas cathepsin D, PDZK1, and cyclin D1 are not. Similar associations have been found at the mRNA level using microarray analysis of tumors (**Tables 6** and **7**). To date the only estrogen-regulated gene product whose expression has been shown to be predictive of

Table 6

Summary of Genes Frequently Found to be Regulated by Estrogens in Estrogen-Responsive Breast Cancer Cell Lines, Using Protein Gel Electrophoresis, Differential Hybridization, Differential Display, Subtraction Hybridization, Serial Analysis of Gene Expression, and Microarray Analysis

Gene	Date	Guess/Serendipity Identified	Guess/Serendipity Regulated	Protein Gel Electrophoresis Identified	Protein Gel Electrophoresis Regulated	Differential Hybridization Identified	Differential Hybridization Regulated	Differential Display Identified	Differential Display Regulated	Subtraction Hybridization Identified	Subtraction Hybridization Regulated	Serial Analysis of Gene Expression Identified	Serial Analysis of Gene Expression Regulated	Microarray Identified	Microarray Regulated	Breast tumors: Association with estrogen receptor expression	Breast tumors: Association with estrogen receptor RNA expression by microarray analysis	Breast tumors: Predictive of response to endocrine therapy
Estrogen Receptor	1988	✓	-/+											✓	-/+	Yes	Yes	Yes
Progesterone receptor	1975	✓	+													Yes	Yes	Yes
Cathepsin D	1979			✓	+	✓	+					✓	+			No	No	No
TFF1	1982					✓	+			✓	+			✓	+	Yes	Yes	Yes
TFF3	1997	✓	+											✓	+	Yes	Yes	N.D.
pLIV1	1988					✓	+									Yes	Yes	No
Stanniocalcin 2												✓	+			Yes	Yes	ND
Hsp 27	1981			✓	+	✓	+							✓	+	Yes	Yes	ND
PDZK1	2000													✓	+	No	No	ND
Cyclin D1	2000											✓	+		+	No	Yes	ND

+, upregulation; −, downregulation; ND, not done.

Table 7
Association of the Expression of Specific Genes With That of the Estrogen Receptor in Breast Tumors

Gene	Breast cancer cell lines — Regulated	Breast cancer cell lines — Ass.	Bertucci et al (57) Ass.	Rank	Perou et al (58) Ass.	Rank	Gruvberger et al (59) Ass.	Rank	West et al (60) Ass.	Rank	Sorlie et al (50) Ass.	Rank	Finlin et al (55) Ass.	Rank	Bertucci et al (57) Ass.	Rank	Bouras et al (53) Ass.	Rank	Van't Veer et al (62) Ass.	Rank	Perez-Enciso (49)[a] Ass.	Rank
Estrogen receptor (ESR1)	Yes	-/+			+	M	+	1.	+	2.	+		++	M	+				+	4.	+	3.
Progesterone receptor (PgR)	Yes	+																	(+)			
TFF1	Yes	+	+		+		+		+	1	+	M	+		+				+		+	10.
TFF3	Yes	+			+		+	2	+	4	+	M	+	M					+			
pLIV1	Yes	+			+				+	25	+		+						+	19.		
Stanniocalcin 2	Yes	+															+					
IGF2	Yes	+	+	10	+		+	11			+											
IRS1	Yes	+					+	16														
IGFBP1																			+	45.		
IGFBP4									+	41							+		+			
Hsp 27	Yes	+					+	15	+	39									+			
Cyclin D1																						
GATA3	No	+	+	1	+	M	+	3	+	8	+	M	+		+				+	1.		
HNF3α					+	M			+	12	+	M	+						+	6.	+	20.
Xbox 1	Yes	+	+	8	+	M			+	25	+	M	+		+		+		+	15.		
MYB	?	+	+	3					+	8					+				+	23.		
hepsin			+		+				+	8												
Lutheran blood group			+		+				+	31												
ErbB3																			+	12.	+	
CRAB3			+	7											+							
BCL2							+		+	32					+				+	46.	+	
CRIP1							+	12.	+	29												

[a]The study of Perez-Enciso and Tenenhaus is a reanalysis of the data obtained by Perou et al. (58).

Columns 2 and 3 indicate whether expression of a specific gene is regulated in breast cancer cell lines. The four most important studies are shown in boldface.

Ass., expression associated with that of the estrogen receptor mRNA; Rank, the ranking of the expression of the gene in association of that of the estrogen receptor gene; +, increased expression; -, decreased expression; M, mentioned by the authors in the text; ?, equivocal.

response to endocrine therapy of breast cancer patients apart from the steroid receptors is TFF1.

2.7.2. Tumors

Bertucci et al. *(57)* undertook one of the first studies to profile gene expression in primary breast cancers. They analyzed the expression of 176 candidate genes in 34 breast cancers that had shown a differential outcome in response to chemotherapy. Differential expression was observed in estrogen receptor-positive and -negative tumors, with expression of GATA-3 being most highly correlated with that of the estrogen receptor (*see* **Table 7**).

Perou et al. *(58)* analyzed patterns of expression of 8102 genes in breast tumors from 42 individuals. Twenty of these patients had received doxorubicin therapy before surgery, and the expression profile may have been altered by this neoadjuvant therapy. Nevertheless, estrogen receptor mRNA expression was concordant with direct clinical measurement of estrogen receptor protein in the tumors and was significantly associated with that of GATA-3, X-box binding protein-1, and hepatocyte nuclear factor-3α. The data of Perou et al. *(58)* was subsequently reanalyzed *(49)* using partial least squares discriminant analysis. This reanalysis reinforced the association of GATA-3 expression with that of the estrogen receptor but also identified Pescadillo 1 as the third most important gene. Pescadillo 1 had not been identified by Perou et al. *(58)*, but had previously been identified by Charpentier et al. *(47)*.

Gruvberger et al. *(59)* profiled 58 node-negative breast cancers for 6728 sequence-verified cDNA clones in an important study and identified genes whose expression was associated with estrogen receptor expression. Fifty genes were ranked. Of note, *TFF3*, *GATA-3*, and stanniocalcin, which had been identified by Bouras et al. *(53)*, were ranked 2, 3, and 21 respectively. *TFF3* ranked second only after the estrogen receptor.

West et al. *(60)* used microarrays to distinguish patterns of gene expression in 18 estrogen receptor-positive and 20 estrogen receptor-negative breast tumors. *TFF1* and *TFF3* were ranked 1 and 4, respectively. Cytochrome P450 subfamily IIB and *LIV-1*, which had been identified as estrogen-regulated proteins in the ZR-75-1 cell line, ranked 3 and 25, respectively, and GATA-binding protein 3, which was ranked 3 in the study of Gruvberger et al. *(59)*, was ranked 32.

Sørlie et al. *(50)*, in an extension of the study of Perou et al. *(58)*, analyzed 78 breast cancers. As in the earlier study, the majority of the patients had been treated with doxorubicin monotherapy before surgery. Interestingly, this study subdivided the luminal epithelial/estrogen receptor-positive group into two subgroups, with differing expression profiles, having a significantly different outcome. Luminal subtype A had the highest expression of estrogen receptor,

GATA-3, X-box binding protein-1, hepatocyte nuclear factor-3α, *TFF3*, and *LIV-1*. Bertucci et al. *(61)*, in a more extensive study than that published in 2000, analyzed the expression of approx 1000 genes in 55 tumors and 11 cell lines. The tumors were poor-prognosis primary breast cancers treated with adjuvant chemotherapy. This study identified four clusters of genes whose expression refined the prognostic classification derived in the study published in 2000 *(57)*. Cluster I included the estrogen receptor, *MYB*, and *MUC1* and the transcription factors GATA-3, XPB1, ILF1, ELF1 BS69, GL13, and PBX1. The expression of some of these has previously been associated with estrogen receptor status. Bouras et al. *(53)* profiled the expression of 10,000 genes and 25,000 expressed sequence tag clusters in 13 estrogen receptor-positive and 12 estrogen receptor-negative tumors. The study focused on the association of stanniocalcin-2 expression with the estrogen receptor. It found that stanniocalcin-2 was associated with estrogen receptor expression, its mRNA levels were correlated with estrogen receptor mRNA levels, and, in separate experiments on MCF-7 cells, stanniocalcin-2 levels were induced threefold by estrogen.

van't Veer et al. *(62)* used DNA microarray analysis to determine the expression of 25,000 human genes in 117 young patients to identify a poor-prognosis gene signature. As part of this study, an estrogen receptor signature was identified, and 21 genes identified by Gruvberger et al. *(59)* as being associated with the estrogen receptor were present in the 550 estrogen receptor signature genes listed by van't Veer et al. *(62)*.

3. Characteristics of Estrogen-Regulated and Estrogen Receptor-Associated Genes

This section summarizes the available information on the estrogen-regulated genes identified most frequently in breast cancer cells. The associations of the expression of the gene products with the estrogen receptor and the value of the expression of the genes in the prediction of patient response to endocrine therapies are listed in **Table 6**. Also covered are the three genes identified most frequently as associated with expression of the estrogen receptor-α gene in breast tumors, using microarray technology (*see* **Table 7**). It reviews the current known functions of the gene products and relates these to their possible roles in breast tumor cells.

3.1. Hsp27

Heat shock proteins allow cells to survive and recover from stressful conditions. Hsp27 belongs to the group of small heat shock proteins and was originally identified as being regulated by estrogen in MCF-7 cells using double isotope labeling *(15)*. Hsp27 has been investigated as a prognostic marker in breast and other cancers. Its expression in breast tumors is associated with estrogen and progesterone receptor status, but it currently appears to have little prognostic value apart from being modestly associated with shorter disease-free survival in estrogen receptor-positive untreated lymph node-negative patients *(63,64)*.

3.2. Cathepsin D

Cathepsin D is an aspartyl protease that is normally localized in lysosomes and is involved in protein catabolism. It can be secreted from breast cancer cells, and its expression is regulated by estrogen *(18)*. It is transcribed from two promoters, one of which is estrogen-regulated *(65)*. The importance of cathepsin D in breast cancer invasion and metastasis has been extensively reviewed *(66)*. Cathepsin D expression does not appear to be highly dependent on the estrogen receptor in vivo, it is a marker of poor prognosis, and it appears to be involved in tumor growth and metastasis *(33)*.

3.3. TFF1 and TFF3

TFF1 has been identified as an estrogen regulated mRNA by several groups *([22,23,24,25]*; *see* **Tables 1**, **2**, **4**, and **5**) and was previously referred to as pS2, pNR-2, and BCE1. TFFs share homology within a conserved trefoil domain of 42 to 43 amino acids. The trefoil motif contains several well-conserved features including six cysteine residues with essentially conserved spacing. Three human TFFs have been identified: TFF1, TFF2 and TFF3. TFF1 and TFF3 each contain one trefoil domain and are 60 and 59 amino acids long, respectively, whereas TFF2 contains two trefoil domains in a single chain of 106 amino acids.

TFF1, TFF2, and TFF3, are expressed in breast cancer. Somewhat surprisingly, the principle site of expression of trefoil proteins in normal tissues is the gastrointestinal tract, where they are involved in the protection and repair of the mucosa *(67)*. TFF1 expression in breast cancer is variable and is associated with a good prognosis, estrogen receptor positivity, low grade, and response to endocrine therapy *(67,68)*. The biological function of TFF1 in breast cancer is not fully understood. It may be an estrogen-regulated autocrine motogen, as recombinant TFF1 stimulates the migration of breast cancer cells *(30)*. The observation that TFF1 stimulates cell movement is at odds with its value as a good prognostic marker in breast cancer. However, its regulation by estrogen means that it is expressed in well-differentiated, estrogen receptor-positive tumors, which are themselves a good prognostic group. Very little is known about TFF3 expression in breast cancer. It is known to be regulated by estrogen in breast cancer cells *(69)*, but is not expressed at high levels in the most commonly used estrogen-responsive cell lines. Its association with estrogen receptor status in many studies on primary tumors, however, marks it out as a protein of considerable potential future interest (*see* **Table 7**).

3.4. LIV1

LIV1 was identified from ZR-75 breast cancer cells. Measurement of the mRNA in breast tumors showed that it is preferentially expressed in lymph node-positive, estrogen receptor-positive small tumors *(70)*. Sequence analysis has suggested that it belongs to a family of zinc-transporting proteins that contain seven transmembrane domains and that it may have metalloproteinase activity *(32)*. There is experimental evidence for the location of LIV1 in the plasma membrane and for zinc-transporting activity but not for metalloproteinase activity. The protein is expressed at very low levels because of a PEST sequence (residues 210–223), which has hampered its study. Its function in breast cancer is unknown, but zinc is an important divalent cation involved in the control of cell turnover.

3.5. Stanniocalcin-2

Stanniocalcin-2 has been identified as an estrogen-regulated protein by SAGE *(47)* and microarray *(53)* analysis in MCF-7 cells, and its expression is associated with that of estrogen and progesterone receptor in primary breast tumors, using *in situ* hybridization to tissue microarrays and to estrogen receptor and TFF1 by immunohistochemistry. Stanniocalcin-2 is a homolog of a glycoprotein antihypercalcemic hormone in bony fish. In fish, stanniocalcin counteracts hypercalcemia by slowing calcium uptake in the gills, increasing phosphate reabsorption in the renal proximal tubules, and inhibiting renal calcium transport. Its role in normal breast physiology is not known, but it has been speculated that it, along with other calcium-mobilizing proteins, may be involved in the delivery of maternal calcium to neonates. It is also interesting to speculate that it may be involved in the development of microcalcification in breast lesions.

3.6. RERG

RERG was identified by Sørlie et al. *(50)* as an estrogen-related novel *ras*-related gene whose expression is associated with estrogen receptor positivity, a slow rate of tumor cell proliferation, and a favorable prognosis. As its name suggests, the RERG protein belongs to the Ras superfamily of GTP-binding proteins that control a diverse array of cellular functions. Like Ras, it has intrinsic GTPase activity but unlike Ras, it lacks COOH-terminal prenylation sequence and is located in the cytoplasm. MCF-7 cells transfected with a RERG expression vector have reduced proliferation both in cell culture and as xenografts in nude mice. It is a conundrum that RERG is an inhibitor of cell proliferation as estrogen itself is necessary for the growth of MCF-7 cells as xenografts, and it universally stimulates the proliferation of estrogen receptor-positive breast cancer cells.

3.7. GATA-3

GATA-3 belongs to the GATA family of transcription factors, which bind to the consensus DNA sequence (A/T)GATA(A/G). The DNA-binding domain comprises one or two zinc finger domains and an adjacent highly basic region. There are six vertebrate GATA-binding transcription factors. GATA-1, -2, and -3 compose one subfamily and are expressed principally in cells of erythroid lineage, whereas GATA-4, -5, and -6 are expressed in endodermally derived tissues *(71,72)*. Numerous target genes for GATA transcription factors have been identified. Given the consensus that GATA-3 is expressed in cells of erythroid lineage, it is surprising that GATA-3 is expressed in breast tumors and even more surprising that its expression is related to that of the estrogen receptor. As both the estrogen receptor and GATA-3 are transcription factors, it is possible that they regulate each others expression; however, Hoch et al. *(54)* showed that expression of GATA-3, although associated with that of the estrogen receptor, is not regulated by estrogen in MCF-7 cells. The estrogen receptor has been reported to bind to GATA-1 in the zinc finger domain, and although no interaction has been reported between GATA-3 and the estrogen receptor, the biological basis for the association between estrogen receptor and GATA-3 expression may derive from an interaction between the two proteins.

3.8. HNF3α (FOXA1)

HNF3α, also known as *FOXA1*, belongs to the hepatocyte nuclear factor-3 *(HNF3)* gene family. The *HNF3* genes are members of the fork head class of DNA-binding proteins, all of which contain a highly conserved 110-amino acid fork head motif, a variant of the helix–turn–helix motif first identified in the *Drosophila* fork-head gene. HNF3α is expressed in embryonic endoderm and adult tissues of endodermal origin including stomach, intestine, liver, and lung. Translocations *(73)* and breakpoints *(74)* within the fork head domain are associated with certain cancers, and HNF3α amplification and overexpression have been reported in esophageal and lung carcinomas *(75)*. Studies on the expression of α-fetoprotein in the liver have suggested that *HNF3α* plays a role in chromatin assembly *(76)*; however, it is not clear why expression of *HNF3α* should be associated with that of the estrogen receptor, and it will be of some interest to identify the genes that are regulated by *HNF3α* in breast cancer cells.

3.9. Human X-Box-Binding Protein-1

Human X-box binding protein-1 (HXBP-1) is identical to tax-responsive element-binding protein 5, and is a basic region–leucine zipper transcription factor that binds to the X2-box in the promoter region of the major histocompatibility complex class II *DRα* and *DPβ* genes and also forms stable heterodimers with the c-Fos protein. *HXBP-1* knockout mice show that this gene plays an important role in the growth of cardiac myocytes and hepatocytes *(77)*, and it is thought to play a role in exocrine gland and skeletal development *(78)*. Like *GATA-3* and *HNF3α*, it was identified as being associated with estrogen receptor status in the majority of breast cancer array studies, although its association was generally ranked lower than that of *GATA-3* (*see* **Table 7**). Its function in breast cancer is not known, but it is interesting to note that cDNA representational difference analysis found that *HXBP-1* expression is reduced in advanced prostate cancer, and that there is an inverse association with histological differentiation *(79)*.

4. Conclusions

Research over the past 25 yr has identified genes that are regulated by steroid hormones in breast cancer cell lines or associated with the expression of the estrogen receptor in breast tumors.

The number of studies that has been performed and the number of hormonally regulated genes identified are testament to the perceived clinical importance of the identification of markers of estrogen responsiveness. Although there is some degree of consensus from the studies, there are many discrepancies (*see* **Tables 6** and **7**).

It is noteworthy that, despite improvements to the methodologies and the sensitivity of methods such as SAGE and microarrays, they have frequently failed to identify known estrogen-regulated genes. Two good examples of this are the progesterone receptor and the docking protein IRS-1, which is involved in IGF-I signal transduction, both of which are known to be regulated by estrogens *(11,14)*. This failure could be because of the low abundance of the proteins or result from the protocols used to generate the two RNA populations that are compared.

There are also discrepancies between the data from cell lines and tumors. This may be in part because of an over-reliance on one cell line. Almost all studies have used the MCF-7 estrogen-responsive breast cancer cell line. The expressions of many known estrogen-regulated genes differ markedly in abundance among different cell lines. A good example of this is the trefoil protein TFF3, which is expressed at very low levels in MCF-7 cells, but at much higher levels in two early-passage breast cancer cell lines *(69)*.

Finally, despite years of endeavor, reliable markers of hormone responsiveness have yet to be identified. In all probability, the expression of no single protein will provide absolute prediction of hormone responsiveness, and it is most probable that hormone responsiveness will be predicted using the expression of a panel of genes using chip based technology.

References

1. Beatson, G. T. (1896) On the treatment of inoperable cases of carcinoma of the mamma: suggestions for a new method of treatment with illustrative cases. *Lancet* **2,** 104–107.
2. Toft, D. and Gorski, J. (1966) A receptor molecule for estrogens: isolation from the rat uterus and preliminary characterization. *Proc. Natl. Acad. Sci. USA* **55,** 1574–1581.
3. Osborne, C. K., Yochmowitz, M. G., Knight, W. A. D., and McGuire, W. L. (1980) The value of estrogen and progesterone receptors in the treatment of breast cancer. *Cancer* **46,** 2884–2888.
4. Jensen, E. V. and Jacobsen, H. I. (1960) Fate of steroidal estrogens in target tissues, in *Biological Activities of Steroids in Relation to Cancer* (Pincus, G., Vollmer, E. P., eds.). Academic, New York, NY, pp. 161–174.
5. Greene, G. L., Closs, L. E., Fleming, H., De Sombre, E. R., and Jensen, E. V. (1977) Antibodies to estrogen receptor: immunochemical similarity of estrophilin from various mammalian species. *Proc. Natl. Acad. Sci. USA* **74,** 3681–3685.
6. Green, S., Walter, P., Kumar. V., et al. (1986) Human oestrogen receptor cDNA: sequence, expression and homology to v-erb-A. *Nature* **320,** 134–139.
7. Clayton, S. J., May, F. E. B., and Westley, B. R. (1997) Insulin-like growth factors control the regulation of oestrogen and progesterone receptor expression by oestrogens. *Mol. Cell. Endocrinol.* **128,** 57–68.
8. Westley, B. R. and May, F. E. B. (1988) Oestrogen regulates oestrogen receptor mRNA levels in an oestrogen-responsive human breast cancer cell line. *Biochem. Biophys. Res. Commun.* **155,** 1113–1118.
9. Donaghue, C., Westley, B. R., and May, F. E. B. (1999) Selective promoter usage of the human estrogen receptor-alpha gene and its regulation by estrogen. *Mol. Endocrinol.* **13,** 1934–1950.
10. McGuire, W. L. and Horwitz, K. B. (1978) Progesterone receptors in breast cancer, in *Hormones, Receptors and Breast Cancer* (McGuire, W. L., ed.). Raven, New York, NY, pp. 31–42 .
11. May, F. E. B., Johnson, M. D., Wiseman, L. R., Wakeling, A. E., Kastner, P., and Westley, B. R. (1989) Regulation of progesterone receptor mRNA by estradiol and antioestrogens in breast cancer cell lines. *J. Steroid Biochem.* **33,** 1035–1041.
12. Elledge, R. M., Green, S., Pugh, R., et al. (2000) Estrogen receptor (ER) and progesterone receptor (PgR) by ligand-binding assay compared with ER, PgR and pS2 by immunohistochemistry in predicting response to tamoxifen in metastatic breast cancer: a Southwest Oncology Group Study. *Int. J. Cancer* **89,** 111–117.
13. Stewart, A. J., Johnson, M. D., May, F. E. B., and Westley, B. R. (1990) Role of type I insulin-like growth factor receptor in the estrogen-stimulated proliferation of human breast cancer cells. *J. Biol. Chem.* **265,** 21,172–178.

14. Molloy, C. A., May, F. E. B., and Westley, B. R. (2000) Insulin receptor substrate-1 expression is regulated by estrogen in the MCF-7 human breast cancer cell line. *J. Biol. Chem.* **275,** 12,565–12,571.
15. Edwards, D. P, Adams, D. J., and McGuire, W. L. (1981) Estradiol stimulates synthesis of a major intracellular protein in a human breast cancer cell line (MCF-7). *Breast Cancer Res. Treat.* **1,** 209–223.
16. Faucher, C., Capdevielle, J., Canal, I., et al. (1993) The 28-kDa protein whose phosphorylation is induced by protein kinase C activators in MCF-7 cells belongs to the family of low molecular mass heat shock proteins and is the estrogen-regulated 24-kDa protein. *J. Biol. Chem.* **268,** 15,168–15,173.
17. Westley, B. R. and Rochefort, H. (1980) A secreted glycoprotein induced by estrogen in human breast cancer cell lines. *Cell* **20,** 353–362.
18. Westley, B. and May, F. E. B. (1987) Oestrogen regulates cathepsin D mRNA levels in oestrogen responsive human breast cancer cells. *Nucleic Acids Res.* **15,** 3773–3786.
19. Chalbos, D. and Rochefort, H. (1984) A 250-kilodalton cellular protein is induced by progestins in two human breast cancer cell lines MCF-7 and T47D. *Biochem. Biophys. Res. Commun.* **121,** 421–427.
20. Chalbos, D., Chambon, M., Ailhaud, G., and Rochefort, H. (1987) Fatty acid synthase and its mRNA are induced by progestins in breast cancer cells. *J. Biol. Chem.* **262,** 9923–9926.
21. O'Farrell, P. H. (1975) High resolution two-dimensional electrophoresis of proteins. *J. Biol. Chem.* **250,** 4007–4021.
22. Masiakowski, P., Breathnach, R., Bloch, J., Gannon, F., Krust, A., and Chambon, P. (1982) Cloning of cDNA sequences of hormone-regulated genes from MCF-7 human breast cancer cell line. *Nucleic Acids Res.* **10,** 7895–7903.
23. Prud'homme, J. F., Fridlansky, F., Le Cunff, M., et al. (1985) Cloning of a gene expressed in human breast cancer and regulated by estrogen in MCF-7 cells. *DNA* **4,** 11–21.
24. May, F. E. B. and Westley, B. R. (1986) Cloning of estrogen-regulated messenger RNA sequences from human breast cancer cells. *Cancer Res.* **46,** 6034–6040.
25. May, F. E. B. and Westley, B. R, (1988) Identification and characterization of estrogen-regulated RNAs in human breast cancer cells. *J. Biol. Chem.* **263,** 12,901–12,908.
26. May, F. E. B. and Westley, B. R. (1987) Effects of tamoxifen and 4-hydroxytamoxifen on the pNR-1 and pNR-2 estrogen-regulated RNAs in human breast cancer cells. *J. Biol. Chem.* **262,** 15,894–15,899.
27. Manning, D. L., Daly, R., Lord, P. G., Kelly, K. F., and Green, C. D. (1988) Effects of oestrogen on the expression of a 4.4 kb mRNA in the ZR-75-1 human breast cancer cell line. *Mol. Cell. Endocrinol.* **59,** 205–212.
28. Manning, D. L., Archibald, L. H., and Ow, K. T. (1990) Cloning of estrogen-responsive messenger RNAs in the T-47D human breast cancer cell line. *Cancer Res.* **50,** 4098–4104.

29. Manning, D. L. and Nicholson, R. I. (1993) Isolation of pMGT1: a gene that is repressed by oestrogen and increased by antioestrogens and antiprogestins. *Eur. J. Cancer* **29A**, 759–762.

30. Prest, S. J., May F. E. B., and Westley B. R. (2002) The estrogen-regulated protein, TFF1, stimulates migration of human breast cancer cells. *FASEB J.* **16**, 592–994.

31. May, F. E. B., Church, S. T., Major, S., and Westley, B. R. (2003) The closely related estrogen-regulated trefoil proteins TFF1 and TFF3 have markedly different hydrodynamic properties, overall charge and distribution of surface charge. *Biochemistry* **42**, 8250–8259.

32. Taylor, K. M. and Nicholson, R. I. (2003) The LZT proteins: the LIV-1 subfamily of zinc transporters. *Biochim. Biophys. Acta* **1611**, 16–30.

33. Glondu, M., Liauet-Coopman, E., Derocq, D., Platet, N., Rochefort, H., and Garcia, M. (2002) Down-regulation of cathepsin-D expression by antisense gene transfer inhibits tumour growth and experimental lung metastasis of human breast cancer cells. *Oncogene* **21**, 5127–5134.

34. Kuang, W. W., Thompson, D. A., Hoch, R. V., and Weigel, R. J. (1998) Differential screening and suppression subtractive hybridization identified genes differentially expressed in an estrogen receptor-positive breast carcinoma cell line. *Nucleic Acids Res.* **26**, 1116–1123.

35. Ghosh, M. G., Thompson, D. A., and Weigel, R. J. (2000) *PDZK1* and *GREB1* are estrogen-regulated genes expressed in hormone-responsive breast cancer. *Cancer Res.* **60**, 6367–6375.

36. Liang, P. and Pardee, A. B. (1992) Differential display of eukaryotic messenger RNA by means of the polymerase chain reaction. *Science* **257**, 967–971.

37. Ediger, T. R., Kraus, W. L., Weinman, E. J., and Katzenellenbogen, B. S. (1999) Estrogen receptor regulation of the Na^+/H^+ exchange regulatory factor. *Endocrinology* **140**, 2976–2982.

38. Stephen, R., Corcoran, D., and Darbre, P. D. (1998) A novel oestrogen-regulated gene in human breast cancer cells identified by differential display. *J. Mol. Endocrinol.* **20**, 375–380.

39. Thompson, D. A. and Weigel, R. J. (1998) Characterization of a gene that is inversely correlated with estrogen receptor expression (*ICERE-1*) in breast carcinomas. *Eur. J. Biochem.* **252**, 169–177.

40. Lapointe, J. and Labrie, C. (1999) Identification and cloning of a novel androgen-responsive gene, uridine diphosphoglucose dehydrogenase, in human breast cancer cells. *Endocrinology* **140**, 4486–4493.

41. Hamilton, J. A., Callaghan, M. J., Sutherland, R. L., and Watts, C. K. (1997) Identification of *PRG1*, a novel progestin-responsive gene with sequence homology to 6-phosphofructo-2-kinase/fructose-2,6-bisphosphatase. *Mol. Endocrinol.* **11**, 490–502.

42. Miller, M. M., James, R. A., Richer, J. K., Gordon, D. F., Wood, W. M., and Horwitz, K. B. (1997) Progesterone regulated expression of flavin-containing-containing monooxygenase 5 by the B-isoform of progesterone receptors: implications for tamoxifen carcinogenicity. *J. Clin. Endocrinol. Metab.* **82**, 2956–2961.

43. Purmonen, S., Ahola, T. M., Pennanen, P., et al. (2002) HDLG5/KIAA0583, encoding a MAGUK-family protein, is a primary progesterone target gene in breast cancer cells. *Int. J. Cancer,* **102**, 1–6.

44. Ahola, T. M., Purmonen, S., Pennanen, P., Zhuang, Y. H., Tuohimaa, P., and Ylikomi, T. (2002) Progestin upregulates G-protein-coupled receptor 30 in breast cancer cells. *Eur. J. Biochem.* **269**, 2485–2490.

45. Kester, H. A., van der Leede, B. M., van der Saag, P. T., and van der Burg, B. (1997) Novel progesterone target genes identified by an improved differential display technique suggest that progestin-induced growth inhibition of breast cancer cells coincides with enhancement of differentiation. *J. Biol. Chem.* **272**, 16,637–16,643.

46. Inadera, H., Hashimoto, S., Dong, H. Y., et al. (2000) WISP2 as a novel estrogen-responsive gene in human breast cancer cells. *Biochem. Biophys. Res. Commun.* **275**, 108–114.

47. Charpentier, A. H., Bednarek, A. K., Daniel, R. L., et al. (2000) Effects of estrogen on global gene expression: identification of novel targets of estrogen action. *Cancer Res.* **60**, 5977–5983.

48. Seth, P., Krop, I., Porter, D., and Polyak, K. (2002) Novel estrogen and tamoxifen induced genes identified by SAGE (Serial Analysis of Gene Expression) *Oncogene* **21**, 836–843.

49. Perez-Enciso, M. and Tenenhaus, M. (2003) Prediction of clinical outcome with microarray data: a partial least squares discriminant analysis (PLS-DA) approach. *Hum Genet.* **112**, 581–592.

50. Sorlie, T., Perou, C. M., Tibshirani, R., et al. (2001) Gene expression patterns of breast carcinomas distinguish tumor subclasses with clinical implications. *Proc. Natl. Acad. Sci. USA* **98**, 10,869–10,874.

51. van de Vijver, M. J., He, Y.D., van't Veer, L. J., et al. (2002) A gene-expression signature as a predictor of survival in breast cancer. *N. Engl. J. Med.* **347**, 1999–2009.

52. Soulez, M. and Parker, M. G. (2001) Identification of novel oestrogen receptor target genes in human ZR-75-1 breast cancer cells by expression profiling. *J. Mol. Endocrinol.* **27**, 259–274.

53. Bouras, T., Southey, M. C., Chang, A. C., et al. (2002) Stanniocalcin 2 is an estrogen-responsive gene coexpressed with the estrogen receptor in human breast cancer. *Cancer Res.* **621**, 289–295.

54. Hoch, R.V., Thompson, D. A., Baker, R. J., and Weigel, R. J. (1999) GATA-3 is expressed in association with estrogen receptor in breast cancer. *Int. J. Cancer.* **84**, 122–128.

55. Finlin, B. S., Gau, C. L., Murphy, G. A., et al. (2001) RERG is a novel ras-related, estrogen-regulated and growth-inhibitory gene in breast cancer. *J. Biol. Chem.* **276**, 42,259–42,267.

56. Inoue, A., Yoshida, N., Omoto, Y., et al. (2002) Development of cDNA microarray for expression profiling of estrogen-responsive genes. *J. Mol. Endocrinol.* **29**, 175–192.

57. Bertucci, F., Houlgatte, R., Benziane, A., et al. (2000) Gene expression profiling of primary breast carcinomas using arrays of candidate genes. *Hum. Mol. Genet.* **9,** 2981–2991.

58. Perou, C. M., Sorlie, T., Elsen, M. B., et al. (2000) Molecular portraits of human breast tumours. *Nature* **406,** 747–752.

59. Gruvberger, S., Ringner, M., Chen, Y., et al. (2001) Estrogen receptor status in breast cancer is associated with remarkably distinct gene expression patterns. *Cancer Res.* **61,** 5979–5984.

60. West, M., Blanchette, C., Dressman, C., et al. (2001) Predicting the clinical status of human breast cancer by using gene expression profiles. *Proc. Natl. Acad. Sci. USA* **98,** 11,462–11,467.

61. Bertucci, F., Nasser, V., Granjeaud, S., et al. (2002) Gene expression profiles of poor-prognosis primary breast cancer correlate with survival. *Hum. Mol. Genet.* **11,** 863–872.

62. van't Veer, L. J., Dai, H., van de Vijver, M. J., et al. (2002) Gene expression profiling predicts clinical outcome of breast cancer. *Nature* **415,** 530–536.

63. Ciocca, D. R., Oesterreich, S., Chamness, G. C., McGuire, W. L., and Fuqua, S. A. (1993) Biological and clinical implications of heat shock protein 27,000 (Hsp27): a review. *J. Natl. Cancer Inst.* **85,** 1558–1570.

64. Oesterreich, S., Hilsenbeck, S. G., Ciocca, D. R., et al. (1996) The small heat shock protein HSP27 is not an independent prognostic marker in axillary lymph node-negative breast cancer patients. *Clin. Cancer Res.* **2,** 1199–1206.

65. May, F. E. B., Smith, D. J., and Westley, B. R. (1993) The human cathepsin D-encoding gene is transcribed from an estrogen-regulated and a constitutive start point. *Gene* **134,** 277–282.

66. Westley, B. R. and May, F. E. B. (1996) Cathepsin D and breast cancer. *Eur. J. Cancer* **32,** 15–24.

67. Ribieras, S., Tomasetto, C., and Rio, M. C. (1998) The pS2/TFF1 trefoil factor, from basic research to clinical applications. *Biochim. Biophys. Acta* **1378,** F61–F77.

68. Henry, J. A., Piggott, N. H., Mallick U. K., et al. (1991) pNR-2/pS2 immunohistochemical staining in breast cancer correlation with prognostic factors and endocrine response. *Br. J. Cancer* **63,** 615–622.

69. May, F. E. B. and Westley, B. R. (1997) Expression of human intestinal trefoil factor in malignant cells and its regulation by oestrogen in breast cancer cells. *J. Pathol.* **182,** 404–413.

70. Manning, D. L., Robertson, J. F., Ellis, I. O., et al. (1994) Oestrogen-regulated genes in breast cancer: association of pLIV1 with lymph node involvement. *Eur. J. Cancer* **30,** 675–678.

71. Parry, P., Wei, Y., and Evans, G. (1994) Cloning and characterization of the t(X;11) breakpoint from a leukemic cell line identify a new member of the fork head gene family. *Genes Chromosomes Cancer* **11,** 79–84.

72. Galili, N., Davis, R. J., Fredericks, W. J., et al. (1993) Fusion of a fork head domain gene to PAX3 in the solid tumour alveolar rhabdomyosarcoma. *Nat. Genet.* **5,** 230–235.

73. Lin, L., Miller, C. T., Contreras, J. I., et al. (2002) The hepatocyte nuclear factor 3 alpha gene, HNF3alpha (FOXA1), on chromosome band 14q13 is amplified and overexpressed in esophageal and lung adenocarcinomas. *Cancer Res.* **62,** 5273–5279.

74. Crowe, A. J., Sang, L., Li, K. K., Lee, K. C., Spear, B. T., and Barton, M. C. (1999) Hepatocyte nuclear factor 3 relieves chromatin-mediated repression of the alpha-fetoprotein gene. *J. Biol. Chem.* **274,** 25,113–25,120.

75. Patient, R. K. and McGhee, J. D. (2002) The GATA family (vertebrates and invertebrates). *Curr. Opin. Genet. Dev.* **12,** 416–422.

76. Lowry, J. A. and Atchley, W. R. (2000) Molecular evolution of the GATA family of transcription factors: conservation within the DNA-binding domain. *J. Mol. Evol.* **50,** 103–115.

77. Masaki, T., Noguchi, H., Kobayashi, M., Yoshida, M., and Takamatsu, K. (2000) Isolation and characterisation of the gene encoding mouse tax-responsive element-binding protein (TREB) 5. *DNA Res.* **7,** 187–193.

78. Reimold, A. M., Ponath, P. D., Li, Y. S., et al. (1996) Transcription factor B cell lineage-specific activator protein regulates the gene for human X-box binding protein 1. *J. Exp. Med.* **183,** 393–401.

79. Takahashi, S., Suzuki, S., Inaguma, S., et al. (2002) Down-regulation of human X-box binding protein 1 (hXBP-1) expression correlates with tumor progression in human prostate cancers. *Prostate* **50,** 154–161.

26

Sequencing of the Tumor Suppressor Gene *TP 53*

Barbro Linderholm, Torbjörn Norberg, and Jonas Bergh

Summary

The tumour suppressor gene, *TP 53* (commonly also called *p53*) has multiple, important cellular functions involving control of apoptosis, downstream cell cycle regulation via p21 and cyclin dependent kinases, and control of tumour angiogenesis. Somatic mutation of *TP 53* is considered to be the most common genetic mutation in human cancer. Mutations of the gene are associated with drug resistance and poor patient prognosis in human cancers. Immunohistochemistry to detect mutated *TP 53* is unreliable and molecular biology approaches are therefore preferable for its assessment. This chapter describes protocols for the 'gold standard', but perhaps complex and time consuming, methods for sequencing *TP 53*, by cDNA and genomic based sequencing techniques.

Key Words: *TP 53*, *p53*, molecular biology, cDNA, PCR, genomic based sequencing, microdissection

1. Introduction

This chapter will describe sequencing of the tumor suppressor gene *TP 53*, previously commonly known as *p53*. We have chosen to describe this method, as molecular analyses of this gene have resulted in the most accurate results *(1)*. The gene was initially described to function as an oncogene, but later studies have clearly revealed that *TP 53* is a tumor suppressor gene. The gene is located to the short arm of chromosome 17, band 13.1 *(2,3)*. The gene consists of 11 exons, with larger intron regions between exons 1 and 2, 9 and 10, and 10 and 11. Exon 1 is noncoding. Only 14% of reported studies have analyzed all coding exons *(1)*. Some 40% of the studies have only analyzed exons 5 through 8 *(1)*. In this review, the authors also show that studies of exons 4–10 will result in the detection of more than 99% of *TP 53* mutations *(1)*. Sequencing from genomic DNA compared with complementary (c)DNA will increase the workload, but the former will give the most complete picture of the *TP 53* status *(4)*. The translated protein contains 393 amino acids (aa). The protein

From: *Methods in Molecular Medicine, Vol. 120: Breast Cancer Research Protocols*
Edited by: S. A. Brooks and A. L. Harris © Humana Press Inc., Totowa, NJ

contains three principal domains: transactivation, aa 1–42; DNA binding, aa 100–293; and oligomerization, aa 319–393 *(5)*. The protein is organized as a tetramer *(6)*. Ultraviolet light, carcinogens, radiation, and cytostatics can activate normal thymidine phosphorylase (TP). The oncogene *Mdm-2* binds to the amino terminal of *TP 53 (7)*, followed by downregulation of *TP 53*.

TP 53 has multiple important cellular functions involving control of apoptosis and downstream cell cycle regulation via p21 and the cyclin-dependent kinases, as well as involvement in the control of tumor angiogenesis *(1,8)*. TP can be inactivated by binding to several viral oncoproteins: adenovirus protein E1B, E6 of human papilloma virus, X of hepatitis B, and large T-antigen from SV40 *(9)*. Germ line (as part of the Li-Fraumeni syndrome) or somatic mutations also result in altered or loss of *TP 53* function. The somatic mutation of the *TP 53* gene is considered to be the most common genetic alteration in human cancer *(19)*. A small, intrapatient breast cancer study revealed new and further *TP 53* mutations during tumor progression *(11)*. *TP 53* mutations have been demonstrated to be associated with worse prognosis and drug resistance for a long list of human cancers *(1,12,13)*.

1.1. Methods for TP 53 Determination

Immunohistochemistry, the subject of Chapter 15, is probably the most common method used. This method contains too many shortcomings to be recommended. Several studies have revealed inferior results with immunohistochemistry compared with molecular biological techniques *(14–17)*. Immunohistochemistry misses 11.3% of the frameshift mutation and 7.5% of the nonsense mutations in comparison with the *p53* database *(1)*. In addition to this, a rather high rate of false positivity is recorded by immunohistochemistry, likely because of activation of wild-ype *TP 53* detected as a weak immunohistochemical labeling *(15)*. The luminometric method for protein-based *TP 53* determinations suffers from the same type of shortcomings as immunohistochemistry *(18)*.

1.2. Short List of Methods for TP 53 Determination

1.2.1. RNA/DNA-Based Methods for Screening

1. Single-strand conformation polymorphism.
2. Dideoxy fingerprinting.
3. Heteroduplex analysis.
4. Denaturing high-performance liquid chromatography.
5. Denaturant gradient gel electrophoresis.
6. Constant denaturant gel electrophoresis.
7. Chemical cleavage of mismatch or hydroxylamine/tetroxide.
8. Enzymatic mutation detection.

1.2.2. Detection of Specific Mutation Positions

1. Ligase chain reaction.
2. DNA minisequencing.
3. Oligonucleotide arrays.
4. Allele-specific oligonucleotide hybridization.
5. Oligonucleotide ligation assay.
6. Complete sequencing from cDNA or genomic DNA.

1.2.3. Protein-Based Methods

1. Immunohistochemistry.
2. Luminometric immunoassay.

In this chapter, therefore, we will only describe the sequencing of *TP 53* as the present "gold standard" for *TP 53* determinations. On the downside, the present standard sequencing procedures are considered to be complex, time-consuming, and labor-intensive. Accordingly, rapid chip-based and functional yeast assays are presently being explored with an aim to overcome these problems *(19,20)*.

The methods for cDNA- and genomic-based sequencing are herein described.

2. Materials

1. RNeasy Mini kit, Qiagen (VWR International, Stockholm, Sweden).
2. β-Mercaptoethanol (β-ME) must be added to Buffer RLT (Qiagen) before use. (**Caution:** β-ME is toxic; dispense in a fume hood and wear appropriate protective clothing.) Add 10 μL of β-ME per 1 mL of Buffer RLT. Buffer RLT is stable for 1 mo after addition of β-ME.
3. Buffer RPE (Qiagen) is supplied as a concentrate. Before using for the first time, add 4 vol of ethanol (99%), as indicated on the bottle, to obtain a working solution. Place a piece of dry ice on a Styrofoam™ plate.
4. 14.3 *M* β-ME solution.
5. Diethyl pyrocarbonate-treated water.
6. RNA guard (Amersham Biosciences, Uppsala, Sweden).
7. Moloney murine leukemia virus reverse transcriptase (200 U, Amersham Biosciences).
8. 1 *M* Tris-HCl (pH 8.3) stock solution.
9. 1 *M* Tris-HCl (pH 7.5) stock solution.
10. Ethylenediaminetetraacetic acid.
11. Dithiothreitol (Amersham Biosciences).
12. Dexoxycytidine 5'-triphosphate, deoxyadenosine 5'-triphosphate, deoxythymidine 5'-triphosphate, deoxyinosinlate 5'-triphosphate, deoxyguanosine 5'-triphosphate (Amersham Biosciences).
13. pd[N]$_6$ Random primers (Amersham Biosciences).

14. 2X cDNA mix: 90 mM Tris-HCl (pH 8.3), 138 mM KCl, 18 mM MgCl$_2$, 30 mM dithiothreitol, 3.6 mM dexoxycytidine 5'-triphosphate, deoxyadenosine 5'-triphosphate, deoxythymidine 5'-triphosphate, and deoxyinosinlate 5'-triphosphate, 0.9 mM deoxyguanosine 5'-triphosphate, and 0.152 A260 U of pd[N]$_6$ random primers (approx 2.5 pmol of primers).
15. Superfrost® glass slides.
16. Xylene.
17. Myers solution.
18. QIAamp DNA minikit, (VWR International).
19. 10X PCR Buffer II (PerkinElmer, Stockholm, Sweden).
20. 25 mM MgCl$_2$ (PerkinElmer).
21. 4 U of *Taq* Gold DNA polymerase (PerkinElmer) solution.
22. 1% Agarose gels containing 5 µg/mL of ethidium bromide.
23. Reference standard in gels: 100-bp ladder (Amersham Biosciences.
24. Autoload kit (Amersham Biosciences).
25. ALF Express™ (Amersham Biosciences).
26. Reprogel, acrylamide gel solution (Amersham Biosciences).
27. Primers. Polymerase chain reaction (PCR) and DNA sequencing primers are synthesized based on the cDNA sequence of the *p53* messenger RNA. Four sets of primers should be used to cover the entire protein-coding region of the *p53* cDNA.
   a. PCR Primers:
   • Fragment 1 (B = biotin-labeled): B-5'-GAC ACG CTT CCC TGG ATT GGC-3' and 5'-GCA AAA CAT CTT GTT GAG GGC A-3'. Covers the entire sequence of exons 2,3, and 4, plus parts of exons 1 and 5.
   • Fragment 2: B-5'-GTT TCC GCT TGG GCT TCT TGC A-3' and 5'-GGT ACA GCT AGA GCC AAC CTC-3'. Covers the entire sequence of exons 5 and 6, plus parts of exons 4 and 7.
   • Fragment 3: 5'-TGG CCC CTC CTC AGC ATC TTA-3' and B-5'-CAA GGC CTC ATT CAG CTC TC-3'. Covers the entire sequence of exons 6–9 plus parts of exons 5 and 10.
   • Fragment 4: 5'-CGG CGC ATA GAG GAA GAG AAT-3' and B-5'-CGC ACA CCT ATT GCA AGC AAG GG-3'. Covers the entire sequence of exons 9, 10 and 11 plus part of exon 8.
   b. DNA sequencing primers (Cy5-labeled):
   • Fragment 1: –5'-CAG GGG AGT ACG TGC AAG TCA CAG-3'.
   • Fragment 2: F-5'-GCC AAC CTC AGG CGG CTC ATA-3'.
   • Fragment 3: F-5'-CGA GTG GAA GGA AAT TTG CGT-3'.
   • Fragment 4: F-5'-GGG GAG CCT CAC CAC GAG CTG-3'.

3. Methods

3.1. RNA Extraction

The procedure is basically as described in the kit-supplied protocol, with minor modifications (*see* **Note 1**).

During this procedure, care should be taken to avoid thawing of the specimen in order to avoid RNA degradation. This is important if repeated RNA preparation proved to be necessary.

Note: Perform the extraction in a designated area, preferably a laminar air flow bench.

1. Place a 1.5-mL polypropylene microcentrifuge tube containing 500 µL of Buffer RLT on wet ice.
2. Place a disposable Petri dish on dry ice (*see* **Note 2**) and carefully transfer the tumor onto the dish using forceps. Wash the forceps between samples by dipping in 99% ethanol and flame it briefly over a Bunsen burner.
3. Cut a section of frozen tumor specimen (5 × 2 × 2 mm) using a disposable scalpel; cut the section into smaller pieces with the scalpel, and transfer into the Buffer RLT-containing tube.
4. Homogenize the sample with a conventional rotor–stator homogenizer (Polytron 1200C; Kinimatica, Bethlehem, PA) until the sample is uniformly homogeneous (usually 10–20 s) (*see* **Note 3**).
5. Centrifuge the tissue lysate for 3 min at maximum speed using a microcentrifuge. Carefully transfer the supernatant to a new microcentrifuge tube (not kit-supplied) by pipetting (*see* **Note 4**). Use only this supernatant (lysate) in subsequent steps. In some preparations, very small amounts of insoluble material will be present, making the pellet invisible.
6. Add 1 vol (500 µL) of 70% ethanol to the cleared lysate, and mix immediately by pipetting. *Do not centrifuge.* If some lysate is lost during **steps 4** and **5**, adjust volume of ethanol accordingly. A precipitate may form after the addition of ethanol, but this will not affect the RNeasy procedure.
7. Apply the sample, including any precipitate that may have formed, to an RNeasy mini column placed in a 2-mL collection tube (kit-supplied). Close the tube gently, and centrifuge for 15 s at 8000*g*. Discard the flowthrough. Reuse the collection tube for **step 8**.
8. Add 700 µL of Buffer RW1 (Qiagen) to the RNeasy column. Close the tube gently, and centrifuge for 15 s at 8000*g* to wash the column. Discard the flowthrough and collection tube.
9. Transfer the RNeasy column into a new 2-mL collection tube (kit-supplied). Pipet 500 µL of Buffer RPE onto the RNeasy column. Close the tube gently, and centrifuge for 15 s at 8000*g* to wash the column. Discard the flowthrough. Reuse the collection tube for **step 10**.
10. Add another 500 µL of Buffer RPE to the RNeasy column. Close the tube gently, and centrifuge for 2 min at 8000*g* to dry the RNeasy silica gel membrane. It is important to dry the RNeasy silica gel membrane, because residual ethanol may interfere with downstream reactions.
11. To elute, transfer the RNeasy column to a new 1.5-mL collection tube (kit-supplied). Pipet 50 µL of RNase-free water directly onto the RNeasy silica gel membrane. Close the tube gently, and centrifuge for 1 min at 8000*g* to elute the RNA.

3.2. cDNA Synthesis

Prepare the 2X cDNA mix. The mix can be stored at –20°C for several months.

1. Heat to denature the RNA sample at 90°C for 3 min.
2. Chill on wet ice for 3 min.
3. Prepare a cDNA reaction mixture: transfer 25 µL of a given RNA sample to a microcentrifuge tube containing:
    a. 10 µL of Moloney leukemia virus reverse transcriptase (200 U, Amersham Biosciences).
    b. 2.5 µL of RNA guard (62.5 U).
    c. 37.5 µL of 2X cDNA mix to yield a final volume of 75 µL.
4. Incubate the cDNA mixture for 1 h at 37°C.
5. Heat-denature the reaction products at 90°C for 3 min and store at –20°C.

3.3. Genomic DNA-Based Analysis

3.3.1. Microdissection for DNA-Based Sequencing

1. Prepare 16-µm-thick slice of representative formalin fixed paraffin embedded tumor and place on Superfrost glass slide.
2. Incubate at 58°C overnight in a lab oven.
3. Incubate the section in xylene twice for 15 min each, may be repeated twice.
4. Rinse twice in 99% alcohol, twice in 95% alcohol, and finally, twice in 70% alcohol.
5. Place in Myers solution for 50–60 s.
6. Put the slides in distilled water for 10 min. It is also possible to store it in distilled water for a maximum of 24 h.
7. Number 1.5-mL tubes and fill with 50 µL of ultrapure water.
8. Microdissect tumor cell clusters by scraping off areas on the glass slide, using a microscope and a syringe needle (*see* **Note 5**).
9. Transfer the tumor clusters to tubes and store in a microcentrifuge refrigerator until preparation of DNA.

3.3.2. DNA Preparation From Microdissected Material (QIAamp DNA minikit, VWR International) (see **Note 6**)

1. Put the samples on the lab bench.
2. Add 180 µL of ATL lysis buffer (Qiagen).
3. Add 20 µL of proteinase K stock.
4. Vortex.
5. Incubate in 56°C for 1–4 h, vortex occasionally.
6. Centrifuge briefly.
7. Add 200 µL of AL buffer (Qiagen), vortex.
8. Incubate for 10 min in 70°C, centrifuge briefly.
9. Transfer the total content of the tubes to a column.

10. Centrifuge 8000*g* for 1 min.
11. Put the column in a new clean tube. Discard the old tube.
12. Open carefully the top of the column and add 500 μL of AW1 (wash) buffer (Qiagen).
13. Centrifuge 8000*g* for 1 min.
14. Put the column in a new clean tube. Discard the old tube.
15. Carefully open the top of the column and add 500 μL of AW2 (wash) buffer (Qiagen).
16. Centrifuge 14,000*g* for 3 min.
17. Put the column in a new clean tube with the top cut off.
18. Carefully open the top of the column, add 200 μL of AE (elution) buffer (Qiagen).
19. Incubate in room temperature for 1 min.
20. Centrifuge 8000*g* for 1 min.
21. Remove the eluate to a new numbered tube.
22. Store the eluate at –70°C.

3.4. Polymerase Chain Reaction

*3.4.1. cDNA-Based Analysis (see **Note 7**)*

1. Mix together in individual 0.2-mL PCR tubes (PerkinElmer).
   a. 5 μL of 10X PCR Buffer II (PerkinElmer).
   b. 1 μL (5 pmol) each of the 5' primer and the 3' primer (one of them being biotinylated).
   c. 2 μL of 25 m*M* MgCl$_2$ solution.
   d. 35.6 μL of dH$_2$O.
   e. 0.4 μL of *Taq* Gold DNA polymerase (4 U).
2. Add 5 μL of a given cDNA preparation or negative-control template to specific tubes, yielding total PCR reaction volumes of 50 μL.
3. Incubate the reaction mixtures in a PCR machine programmed to carry out a 5-min hold at 94°C, followed by 38 temperature cycles with the profile: 94°C for 15 s, 58°C for 30 s, and 72°C for 45 s.
4. Provide a 5-min incubation at 72°C after conclusion of the thermocycling program, followed by incubation at 22°C.

3.4.2. Genomic DNA-Based Analysis

The PCR reaction is conducted in a two-step fashion, a so-called "nested approach," with slightly different protocols for the individual fragments.

Exon 4 is divided into two fragments to improve success rate in sequencing.

3.4.2.1. PCR 1 FOR ALL FRAGMENTS: EXONS 4:1, 4:2, AND 5–8 (*SEE* **NOTE 8**)

1. Mix in individual 0.2-mL PCR tubes (Perkin-Elmer):
   a. 5 μL of PCR Buffer II
   b. 5 μL of 1.5-m*M* MgCl$_2$ solution.
   c. 3 μL of 0.2-m*M* deoxynucleotide 5'-triphosphate (dNTP) mix.

    d. 1 µL of each primer (10 pmol each).
    e. 29.7 µL of ultrapure water.
    f. 5 µL of DNA sample.
    g. 0.3 µL of *Taq* Gold DNA polymerase.
2. Incubate the reaction mixtures in a PCR machine programmed to carry out a 10-min hold at 95°C, followed by 30 temperature cycles with the profile: 95°C for 45 s, 59°C for 45 s, and 72°C for 45 s.
3. Provide a 5-min incubation at 72°C after conclusion of the thermocycling program, followed by incubation at 22°C.

3.4.2.2. PCR 2: EXON 4:1 (*SEE* NOTE 9)

1. Mix in individual 0.2-mL PCR tubes (PerkinElmer)
    a. 5 µL of PCR Buffer II.
    b. 3 µL of 1.5-mM MgCl$_2$ solution.
    c. 3 µL of 0.2-mM dNTP mix.
    d. 1 µL of each primer (10 pmol each).
    e. 34.4 µL of ultrapure water.
    f. 2 µL of PCR 1.
    g. 0.6 µL of *Taq* Gold DNA polymerase.
2. Incubate the reaction mixtures in a PCR machine programmed to carry out a 10-min hold at 95°C, followed by 40 temperature cycles with the profile: 95°C for 45 s, 59°C for 45 s, and 72°C for 45 s.
3. Provide a 5-min incubation at 72°C after conclusion of the thermocycling program, followed by incubation at 22°C.

3.4.2.3. PCR 2: EXONS 4:2, 5, 6, AND 8 (*SEE* NOTE 9)

1. Mix in individual 0.2-mL PCR tubes (PerkinElmer):
    a. 5 µL of PCR Buffer II.
    b. 5 µL of 1.5-mM MgCl$_2$ solution.
    c. 3 µL of 0.2-mM dNTP mix.
    d. 1 µL of each primer (10 pmol each).
    e. 32.7 µL of ultrapure water.
    f. 2 µL of PCR 1.
    g. 0.3 mL of *Taq* Gold DNA polymerase.
2. Incubate the reaction mixtures in a PCR machine programmed to carry out a 10-min hold at 95°C, followed by 40 temperature cycles with the profile: 95°C for 45 s, 59°C for 45 s, and 72°C for 45 s.
3. Provide a 5-min incubation at 72°C after conclusion of the thermocycling program, followed by incubation at 22°C.

3.4.2.4. PCR 2: EXON 7 (*SEE* NOTE 9)

1. Mix in individual 0.2-mL PCR tubes (PerkinElmer):
    a. 5 µL of PCR Buffer II.
    b. 5.5 µL of 1.5-mM MgCl$_2$ solution.
    c. 3 µL of 0.2-mM dNTP mix.

    d. 1 μL of each primer (10 pmol each).
    e. 32.2 μL of ultrapure water.
    f. 2 μL of PCR 1.
    g. 0.8 μL of *Taq* Gold DNA polymerase.
2. Incubate the reaction mixtures in a PCR machine programmed to carry out a 10-min hold at 95°C, followed by 40 temperature cycles with the profile: 95°C for 45 s, 59°C for 45 s, and 72°C for 45 s.
3. Provide a 5-min incubation at 72°C after conclusion of the thermocycling program, followed by incubation at 22°C.

3.5. Primers

PCR and DNA sequencing primers are synthesized based on the DNA sequence of the *p53* gene. Sets of primers should be used to cover exons 4–8 of the *p53* gene.

By linking a common sequence tag, the M13 universal (boldfaced section of primers), a common sequencing primer can be used for all fragments.

3.5.1. Exon 4:1, PCR 1

1. HEAN71: 5'-CTG GGA CCT GGA GGG CTG GG-3'.
2. p53e4r1B: 5'-B-CTG GGA AGG GAC AGA AGA T-3'.

3.5.2. Exon 4:2, PCR 1

1. BECE5B: 5'-B-ATA CGG CCA GGC ATT GAA GT-3'.
2. BECE3: 5'-AGA GGA ATC CCA AAG TTC CA-3'.

3.5.3. Exon 4:1, PCR 2

1. BECE4T: 5'-**AGT CAC GAC GTT GTA AAA CGA CGG CCA GT**C TGA GGA CCT GGT CCT CTG AC-3'.
2. p53e4r1B: 5'-B-CTG GGA AGG GAC AGA AGA T-3'.

3.5.4. Exon 4:2, PCR 2

1. BECE5B: 5'-B-ATA CGG CCA GGC ATT GAA GT-3'.
2. p53e4f2T: 5'-AGT CAC GAC GTT GTA AAA CGA CGG CCA GTG CTC CCA GAA TGC CAG AG-3'.

3.5.5. Exon 5, PCR 1

1. RIT596: 5'-GGA GGT GCT TAC ACA T-3'.
2. HEAN56: 5'-GAG GCC TGG GGA CCC TGG GC-3'.

3.5.6. Exon 5, PCR 2

1. RIT597T: 5'-**AGT CAC GAC GTT GTA AAA CGA CGG CCA GT**T TCA CTT GTG CCC TGA CTT-3'.
2. HEAN55B: 5'-B-ACC AGC CCT GTC GTC TCT CC-3'.

3.5.7. Exon 6, PCR1

1. HEAN50: 5'-CGG AGG GCC ACT GAC AAC CA-3'.
2. HEAN77: 5'-GCC TGG AGA GAC GAC AGG GC-3'.

3.5.8. Exon 6, PCR 2

1. HEAN78T: 5'-**AGT CAC GAC GTT GTA AAA CGA CGG CCA GT**T TGC CCA GGG TCC CCA GGC C-3'.
2. HEAN45B: 5'-B-CTT AAC CCC TCC TCC CAG AG-3'.

3.5.9. Exon 7, PCR1

1. HEAN57: 5'-TGC TTG CCA CAG GTC TCC CC-3'.
2. HEAN60: 5'-CGG CAA GCA GAG GCT GGG GC-3'.

3.5.10. Exon 7, PCR 2

1. HEAN58T: 5'-**AGT CAC GAC GTT GTA AAA CGA CGG CCA GT**C GCA CTG GCC TCA TCT TGG G-3'.
2. HEAN59B: 5'-B-CAG CAG GCC AGT GTG CAG GG-3'.

3.5.11. Exon 8, PCR1

1. HEAN61: 5'-ACA GGT AGG ACC TGA TTT CC-3'.
2. HEAN64: 5'-TGA ATC TGA GGC ATA ACT GC-3'.

3.5.12. Exon 8, PCR 2

1. HEAN62B: 5'-B-GCC TCT TGC TTC TCT TTT CC-3'.
2. e8RT: 5'-**AGT CAC GAC GTT GTA AAA CGA CGG CCA GT**T CT CCA CCG CTT CTT GTC-3'.

3.6. Agarose Gel Electrophoresis and Quality Control

To control for contamination of PCR products that might have originated during the steps preceding DNA sequencing, negative-control samples for both RNA isolation and cDNA preparation steps should be run on agarose gel electrophoresis. Negative controls consist of not adding tissue to RNA extraction tubes or not adding RNA to cDNA reaction mixtures. The presence of amplified DNA in negative-control sample tubes should result in the conclusion that all samples might be contaminated, and the corresponding batch of samples should be discarded.

1. Perform electrophoresis on 5-μL aliquots of relevant PCR products.
2. Separate on 1% agarose gel containing 5 μL/mL of ethidium bromide.
3. Reference standard: 100-bp ladder (0.2 μg, Amersham Biosciences).

3.7. Sequence Analysis of PCR Products, Using Solid-Phase Sequencing and an Automated DNA Sequencer

1. Transfer the PCR product (40 µL) to a 10-well plate containing 80 µL of BW buffer (1 m*M* NaCl, 5 m*M* Tris-HCl [pH 7.5], and 0.5 m*M* ethylenediamine-tetraacetic acid) in each well. Mix by pipetting and be sure to avoid bubbles. Insert the combs, with the flat side facing away from the operator, and dip a couple of times. Leave at room temperature for at least 60 min, dipping occasionally will improve the capture.
2. Move the comb to a Petri dish containing 0.1 *M* of NaOH and incubate for 5 min. Wash the comb once in 10 m*M* Tris-HCl (pH 7.5).
3. Add 104 µL of water, 12 µL of 10X annealing buffer, 4 µL of a 1-pmol/µL Cy5-labeled sequencing primer to a new slot in a 10-well plate and insert the comb. Heat the annealing mix to 65°C for 5 min, and then leave at room temperature to cool.
4. Dispense 20 µL of sequence mix in each well of a 40-well plate (keeping the plate on ice) just before inserting the comb, with the flat side facing away from the operator. Incubate 5 min at 42°C, and then place on ice.
   Sequence mix:
   a. 2 µL of 10X annealing buffer.
   b. 1 µL of extension buffer.
   c. 1 µL of dimethyl sulfoxide.
   d. 4 µL of d/ddNTP mix.
   e. 11 µL of water.
   f. 1 µL (2 U) of T7 polymerase diluted in enzyme dilution buffer.

Make master mixes for each d/ddNTP and store on ice. Add enzyme as late as possible.

5. Rinse the wells on an ALF Express gel prewarmed to 55°C and load 100% formamide stop solution to each well with a syringe. Insert the comb with the flat side facing away from the operator and leave for 10 min. Remove the comb carefully; start the ALF Express.

3.8. Sequencing Evaluation and Verification

Evaluation of the *p53* sequences can be performed with the aid of a sequence analysis software (Mutation Analyzer, version 1.0; Amersham Biosciences) that compares the wild-type *p53* sequence with the sequences obtained from the sample analysis.

Confirm all mutations by reamplification of the relevant samples and resequencing the newly prepared PCR products.

4. Notes

1. When performing RNA extraction for the cDNA-based analysis, it is necessary to always "extract" a negative control (tumor-negative sample) in order to detect possible contamination.

2. To avoid degradation, always use clean tubes directly taken from the plastic container; be sure to wear gloves when handling the materials at all steps. Let the plastic cool for a few seconds (10–20) before transferring the tumor sample. A visible "white spot" will form in the Petri dish when it is cold. Discard and replace the Petri dish and scalpel between samples.

3. Clean the knives carefully between samples by running repeatedly the homogenizer in a glass beaker containing 70% ethanol for 2 to 3 s; repeat the procedure in a new container with 70% ethanol. Let the knives dry shortly before processing the next sample.

4. Be sure to use filtered pipet tips.

5. Use a new syringe needle for *each* sample when microdissecting for DNA-based sequencing.

6. DNA preparation from microdissected material (QIAamp DNA minikit, VWR International): remember to extract a negative control.

7. When performing the PCR for the cDNA-based analysis, if possible, make a master mix for each primer pair. Always include negative controls, both the negative RNA control as well as negative PCR control. Always strive to have fresh primers of good quality to increase the success rate of the PCR. This is especially important for modified primers (biotin).

8. For the genomic DNA-based analysis, running PCR 1 for all fragments (4:1, 4:2, and 5–8): remember to always include negative controls, both the negative DNA control as well as negative PCR control.

9. For PCR 2 (exons 4:1, 4:2, 5, 6, 8, and exon 7): always include negative controls, both the two PCR 1 negative controls, as well as negative PCR control.

References

1. Soussi, T. and Beroud, C. (2001) Assessing *TP53* status in human tumours to evaluate clinical outcome. *Nat. Rev. Cancer* **1,** 233–240.

2. McBride, O., Merry, D., and Givol, D. (1986) The gene for human p53 cellular tumor antigen is located on chromosome 17 short arm (17p13). *Proc. Natl. Acad. Sci. USA* **83,** 130–134.

3. Miller, C., Mohandas, T., Wolf, D., Prokocimer, M., Rotter, V., and Koeffler, H. (1986) Human p53 gene localized to short arm of chromosome 17. *Nature* **319,** 783–784.

4. Williams, C., Norberg, T., Ahmadian, A., et al. (1998) Assessment of sequence-based *p53* gene analysis in human breast cancer: messenger RNA in comparison with genomic DNA targets. *Clin. Chem.* **44,** 455–462.

5. Kirsch, D. G. and Kastan, M. B. (1998) Tumor-suppressor p53: implications for tumor development and prognosis. *J. Clin. Oncol.* **16,** 3158–3168.

6. Friedman, P. N., Chen, X., Bargonetti, J., and Prives, C. (1993) The p53 protein is an unusually shaped tetramer that binds directly to DNA. *Proc. Natl. Acad. Sci. USA* **90,** 3319–3323.

7. Kussie, P. H., Gorina, S., Marechal, V., et al. (1996) Structure of the MDM2 oncoprotein bound to the p53 tumor suppressor transactivation domain. *Science* **274,** 948–953.

 8. Linderholm, B. K., Lindahl, T., Holmberg, L., et al. (2001) The expression of vascular endothelial growth factor correlates with mutant *p53* and poor prognosis in human breast cancer. *Cancer Res.* **61,** 2256–2260.
 9. Harris, C. C. (1996) Structure and function of the p53 tumor s-uppressor gene: clues for rational cancer therapeutic strategies. *J. Natl. Cancer Inst.* **88,** 1442–1455.
10. Soussi, T., Dehouche, K., and Beroud, C. (2000) p53 website and analysis of *p53* gene mutations in human cancer: forging a link between epidemiology and carcinogenesis. *Hum. Mutat.* **15,** 105–113.
11. Norberg, T., Klaar, S., Karf, G., Nordgren, H., Holmberg, L., and Bergh, J. (2001) Increased p53 mutation frequency during tumor progression-results from a breast cancer cohort. *Cancer Res.* **61,** 8317–8321.
12. Bergh, J., Norberg, T., Sjögren, S., Lindgren, A., and Holmberg, L. (1995) Complete sequencing of the *p53* gene provides prognostic information in breast cancer patients, particularly in relation to adjuvant systemic therapy and radiotherapy. *Nat. Med.* **1,** 1029–1034.
13. Bergh, J. (1999) Clinical studies of p53 in treatment and benefit of breast cancer patients. *Endocr. Relat. Cancer* **6,** 51–59.
14. Fisher, C. J., Gillett, C. E., Vojtesek, B., Barnes, D. M., and Millis, R. R. (1994) Problems with p53 immunohistochemical staining: the effect of fixation and variation in the methods of evaluation. *Br. J. Cancer* **69,** 26–31.
15. Sjögren, S., Inganäs, M., Norberg, T., et al. (1996) The *p53* gene in breast cancer: prognostic value of complementary DNA sequencing versus immunohistochemistry. *J. Natl. Cancer Inst.* **88,** 173–182.
16. Chappuis, P. O., Estreicher, A., Dieterich, B., et al. (1999) Prognostic significance of *p53* mutation in breast cancer: frequent detection of non-missense mutations by yeast functional assay. *Int. J. Cancer* **84,** 587–593.
17. Duddy, P. M., Hanby, A. M., Barnes, D. M., and Camplejohn, R. S. (2000) Improving the detection of p53 mutations in breast cancer by use of the FASAY, a functional assay. *J. Mol. Diag.* **2,** 139–144.
18. Norberg, T., Lennerstrand, J., Inganas, M., and Bergh, J. (1998) Comparison between p53 protein measurements using the luminometric immunoassay and immunohistochemistry with detection of p53 gene mutations using cDNA sequencing in human breast tumors. *Int. J. Cancer* **79,** 376–383.
19. Ahrendt, S. A., Halachmi, S., Chow, J. T., et al. (1999) Rapid p53 sequence analysis in primary lung cancer using an oligonucleotide probe array. *Proc. Natl. Acad. Sci. USA* **96,** 7382–7387.
20. Bonnefoi, H., Ducraux, A., Movarekhi, S., et al. (2002) p53 as a potential predictive factor of response to chemotherapy: feasibility of p53 assessment using a functional test in yeast from trucut biopsies in breast cancer patients. *Br. J. Cancer* **86,** 750–755.

27

Expression Profiling Using cDNA Microarrays

Chris Jones, Peter Simpson, Alan Mackay, and Sunil R. Lakhani

Summary

Microarray technology is revolutionizing the assessment of gene expression in human disease. Coupled with the publication of the human genome, it is becoming possible to measure the relevant levels of all 30,000–40,000 human genes in a single experiment. The applications of these methods to breast cancer research are helping us to both further our understanding of the biology of mammary tumorigenesis, as well as providing novel subclassifications of breast cancer of direct clinical relevance. Unbiased RNA amplification techniques are allow the study of small biopsy samples as well as archival pathology specimens, increasing our molecular understanding, and providing real hope for the clinical application of gene expression profiling.

Key Words: Gene expression; cDNA; microarray; hybridization; RNA; amplification; microdissection.

1. Introduction

The advent of cDNA microarray technology has provided researchers for the first time with the means to probe the relative expression levels of the 30,000–40,000 human genes identified by the Human Genome Project. Although the applications of this technology in the postgenomic world are extensive, the early focus of such studies has been to examine the transcriptional profiles human tumors, with a view to understanding the inherent biology of the disease, as well as uncovering potential new avenues for diagnosis, prognostication, and therapeutic intervention.

Complementary (c)DNA microarray experiments are based on the differential labeling of two different RNA samples, cohybridized to glass slides containing thousands of spotted strands of cDNA, each representing an individual gene. Measurement of the relative levels of each labeled RNA binding to the spots gives an indication of relative gene expression for thousands of genes in a single experiment (*1*). Numerous different types of platforms are available, and include cDNA fragments spotted onto a glass or silicon support, generated

From: *Methods in Molecular Medicine, Vol. 120: Breast Cancer Research Protocols*
Edited by: S. A. Brooks and A. L. Harris © Humana Press Inc., Totowa, NJ

in-house, obtained via academic collaborations, or purchased from a number or commercial suppliers. Oligonucleotide arrays, such as those generated *in situ* by ortholithography (Affymetrix) *(2)*, or by ink-jet spotting of long (80-mer) oligonucleotides *(3)*, form an analogous system not covered in this chapter. Chapter 28 describes an alternative approach of using filter cDNA microarrays.

The application of these techniques to breast cancer has provided a framework for novel molecular classifications of invasive breast tumors *(4,5)*, as well as identifying groups of patients with different prognoses, and hence requiring different therapeutic management *(6,7)*. The promise of utilizing microarray-based expression profiling for molecular diagnostics is one that is already beginning to bear fruit; there can be little doubt that the study of a wide range of breast tumors and premalignant breast lesions in this way will lead to improved and earlier identification of patients who would benefit from different treatment options. Global profiling strategies will hopefully aid the unraveling of the basic biology of breast tumorigenesis and drive the development of novel therapies to underpin the new diagnostic capabilities of the technology.

This chapter aims to introduce the basic methodology for carrying out a microarray experiment, from isolation of RNA through hybridization, obtaining, and normalizing the raw data for downstream high-level statistical analysis. The field of cDNA microarrays is one of the most hotly studied techniques in molecular biology; the explosion in options for carrying out microarray experiments and the interpretation of them means that a comprehensive review is beyond the scope of this chapter. Instead, the reader is directed to the excellent protocols manual *(8)* and collection of reviews *(9,10)*.

An important initial factor to consider before a microarray study is undertaken is the experimental design. Too many microarray experiments are being carried out without due consideration to design, and with too few (if any) replications, and efforts are being made to communicate sound experiment design to investigators worldwide *(11)*. One of the benefits of the standards being issued for microarray experimental publishing—the minimum information about a microarray experiment *(12)*—is the open, on-line availability of all primary data. With correct experimental design, cross-comparisons among labs and large meta-analysis should be possible; however, defining a universal reference against which all experiments could be compared is proving problematic (*see* **Note 1**). The correct choice of reference RNA for an individual experiment nonetheless remains a critical decision for any group.

2. Materials

1. Trizol reagent (cat. no. 15596-026; Invitrogen, UK).
2. 0.1% Diethyl pyrocarbonate (DEPC) dissolved in double distilled (dd)H_2O.

3. 75% Ethanol (made up with DEPC ddH$_2$O).
4. PicoPure RNA Isolation kit (KIT0202; Arcturus, Mountainview, CA).
5. RiboAmp RNA Amplification kit (KIT0201, Arcturus).
6. Deoxynucleotide 5'-triphosphate (dNTP) mix: 25 m*M* deoxyadenosine 5'-triphosphate, deoxythymidine 5'-triphosphate, deoxyguanosine 5'-triphosphate, and 10 m*M* of dexoxycytidine 5'-triphosphate (dCTP).
7. Superscript II, 200 U/μL (cat no. 18064-014, Invitrogen).
8. dCTP-Cy3, dCTP-Cy5, 1 m*M* stock (cat. nos. PA53021, PA55021; Amersham, UK).
9. Anchored oligo-dT$_{17}$ (2 μg/μL).
10. AutoSeq G-50 columns (cat. no. 27-5340-02, Amersham).
11. PolyA DNA, 2 μg/μL (cat. no. P0887; Sigma, UK).
12. Cot1 DNA, 2 μg/μL (cat. no. 15279-011, Invitrogen).
13. Hybridization buffer: 5X saline–sodium citrate (SSC), 6X Denhardt's solution, 60 m*M* Tris-HCl (pH 7.6), 0.12% sarkosyl, 48% deionised formamide, filter-sterilized.
14. 25 × 60-mm cover slips (406/0188/87; BDH, Poole, UK).
15. Wash solution 1: 2X SSC, filter sterilized.
16. Wash solution 2: 0.1X SSC, 0.1% sodium dodecyl sulfate (SDS), filter-sterilized.
17. Wash solution 3: 0.1X SSC, filter-sterilized.

3. Methods

3.1. RNA Extraction

The success of a microarray experiment depends to a large degree on the quality of the RNA used. Contaminated RNA will label inefficiently and may lead to high background during hybridization, whereas RNA degradation may lead to 3' or size-biased labeling. Accurate and sensitive estimation of the relative amounts of messenger (m)RNA therefore depends on the ability of the investigator to generate RNA preparations that are pure and undamaged.

3.1.1. Cultured Cells and Mammalian Tissue Preparations

Cells grown in monolayers can be collected by scraping and centrifugation or by lysing them *in situ*. Collect cells grown in suspension by centrifugation. Remove the medium and wash in ice-cold phosphate-buffered saline before beginning extraction.

1. Tissue samples: homogenize in 15-mL polypropylene tube containing 1 mL of Trizol reagent per 100 mg of tissue.
2. Cultured cells: add 1 mL of Trizol reagent per 10^7 cells in a 15-mL polypropylene tube, and vortex vigorously for 1 min at room temperature.
3. Add 0.2 mL of chloroform per 1 mL of Trizol reagent used, mix vigorously for 15–20 s, and incubate at room temperature for 2–3 min.
4. Centrifuge the samples at 12,000*g* for 15 min at 4°C.
5. Transfer the aqueous upper phase to a new 2-mL microcentrifuge tube and add 0.5 mL isopropanol per 1 mL of Trizol reagent used. Mix by inversion.

6. Incubate at room temperature for 10 min and centrifuge at 12,000*g* for 15 min at 4°C. The RNA should now be seen as a pellet at the bottom of the tube.

7. Remove supernatant carefully by aspiration, and wash pellet once with 75% ethanol, adding at least 1 mL of ethanol per 1 mL of Trizol reagent used. Vortex and centrifuge at 7,500*g* for 5 min at 4°C.

8. Remove supernatant and air-dry the RNA pellet. Resuspend in 50–100 µL DEPC H₂O and incubate at 55–60°C until pellet is completely redissolved.

9. Quantitate total RNA (*see* **Note 2**) using spectrophotometer, and assess quality by electrophoresis of 2 µg of the sample in a 1% agarose 1X Tris borate ethylenediaminetetraacetic acid RNA gel. The 28S and 18S species of ribosomal RNA (rRNA) should be clearly visible after ultraviolet illumination, as should a more-diffuse, fast-migrating band composed of transfer RNA and 5S rRNA. For undegraded RNA, the 28S rRNA band should be stained at approximately twice the intensity of the 18S band, and no smearing of either band should be visible. This may be conveniently quantitated using an Agilent (UK) 2100 Bioanalyzer, if available.

10. Add 3X vol of 100% ethanol to aqueous sample and store at –70°C.

3.1.2. Pathology Specimens

It is often desirable to obtain a pure population of breast cancer cells directly from pathology specimens to investigate directly gene expression in different breast lesions without contamination from surrounding cell types. There are a number of different microdissection systems available (laser-assisted microdissection and isolation of DNA and RNA is the subject of Chapter 8; *see* **Note 3**), and a variety of RNA extraction procedures that could be applied to them. This protocol describes the use of the Arcturus (UK) PixCell Laser Capture Microdissection (LCM) instrument, and associated PicoPure RNA isolation kit.

1. Add 50 µL extraction buffer XB to a 0.5-mL microcentrifuge tube, insert the CapSure LCM cap, and invert the assembly. Flick down the tube to ensure all extraction buffer is covering the cap.

2. Incubate at 42°C for 30 min.

3. Centrifuge assembly at 800*g* for 2 min to collect the cell extract.

4. Precondition the RNA purification column. Add 50 µL extraction buffer XB on the purification column membrane. Incubate at room temperature for 5 min and centrifuge at 16,000*g* for 1 min.

5. Add 50 µL of 70% ethanol to the cell extract, and mix well by pipetting up and down.

6. Add cell extract/ethanol to the preconditioned purification column. Centrifuge at 8000*g* for 1 min.

7. Add 50 µL of wash buffer W1 to the column and centrifuge at 8000*g* for 1 min.

8. Add 50 µL of wash buffer W2 to the column and centrifuge at 8000*g* for 1 min.

9. Add another 50 µL of wash buffer W2 to the column and centrifuge at 8000*g* for 2 min.

10. Transfer the column to a clean microfuge tube and add 11 μL of elution buffer EB. Incubate at room temperature for 1 min and centrifuge at 16,000*g* to elute the RNA. Repeat this step for less than 1000 cells, collecting elute in the same tube.
11. The sample may be used immediately or stored at –80°C until required.

3.2. Amplification of Small Quantities of mRNA From Pathological Specimens

Microarray studies require microgram quantities of probe per array hybridization and multiple experiments per study. In order to generate enough RNA from small quantities of (microdissected) pathological specimens, amplification of starting material can generate sufficient quantities of antisense RNA (aRNA) for microarray hybridization. Although there are a number of different methods available for RNA amplification (*see* **Note 4**), care must be taken to ensure that there is minimal bias in order to get an accurate representation of all expressed transcripts in a cell population. This method describes a linear amplification process using the Arcturus RiboAmp kit. The RiboAmp kit utilizes a five-step process for the linear amplification of mRNA. A first-strand synthesis reaction yields cDNA complementary to the mRNA; a second-strand reaction yields double-stranded cDNA, which is column-purified. An in vitro transcription reaction yields aRNA, which is also then column-purified.

1. Add 1 μL of Primer A to 10-μL RNA sample, incubate at 70°C for 10 min, and then chill the sample at 4°C for 1 min.
2. Add 7 μL of 1st Strand Master Mix and 2 μL of 1st Strand Enzyme Mix to each sample and incubate at 42°C for 1 h.
3. Incubate the sample at 70°C for 10 min, and then chill the sample at 4°C for 1 min.
4. Add 2 μL of 1st Strand Nuclease Mix, and incubate at 37°C for 30 min.
5. Heat the sample to 95°C for 5 min, and then chill the sample at 4°C for 1 min.
6. Add 1 μL of Primer B, heat the sample to 95°C for 2 min, and then chill the sample at 4°C for 2 min.
7. Add 29 μL of 2nd Reaction Master Mix and 1 μL of 2nd Reaction Enzyme Mix, and incubate at 25°C for 10 min, 37°C for 30 min, 70°C for 15 min, and then chill the sample at 4°C for up to 30 min.
8. Add 50 μL of DNA binding buffer DB to a DNA/RNA Purification Column, and incubate at room temperature for 5 min.
9. Centrifuge at 16,000*g* for 1 min. Discard flowthrough and reinsert column in the collection tube.
10. Add 250 μL of DNA binding buffer DB to the second-strand synthesis sample tube, and add entire sample volume to the purification column.
11. Centrifuge at 10,000*g* for 1 min. Discard flowthrough and reinsert column in the collection tube.
12. Add 250 μL of DNA Wash Buffer DW to the column and centrifuge at 16,000*g* for 2 min. Discard flowthrough and collection tube.

13. Place column into a microcentrifuge tube and add 50 μL of DNA Elution Buffer DE to the column. Incubate at room temperature for 1 min, and then centrifuge at 16,000*g* for 1 min. Discard the column and retain the elute.

14. Concentrate the sample to a target volume of 8 μL, using a SpeedVac for approx 14 min.

15. Add 4 μL of in vitro transcription (IVT) buffer, 6 μL of IVT Master Mix, and 2 μL of Enzyme Mix to each sample and incubate at 42°C for 4 h. Cool sample to 4°C.

16. Add 1 μL of DNase Mix and incubate at 37°C for 15 min. Cool sample to 4°C.

17. Add 50 μL of RNA Binding Buffer RB to a new DNA/RNA purification column, and incubate at room temperature for 5 min.

18. Centrifuge at 16,000*g* for 1 min. Discard flowthrough and reinsert column in the collection tube.

19. Add 120 μL of RNA Binding Buffer RB to the IVT reaction sample and add entire sample volume to the column.

20. Centrifuge at 10,000*g* for 1 min. Discard flowthrough and reinsert column in the collection tube.

21. Add 200 μL of RNA Wash Buffer RW to the column and centrifuge at 10,000*g* for 1 min.

22. Discard the flowthrough and return column to the original collection tube. Add 200 μL of fresh RNA Wash Buffer RW to the column, and centrifuge at 16,000*g* for 2 min. Discard the flowthrough and the used collection tube.

23. Place column into a microcentrifuge tube and add 50 μL of RNA Elution Buffer RE to the column. Incubate at room temperature for 1 min, and then centrifuge at 16,000*g* for 1 min. Discard the column and retain the eluted material.

24. The purified aRNA is ready for use in a labeling reaction or for use in a second round of amplification.

3.3. cDNA Labeling

Most labeling protocols are based on reverse transcription of mRNA, either from highly purified poly(A) mRNA or total RNA extracts (*see* **Note 5**). The direct synthesis of fluorochrome-labeled first-strand cDNA is carried out in a reaction catalyzed by reverse transcriptase that contains mRNA as a template, dye-conjugated deoxynucleotide triphosphates as substrates, and either oligo(dT)$_{12-18}$ or anchored oligo(dT)$_{12-18}$ (*see* **Note 6**) as a primer. There are alternatives to the enzyme (SuperScript II), and cyanine dyes given in this protocol, although these are the standard combination in labeling for microarray experiments.

1. Precipitate 25–100 μg of total RNA (or 1 μg poly [A] mRNA) by adding 1/40 volume of 3-*M* sodium acetate to the RNA preparation in 75% ethanol, and incubating at −70°C for 20–30 min.

2. Centrifuge at 12,000*g* to pellet the RNA. Remove the supernatant and add 100 μL of 70% ethanol DEPC ddH$_2$O to wash the pellet.

3. Centrifuge at 12,000g for 10 min, remove supernatant, and air-dry.
4. Resuspend RNA pellet in 12.9 µL of DEPC ddH$_2$O and add 2.5 µL of anchored oligo-dT$_{17}$. Incubate the mixture at 70°C for 10 min and snap chill on ice.
5. Add the following to the mixture: 6.0 µL of 5X first-strand buffer, 3 µL of 0.1-M dithiothreitol, 0.6 µL of dNTP mix, 3 µL of dCTP-Cy3 or dCTP-Cy5, and 2 µL of SuperScript II.
6. Incubate at 42°C for 2 h.
7. Add 1.5 µL of 1-M NaOH and incubate at 70°C for 20 min to hydrolyze the RNA.
8. Add 1.5 µL of 1-M HCl to neutralize the reaction.
9. Resuspend resin in AutoSeq column by vortexing gently. Loosen cap a one-quarter turn and snap off the bottom closure.
10. Place column in 1.5-mL microfuge tube, prespin at 2000g for 1 min. Blot any excess fluid from the column.
11. Place column in new 1.5-mL tube and slowly apply sample to the center of the angled surface of the compacted resin bed, being careful not to disturb the resin. Spin column for 1 min at 2000g. Resulting flow-through should be approx 33 µL in volume and be faintly colored pink or blue depending on which Cy dye has been incorporated.
12. Two to three microliters of the sample of Cy5-labelled cDNA can be removed for checking the quality of labeling by running on a 2% agarose 1X Tris acetate ethylenediaminetetraacetic acid gel, and scanning on a fluorescence scanner. Successful labeling produces a dense smear of labeled cDNA from 400 to more than 1000 nucleotides in length, with a minimum of low-molecular-weight transcripts.

3.4. Hybridization and Post-Hybridization Washing

The protocols below refer to those optimized by the Sanger Institute for their 10,000 clone Hver 1.2.1 microarrays, and may not be entirely applicable to all cDNA microarray platforms.

3.4.1. Prehybridization

Prehybridization is used to wash unbound DNA from the slide before addition of the target, as well as block reactive groups on the surface of the slide (e.g., free amine groups) that can bind labeled target DNA nonspecifically.

1. Incubate microarray slide at 47°C for 2–4 h in hybridization buffer, either 50 µL under a 25 × 60-mm cover slip, or 50 mL in a Coplin jar.
2. Centrifuge microarray slides in individual 50-mL polypropylene tubes at 800g for 2 min to dry.

3.4.2. Hybridization

The following protocol refers to the conventional method of hybridizing microarrays under cover slips and in humidified chambers, although other commercial alternatives are now available (*see* **Note 7**).

1. Combine the two single-stranded (ss) cDNA samples as follows: 33 μL of ss cDNA sample 1 (Cy3-labeled), 33 μL of ss cDNA sample 2 (Cy5-labeled), 4 μL of poly (A) DNA, 4 μL of human Cot1 DNA, 7.4 μL of 3-*M* sodium acetate (pH 5.2), and 243 μL of 100% ethanol.
2. Precipitate ss cDNA, poly(A), and Cot1 DNA at −70° for 20 min.
3. Centrifuge at 12,000*g* to pellet the RNA. Remove the supernatant and add 100 μL of 70% ethanol DEPC ddH$_2$O to wash the pellet.
4. Centrifuge at 12,000*g* for 10 min, remove supernatant, and air-dry.
5. Resuspend pellet in 40 μL of hybridization buffer and add 8 μL of ddH$_2$O to bring final volume to 48 μL.
6. Incubate cDNA mixture at 100°C for 5 min. Allow to cool to room temperature and centrifuge briefly to remove evaporated liquid from the lid of tube.
7. Apply quickly, but carefully, 48 μL of sample in hybridization buffer to center of cover slip, avoiding air bubbles. Press down gently the inverted slide-containing array onto cover slip, ensuring entire array area is covered. Any small air bubbles will gradually disappear during the hybridization.
8. Place microarray slide in a humid chamber to prevent buffer from evaporating during hybridization.
9. Incubate at 47°C for 12–24 h.

3.4.3. Post-Hybridization Washing

Washing of the arrays can be critical for generating crisp microarray images with a high signal-to-nose ratio, and without artifactual background obscuring some or all of the array (*see* **Note 8**). Washes are generally performed at room temperature, as in the following protocol; however, some investigators perform the early wash steps at temperatures up to 55°C. The optimal wash temperature for a particular array should be determined empirically.

1. Remove microarray from humid chamber and place quickly in a 50-mL polypropylene tube containing wash solution 1. Do not remove cover slip at this stage; it should slide off the array within 10–15 s of being placed in the wash solution, at which point it can be carefully removed without scraping against the microarray slide. Wash on a rocking platform at room temperature for 10 min.
2. Transfer microarray into a clean Falcon tube containing wash solution 2. Wash on a rocking platform at room temperature for 10 min.
3. Repeat **step 2**.
4. Transfer microarray in slide rack to wash solution 3. Wash on a rocking platform at room temperature for 10 min.
5. Repeat **step 4** three more times.
6. Transfer the microarray in a slide rack to a centrifuge quickly and spin at 800*g* for 2 min to dry the microarray slides.

3.5. Scanning and Analysis

The means by which a microarray slide is scanned to generate a high-resolution image and the way in which the image is extracted to generate the raw fluorescence intensity values for both red and green channels will have a substantial impact on subsequent analyses. A large number of commercial scanners and both commercial and free software programs are available for the scanning and analysis of a cDNA microarray slide. Although it beyond the scope of this chapter to review and compare them all *(8–10)*, the following sections will hopefully highlight some of the most salient issues involved in this key part of the experiment.

3.5.1. Image Analysis

In a microarray experiment, hybridized microarray slides are imaged in a microarray scanner to produce red and green fluorescence intensity measurements over a large collection of pixels that collectively cover the array. Fluorescence intensities correspond to the levels of hybridization of the two targets to the probes spotted on the slide. These fluorescence intensity values are stored as 16-bit images that are typically described as the "raw" data.

The processing of scanned microarray images can be separated into three major tasks. *Addressing*, or *gridding*, is the process of assigning coordinates to each of the spots, and it is the automation of this part of the procedure that permits high-throughput analysis. *Segmentation* allows the classification of pixels either as foreground, i.e., within a printed DNA spot, or background. This is a key factor in the generation of log ratio of intensities, and the choice of method available for different hardware/software may vary, and make cross-platform comparisons problematic. *Intensity extraction* involves calculating, for each spot on the array, red and green foreground fluorescence intensity pairs, background intensities, and possibly, quality measures. The choice of background correction method is reported to have a larger impact on the log ratio of intensities than the segmentation method used, and a widely accepted way to correct spot intensities for background has yet to emerge. Some researchers have suggested that no background adjustment is preferable; although, this appears to reduce the ability to identify differentially expressed genes.

3.5.2. Normalization

The first step in dealing with the extracted fluorescence intensity values is to correct for systematic differences in the relative intensity of each channel. Normalization also aims to correct for other differences in intensities among samples on the same slide, or among slides, that do not represent true biological variation among the samples. In particular, dye bias, where red intensities often tend to be lower than the green intensities because of the relatively lower incorporation of Cy5 nucleotides, must be corrected for. Furthermore, overall spot intensities can vary because of differences in the location on the array, the sample plate origin, the arraying pins used, and the slide-scanning parameters.

As well as normalization based on a global adjustment of intensity values, approaches that take into account systematic biases that may appear in the data. It is apparent that the log ratio values can have a systematic dependence on intensity, and a locally weighted linear regression (lowess) normalization is frequently used to correct for such intensity-dependent effects.

Although there is, as yet, no consensus for a globally applicable normalization strategy, it is clear that it is necessary to normalize fluorescence intensities both within and among slides before performing further analysis of data to minimize false positives and to identify genes that are truly differentially expressed between the two samples.

4. Notes

1. Although there is no current consensus of references, Brown and Botstein's groups at Stanford University have described a pool of RNA derived from 11 diverse human tumor cell lines *(13)*. This approach has the advantage of generating large amounts of renewable material; however, tight control is required to minimize batch-to-batch variation. Stratagene (UK) produced a commercially available reference RNA based on 10 tumor cell lines; however, little is known about the cell culture conditions or provenance. Other sources of reference RNA include a pool of all experimental samples *(6)*, as well as labeled oligonucleotides *(14)* and even genomic DNA *(15)*.

2. For many cDNA microarray experiments, it is desirable to utilize mRNA for labeling. Poly (A) selection of mRNA can be performed on total RNA using the Oligotex mRNA kit (cat. no. 70022, Qiagen).

3. Other microdissection systems include laser pressure catapulting using the P.A.L.M. instrument (P.A.L.M. Microlaser Technologies, Bernried, Germany) and the Leica LS AMD (Bucks, UK) microdissection platform. These technologies work in different ways to the Arcturus LCM method, but can be considered analogous for their ability to generate pure populations of breast cells for microarray analysis.

4. Two basic approaches have been taken toward RNA amplification to allow microarray profiling to be performed on small clinical samples and histological materials. Linear T7 amplification using allows a 2000–10,000-fold amplification of input RNA into aRNA without affecting the representation or distribution of expressed cDNA *(16)*. PCR-based amplification using a combination of antisense RNA amplification and template switching primers (Clontech, Palo Alto, CA) allows amplification of 10,000–100,000 times without bias *(17)*. Newer methods include single-primer amplification, which reduces the input material required to 30 ng without affecting representation *(18)*, and global RT-PCR based procedure *(19)*, which claims to allow microarray analysis from 1 million-fold less input RNA. Indeed, amplification methods now perhaps allow the microarray analysis of single cells.

5. An alternative method to direct labeling, called indirect or amino allyl labeling, circumvents the need to incorporate bulky fluorescent dyes during reverse tran-

scription. In this method, an amino allyl deoxyuridine 5'-triphosphate can be coupled to a reactive *N*-hydroxysuccinimydl ester fluorescent dye after reverse transcription *(20)*. Although this technique is longer than direct labeling, reports of better sensitivity, decreased dye bias and reduced cost are making it more attractive for many researchers.

6. Anchored primers are a mixture of four synthetic oligonucleotides, consisting of an oligo(dT) backbone and an A, G, or C residue in the 3'-terminal position. Priming with an anchored primer ensures that cDNA synthesis is initiated at the 5' end of the poly (A) tract of the mRNA. This method of priming is recommended if the hybridization probes on the microarrays correspond to the 3' ends of the transcripts.

7. Hybridizing under cover slips is known to occasionally give problems associated with uneven probe distribution, and a variety of commercial alternatives have emerged. These vary from ones based on a simple vibrating temperature-controlled platform to ones based on complex systems of probe application and mixing. One common problem with such systems is the large volume of probe required, with the dilution necessary which gives rise to loss of signal.

8. The three most critical aspects of the wash procedure as are follows. First, the cover slip must be removed early in the wash protocol, and without having to manipulate it manually to remove it from the array slide. Excessive drying during the hybridization process may lead to difficulty in removing the cover slip, and this should avoided. Second, excessive amounts of SDS should not be used in the wash solutions, as this can lead to general background problems because of the autofluorescence of SDS solutions. Adequate post-SDS stage washing should be performed. Finally, the slides must not be allowed to dry out at any stage during the washing procedure.

Acknowledgments

We would like to thank the Sanger Institute Microarray Facility and the Breakthrough Toby Robins Breast Cancer Research Centre Microarray Lab for providing assistance with microarray experimental design, protocols, and analysis.

References

1. Schena, M., Shalon, D., Davis, R. W., and Brown P. O. (1995) Quantitative monitoring of gene expression patterns with a complementary DNA microarray. *Science* **270**, 467–470.
2. Lockhart, D. J., Dong, H., Byrne, M. C., et al. (1996) Expression monitoring by hybridization to high-density oligonucleotide arrays. *Nat. Biotechnol.* **14**, 1675–1680.
3. Hughes, T. R., Mao M., Jones, A. R., et al. (2001) Expression profiling using microarrays fabricated by an ink-jet oligonucleotide synthesizer. *Nat. Biotechnol.* **19**, 342–347.
4. Perou, C. M., Sorlie, T., Eisen, M. B., et al. (2000) Molecular portraits of human breast tumours. *Nature* **406**, 747–752.

5. Sorlie, T., Perou, C. M., Tibshirani, R., et al. (2001) Gene expression patterns of breast carcinomas distinguish tumor subclasses with clinical implications. *Proc. Natl. Acad. Sci. USA* **98**, 10,869–10,874.

6. van't Veer, L. J., Dai, H., van de Vijver, M. J., et al. (2002) Gene expression profiling predicts clinical outcome of breast cancer. *Nature* **415**, 530–536.

7. van de Vijver, M. J., He, Y. D., van't Veer, L. J., et al. (2002) A gene-expression signature as a predictor of survival in breast cancer. *N. Engl. J. Med.* **347**, 1999–2009.

8. Bowtell, D. D. and Sambrook, J. F. (2002) *DNA Microarrays: a Molecular Cloning Manual.* Cold Spring Harbor Laboratory Press, Cold Spring Harbor, NY.

9. The chipping forecast (1999) *Nat. Genet.* **21(Suppl)**.

10. The chipping forecast II (2002) *Nat. Genet.* **32(Suppl)**.

11. Churchill, G. A. (2002) Fundamentals of experimental design for cDNA microarrays. *Nat. Genet.* **32(Suppl)**, 490–495.

12. Brazma, A., Hingamp, P., Quackenbush, J., et al. (2001) Minimum information about a microarray experiment (MIAME)-toward standards for microarray data. *Nat. Genet.* **29**, 365–371.

13. Perou, C. M., Jeffrey, S. S., van de Rijn, M., et al. (1999) Distinctive gene expression patterns in human mammary epithelial cells and breast cancers. *Proc. Natl. Acad. Sci. USA* **96**, 9212–9217.

14. Hill, A. A., Brown, E. L., Whitley, M. Z., Tucker-Kellogg, G., Hunter, C. P., and Slonim, D. K. (2001) Evaluation of normalization procedures for oligonucleotide array data based on spiked cRNA controls. *Genome Biol,* **2**, RESEARCH0055.

15. Talaat, A. M., Howard, S. T., Hale, W. T., Lyons, R., Garner, H., and Johnston, S. A. (2002) Genomic DNA standards for gene expression profiling in *Mycobacterium tuberculosis. Nucleic Acids Res.* **30**, e104.

16. Phillips, J. and Eberwine, J. H. (1996) Antisense RNA amplification: a linear amplification method for analyzing the mRNA population from single living cells. *Methods* **10**, 283–288.

17. Wang, E., Miller, L. D., Ohnmacht, G. A., Liu, E. T., and Marincola, F. M. (2000) High-fidelity mRNA amplification for gene profiling. *Nat. Biotechnol.* **18**, 457–459.

18. Smith, L., Underhill, P, Pritchard, C., et al. (2003) Single primer amplification (SPA) of cDNA for microarray expression analysis. *Nucleic Acids Res.* **31**, E9–E9.

19. Iscove, N. N., Barbara, M., Gu, M., Gibson, M., Modi, C., and Winegarden, N. (2002) Representation is faithfully preserved in global cDNA amplified exponentially from sub-picogram quantities of mRNA. *Nat. Biotechnol.* **20**, 940–943.

20. Manduchi, E., Scearce, L. M., Brestelli, J. E., Grant, G. R., Kaestner, K. H., and Stoeckert, Jr., C. J. (2002) Comparison of different labeling methods for two-channel high-density microarray experiments. *Physiol. Genomics* **10**, 169–179.

28

Gene Expression Analysis Using Filter cDNA Microarrays

Peter Simpson, Chris Jones, Alan Mackay, and Sunil R. Lakhani

Summary

The analysis of gene expression patterns by filter-based complementary (c)DNA microarray remains an important technique in the molecular biology laboratory, despite the development of large-scale cDNA microarray analysis (*see* Chapter 27). This chapter provides an overview of the methods necessary to carry out the production of membrane-based cDNA arrays and the subsequent synthesis and hybridization of radiolabeled cDNA probes.

Key Words: cDNA microarray; gene expression; hybridization; radioactive probe; RNA.

1. Introduction

Microarray analysis of gene expression on filter-based supports has been superseded by technological advances in the development of larger-scale analysis utilizing glass complementary (c)DNA microarrays and fluorescent detection methods *(1–4)*, which are the subject of Chapter 27. However, the cost and time necessary to develop in-house glass microarray facilities and the cost of performing individual experiments is often inaccessible to an academic molecular biology lab. Thus, membrane cDNA arrays remain an important facility in the study of gene-expression patterns *(5–8)*.

A molecular biology lab already performing hybridizations, such as Southern and Northern blotting, can easily set up filter cDNA microarray experiments, because the principles are essentially the same. Complex cDNA probes are labeled with radioactive deoxynucleotide 5'-triphosphate (dNTP) rather than Cy3- or Cy5-labeled deoxyuridine 5'-triphosphate, which is not only cheaper, but provides enhanced sensitivity over fluorescent dyes. Smaller amounts of RNA can therefore be used for each experiment (typically 5–25 µg rather than 25–100 µg), enabling more replicate hybridizations to be performed. Both test and reference RNA populations are labeled with the same radioactive

From: *Methods in Molecular Medicine, Vol. 120: Breast Cancer Research Protocols*
Edited by: S. A. Brooks and A. L. Harris © Humana Press Inc., Totowa, NJ

molecule, thus avoiding labeling bias that occurs during incorporation of the different fluorescent dyes. Hybridization is either visualized by phosphorimaging or by autoradiography. Filter cDNA arrays can also be stripped of labeled probe and therefore reanalyzed three to five times with reproducible results.

Filter arrays purchased from commercial sources provide a useful resource of clone collections specific to human, mouse, and rat and containing 100–5000 sequence-verified cDNA clones, for example Atlas™ arrays (www.clontech.com), GeneFilters® microarrays (www.resgen.com), and Panorama™ gene arrays (www.sigma-genosys.com). Optimized protocols and reagents ensure that successful gene expression profiling is usually reliant only on the quality of RNA available.

The focus of this chapter, however, will be on how filter cDNA arrays, produced in-house, can provide the opportunity to analyze a unique collection of genes of particular relevance to the user's research program. The preparation and characterization of a set of cDNA clones is, in itself, a significant amount of work, and so detailed protocols for these steps are not covered in this chapter, although some important issues to consider are discussed briefly. During the creation of the cDNA library, it may be appropriate to incorporate steps of normalization of messenger RNA/cDNA abundance and/or subtractive hybridization (9) in order to minimize the repetitious cloning of abundantly expressed sequences and to maximize both the cloning of lower abundant sequences and the detection of differentially expressed genes (10,11). Individual cloned cDNA fragments are processed by polymerase chain reaction (PCR) using PCR primers specific for sequences either side of the multiple cloning site into which the library was cloned (e.g., M13 forward and reverse primers, T3 and T7 universal primers). Amplified cDNA clones can be purified using any number of commercially available systems and should be analyzed by agarose gel electrophoresis to ensure the presence of single amplified clones and to assess yield. Sequence verification is necessary to again minimize the repetition of sequences arrayed, but critically, to ensure cloned cDNA fragments show minimal sequence similarity to other genes, as gene families and conserved sequences give rise to difficulties in these systems.

Filter arrays can be produced by a number of means depending on the sophistication of array desired and the technology and finances available. A basic slot or dot blotting apparatus can create reasonable 48- or 96-spot arrays; alternatively, handheld (12) or automated spotters (5,8) can produce filters of the same or higher density. It is necessary to produce multiple replicates of each filter for simultaneous comparison of the same gene set with different RNA samples. Filters should be produced to contain multiple positive-control spots consisting of housekeeping genes (and sometimes genomic DNA) and negative-control spots containing no DNA (and containing plasmid DNA) to assess the quality of hybridization and assist analysis. It is also useful, where appropriate, to include genes that are already known to be differentially expressed (both up- and downregulated) in the system being investigated.

2. Materials

1. PCR products of cloned cDNA library prepared in 96-well PCR plates at approx 50 ng DNA in 25 µL (*see* **Note 1**).
2. 5–25 µg Total RNA from test and reference sources, prepared as described in Chapter 27.
3. 96-Well dot-blotting apparatus (cat. no. 170-3938; Bio-Rad, UK) and vacuum manifold.
4. Hybond-N⁺ positively charged nylon membrane (cat. no. RPN203B; Amersham Biosciences, UK) and clean, flat-edge forceps for handling.
5. Ultraviolet (UV) transilluminator (254 nm).
6. Water bath or thermal cycler.
7. Shaking water bath.
8. Rotating hybridization oven and glass hybridization tubes (Hybaid, UK).
9. PhosphorImaging system (Molecular Dynamics, Sunnyvale, CA).
10. 3000 Ci/mmol [α-^{32}P] of deoxycytidine 5'-triphosphate (dCTP) or [α-^{33}P] of dCTP (cat. no. 33004X or 58201; ICN Biomedicals, Belgium).
11. 10X dNTP mix: deoxyadenosine 5'-triphosphate, deoxyguanosine 5'-triphosphate, and deoxythymidine 5'-triphosphate, each at 10 mM and dCTP at 60 µM.
12. Anchored oligo(dT)$_{10-20}$ primer (1 µg/µL) (*see* **Note 6** in Chapter 27).
13. SuperScript™ II RNase H–reverse transcriptase (200 U/µL), 5RPN203B First Strand buffer and 0.1 M dithiothreitol ([DTT] cat. no. 18064-014; Invitrogen, UK).
14. RNAseOUT™ recombinant ribonuclease inhibitor, 40 U/µL (cat. no. 10777-019, Invitrogen).
15. 10 mg/mL salmon sperm DNA (cat. no. 15632-011, Invitrogen).
16. Auto-Seq G-50 columns (cat. no. 27-5340-02, Amersham Biosciences).
17. 0.1% (v/v) diethylpyrocarbonate ([DEPC] cat. no. UKD5758; Sigma, UK)-treated double distilled (dd)H$_2$O: dissolve 1 mL of DEPC in 1 L of ddH$_2$O in a fume cupboard. Autoclave solution to inactive DEPC and store at room temperature. **Caution:** DEPC is toxic and a potential carcinogen; wear suitable protective clothing, always handle in a chemical fume hood, and take care when opening bottle in case of pressure build uppossible splattering.
18. 1 M NaOH solution: prepare and use with care. Wear suitable protective clothing (gloves and face mask).
19. 1 M HCl: prepare and use with care. Wear suitable protective clothing (gloves, goggles) and work in chemical fume hood.
20. 20X Saline–sodium citrate (SSC) stock solution: prepare 500 mL of 3 M NaCl and 0.3 M Na$_3$-citrate. Autoclave and store at room temperature. It is stable for at least 6 mo.

21. 20% (w/v) Sodium dodecyl sulfate (SDS) stock solution: prepare 500 mL of a 10% (w/v) SDS solution. Avoid inhaling SDS by wearing a facemask when weighing out powder. This does not require autoclaving. Store at room temperature and it is stable for 1 yr.

22. 50X Denhardt's reagent: 1% (w/v) Ficoll 400, 1% (w/v) bovine serum albumin, and 1 % (w/v) polyvinylpyrrolidone; filter sterilize and store 20-mL aliquots at –20°C.

23. 50% (w/v) Dextran sulfate: prepare in a vessel (e.g., 30-mL Universal) that will be used to store solution, because it is viscous and difficult to pipet. Add dextran sulfate to sterile, distilled water; solution will require vigorous mixing and warming to 50°C will aid dissolving. Store at –20°C.

24. Denaturing solution: prepare 500 mL of 1.5 M NaCl and 0.5 M NaOH. There is no need to autoclave this solution. It is stable for several days during membrane preparation. Store at room temperature.

25. Neutralizing solution: prepare 500 mL of 1.5 M NaCl, 0.5 M Tris-HCl (pH 7.2), and 1-mM ethylenediaminetetraacetic acid. There is no need to autoclave this solution. It is stable for several days during membrane preparation. Store at room temperature.

26. Prehybridization buffer: 5X SSC, 5X Denhardt's reagent, 0.5% (w/v) SDS, and 100 µg/mL of denatured salmon sperm DNA. Prepare freshly. It is sufficient for 25 mL per hybridization tube.

27. Hybridization buffer: prepare as for prehybridization buffer, but containing 10% (w/v) dextran sulfate. Prepare freshly.

28. Wash solution 1: 2X SSC and 0.1% (w/v) SDS solution. Prewarm overnight before washing in water bath set to 68°C.

29. Wash solution 2: 1X SSC and 0.1% (w/v) SDS solution. Prewarm overnight before washing in water bath set to 68°C.

30. Wash solution 3: 0.1X SSC and 0.1% (w/v) SDS solution. Prewarm overnight before washing in water bath set to 68°C.

31. Wash solution 4: 0.1X SSC, 0.1% (w/v) SDS, 0.2 M Tris-HCl (pH 7.5).

32. Stripping solution: 0.4 M NaOH.

3. Methods

3.1. Production of Filter cDNA Arrays

1. Denature PCR products at 95°C for 10 min and rapidily cool on ice (*see* **Note 2**).

2. Set up the dot or slot blotting apparatus containing a piece of Hybond-N+ nylon membrane cut to the size of the apparatus and prewetted in 10X SSC. For orientation purposes, cut off a designated corner of the filter and label DNA side of membrane in pencil. Connect apparatus to a vacuum manifold.

3. Add 25 µL of 20X SSC to the DNA and mix by pipetting up and down. Carefully apply to apparatus ensuring all DNA solution is expelled from pipet tips; use vacuum to draw DNA through onto the membrane (*see* **Note 3**).

4. Add 100–200 µL of 10X SSC to the wells of the 96-well plate and apply to dot blotting apparatus; apply vacuum (*see* **Note 3**).

5. Add a further 200 μL of 10X SSC directly to dot blotting apparatus, apply vacuum, and leave for additional 5 min after all DNA/SSC solution has drawn through onto the membrane (*see* **Note 3**).
6. On a workbench, lay down a piece of Saran Wrap™ with two piles of two to three pieces of filter paper cut to a size slightly larger than membrane being created. Soak the first pile with denaturing solution and second pile with neutralizing solution.
7. Remove the membrane from the apparatus and place it, DNA-side up, onto filter paper soaked in denaturing solution for 5 min.
8. Place membrane, DNA-side up, on filter paper soaked in neutralizing solution for 1 min.
9. Place membrane, DNA-side up, on dry filter paper and leave to air-dry for 1 h at room temperature.
10. Crosslink DNA to the membrane by exposing DNA side of membrane directly to UV light source (254 nm) for approx 1 min (*see* **Note 4**).
11. Store cDNA filters, wrapped in Saran Wrap, at room temperature.

3.2. Preparation of Radioactively Labeled cDNA Probe

As with fluorescent labeling of cDNA during first-strand cDNA synthesis (*see* Chapter 27), this protocol is based on reverse transcription of messenger RNA with the direct incorporation of a radioactively labeled dCTP molecule. Either ^{32}P or ^{33}P isotopes are suitable for this application, although ^{33}P is probably the choice compound, as the associated exposure risks are reduced. Because the maximum energy emission of ^{33}P is less than that for ^{32}P (0.25 MeV vs 1.71 MeV; *see* ICN catalog for more information), then a longer exposure time to detect hybridization signal may be required.

Caution: Because the target RNA is radioactively labeled, all the remaining steps involve handling of radioactivity. It is imperative that local radiation rules are strictly adhered to, and that inexperienced users be properly trained to use these isotopes safely.

1. In a 0.5-mL microcentrifuge tube, safely add 5–25 μg of total RNA, 1 μL of anchored oligo(dT)$_{10-20}$ primer, and DEPC ddH$_2$O to a total volume of 11 μL. Mix the contents of the tube well by pipetting and spin briefly in a microcentrifuge.
2. Incubate at 70°C for 10 min, and then rapidly cool on ice for 2–5 min.
3. To the RNA, add the following: 6 μL of 5X first-strand buffer, 3 μL of 10X dNTP mix, 3 μL of 0.1-M DTT, 1 μL of RNAseOUT, 5 μL of [α-^{33}P] dCTP (3000 Ci/mmol), and 1 μL of Superscript II. Mix the contents well by pipetting and spin briefly in a microcentrifuge.
4. Incubate the reaction mixture at 42°C for 60 min.
5. Spin tubes briefly in a microcentrifuge. Add a further 1 μL of reverse transcriptase to each reaction, mix well by pipetting, and incubate for a further 60 min at 42°C.
6. To hydrolyze the RNA, add 1.5 μL of 1 M NaOH solution to the reaction and

incubate at 70°C for 20 min.

7. Add 1.5 µL of 1 M HCl to neutralize the solution.

8. Resuspend resin in an AutoSeq column by vortexing gently. Loosen cap a one-quarter turn and snap off the bottom closure.

9. Place column in 1.5-mL microfuge tube; prespin at 2000g for 1 min. Blot any excess fluid from the column.

10. Place column in new 1.5-mL tube and slowly apply sample to the center of the angled surface of the compacted resin bed, being careful not to disturb the resin.

11. Spin column for 1 min at 2000g.

12. Measure the incorporation of [α-^{33}P] dCTP into newly synthesized cDNA by counting 1 µL in a scintillation counter. The probe ought to be in the region of 10^6 cpm/mL of hybridization buffer.

3.3. Hybridization, Washing, and Detection

Note: At any point during or after hybridization *do not* let the membranes dry out. If this occurs, it will not be possible to remove any hybridization signal from the membranes, thus rendering them unusable.

1. Place membranes in hybridization tube so that DNA side is facing center of the tube and add 25 mL of prehybridization solution. Place tubes in rotating hybridization oven and incubate for 2–4 h (*see* **Note 5**).

2. Denature labeled probe by incubating in boiling water bath for 10 min. Quench on ice, spin briefly in microcentrifuge, and add to 5–10 mL of hybridization buffer (*see* **Note 6**).

3. Replace prehybridization buffer with hybridization buffer and incubate overnight in a rotating hybridization oven.

4. Pour hybridization solution carefully down designated radioactivity disposal sink with plenty of running water.

5. Rinse hybridized membranes carefully by adding approx 25 mL of wash solution 1 into tube, close lid, invert tube, and carefully dispose down radioactivity disposal sink with plenty of running water.

6. Remove hybridized membranes from hybridization tubes, using forceps, and place into a plastic container (sandwich box with lid), immediately pour wash solution 1 over membrane, seal box, and place into water bath (prewarmed to 68°C). Place a heavy object on top of the box and proceed to wash the membrane in the shaking water bath for 30 min.

7. Dispose of wash solution down sink with plenty of running water and repeat washing steps with wash solutions 2 and 3 (*see* **Note 7**).

8. Once washed, wrap membranes in Saran Wrap such that DNA side is wrinkle-free.

9. Tape membrane to PhosphorImager base plate and wipe so other exposed surface and surrounding plate is dry. Expose to a storage phosphorimaging screen for 1–7 d. Scan the screen using a PhosphorImaging system (*see* **Note 8**).

10. Further washing of membranes may be necessary, depending on background signal detected.

3.4. Stripping Membranes

If hybridized membranes have not been left to dry out, the radiolabeled target can be removed allowing membranes to be reprobed several times. Membranes that have dried are useless for further experiments.

1. Incubate membrane in stripping solution for 30 min at 45°C.
2. Incubate in 2 charges of wash solution 4, for 15 min each, incubation at room temperature.
3. Alternatively, boil a solution of 0.5% (w/v) SDS and pour over membranes; incubate with agitation until solution cools to room temperature.
4. Assess efficiency of stripping by exposing to phosphorimaging screen for normal length of time.
5. If stripping is satisfactory, store membranes sealed in Saran Wrap until further use.

3.5. Data Acquisition and Analysis

Software available to analyze filter cDNA microarray data include ImageQuaNT® (Molecular Dynamics) and Molecular Analyst™ (Bio-Rad). AtlasImage™ software (Clontech) has also been developed specifically for the analysis of information obtained through hybridization to Atlas cDNA microarrays, although it is not a necessity to purchase this software to utilize these membranes.

The intensity of the hybridization signal for each feature or spot on the array is processed in a manner similar to that described earlier for cDNA microarray on glass slides with fluorescently labeled probes (*see* Chapter 27). The main difference is that in this case, raw expression data for a single experimental sample are processed before being compared with other samples, as opposed to fluorescent methods, where it is the ratio of expression between a test and a reference sample that is first calculated and then processed.

The features on an array are detected by a dedicated grid system specific for the format of the array and the hybridization intensity within each area, or grid, is quantified. These raw data are processed by means of background removal in which the hybridization intensity of negative control spots and/or the local area surrounding each spot is subtracted from the intensity data for each spot. Images of hybridized membranes with little or no background, which is even across the whole membrane, are much easier to analyze, suggesting efficient prehybridization and thus stringent washing to block and remove nonspecific hybridization signal is imperative. Data are normalized to help control for inevitable intra- and interexperimental variation introduced by different efficiencies in probe labeling, filter hybridization, and washing. Here, the raw data for a specific group of positive control genes, or more accurately the total raw data for all genes across the array, are compared among membranes. Differences are accounted for to allow accurate comparisons to be made among the relative levels of expression of all genes in different populations of cells.

Obtaining accurate gene expression measurements is improved by preparing membranes with each gene present in duplicate (as a minimum) and by performing multiple repeat hybridizations for each experimental sample.

4. Notes

1. DNA can be prepared in 0.5-mL microcentrifuge tubes or in 96-well plates; the latter provides a much more efficient means of handling the DNA, particularly if a 96-well dot blotting apparatus is being used. Multichannel pipets can be utilized for transferring, mixing, and applying DNA/SSC solutions to the membranes.

2. A Stratacooler® 96 benchtop cooler (cat. no. 400013, Stratagene) is very useful for the purpose of snap cooling DNA in a 96-well plate and although expensive, is much more effective than using a bucket of ice.

3. It is critical that all DNA/wash solution (10X SSC) is applied to the membrane so that accurate measures of differential expression across replicate filters can be made.

4. Loss of hybridization signal is observed with suboptimal crosslinking of DNA to membrane. If necessary, perform experiments to optimize amount of UV irradiation required to crosslink DNA efficiently. As an alternative to using a UV transilluminator, a UV crosslinker (Amersham Bioscience or Stratagene) can be used to crosslink DNA to the membrane. Subject membrane, DNA-side up, to UV exposure (wavelength 254 nm) of 70,000 $\mu J/cm^2$; this is an optimized preset mode for Hybond-N$^+$ nylon membranes.

5. Multiple membranes can be simultaneously hybridized with the same labeled target in the same hybridization tube. Either prepare a sandwich of membranes separated by nylon mesh membrane or position membranes edge to edge in the hybridization tube so that they do not overlap. However, be aware that membranes tend to move around both before and during hybridization; thus, if two membranes overlap during hybridization, then reduced access of labeled probe to mobilized target will yield suboptimal hybridization signal. Additionally, membranes at the bottom of a sandwich may also give weaker, and possibly uneven, hybridization signal.

6. The volume of hybridization buffer and washing solutions used depends on size and number of filters used. Typically, 5 mL of hybridization buffer is sufficient for a single 12 × 8-cm membrane in a small hybridization tube; any more and the labeled probe is diluted, and any less and the membrane may dry out. If multiple membranes are being simultaneously hybridized in the same hybridization tube, 10 mL of hybridization buffer is probably more appropriate. For each washing step, 200–400 mL should be sufficient, although this also depends on the size of box being used to perform washes.

7. Stringency of washing of membranes should be high to minimize nonspecific and background hybridization signals, thereby maximizing the signal-to-noise

ratio. Thus, multiple high-temperature (68°C) and low-salt concentration (0.1X SSC) washes should be performed. It is important however, to check hybridization signal between washes, using a Geiger counter to monitor the effectiveness of hybridization and washing procedures. If in doubt, expose membranes to phosphorimaging screen overnight as described; if the background signal is high, then rewash, or if specific gene hybridization signal is low, perform a longer exposure to phosphorimaging screen. Again, it is critical that membranes do not dry out at any stage.

8. If there is no access to phosphorimaging facilities, then use of autoradiographic film (cat. no. 895 2855; Kodak, UK) is suitable, although it suffers from reduced dynamic range of hybridization signal relative to phosphorimaging systems. In such cases, place membrane, covered in Saran Wrap and wiped dry, into a film cassette. In a dark room, cut piece of autoradiographic film to size slightly larger than membrane, cut corner of the film for orientation purposes, and overlay membrane. Place an intensifying screen over film, close cassette, and store at –80°C. After one night, remove cassette from –80°C, allow to equilibrate to room temperature for 30–60 min and then, in the dark room, place film into developer solution (cat. no. 190-0943, Kodak) until hybridization signal is visible then into fixing solution (cat. no. 190-1875, Kodak) until film becomes transparent, rinse film in water, and air-dry.

Acknowledgments

The authors would like to thank Dr. Mike Davies at the Clatterbridge Cancer Research Institute, Wirral, UK, and Dr. Roger Barraclough of the School of Biological Sciences, University of Liverpool, UK, for assistance with protocol development.

References

1. Schena, M., Shalon, D., Davis, R. W., and Brown, P. O. (1995) Quantitative monitoring of gene expression patterns with a complementary DNA microarray. *Science* **20,** 467–470.
2. Sorlie, T., Perou, C. M., Tibshirani, R., et al. (2001) Gene expression patterns of breast carcinomas distinguish tumor subclasses with clinical implications. *Proc. Natl. Acad. Sci. USA* **98,** 10,869–10,874.
3. Perou, C. M., Sorlie, T., Eisen, M. B., et al. (2000) Molecular portraits of human breast tumours. *Nature* **406,** 747–752.
4. van't Veer, L. J., Dai, H., van de Vijver, M. J., et al. (2002) Gene expression profiling predicts clinical outcome of breast cancer. *Nature* **415,** 530–536.
5. Maier, E., Meier-Ewert, S., Ahmadi, A. R., Curtis, J., and Lehrach, H. (1994) Application of robotic technology to automated sequence fingerprint analysis by oligonucleotide hybridisation. *J Biotechnol.* **35,** 191–203.
6. Zhao, N., Hashida, H., Takahashi, N., Misumi, Y., and Sakaki, Y. (1995) High-density cDNA filter analysis: a novel approach for large-scale, quantitative analysis of gene expression. *Gene* **156,** 207–213.

7. Pietu, G., Alibert, O., Guichard, V., et al. (1996) Novel gene transcripts preferentially expressed in human muscles revealed by quantitative hybridization of a high-density cDNA array. *Genome Res.* **6,** 492–503.

8. Becker, K. G., Wood III, W. H., and Cheadle, C. (2003) Membrane-based spotted cDNA arrays, in *DNA Microarrays: a Molecular Cloning Manual.* Cold Spring Harbor Laboratory Press, Cold Spring Harbor, NY, p. 289.

9. Diatchenko, L., Lau, Y. F., Campbell, A. P., et al. (1996) Suppression subtractive hybridization: a method for generating differentially regulated or tissue-specific cDNA probes and libraries. *Proc. Natl. Acad. Sci. USA* **93,** 6025–6030.

10. Kuang, W. W., Thompson, D.A., Hoch, R.V., and Weigel, R. J. (1998) Differential screening and suppression subtractive hybridization identified genes differentially expressed in an estrogen receptor-positive breast carcinoma cell line. *Nucleic Acids Res.* **26,** 1116–1123.

11. Yang, G. P., Ross, D. T., Kuang, W. W., Brown, P. O., and Weigel, R. J. (1999) Combining SSH and cDNA microarrays for rapid identification of differentially expressed genes. *Nucleic Acids Res.* **27,** 1517–1523.

12. Schummer, M., Ng, W., Nelson, P. S., Bumgarner, R. E., and Hood, L. (1997) Inexpensive handheld device for the construction of high-density nucleic acid arrays. *Biotechniques* **23,** 1087–1092.

V

STUDYING CANCER CELL BEHAVIOR IN VITRO AND IN VIVO

29

Methods to Analyze the Effects of the Urokinase System on Cancer Cell Adhesion, Proliferation, Migration, and Signal Transduction Events

Ute Reuning, Manfred Schmitt, Birgit Luber, Veronika Beck, and Viktor Magdolen

Summary

For cellular-invasive processes during a variety of physio- and pathophysiological events, including cancer, a fine-tuned balance between the formation and loosening of cell adhesive contacts has to occur, implicating the action of pericellular proteases; among those, the serine protease, urokinase-type plasminogen activator (uPA), its inhibitor PAI-1, and its cellular receptor uPA-R (CD87). Apart from its proteolytic functions, the uPA system is endowed with properties affecting the proliferative, adhesive, and migratory cellular phenotype. These events depend on signal transduction pathways known to be activated downstream of uPA/uPA-R cell surface interaction and require physical and functional cooperation and crosstalk with cell adhesion and signaling receptors of the integrin superfamily.

This chapter focuses on the description of several in vitro cell biological assay systems suitable for studying (cancer) cell behavior with respect to cell proliferation, cell adhesion, and cell motility, e.g., as a function of uPA-R/integrin-mediated effects.

Key Words: Urokinase system; integrins; extracellular matrix; cell adhesion; cell proliferation; cell migration; time lapse video microscopy; signal transduction, MAPK.

1. Introduction

Tumor invasion and metastasis are linked to the capacity of tumor cells to coordinate a series of biological events implicated in the formation and degradation of structural extracellular matrix (ECM) proteins. By this mechanism, tumor cells cross tissue boundaries, disseminate to various compartments of the body, adhere to distant tissue elements, and eventually form metastases. These complex processes require the concerted and regulated expression of pericellular proteolytic enzymes, mitogens, adhesion receptors (integrins), and ECM components.

From: *Methods in Molecular Medicine, Vol. 120: Breast Cancer Research Protocols*
Edited by: S. A. Brooks and A. L. Harris © Humana Press Inc., Totowa, NJ

Many tumor cells exhibit increased levels of components of the urokinase-type plasminogen activator (uPA) system, encompassing plasmin(ogen), the plasminogen activators uPA and tissue-type plasminogen activator, the plasminogen activator inhibitors (PAIs) type 1 and 2, and the uPA receptor uPAR (CD87) *(1,2)*.The serine protease uPA interacts with the cell surface glycosylphosphatidylinositol-anchored high affinity uPAR, resulting in effective conversion of plasminogen into the serine protease plasmin. Plasmin, in turn, degrades ECM proteins and activates the zymogen pro-uPA into enzymatically active uPA, as well as other ECM degrading enzymes *(3)*. In solid malignant tumors, the proteolytic activity of uPA is controlled by PAI-1. PAI-1 is also required for efficient tumor cell invasiveness *(4)*. Indeed, in patients afflicted with a variety of cancers, elevated tumor tissue antigen levels of uPA, PAI-1, and uPAR are present. Elevation of these proteolytic factors indicates a poor prognosis; such patients experience an early onset of disease recurrence because of metastasis formation and, thus, reduced life expectancy *(1,2)*. Methods for quantification of uPA and its inhibitor PAI-1 in tissue extracts by enzyme-linked immunosorbent assay (ELISA) are described in Chapter 19.

The interaction of uPA with cell surface uPAR and the (patho)physiological consequences arising thereof have stimulated intensive research in recent years *(5)*. In fact, it was shown that uPA in concert with its receptor uPAR exerts certain biological effects, apart from its role in the blood-clotting system and its fibrinolytic properties. These processes are induced by uPA/uPAR-triggered intracellular signal transduction events, ultimately leading to alterations in cell proliferation, adhesion, and migration *(2)*. As such, uPA has been identified as a protease with a growth factor-like, cell-directed function *(2,6)*. The mitogenic activity of uPA is based on the interaction of uPAR with uPA, independent of its proteolytic activity. Moreover, in order to proliferate and to initiate DNA synthesis, cancer cells require an appropriate substratum on which to adhere and spread. Interestingly, the uPA system is also involved in cellular adhesion by virtue of the ability of uPAR and PAI-1 to bind to the ECM component vitronectin *(7)*. Within this adhesion scenario, uPA and PAI-1 compete mutually and with adhesion receptors of the integrin superfamily for vitronectin binding, thereby regulating the adhesive phenotype of cancer cells.

Because uPAR is a glycosylphosphatidylinositol-anchored cell surface receptor lacking a transmembrane domain, at first sight it appears as a very unlikely candidate for intracellular signal transmission, but as a matter of fact, the uPA/uPAR-system is also implicated in cell migratory events via transmission of intracellular signals, for instance, resulting in specific protein-phosphorylation events *(8,9)*. Current research aims at establishing the molecular basis of the uPA/uPAR-mediated signaling pathway and focuses on the identification of cooperating transmembrane adaptors and downstream signaling molecules.

Owing to its multifunctional potential, the uPA system emerged as a prominent new target for antimetastatic therapy. On one hand, approaches directly aim at the suppression of uPA/uPAR-mediated enzymatic activity by using specific active site uPA inhibitors *(10)*, on the other, uPA/uPAR-triggered intracellular signaling, and biological events arising thereof are targeted by competitive molecules interrupting uPA/uPAR interaction *(11)*.

In this chapter, we describe basic methods to determine the effects of the uPA/uPAR system on the proliferative, adhesive, and motile phenotype of cancer cells. In the following text, selected classical methods for determining protein phosphorylation events as well as signaling molecules (e.g., of the mitogen-activated protein [MAP] kinase family) occurring within the uPA/uPAR signaling cascade are outlined. (For further assays measuring expression and activity of other signaling molecules related to the uPA/uPAR-triggered signaling pathway, *see* **refs.** *12* and *13*). The described assay protocols for the evaluation of cell proliferation, adhesion, migration, and signal transduction may be used for the analyses of the effects of uPA on breast cancer cells, as well as for the investigation of other cells or the cell-directed effects of other stimulants.

2. Materials

2.1. Cell Proliferation Assays

2.1.1. Cell Counting

1. Cell culture instruments: cell incubator, laminar flow cabinet, and pipets.
2. Cell culture material: cell culture flasks, 24-well cell culture plates, and sterile 15-mL Falcon tubes (Becton-Dickinson, Heidelberg, Germany).
3. Cell culture medium: Dulbecco's modified Eagle medium (DMEM), fetal calf serum (FCS), penicillin/streptomycin (1000 U), 10 mM of 4-2-hydroxyethyl-1-piperazineethanesulfonic acid (HEPES), 50 mM arginine, and 272 mM asparagine solutions (Gibco, Karlsruhe, Germany).
4. 0.05% (w/v) ethylendiaminetetraacetate (EDTA).
5. Phosphate-buffered saline (PBS), Gibco.
6. 0.4% (w/v) Trypan blue (Sigma, Deisenhofen, Germany).
7. Neubauer hemocytometer.
8. Latex or plastic gloves.

2.1.2. 3-(4,5-Dimethylthiazol-2-yl)-2,5-Diphenyltetrazoliumbromid (MTT) Assay

1. Cell culture instruments: cell incubator and laminar flow cabinet.
2. Cell culture material: cell culture flasks, sterile 96-well cell culture plates, and sterile 15-mL Falcon tubes.
3. Cell culture medium and solutions: *see* **step 3** in **Subheading 2.1.1.**

4. 0.05% (w/v) EDTA.
5. Purified high-molecular-weight uPA (Curasan, Kleinostheim, Germany).
6. 3-(4,5-Dimethylthiazol-2-yl)-2,5-diphenyltetrazoliumbromid (MTT) (Sigma).
7. Dimethyl sulfoxide (DMSO) (Sigma).
8. ELISA plate reader (570 nm, e.g., Titertek Multiscan; ICN/Flow Laboratories, Meckenheim, Germany).
9. Latex or plastic gloves.

2.1.3. Determination of DNA Synthesis by Incorporation of [³H]-Methyl Thymidine

1. Cell culture instruments: cell incubator and laminar flow cabinet.
2. Cell culture material: cell culture flasks, sterile 96-well cell culture plates, and sterile 15-mL Falcon tubes.
3. Cell culture medium and solutions: *see* **step 3** in **Subheading 2.1.1.**
4. 0.05% (w/v) EDTA.
5. Purified high-molecular-weight uPA (Curasan).
6. [³H]-Methyl thymidine (25 µCi/mL [25 Ci/mmol]; Amersham, Freiburg, Germany).

2.1.3.1. CELL HARVESTING USING A CELL HARVESTER INSTRUMENT

1. Cell Harvester 96 (TomTec, Orange, CA).
2. Fiberglass filter (Printed Filtermat A; Wallac, Turku, Finland).
3. Wax (MeltiLex™, Wallac).
4. Microsealer (cat. no. 1495-021, TomTec).
5. 1450 Microbeta Plus Liquid Scintillation Plate Counter (Wallac).

2.1.3.2. MANUAL CELL HARVESTING

1. 10% (v/v) trichloroacetic acid ([TCA]; Sigma).
2. Solubilization buffer: 0.1 *N* NaOH and 1% (w/v) sodium dodecyl sulfate (SDS).
3. Bicinchoninic acid protein determination kit (Pierce, Rockford, IL).
4. Neubauer hemocytometer.
5. Liquid scintillation vials.
6. Scintillation liquid (Quickszint 2000, ICN/Flow Laboratories).
7. Liquid scintillation counter.

2.2. In Vitro Cell Adhesion Assays

2.2.1. Cell–Matrix Adhesion

1. Cell culture instruments: cell incubator and laminar flow cabinet.
2. Cell culture material: cell culture flasks, sterile 96-well cell culture plates, and sterile 15-mL Falcon tubes.
3. Cell culture medium and solutions: *see* **step 3** in **Subheading 2.1.1.**
4. 0.05% (w/v) EDTA.
5. Purified ECM proteins: e.g., vitronectin, fibronectin (Becton-Dickinson), collagens (Sigma).

6. Hexosaminidase substrate buffer: 100 mM sodium citrate (pH 5.0), 0.5% (v/v) Triton X-100, and 15 mM *p*-nitrophenyl-*N*-acetyl-β-D-glucosaminide (Sigma).
7. Stop buffer: 0.2 M NaOH, 5 mM of EDTA.
8. Cell culture grade bovine serum albumin ([BSA]; Gibco).
9. ELISA plate reader (405 nm, e.g., Titertek Multiscan; ICN/Flow Laboratories).

2.2.2. Cell–Cell Adhesion

1. Cell culture instruments: cell incubator and laminar flow cabinet.
2. Cell culture material: cell culture flasks, sterile 96-well cell culture plates, and sterile 15-mL Falcon tubes.
3. Cell culture medium and solutions: *see* **step 3** in **Subheading 2.1.1.**
4. 0.05% (w/v) EDTA.
5. Sterile 96-well cell culture plates for fluorimeter measurements (Optical Btn-Plt, polymer base (with lid) cell culture plates [no. 165305], Nunc, Wiesbaden, Germany).
6. Lipophilic tracer 3,3'-dioctadecycloxacarbocyanine perchlorate ([DiO]; Molecular Probes, Eugene, OR).
7. DMSO.
8. Victor plate fluorimeter (PerkinElmer, Shelton, CT).

2.3. Cell Motility Assay

1. Cell culture instruments: cell incubator and laminar flow cabinet.
2. Cell culture material: cell culture flasks, sterile 96-well cell culture plates, and sterile 15-mL Falcon tubes.
3. Cell culture medium and solutions: *see* **step 3** in **Subheading 2.1.1.**
4. 0.05% (w/v) EDTA.
5. PBS.
6. 3.5-cm Cell culture Petri dishes with a glass bottom (cat. no. P35G-0-14-C-gm; MatTek, Ashland, MA).
7. Purified ECM proteins (vitronectin, fibronectin, collagens; Becton-Dickinson, Gibco).
8. Axiovert confocal laser-scan microscope LSM 510 with lens PNF ×20/0.4 PH2, using a helium–neon laser at 543 nm for the transmission scanning mode (Zeiss, Göttingen, Germany).
9. Laser-scan microscope software (Zeiss, LSM 5 Image Browser) for semiautomatic tracking of cell nuclei.
10. Microscope-coupled incubation chamber (Zeiss), which is temperature and CO_2-controlled and allows constant temperature of 37°C and 5% (v/v) CO_2.

2.4. Detection of Tyrosine-Phosphorylated Proteins by Western Blot Analysis

1. Protein sample in lysis buffer: 50 mM HEPES (pH 7.5), 150 mM NaCl, 1 mM of EDTA, 10% (v/v) glycerol, and 1% (v/v) Triton X-100. Add the following components freshly: 10 mM sodium fluoride, 1 mM sodium orthovanadate, 10 µg/mL of aprotinin, and 1 mM phenylmethylsulfonyl fluoride.

2. Standard SDS electrophoresis buffer, 10–12% (w/v) SDS-polyacrylamide gels.
3. Sample buffer: 62.5 m*M* Tris-HCl (pH 6.8), 2% (w/v) SDS, 10% (v/v) glycerol, 50 m*M* of dithiothreitol, and 0.1% (w/v) bromophenol blue.
4. Transfer buffer: 25 m*M* Tris, 0.2 *M* glycine (pH 8.5), and 20% (v/v) ethanol.
5. Blocking buffer: PBS containing 3% (w/v) nonfat dry milk (Merck, Darmstadt, Germany).
6. Dilution buffer for primary and secondary antibodies: use blocking buffer (*see* **step 5**).
7. Primary antibody: monoclonal antibodies directed to phosphotyrosine (e.g., from Upstate Biotechnology, Charlottesville, VA).
8. Secondary antibody: horseradish peroxidase-conjugated goat antimouse immunoglobulin (Ig)G (e.g., from Santa Cruz Biotechnology, Santa Cruz, CA).
9. Wash buffer: PBS containing 0.05% (v/v) Tween-20.
10. Nitrocellulose (Schleicher & Schuell, Dassel, Germany) or polyvinylidene fluoride membranes (SD 1300; Pall, Dreieich, Germany).
11. Plastic container.
12. Blotting paper (Whatman, Maidstone, UK).
13. Chemiluminescence (ECL) detection reagent kit (Amersham).

2.5. Detection of (Activated) MAP Kinase by Western Blot Analysis

1. Protein sample in lysis buffer: *see* **Subheading 2.4.**
2. Standard SDS electrophoresis buffer, 10–12% (w/v) SDS-polyacrylamide gels.
3. Sample buffer: 62.5 m*M* Tris-HCl (pH 6.8), 2% (w/v) SDS, 10% (v/v) glycerol, 50 m*M* dithiothreitol, and 0.1% (w/v) bromophenol blue.
4. Transfer buffer: 25 m*M* Tris, 0.2 *M* glycine (pH 8.5), and 20% (v/v) ethanol.
5. Blocking buffer: Tris-buffered saline (TBS): 10 m*M* Tris-HCl (pH 7.5), 140 m*M* NaCl, 5% (w/v) nonfat dry milk; while stirring, add 0.1% (v/v) Tween-20.
6. Primary antibodies: polyclonal rabbit antibody directed to p44/p42 MAP kinase and polyclonal rabbit antibody directed to phospho-p44/p42 MAP kinase (e.g., from New England BioLabs, Beverly, MA).
7. Secondary antibody: horseradish peroxidase-conjugated goat antirabbit IgG (e.g., from Santa Cruz Biotechnology).
8. Dilution buffer for primary antibody directed to p44/p42 MAP kinase: TBS, 0.1% (v/v) Tween-20, and 5% (w/v) BSA.
9. Dilution buffer for primary antibody directed to phospho-p44/p42 MAP kinase: TBS, 0.1% (v/v) Tween-20, and 5% (w/v) nonfat dry milk powder.
10. Dilution buffer for secondary antibodies: use blocking buffer (*see* **step 5**).
11. Wash buffer: TBS and 0.1% (v/v) Tween-20.
12. Nitrocellulose (Schleicher & Schuell) or polyvinylidene fluoride membranes (Pall).
13. Plastic container.
14. Blotting paper (Whatman).
15. ECL detection reagent kit (Amersham).

3. Methods

3.1. Cell Proliferation Assays

For the evaluation of cell proliferation, any of the three following experimental approaches may be chosen.

3.1.1. Cell Counting

1. Seed cells in 24-well cell culture plates at a density of 2.5×10^4 cells/well and incubate overnight in DMEM containing 10% (v/v) FCS.
2. After 24 h, wash cells twice in FCS-free medium and change the cell culture medium to starvation medium containing 0.5% (v/v) FCS. Cultivate for another 24 h.
3. Add purified uPA (1–10 nM) in fresh DMEM, containing 0.5% (v/v) FCS and cultivate cells for distinct time intervals.
4. Thereafter, wash cell monolayers once in PBS.
5. Detach cells in 0.05% (w/v) EDTA and centrifuge at 1000g.
6. Resuspend cell pellet in 400 μL of DMEM on inclusion of 100 μL of the dye Trypan blue (0.4% [w/v]) in order to identify nonviable blue-stained cells.
7. Fill Neubauer hemocytometer with the cell suspension and count cell numbers; in case cell suspensions are too dense for reliable counting by a Neubauer hemocytometer, dilute cell suspension further for adequate and countable amount of cells; repeat counting twice.
8. Plot data as cell number over time of (uPA) stimulation of cells.

3.1.2. MTT Assay

The MTT assay (adapted from **ref. *14***) uses the linear correlation of the enzymatic conversion of MTT into a blue formazan product, elicited by mitochondrial dehydrogenases, to cell number.

1. Suspend cells at a density of 5×10^5 per mL of DMEM containing 10% (v/v) FCS (*see* **Subheading 2.1.1.**). Transfer 50 μL each to wells of a 96-well, flat-bottom cell culture plate. Incubate cells for 24 h at 37°C in a humidified 5% (v/v) CO_2 atmosphere.
2. After 24 h, wash cells in FCS-free medium and replace the 10% FCS-containing medium by a starvation medium containing 0.5% (v/v) FCS, only. Incubate for 24 h at 37°C.
3. Prepare a stock solution of 2 mg of MTT/mL in DMEM (*see* **Note 1**), without phenol red, under sterile conditions. Filter MTT solution through a 0.2-μm filter and store the ready-to-use solution at 2–8°C for frequent use or, alternatively, frozen at –20°C for an extended period of storage.
4. Rinse cells with FCS-free DMEM and add 100 μL of uPA (or any other stimulant) containing fresh starvation medium supplemented with 0.5% (v/v) FCS. As a control, use cells which received DMEM containing 0.5% (v/v) FCS, only.

5. Allow cells to incubate at 37°C for distinct time intervals.
6. After distinct time intervals, add 20 μL of MTT and incubate cells for another 2 h at 37°C.
7. At the end of incubation period, aspirate the medium and let the formed violet formazan crystals dry under the laminar flow.
8. Solubilize formazan crystals in DMSO (*see* **Note 2**).
9. Conduct spectrophotometrical measurements in a plate reader at 570 nm; absorbance reading is directly proportional to cell number (as few as 1000 cells/well can be detected; *see* **Note 3**).
10. Perform assays in quadruplicate.

3.1.3. Determination of DNA Synthesis by Incorporation of [^{3}H]-Methyl Thymidine

In order to determine cellular DNA synthesis as a measure of cell proliferation, [^{3}H]-methyl thymidine is added to cells and its incorporation into cells taken as a measure of the rate of new DNA synthesis.

1. Seed cells at a density of 2×10^4 per well (200 μL) in a 24-well flat bottom cell culture plate (in quadruplicates) in DMEM containing 10% (v/v) FCS. Incubate for 24 h at 37°C.
2. Wash cells in FCS-free DMEM and replace the 10% FCS-containing medium by starvation medium containing 0.5% (v/v) FCS. Incubate for 24 h at 37°C.
3. Add uPA (or any other stimulant) in fresh starvation medium and cultivate cells at 37°C for different time intervals (e.g., ranging from 2 to 96 h). As a control, use cells that received 0.5% (v/v) FCS-containing medium only.
4. After distinct periods of cell stimulation, aspirate medium and wash cells once in PBS.
5. Add 300 μL of [^{3}H]-methyl thymidine (25 μCi/mL [25 Ci/mmol]) (*see* **Note 4**) in DMEM containing 0.5% (v/v) FCS. Incubate cells for another 6 h at 37°C.

Two methods for processing of cells and determination of the incorporated radiotracer can be applied.

3.1.3.1. MANUAL PROCESSING

1. Aspirate medium and wash wells containing the cells three times with PBS.
2. Detach cells by 0.05% (w/v) EDTA. Resuspend cell pellets in PBS.
3. Precipitate cell suspensions with 10% (v/v) TCA (30 min, 4°C).
4. Wash cell precipitates in PBS and dissolve the TCA-insoluble fraction in 1 mL of 0.1 *N* NaOH and 1% (w/v) SDS. Incubate overnight.
5. Transfer the dissolved TCA-precipitated cell pellets or aliquots thereof into liquid scintillation vials. Add 3 mL scintillation fluid.
6. Determine incorporated radioactivity in a liquid scintillation counter.

3.1.3.2. Cell Harvesting Using a Cell Harvester Instrument

1. By use of a cell harvester instrument, transfer cell lysates onto a fiberglass filter (Printed Filtermat A, Wallac).
2. Thereafter, rinse the cell harvester three times with PBS.
3. Melt wax (MeltiLex, Wallac) over the filters in a Microsealer (TomTec).
4. Measure the sealed plates in a liquid scintillation plate counter (e.g., 1450 Microbeta Plus) in order to determine the [^{3}H]-methyl thymidine incorporated in cellular DNA.
5. Measure protein content (BCA protein reagent kit, Pierce).
6. Normalize counts per minute (cpm) values obtained to the protein concentration of the cell lysates harvested in parallel or cell counts of parallel wells and express data as thymidine incorporation per protein or, alternatively, per cell (*6*).

3.2. In Vitro Cell Adhesion Assays

3.2.1. Cell–Matrix Adhesion

The following simple, but sensitive, adhesion assay format (*15*) utilizes the linear correlation of the activity of the ubiquitous lysosomal enzyme *N*-acetyl-β-D-hexosaminidase to cell numbers. Hereby, the chromogenic substrate *p*-nitrophenol-*N*-acetyl-β-D-glucosamide is used, which is consumed by hexosaminidase.

1. Coat 96-well flat-bottomed cell culture plates with a cell adhesion supporting purified ECM protein, such as vitronectin, fibronectin, or collagen, depending on the cell type; dilute the ECM proteins to a concentration of 10 µg/mL PBS and add 50–75 µL of this solution to each well. Incubate the plate overnight at 4°C or for 2 h at room temperature. Aspirate the coating solution and wash once with PBS.
2. Block plates for 2 h at room temperature in PBS containing 2% (w/v) BSA.
3. Wash coated wells once in PBS and immediately transfer 50 µL of cell suspension at a density of 5×10^4 cells/well.
4. After 45–60 min (or whatever time the cell type to be tested needs for proper adhesion), remove nonadherent cells by two washes in PBS (at 37°C).
5. Thereafter, add 50 µL/well of hexosaminidase substrate in substrate buffer. Incubate plate for 1 h at 37°C.
6. Terminate the reaction by addition of 50 µL of stop buffer to each well.
7. Follow colorimetric development of the chromogenic substrate by photometric measurement in a plate reader at 405 nm.
8. Set up standard curve by placing 3000–100,000 cells per well. However, treat those cells like the adherent cells, without prior washing.

3.2.2. Cell–Cell Adhesion: Fluorescent Labeling of Cells

Cell membranes provide a convenient conduit for loading living cells with lipophilic dyes, which are tolerated by the cells in high concentration. Lateral diffusion of the dye within the cell membrane allows staining of the entire cell. Labeling can be performed with either adherent cells or cells in suspension.

1. Transfer 50 μL of unlabeled cells (10^6/mL) to wells of an ECM-coated fluorimeter 96-well plate (Optical Btn-Plt, polymer base [with lid] cell culture plates [cat. no. 165305]) and cultivate plate for 1–2 d in order to achieve a 100% confluent monolayer.
2. Culture different type of cells in culture flasks.
3. Prepare stock solutions of the lipophilic tracer DiO in DMSO at concentrations ranging from 1–2.5 mg/mL (*see* **Note 5**).
4. Add DiO ranging from 1:250 to 1:1000 dilution into the cell culture flasks. Maximal labeling is achieved after 2 h, even though somewhat longer incubation periods do not affect cellular viability (*see* **Note 6**).
5. Detach DiO-labeled cells in 0.05% (w/v) EDTA and centrifuge at 1000*g*. Rinse once in PBS.
6. Resuspend cell pellet in fresh cell culture medium.
7. Plate DiO-labeled cells at a density of $1–5 \times 10^4$ per well on top of the monolayers described in **step 1**.
8. Allow DiO-labeled cells to adhere to the monolayer cells (1 h), depending on the cell type used.
9. Wash gently the plate five times in PBS to discard nonadherent cells.
10. Determine number of fluorescent DiO-labeled cells adherent to the monolayer cells in a plate fluorimeter (DiO excitation wavelength: 484 nm, emission wavelength: 501 nm).
11. In parallel, establish a standard curve with fluorescent DiO-labeled cells in suspension in order to correlate fluorescence intensity with cell number.

3.3. Cell Motility Monitored by Time-Lapse Video Microscopy

1. Coat the glass bottom of a specialized cell culture Petri dish with purified ECM protein(s) as described under **Subheading 3.2.1.** Usually, beforehand, different ECM proteins should be tested to select the most suitable adhesion matrix for the respective cell type to be tested in the cell motility assay.
2. Wash the cell culture dishes two times with PBS. Subsequently block with PBS containing 2% (w/v) BSA (2 h, room temperature) to minimize nonspecific cell adherence.
3. After another wash in PBS, seed cells at a density of 2×10^5 per 3.5-cm cell culture Petri dish. Incubate dish for 2 h at 37°C under 5% (v/v) CO_2. This timeframe allows cells to attach to the dish before time-lapse video microscopy is started.
4. Cover Petri dish with a glass lid and transfer it to the table of the temperature- and CO_2-controlled incubation chamber of the microscope.
5. Phase-contrast transmission images are taken automatically every third minute up to 10 h and stored on a computer disk. For statistical reasons, a minimum of 40 cells should be visible in the area of observation.
6. The number of motile cells is determined and the individual cell speed measured by drawing outlines of cells on a transparency sheet that is fixed to the computer screen. Cells that leave the observation field or that divide during the observation time are not considered.

7. Semiautomatic tracing of cell nuclei using the Zeiss laser-scanning microscope software allows determination of the individual cell speed. Random cell movement of cells is assessed semiautomatically by tracing the cell nuclei during time of observation. The calculation of the cell speed is based on displacement of an individual cell divided by the time of recording.

3.4. Detection of Tyrosine-Phosphorylated Proteins by Western Blot Analysis

1. Plate cells into 6-well cell culture dishes, change medium, and add uPA as described under **Subheading 3.1.1.**
2. At distinct time intervals (ranging from 5 min to 24 h), wash cells in PBS and lyse them for 5 min on ice, using cell lysis buffer (*see* **Note 7**).
3. Determine protein concentration in cell lysates (BCA protein reagent kit, Pierce).
4. Perform standard SDS polyacrylamide gel electrophoresis using 10–12% (w/v) polyacrylamide gels (methods are given in Chapter 17).
5. For sample preparation, add 10–50 µg of protein of cell lysates into conical, 1-mL test tube (e.g., from Eppendorf, Hamburg, Germany) and supplement with 10–15 µL of sample buffer.
6. Heat samples for 3 min at 95°C.
7. Load samples onto the SDS polyacrylamide gel and perform gel electrophoresis at 120 V.
8. According to standard protocols (*see* Chapter 17), transfer proteins from the gel onto nitrocellulose or PVDF membrane at 100 mA for 2 h in transfer buffer.
9. Incubate blots for 2 h at room temperature in PBS containing 2% (w/v) BSA (*see* **Note 8**).
10. Incubate membrane with phosphotyrosine-directed monoclonal antibodies in PBS 1% (w/v) BSA (2 h, room temperature). Use gentle agitation.
11. Wash the membrane three times in PBS plus 0.1% (v/v) Tween-20 (10 min, room temperature).
12. Incubate membrane with horseradish peroxidase-conjugated goat antimouse IgG (1:1,000) (45 min, room temperature).
13. Detect bound antibodies by ECL; for this, mix equal volumes of the Luminol reagent and the oxidizing reagent for ECL detection.
14. Incubate membrane in this solution and agitate gently for 1 min. Discard excess liquid.
15. Position the membrane with the protein side up in a sheet protector and expose it to X-ray film in a dark room for varying times, ranging from 15 s to 30 min (*see* **Note 9**).

3.5. Detection of (Activated) MAP Kinase by Western Blot Analysis

1. Prepare cell lysates and perform electrophoresis as described in **Subheading 3.4.**
2. Mix cell lysates (10–50 µg protein) with 10–15 µL of sample buffer.
3. After transfer, wash nitrocellulose membrane with TBS for 5 min at room temperature.

 4. Incubate membrane in blocking buffer (TBS plus 5% [w/v] nonfat dry milk). While stirring, add 0.1% (v/v) Tween-20.
 5. Wash membrane three times, 5 min each, in TBS containing 0.1% (v/v) Tween-20.
 6. Add primary antibody directed to p44/42 MAP kinase (in TBS containing 0.1% [v/v] Tween-20 and 5% [w/v] BSA); for those directed to phospho-p44/42 MAP kinase, incubate in TBS containing 0.1% (v/v) Tween-20, 5% (w/v) nonfat dry-milk powder. Incubate overnight at 4°C.
 7. Wash membrane three times, 5 min each, in wash buffer.
 8. Incubate membrane with horseradish peroxidase-conjugated secondary antibody at a 1:2,000 dilution in blocking buffer (1 h, room temperature).
 9. Wash membrane three times, 5 min each, in TBS containing 0.1% (v/v) Tween-20.
10. Detect bound antibodies by ECL as described in **Subheading 3.4.**

4. Notes

 1. MTT assay. **Caution:** Avoid any direct contact of MTT with eyes or skin. The reagent is an irritant.
 2. **Caution:** DMSO is an organic solvent. Handling should be performed using a fume hood and, on completion of the assay, the contents of the plate be dumped into an organic waste disposal.
 3. The colored formazan product is stable at 4°C, and absorbance can be recorded several days later. To do so, store the plate in a humidified atmosphere to avoid evaporation during storage. The ability of cells to convert the tetrazolium in the dye solution to the formazan product varies among different cell types and strongly depends on their metabolic capacity. Most eukaryotic cells in culture reduce the tetrazolium sufficiently to perform the assay accurately, even at low cell numbers. The culture conditions used to grow the cells can affect the results. Therefore, it is recommended to consider the culture conditions when analyzing results of proliferation assays. Care should be taken to avoid bubble formation after the formazan product has been solubilized, because bubbles in the liquid may interfere with the spectrophotometrical recording.
 4. Work safely with tritium-containing substances. Radioactive half-life is 12.4 yr. Tritiated thymidine is regarded as more toxic than tritiated water, partly because the activity is concentrated in cell nuclei. Because of its low β-energy, tritium cannot be monitored directly; therefore, regular swabbing and counting of the work area is advisable. Tritium can be absorbed through the skin; therefore, gloves must always be worn. (Information taken from Amersham Biosciences website: www4.amershambiosciences.com.)
 5. **Caution:** DiO may precipitate from the stock solution after several hours. Sonication may help in this case.
 6. DiO labeling does not appreciably affect cell viability or basic cell physiological properties. In general, the dye does not transfer from labeled to unlabeled cells. The dye is weakly fluorescent in water, but highly fluorescent and photostable when incorporated into cell membranes. For adherent cells, labeling in the adhesive state results in improved viability compared with labeling performed in cell suspension.

7. Viscosity resulting from DNA can be reduced somewhat by boiling the samples for 5 min and/or by shearing the sample by passing it several times through a 22-gage needle.

8. Wear gloves and transfer the membrane blot from one procedure step to another using clean forceps.

9. Because of the kinetics of the detection reaction, the signal on ECL development is most intense immediately after the addition of the ECL reagent and declines over the following 2 h.

References

1. Schmitt, M., Harbeck, N., Thomssen, C., et al. (1997) Clinical impact of the plasminogen activation system in tumor invasion and metastasis: prognostic relevance and target for therapy. *Thromb. Hemost.* **78,** 285–296.

2. Reuning, U., Magdolen, V., Wilhelm, O., et al. (1998) Multifunctional potential of the plasminogen activation system in tumor invasion and metastasis. *Int. J. Oncol.* **13,** 893–906.

3. Mazar, A. P. (2001) The urokinase plasminogen activator receptor (uPAR) as a target for the diagnosis and therapy of cancer. *Anticancer Drugs* **12,** 387–400.

4. Andreasen, P. A., Egelund, R., and Petersen, H. H. (2000) The plasminogen activation system in tumor growth, invasion, and metastasis. *Cell. Mol. Life Sci.* **57,** 25–40.

5. Ossowski, L., Aguirre-Ghiso, J. A. (2000) Urokinase receptor and integrin partnership: coordination of signaling for cell adhesion, migration, and growth. *Curr. Opin. Cell Biol.* **12,** 613–620.

6. Fischer, K., Lutz, V., Wilhelm, O., et al. (1998) Urokinase induces proliferation of human ovarian cancer cells: characterization of structural elements required for growth factor function. *FEBS Lett.* **438,** 101–105.

7. Chapman, H. A. and Wei, Y. (2001) Protease crosstalk with integrins: the urokinase receptor paradigm. *Thromb. Haemost.* **86,** 124–129.

8. Kjoller, L. (2002) The urokinase plasminogen activator receptor in the regulation of the actin cytoskeleton and cell motility. *Biol. Chem.* **383,** 5–19.

9. Yebra, M., Goretzki, L., Pfeifer, M., and Mueller, B. M. (1999) Urokinase-type plasminogen activator binding to its receptor stimulates tumor cell migration by enhancing integrin-mediated signal transduction. *Exp. Cell Res.* **250,** 231–240.

10. Magdolen, V., Arroyo de Prada, N., Sperl, S., et al. (2000) Natural and synthetic inhibitors of the tumor-associated serine protease urokinase-type plasminogen activator. *Adv. Exp. Med. Biol.* **477,** 331–341.

11. Muehlenweg, B., Sperl, S., Magdolen, V., Schmitt, M., and Harbeck, N. (2001) Interference with the urokinase plasminogen activator system: a promising therapy concept for solid tumours. *Expert Opin. Biol. Ther.* **1,** 683–691.

12. Kusch, A., Tkachuk, S., Haller, H., et al. (2000) Urokinase stimulates human vascular smooth muscle cell migration via a phosphatidylinositol 3-kinase-Tyk2 interaction. *J. Biol. Chem.* **274,** 24,059–24,065.

13. Dumler, I., Kopmann, A., Wagner, K., et al. (2000) Urokinase induces activation and formation of Stat4 and Stat1-Stat2 complexes in human vascular smooth muscle cells. *J. Biol. Chem.* **275,** 39,466–39,473.

14. Carmichael, J., DeGraff, W. G., Gazdar, A. F., Minna, J. D., and Mitchell, J. B. (1987) Evaluation of a tetrazolium-based semiautomated colorimetric assay: assessment of chemosensitivity testing. *Cancer Res.* **47,** 936–942.

15. Landegren, U. (1984) Measurement of cell numbers by means of the endogenous enzyme hexosaminidase. Applications to detection of lymphokines and cell surface antigens. *J. Immunol. Meth.* **67,** 379–388.

30

Phospho-Specific Antibodies as a Tool to Study In Vivo Regulation of BRCA1 After DNA Damage

Kum Kum Khanna, Magtouf Gatei, and Gordon Tribbick

Summary

Phospho-specific antibodies have become very useful reagents for study of signal transduction pathways. This chapter describes the production of phospho-specific antibodies and their use to assess individual phosphorylation events in vivo in cells. The first step involves the synthesis of peptides (12–15 residues), where the phosphorylation site is centrally located, and a cysteine residue is incorporated at either the N- or C-terminus of the peptide to facilitate coupling it to an immunogenic carrier protein. No special immunization protocols are required to generate phospho-specific antibodies. Typically, animals of choice are immunized twice, several weeks apart, and enzyme-linked immunosorbent assay is used to determine the relative titer of sera against phosphorylated and nonphosphorylated peptides. Where the titer against phosphorylated peptides is much greater than nonphosphorylated peptides, the sera can be used at appropriate dilutions without further processing. In case a significant level of antibodies specific to the nonphosphorylated peptide is present in the antisera, an enhancement step is used to obtain a useful phospho-specific antibody. Although these enhanced antisera are suitable for many applications, there may be circumstances where affinity-purified antibodies are required. These antibodies can be used to detect a particular phosphorylation event in vivo using Western blotting, immunoprecipitation, and immunofluorescence.

Key Words: Immunization; antiphospho-specific antibodies; purification; Western blotting; immunoprecipitation; immunofluorescence.

1. Introduction

Antiphospho-specific antibodies have become very useful reagents in the study of signal transduction pathways. For DNA damage signaling, protein phosphorylation cascades are used as the principle means for the transduction of signals originating at sites of DNA damage, each phosphorylated sequence providing a binding moiety and activation for proteins involved in the next stage in the cascade of protein binding and phosphorylation. In mammals, the breast cancer-1 (BRCA1) protein functions as a critical regulator of the DNA

From: *Methods in Molecular Medicine, Vol. 120: Breast Cancer Research Protocols*
Edited by: S. A. Brooks and A. L. Harris © Humana Press Inc., Totowa, NJ

damage response. The key finding that linked BRCA1 to the DNA damage response pathway was its colocalization with Rad51, the eukaryotic equivalent of bacterial recA, which has been implicated in the homology directed repair of double-stranded breaks *(1)*. Following DNA damage, BRCA1 and its associated proteins relocalize to the sites of postreplicative repair and colocalize with proliferating cell nuclear antigen (PCNA). BRCA1 is also associated with Rad50, Mre11, and Nbs1, which are all involved in detection and repair of double-strand breaks. Functional data from the study of *Brca1-* and *Brca2-* mutated mice have confirmed the role of these genes in maintaining genomic integrity, with the homozygous mutant cells exhibiting a defect in homology-directed repair of DNA double-stranded breaks and sensitivity to ionizing radiation.

BRCA1 is hyperphosphorylated in response to DNA damage, and this hyperphosphorylation of BRCA1 can be detected as a change in its electrophoretic mobility after sodium dodecyl sulfate (SDS)-polyacrylamide gel electrophoresis and Western blotting with anti-BRCA1 antibody. In terms of studying damage-induced phosphorylation of BRCA1, we first had to determine the kinase(s) responsible for BRCA1 mobility shift, identify individual residues that are phosphorylated, and raise antiphospho-specific antibodies to validate that each site is phosphorylated in vivo *(2,3)*. Using cells deficient in ataxia telangiectasia-mutated (ATM) kinase, which acts at the top of double-strand break response pathway, we were able to show that ionizing radiation (IR)-induced phosphorylation of BRCA1 is ATM kinase-dependent. ATM kinase-phosphorylated BRCA1 on multiple serine residues in response to IR *(2)*, and we mapped the ATM kinase-dependent sites of phosphorylation in BRCA1 (Ser-1387, S-1423, S-1457, and S-1524). We made phospho-specific antibodies that allowed us to look at particular phosphorylation event on BRCA1 in vivo and allowed us to quantitate it and compare the response to various to damaging agents *(3)*. Using phospho-specific antibodies against BRCA1, we were able to show that IR-induced phosphorylations of BRCA1 are catalyzed by ATM kinase, whereas ultraviolet (UV)-induced phosphorylations of BRCA1 are catalyzed by a related kinase, ATM and Rad3-related kinase. This led us to conclude that although ATM kinase and ATM and Rad3-related kinase phosphorylate an overlapping pool of cellular substrates in vitro, in vivo they are nonredundant kinases that regulate distinct and partially overlapping cellular responses to genotoxic stress.

More recently, we have identified ATM kinase mutations in multiple-case breast cancer families *(4)* and have shown that these mutations severely comprise the kinase activity of mutant ATM kinase. Phosphorylation of BRCA1 in the ATM kinase-heterozygous cell lines after IR was dramatically reduced, as assessed by Western blotting with antiphospho-specific BRCA1 antibodies. Based on these findings, we are currently developing methods to screen for ATM kinase mutations in multiple-case breast cancer families.

This chapter aims to describe production of phospho-specific antibodies and their use to assess site(s) of phosphorylation of BRCA1 in vivo. As the specific sites of phosphorylation in BRCA1 were known, the challenge for us was to make an antipeptide antibody to the phosphorylated peptide sequences that can be used as a probe to identify the state of phosphorylation of the specific site in BRCA1 in vivo.

1.1. Factors Involved in the Production of Antiphosphorylated Peptide Antibodies

For generating an antiphosphorylated peptide antibody, we used 12- to 15-residue peptides, of which the phosphorylation sites are centrally located within the peptide sequences but not at the very N- and C-termini. Although it is possible to raise antibodies to shorter sequences or, indeed, to single residues, the shorter the peptide used as immunogen, the more likely the antipeptide antibody generated will crossreact and bind to related proteins. As peptides are generally not immunogenic in their own right, it is necessary to couple them to immunogenic carrier proteins. To facilitate this coupling, a cysteine residue is incorporated at either the N- or C-terminus of the peptide and reacted to conjugate the peptide to an immunogenic carrier protein. We found that the diphtheria toxoid is most suitable as a carrier; this couples to the peptide using a heterobifunctional reagent, 6-maleimido-caproyl *n*-hydroxy succinimide (MCS).

1.2. Coupling Using MCS

This is one of the best methods to couple a peptide to the carrier protein via a specific amino acid residue in the peptide and to maintain peptide antigenicity (*5*). It relies on the specificity of reaction between a maleimide group and a sulfhydryl group. For this procedure, the peptide to be conjugated must contain one or more fully reduced cysteines. The peptide, generally, will not contain a "natural" cysteine, and a cysteine normally has to be added to the peptide sequence. Assistance in making the choice of where to place the cysteine residue in the peptide can be had by the observing following guidelines. Where the peptide is from an internal sequence of a protein, the cysteine can be positioned at either the N- or the C-terminus of the peptide (*6*). Where the peptide is from the very N-terminus of the protein, the cysteine should be at the C-terminus of the peptide. Conversely, where the peptide represents the very C-terminus of the protein, the cysteine should be at the N-terminus of the peptide.

The reagent MCS is first reacted with the carrier protein to add maleimido groups to lysine side chains. The MCS-activated carrier protein is mixed with peptide (containing cysteines in the fully reduced form), and the maleimido groups react with cysteine sulfhydryl groups to form stable thioether bonds, linking the peptide to the carrier protein. In the procedure we use, we generally aim to couple 1–1.5 peptide molecules per 10,000 Da of carrier protein. The extent of coupling can be accurately determined on a mole–peptide/mole–carrier basis.

1.3. Antibody Generation

No special immunization protocols are required to generate antiphosphorylated peptide antisera. Typically, animals of choice are immunized twice, several weeks apart. The first immunization is with an emulsion of the peptide-carrier conjugate (equivalent to 0.35 mg peptide) with 2 vol of Freund's complete adjuvant, and this is injected subcutaneously. A second similar immunization followed 2 wk later, this time using Freund's incomplete adjuvant. Potent antipeptide sera were obtained 2–4 wk subsequently *(7)*. It is important, however, to understand that other antibodies specific for nonphosphorylated peptide may also be generated. To obtain the most complete information on the specificity of antipeptide antibodies that have been generated, epitope mapping using a set of overlapping peptides can be used; however, this approach was not employed by us; instead we employed an enzyme-linked immunosorbent assay to determine the relative titer of sera against phosphorylated and nonphosphorylated peptide.

1.4. Testing Phosphorylated Peptide Sera

Phosphorylated and nonphosphorylated peptide that have biotin coupled to their N- or C-terminus are immobilized in solid-phase immunoassays by avidin or streptavidin. This method of immobilization is independent of the sequence of the peptide being tested. The sera are titrated on a microtiter plate coated with nonphosphorylated peptide and phosphorylated peptide. Where the titer of specific antiphosphorylated antibody are very much greater than the titer to the nonphosphorylated peptide, the sera can be used at an appropriate dilution, without further processing, to probe for the phosphorylated protein. Even though the antibodies specific for the nonphosphorylated peptide may be present, any low-level binding will not interfere with the interpretation of the data. Where the level of antibodies to the nonphosphorylated peptide is relatively high, or perhaps even greater than the level of antiphosphorylated peptide antibodies, using the antisera at any dilution would result in ambiguous results, i.e., both the phosphorylated and the nonphosphorylated protein sequence would be detected.

1.5. Phosphorylated Peptide Antibody Enhancement

Where a significant level of antibodies specific to the nonphosphorylated peptide is present in the antisera, useful antiphosphorylated peptide antibodies can be obtained using an enhancement process.

To achieve this, the nonphosphorylated analog of the peptide used for the immunization is coupled to thiopropyl-Sepharose 6B (cat. no. 17-0420-01; Amersham Biosciences, Castle Hill, Australia), using the available cysteine residue, following the manufacturer's instructions. After coupling, the gel is incubated with aliquots of the antisera to absorb antibodies specific to the nonphosphorylated peptide sequence. The resultant antiserum will have an enhanced specificity for the phosphorylated peptide sequence. It will still be desirable to test the resultant enhanced antisera to confirm the level of enhancement achieved, and establish the dilution to be used to probe for the phosphorylated protein.

1.6. Affinity Purification of Antiphosphorylated Peptide Antibodies

Although enhanced antisera may be suitable for many applications, there may be circumstances where affinity purified antibodies are required. For example, affinity purification may be required where an unacceptable level of background binding is observed using the enhanced serum, possibly caused by other antibodies present in the serum, or when absence of other proteins is important, such as when direct labeling of the antibody is required. For affinity purification, phosphorylated peptide is coupled to thiopropyl-Sepharose 6B, and the resultant gel is incubated with aliquots of the enhanced serum. After washing away any unabsorbed protein, specific antibodies are eluted from the peptide (adsorbent), usually by the application of general technique, such as low-pH elution. To produce antibodies that are specific to the phosphorylated peptide only, the enhanced antiserum should be used, as the enhancement procedure removes antibodies from the serum that are specific to the nonphosphorylated peptide. It is not advisable to affinity purify phospho-antibodies directly from antiserum without enhancement step, as antibodies specific for both the phosphorylated and nonphosphorylated peptide sequence will be absorbed and subsequently eluted.

1.7. Use of Phospho-Specific Antibodies

These antibodies can be used to detect a particular phosphorylation event in vivo, using Western blotting, immunoprecipitation, and immunofluorescence. Detailed under **Subheading 3.** are the protocols used for detection of DNA damage-induced phosphorylation of BRCA1, using phospho-specific anti-BRCA1 antibodies.

2. Materials

1. RPMI-1640 culture media supplemented with 100 U/mL of penicillin, 100 μg/mL of streptomycin, and 10% fetal calf serum (complete culture medium).
2. Lysis buffer: prepare 100 mL of 50 mM Tris-HCl (pH 7.4), 150 mM NaCl, 2 mM ethylenediaminetetraacetic acid, 2 mM ethylene glycol-*bis*(2-aminoethylether)-N,N,N',N'-tetraacetic acid, 25 mM sodium fluoride, 25 mM β-glycerophosphate, 0.1 mM sodium orthovandate, 0.2% (v/v) Triton X-100, and 0.3% (v/v) Nonidet NP-40. Store at 4°C. Immediately before use, add protease inhibitors: 0.1 mM phenylmethylsulfonyl fluoride, 5 μg/mL of leupeptin, and 1 μg/mL of aprotinin. Keep the lysis buffer in ice for use.
3. Phosphate buffer saline (PBS): prepare 1 L of 0.15 M NaCl, 0.01 M Na_2HPO_4, and 3.16 mM KH_2PO_4, pH 7.5. Autoclave it and store at room temperature. It is stable for several months. Store at 4°C for washing cells.
4. Acrylamide stock solution: usually obtained ready-to-use as 30% unpolymerized acrylamide (29:1 acrylamide:bisacrylamide). Store in a dark bottle at 4°C.
5. Separating gel buffer stock: prepare 100 mL of 1.5 M Tris-HCl (pH 8.8) in distilled (d)H_2O. Store at room temperature. It is stable for several months.
6. Stacking gel buffer stock: prepare 100 mL of 0.5 M Tris-HCl (pH 6.8) in dH_2O. Store at room temperature. It is stable for several months.
7. 10% (w/v) SDS: prepare 100 mL in dH_2O. Use a surgical mask when weighting SDS. Store at room temperature. It is stable for several months.
8. 10% (w/v) ammonium persulfate (APS): prepare 10 mL of 10% APS in dH_2O. Store at –20°C in 0.5-mL aliquots. Before use, keep it in ice for thawing.
9. N,N,N',N'-tetramethylethylenediamine (TEMED): store in a dark bottle at 4°C.
10. Running buffer stock (10X): prepare 1 L of 0.25-M Tris base and 1.92 M glycine in distilled H_2O. Store at room temperature. It is stable for several months.
11. Running buffer (1X): dilute 100 mL of running buffer stock 10X with dH_2O, add 10mL of 10% SDS, and complete with dH_2O to a final volume of 1 L. Store at room temperature.
12. SDS sample buffer (5X): prepare a stock solution of 0.4 mL of 1 mg/mL bromophenol blue, 4 mL of 10% SDS, 2.5 mL of 0.5 M Tris-HCl (pH 6.8), 0.3 mL glycerol, and 1 mL of 14.3-M β-mercaptoethanol. Mix well, aliquot, and store at – 20°C. Before use, thaw, and warm to dissolve the SDS.
13. Tris–glycine transfer buffer stock (10X): prepare 1 L of 0.49 M Tris base and 0.08 M glycine. Store at room temperature. It is stable for several months.
14. Tris–glycine transfer buffer (1X): dilute 100 mL of Tris–glycine transfer buffer stock and 200 mL of methanol with dH_2O, add 3.6 mL of 10% SDS, and complete with dH_2O to a final volume of 1 L. Store at 4°C.
15. Dithiothreitol: prepare 1 M dithiothreitol in dH_2O. Dispense into 100-μL aliquots and store at –20°C.
16. Blocking solution: prepare in PBS containing 0.05% (v/v) Tween-20 and 5% skim milk. It can be used within 7 d if it is stored at 4°C.

17. Fixing solution for immunostaining of cells: prepare 3% (v/v) paraformaldehyde and 2% (w/v) sucrose solution by mixing 10 mL of the 16% paraformaldehyde with 1 g sucrose in a final volume of 50 mL. Aliquot and store frozen.
18. Permeabilizing buffer: 20 mM 4-2-hydroxyethyl-1-piperazineethanesulfonic acid (pH 7.4), 0.5% (v/v) Triton X-100, 50 mM NaCl, 3 mM MgCl$_2$, and 300 mM sucrose. For a 50-mL final volume, mix 1 mL of 1 M 4-2-hydroxyethyl-1-piperazineethanesulfonic acid, 0.25 mL of Triton X-100, 146 mg of NaCl, 28 µL of 5.36-M MgCl$_2$, and 5.13 g of sucrose.

3. Methods

3.1. Preparation of Phospho-Specific Antibodies to BRCA1

These antibodies were generated at Chiron Mimotopes (Melbourne, Australia) and because of commercial restrictions, we are unable to provide detailed information about the protocols. However, we have listed briefly the steps undertaken to ensure that useful phospho-specific antibody is generated.

1. The peptides (12–15 residues) corresponding to BRCA1 phosphorylation sites were synthesized on polyethylene pins that had been radiation grafted with hydroxyethylmethacrylic acid. These crowns were functionalized with Fmoc-protected aminoesters of 4-hydroxymethylphenoxyacetic to yield a free-acid C-terminus on cleavage. A cysteine residue was incorporated at the N-terminus to provide a sulfhydryl group for subsequent coupling of the peptide to an immunogenic carrier protein, diphtheria toxoid, using a maleimide group of the bifunctional reagent MCS. The quality of purified peptide was checked by ion-spray mass spectrometry, and in most instances, the peptide was more than 80% pure.
2. For injection into recipient rabbit, an aliquot of the peptide carrier protein conjugate was emulsified by mixing with 2 vol of Freund's complete adjuvant. The total volume of emulsion was 1 mL (equivalent to 0.32 mg peptide), and this was injected subcutaneously. A second similar immunization dose was emulsified by mixing with Freund's incomplete adjuvant. The first booster dose was given 14 d, following the first immunization. The rabbits were bled 2 and 4 wk later via vein puncture. The blood was incubated at 37°C for 30 min, and then incubated for overnight at 4°C. The sera were collected by centrifugation and stored at –20 to –60°C for use. The sera were tested by enzyme-linked immunosorbent assay for antibodies specificity for the nonphosphorylated and phosphorylated peptide and carrier protein. Microtiter plates were coated with saturating levels of the biotinylated form of the peptide immobilized on an avidin-coated microtiter plate. The antibody titer was defined as the reciprocal of the serum dilution that results in an absorbance of 1.0 above the background.
3. The antiserum was first passed through the nonphosphorylated peptides conjugated to thiopropyl-Sepharose 6B for enrichment of antiphosphorylated peptide antibodies in the serum. The enhanced serum was then incubated with phospho-

rylated peptide conjugated to thiopropyl-Sepharose 6B, and phosphospecific antibodies were eluted from the peptide (absorbent) by the application of general technique, such as low-pH elution.

4. The affinity-purified polyclonal antibodies to BRCA1 (Ser-1387, S-1423, S-1457, and S-1524) were successfully used to recognize the phosphorylated form of BRCA1 in response to DNA damage, using an immunoblotting technique, and these antibodies had negligible reactivity against unphosphorylated BRCA1.

3.2. Protein Samples Preparation

1. Use Epstein–Barr virus-transformed lymphoblastoid cell lines generated from control and ataxia telangiectasia patients (ATM kinase-deficient) to validate ATM kinase dependence of DNA damage-induced phosphorylation of BRCA1.
2. Culture the cells in complete RPMI-1640 culture medium at 37°C in a humidified atmosphere of 5% CO_2 (*see* **Note 1**).
3. Grow the cells to be tested to approx 80% confluence.
4. Treat the cells with either ^{6}Gy of IR using ^{137}Cs γ-ray source or expose to ultraviolet-C light at 80 J/m^2.
5. Incubate the treated cells for the required time after DNA damage.
6. Collect the treated and mock-treated cells.
7. Centrifuge the cells at 200g for 5 min at 4°C.
8. Wash the cell pellets once with cold PBS.
9. Discard supernatant, add lysis buffer (3–4X the cell pellet volume), resuspend, and incubate on ice for 30 min (*see* **Note 2**).
10. Centrifuge (16,000g) in a microfuge for 15 min at 4°C. Collect the supernatant in a new microfuge tube and estimate protein concentration using the Bio-Rad (Hercules, CA) Protein Assay Dye Reagent Concentrate (*see* **Note 3**). Store protein samples at –70°C in aliquots for use.
11. Mix 40 mg of each protein sample with 6 mL of 5X sample buffer. Heat protein samples at 95°C for 5 min in a final volume, up to 30 mL per sample per lane for immunoblotting.

3.3. Gel Preparation

This protocol is for the preparation of two Bio-Rad miniprotean gels (4.2% polyacrylamide; *see* **Notes 5–7**). Generic methods for SDS-polyacrylamide gel electrophoresis and Western blotting are given in Chapter 17.

1. Separating gel: prepare a mixture of 6 mL of dH$_2$O, 1.4 mL of 30% polyacrylamide, 2.5 mL of separating gel buffer stock, and 100 mL of 10% (w/v) SDS.
2. Stacking gel: prepare a mixture of 6.4 mL dH$_2$O, 1 mL of 30% polyacrylamide, 2.5 mL of stacking gel buffer stock, and 100 μL of 10% (w/v) SDS.
3. Add 100 μL of 10% (w/v) APS and 10 μL of TEMED to the separating gel solution. Mix immediately, swirling to avoid bubble formation. Pipet immediately the solution into the assembled glass plates up to 2 cm from the top of the front glass plate and avoid bubble formation.

4. Overlay very slowly and carefully the separating gel solution with dH_2O up to the top of the front glass plate, using a syringe.

5. Leave the gel, without disturbance in a vertical position, to polymerize at room temperature for 30 min.

6. After polymerization is completed, pour off the overlaid H_2O and wash the top of the gel several times with dH_2O to remove any unpolymerized acrylamide. Then, remove any remaining water with the edge of a paper towel.

7. Add 100 µL of 10% (w/v) APS and 10 µL of TEMED to the stacking gel solution. Mix immediately, swirling to avoid bubble formation. Pipet very carefully this solution directly onto the surface of the separating polymerized gel up to the top of the front glass plate.

8. Insert very rapidly and carefully the appropriate combs into the stacking gel solution. Let the gel to stand at room temperature for polymerization, in a vertical position without disturbance, for 20–30 min.

9. These gels can be stored at 4°C in a sealed plastic bag or in 1X running buffer to be used in the next day.

3.4. Gel Running

1. After polymerization is complete, remove the comb carefully from the stacking gel. Using a squirt bottle, wash the wells with dH_2O to remove any unpolymerized acrylamide and air bubbles. Mount the cassette into the gel apparatus and fill with 1X running buffer.

2. Load the samples in the wells by using a Hamilton syringe. Wash the syringe with buffer after each sample is loaded. Load an equal volume of 1X SDS gel sample buffer into any unused wells.

3. Run the stacking gel at 70 V until the protein dye has moved into the separating gel and forming a straight line. Increase the voltage to 90V, until the bromophenol blue runs off the gel completely. For efficient resolution of the BRCA1 band (220 kDa), keep the gel running, until the 200-kDa band of the prestained protein marker (Bio-Rad Prestained Standard, Broad Range) is 1 cm from the bottom of the separating gel. Turn off the current.

3.5. Transfer of Proteins From SDS-Polyacrylamide Gels to Nitrocellulose Filters

1. Wearing gloves, cut three pieces of Whatman 3MM paper and one piece of nitrocellulose filter per gel.

2. Remove the glass plates holding the gels from the cassette and place them in a tray containing transfer buffer for 10 min.

3. Float the nitrocellulose in a tray containing transfer buffer for 5 min and soak the Whatman paper pieces in another tray.

4. Place on one side of gel holder cassettes (Mini Trans-Blot Electrophoretic Transfer Cell, Bio-Rad) one piece of Whatman paper and squeeze out any air bubbles, using glass pipet.

5. By using the second piece of the Whatman paper, transfer the gel to the transfer apparatus. Avoid any trapped air bubbles between the filter and the gel.
6. Place the nitrocellulose filter on the top surface of the gel.
7. Place the third piece of the Whatman paper on the top surface of the nitrocellulose filter and clamp the cassette shut.
8. Assemble in the tank (the gel should be facing the cathode), insert an ice block in the tank, and fill it with cold Tris-glycine 1X transfer buffer. Apply 100 V for 1 h at 4°C. Collect the nitrocellulose filters for immunoblotting process.

3.6. Immunoblotting

See Chapter 17 for detailed methods.

1. Block the nitrocellulose filters in blocking solution for 1 h at room temperature or overnight at 4°C.
2. Incubate the filter with the required primary antibody (0.5–1 μg/mL) in blocking solution for 2 h at room temperature or overnight at 4°C.
3. Wash three times for 10 min each with PBS containing 0.05% Tween-20 at room temperature.
4. Incubate the filters with the secondary antibody in blocking solution for 1.5 h at room temperature.
5. Wash three times with PBS–Tween-20. Develop with the chemiluminescence according to the specifications of the manufacturer.

3.7. Immunofluorescence Staining With Antiphospho-Specific Antibodies

Generic methods for immunohistochemistry are given in Chapter 15.

1. Cells from normal breast epithelial cell line HBL-100 or breast carcinoma cell line MCF-7 are diluted to 3×10^4 cells/mL in RPMI-1640 media and plated in a 6-well plate with cover slips. They are re-fed the next day and then used on the second day with 50% confluency.
2. Treat cells with ice-cold paraformaldehyde solution for 10 min at 4°C.
3. Rinse twice with PBS.
4. Permeabilize 5 min with ice-cold permeabilizing buffer.
5. Rinse twice with PBS.
6. Block with 3% bovine serum albumin (BSA) in PBS at least 1 h (can be left overnight).
7. Incubate with primary antibody in 3% BSA in PBS for 90 min at room temperature. With antiphospho-BRCA1 antibodies, initial titration is done to determine which dilution allows the strongest specific signal; for most antibodies 1:500–1:1000 works well (stock concentration of proteins in enhanced antibody = 2–2.4 mg/mL; enhanced antibody will contain other proteins, so this concentration may not refer to antibody concentration).
8. Rinse twice with 1.5% BSA in PBS.

9. Incubate with secondary antibody conjugated to a fluorescent tag for 60 min.
10. Rinse with BSA in PBS and then three times with PBS.
11. Apply mountant (VectaShield; Vector Laboratories, Franklin Lakes, NJ) and mount the cover slip to slide.

4. Notes

1. RPMI-1640 medium preparation: this medium was obtained as dried mixture from JRH Biosciences (66215 OSA cat. no. 56509), Lenexa, KS. This medium is prepared by dissolving in Milli-Q water as directed by the manufacturer. Sterilize the solution by filtration through a 0.2-μm filter. Add 100 U/mL of penicillin and 100 μg/mL of streptomycin, and store at 4°C. For culture requirements, this medium should be supplemented with 10% fetal calf serum and stored at 4°C. For use, warm the media in a water bath at 37°C. To avoid any contamination, the culture needs to be carried out in a biological safety cabinet. The cells are then incubated in a cell culture incubator with a humidified atmosphere of 5% CO_2, grown to 80% confluence, and then treated with either IR or ultraviolet-C light.
2. It is very convenient to prepare large amount of protein lysates; estimate protein concentrations, aliquot, and store at –70°C to save time and costs of repeating cultures and protein preparation.
3. For accurate protein estimation, we routinely use a protein dye assay (Bio-Rad Protein Assay Dye Reagent Concentrate) as a measure of equal protein loading. Store the bottle at 4°C.
4. There are many types of mini-gel apparatus available commercially. We commonly use polyacrylamide gels apparatus from Bio-Rad Laboratories.
5. **Caution:** acrylamide and bisacrylamide are potent neurotoxic agents and are absorbed through the skin; consult material safety data sheet before using these agents.
6. Gel polymerization by TEMED is inhibited at low pH.
7. Phenylmethylsulfonyl fluoride should be added from the stock solution just before the lysis buffer is used. **Caution:** it is a destructive agent to the mucous membrane of the respiratory tract, eyes, and skin.

References

1 Scully, R. and Livingston, D. M. (2000) In search of the tumour-suppressor functions of BRCA1 and BRCA2. *Nature* **408,** 429–432.
2. Gatei, M., Scott, S., Fillipovitch, I., et al. (2000) Role of ATM in DNA-damage induced phosphorylation of BRCA1. *Cancer Res.* **60,** 3299–3304.
3. Gatei, M., Zhou, B. B., Hobson, K., Shaun, S., Young, D., and Khanna, K. K (2001) ATM and ATR phosphorylate distinct and overlapping sites on Brca1: in vivo assessment using phospho-specific antibodies manner. *J. Biol. Chem.* **276,** 17,276–17,280.
4. Chenevix-Trench, G., Spurdle, A. B., Gatei, M., et al. (2002) Dominant negative ATM mutations in breast cancer families. *J. Natl. Cancer Inst.* **94,** 205–215.
5. Lee, A. C. J., Powell, J. E., Tregear, G. W., Niall, H. D., and Stevens, V. C. (1980)

A method for preparing b-hCG COOH peptide-carrier conjugates of predictable composition. *Mol. Immunol.* **17,** 749.

6. Schaaper, W. M. M., Lankhof, H., Puijk, W., and Meloen, R. H. (1989) Manipulation of antipeptide immune response by varying the coupling of the peptide with the carrier protein. *Mol. Immunol.* **26,** 81–85.

7. Palfreyman, J. W., Aitcheson T. C., and Taylor, P. (1984) Guidelines for the production of polypeptide specific antisera using small synthetic oligopeptides as immunogens. *J. Immunol. Methods* **75,** 383–393.

31

Models of Hormone Resistance In Vitro and In Vivo

Jennifer MacGregor Schafer and V. Craig Jordan

Summary

Estrogen receptor (ER)-positive MCF-7 breast cancer cell lines can be used both in vitro and in vivo to create anti-hormone resistance. Estrogen withdrawal in vitro results in spontaneous growth of MCF-7 cells. Similarly, culture in the selective ER modulators (SERMs) tamoxifen and raloxifene, can result in SERM resistance. This form of anti-hormone resistance is evidenced by SERM-stimulated tumor growth in athymic mice. These tumors are transplantable into successive generations of overiectomized SERM treated mice. However, there is an evolution of drug resistance to anti-hormones. This is evidenced by a change in sensitivity to estrogen. The natural hormone no longer stimulated tumor growth but causes apoptosis and tumor regression.

Key Words: Tamoxifen; raloxifene; estrogen receptor; aromatase inhibitor; athymic mice.

1. Introduction

The use of in vitro and in vivo models of endocrine responsive breast cancer has greatly advanced our understanding hormonal regulation and the development of hormone resistance. In vitro models are extremely valuable, because they can readily be used; they are generally easy to maintain and provide a controlled context within which to test hormone action. The best characterized and most widely used endocrine-responsive breast cancer cells are MCF-7 cells *(1)*, which are estrogen receptor- and progesterone receptor-positive and highly estrogen-responsive *(2)*. In fact, the growth-promoting effects of estrogen and the growth inhibitory effects of antiestrogens were first defined in these cells *(3)*. This cell line has also been used extensively to study the development of drug resistance that occurs after long-term culture in the presence of an antiestrogen *(4,5)*. The method for developing a drug-resistant cell line in vitro will be described in this chapter. Whereas in vitro models of drug resistance provide a valuable tool to study mechanisms, predefined cell culture conditions may influence experimental outcomes; therefore, in vivo models have

From: *Methods in Molecular Medicine, Vol. 120: Breast Cancer Research Protocols*
Edited by: S. A. Brooks and A. L. Harris © Humana Press Inc., Totowa, NJ

been designed that better recreate the milieu in which breast cancer cells become drug resistant.

For the last two decades, athymic-mouse xenograft models of endocrine-responsive human breast cancer have been widely used to study the mechanism of drug resistance. These models were developed by inoculating ovariectomized athymic mice with human breast cancer cells to establish tumors, then treating with various hormones or anti-estrogens to determine the effects on tumor growth. Although a number of endocrine-responsive cell lines are available, again, none is more widely used than the MCF-7 model. MCF-7 human breast cancer cells readily grow into nonmetastatic solid tumors in athymic mice, with estradiol supplementation *(6)*.

Tamoxifen is an established endocrine therapy for the treatment and prevention of breast cancer *(7,8)*. Clinically, tamoxifen, which is tumoristatic, inhibits the growth of hormone-responsive breast tumors; however, after long-term treatment (2–5 yr), some tumors can develop resistance to tamoxifen. Tamoxifen is able to block estrogen-stimulated growth in athymic mice *(9)*; however, extended tamoxifen treatment for greater than 8 mo results in the appearance of estrogen receptor-positive, tamoxifen-stimulated tumors *(10)* that are transplantable *(11–13)*. These tumors require either estrogen or tamoxifen supplementation for growth (**Fig. 1**; *see* **Note 1**).

Over the last two decades, several theories to explain the mechanism of tamoxifen resistance have been advanced, such as mutant estrogen receptors, though many have been disproved; for example, the local metabolism of tamoxifen resulting in conversion to an estrogenic isomer *(14)*. Another possible mechanism has recently been published that shows a possible role for transcription activator protein-1 in development and maintenance of drug resistance. Overexpression of c-*Jun*, either artificially *(15)* or naturally occurring, over a course of antiestrogen treatment *(16)* results in the development of drug resistance by increasing the transcriptional activity of transcription activator protein-1. The involvement of growth factor receptors is also becoming central to the mechanism of drug resistance. The role of the epidermal growth factor family of growth factor receptors hormone-resistant growth and crosstalk with the estrogen receptor are receiving widespread attention. Another question that remains to be answered is what determines whether tumors will exhibit acquired or intrinsic resistance. Acquired resistance occurs over the course of drug treatment. Though an individual may initially respond to a drug, such as tamoxifen, over time, drug resistant develops. Alternatively, intrinsic resistance occurs immediately; in the case of tamoxifen, because either an individual is estrogen receptor-negative or has a nonfunctional estrogen receptor. There are also cases (that are less clear) that may result from increased growth

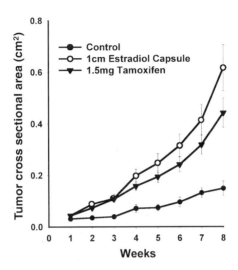

Fig. 1. Growth of retransplanted tamoxifen-stimulated MCF-7 breast cancer tumor over the course of 8 wk. Thirty mice (10 per group) were treated for 8 wk with premenopausal 1-cm 17β-estradiol capsule, 1.5 mg of oral tamoxifen, or no treatment, and measured weekly. Both estrogen and tamoxifen significantly stimulate the growth of these tumors, whereas control tumors grow at a much slower pace.

factor expression, for example. The use of the athymic-mouse xenograft has provided a model to study the progression from hormone-responsive to hormone-resistant and will be described in this chapter.

A recent interesting aspect of acquired drug resistance to tamoxifen is that after 5 yr of tamoxifen treatment, estrogen can act as a tumoricidal agent. This has been shown in vitro by long-term estrogen deprivation of MCF-7 cells, resulting in MCF-7 cells that are growth-inhibited by high-dose estrogen. The mechanism for this phenomenon involves Fas-mediated apoptosis *(17)*. In addition, in xenograft models using these estrogen-deprived MCF-7 cells, high-dose estrogen also inhibits growth. The tumoricidal effects of estrogen are also apparent in the in vivo progression of tamoxifen-treated MCF-7 tumors. Initially, estrogen-stimulated MCF-7 cells are growth-inhibited by tamoxifen, but over time, tamoxifen-stimulated tumors develop that remain responsive to estrogen *(11,18)*. However, during long-term treatment, these tumors cycle through many unique phenotypes, even becoming tamoxifen-stimulated and estrogen-inhibited *(19)*. These xenograft models of drug resistance provide a valuable tool for the investigation into the mechanism of hormone resistance and provide a useful insight into the evolution of endocrine responsive breast cancer in patients.

2. Materials

1. Sterile T75 and T185 polystyrene cell culture flasks.
2. RPMI-1640 cell culture media containing phenol red (cat. no. 11875-093; Invitrogen, Grand Island, NY): under sterile conditions, supplement 500 mL of RPMI-1640 with 10% heat-inactivated fetal bovine serum (cat. no. 12484-028, Invitrogen; heat inactivate at 60°C for 30 min), 2 mM glutamine (cat. no. 12381-018, Invitrogen), 6 ng/mL of bovine insulin (cat. no. 1-6634; Sigma, St. Louis, MO), 5 mL of antibiotic/antimycotic (cat. no. 1524-062, Invitrogen), and 1X nonessential amino acids (cat. no. 12383-014, Invitrogen). Store complete growth media at 4°C.
3. Sterile Hanks buffered salt solution (HBSS): add 500 mL of 10X Hanks buffered saline to 4.5 L of milli-Q water. Stir in 1.75 g of $NaCO_3$, 29.8 g of 4-2-hydroxyethyl-1-piperazineethanesulfonic acid, and 1.75 g of ethylenediamine-tetraacetic acid; adjust pH to 7.38 using 10 N NaOH. Filter sterilize using 0.2-μm pore filter polyethersulfone membrane. Store at 4°C.
4. 0.5% Trypsin (cat. no. 15090-046, Invitorgen): dilute 2.5% trypsin to 0.5% in sterile HBSS under sterile conditions. Store at 0°C.
5. 4-Hydroxytamoxifen ([4-OHT] cat. no. H7904, Sigma) (*see* **Note 2**): prepare a 1-mM solution by dissolving 4-OHT in 100% ethanol. Store at 0°C in a clean amber glass vial with a tight-fitting lid to prevent evaporation, which would alter the concentration.
6. Ovariectomized 4- to 5-wk-old Balb/c nu/nu mice (Harlan Sprague Dawley, Madison, WI).
7. Animal surgical equipment including scissors, forceps, trochar, staple remover, stapler, staples (wound clips), scalpels, and sterile Petri dishes.
8. Sterile field, alcohol swabs, Betadine® swabs, 1-cc syringes, 19- and 22-gage needles, 20-gage × 1.5 gavage needles (cat. no. 9921; Popper and Sons, New Hyde Park, NY), sterile gloves, dry ice, and airtight chamber.
9. Anesthetic: 100 mg/mL of ketamine HCl (cat. no. 301-2025; Fort Dodge Animal Health, Fort Dodge, IA) and 20 mg/mL of xylazine (cat. no. 4401G ; Vetus Animal Health, Westbury, NY), mix 0.3 mL of ketamine with 0.5 mL of xylazine. Ketamine is a controlled substance; therefore, take appropriate precautions. Anesthetic is stable for 1 d.
10. Tamoxifen (cat. no. T-5648, Sigma) is first dissolved in 3 mL of the Tween-80 (cat. no. p8074, Sigma)/polyethylene glycol 400 (cat. no. p3265, Sigma) (add 0.5 mL of Tween-80 to 99.5 mL of the polyethylene glycol 400) and 3 mL of 100% ethanol, followed by vortexing. Ethanol is evaporated under nitrogen before use. After ethanol is evaporated, add 27 mL of 1% carboxymethylcellulose (add 1 g of [medium viscosity] carboxymethylcellulose [cat. no. C-9481, Sigma] to 100 mL of double distilled H_2O. Stir overnight (it takes a long time to dissolve) for a total volume of 30 mL; vortex well. Store at 4°C and wrap in foil. For a final concentration of 0.5 mg/0.05 mL, we usually measure out 300 mg of tamoxifen into a total volume of 30 mL (*see* **Note 3**).

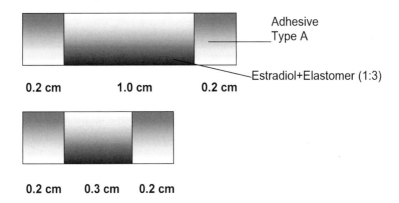

Fig. 2. A diagrammatic representation of estradiol capsules. The 0.2-cm ends are filled with adhesive, whereas the middle section contains the estradiol–elastomer mix. The 0.3-cm capsules deliver a postmenopausal dose of estradiol, whereas the 1-cm capsules deliver a premenopausal dose of estradiol (*see* **Note 4**).

11. 17 β-estradiol capsules. Components: estradiol (cat. no. E-8875, Sigma) Veterinary Silicone Tubing (cat. no. 602-155; Dow Corning, Midland, MI), Surgical Medical Grade Elastomer (Dow Corning, Midland, MI, cat. no. MDX4-4210), and Medical Adhesive Silicone Type A, Factor II (Dow Corning, Midland, MI, cat. no. A100).

   a. Estradiol preparation: weigh the amount of estradiol needed, e.g., weigh 500 mg for 20 1-cm estradiol capsules. Weigh the amount of elastomer needed based on the amount of estradiol in a 1:3 ratio, i.e., 500 mg of estradiol = 1.5 g of elastomer. Mix estradiol and elastomer until it becomes a homogenous paste. Load paste into a 3-cc syringe. Cut tip off screw-cap that comes packaged on the syringe (do not unscrew cap, just cut off the tip), place a 200-μL pipet tip on top of cap, replace plunger, and use.

   b. Capsule preparation: there are two capsule sizes that we use, 1-cm (premenopausal) and 0.3-cm (postmenopausal) (*see* **Note 4**). The following describes measuring of tubing to make the capsule. Add 0.2 cm to each end of the desired length (0.3 or 1.0 cm), i.e., total length used for a 1-cm capsule is 1.4-cm tubing (0.7-cm tubing for a 0.3-cm capsule) (**Fig. 2**). This extra space is for the silastic adhesive that will be put inside to "cap" the ends. Using a marker, measure out the number of capsules (using the method outlined) on tubing and cut with a razor blade. "Inject" estradiol plus elastomer into capsule; do not allow any drug to seep into the 0.2-cm ends. Seal ends with Type A Adhesive; adhesive can be administered with a syringe (put adhesive into a 3-cc syringe with an 18-gage needle; cut needle to 0.5 cm from the base). Adhesive takes about 2 h to dry. Once dry, spray capsules with ethanol and γ-cell irradiate capsules for at least 30 min.

3. Methods

3.1. Development of In Vitro Models of Drug Resistance

3.1.1. Cell Culture

The following protocol uses the standard methods of cell culture and can be applied for the growth of most epithelial breast cancer cell lines that grow in monolayers. For our purposes, we will describe the propagation of the MCF-7 cell line, as it is commonly used in both in vitro and in vivo studies of hormone resistance. All of the procedures in this section take place under sterile conditions.

1. Warm all media, HBSS, and trypsin to 37°C before use.
2. Dispense 2.5×10^{-5} MCF-7 cells (originally obtained from American Type Culture Collection, Rockville, MD) into a T75 tissue culture flask with 10 mL of complete RPMI growth media. Cells grow in a monolayer. Cells should be stored in a 37°C incubator with 5% carbon dioxide.
3. Change media every 2–3 d until cells reach 80% confluence.
4. Once cells are 80% confluent, split cells by first removing RPMI carefully so as not to disrupt the monolayer of cells.
5. Wash cells by incubating with 10 mL of sterile HBSS for 1 min and remove carefully HBSS.
6. Incubate with 0.5 mL of 0.5% trypsin for approx 3 min or until gentle disruption of flask results in release of monolayer.
7. Add 10 mL of complete growth media to inactivate trypsin and resuspend to a single cell suspension by pipetting up and down 10 times.
8. Transfer 1 mL of cell suspension to a new sterile T75 flasks with 9 mL of fresh RPMI for a 1:10 dilution, and continue to grow in a 37°C incubator with 5% CO_2. Repeat process approximately once per week.

3.1.2. Drug Treatment

Developing an in vitro drug resistance model is a relatively simple process, but it takes places gradually over the course of months or years. In our example of MCF-7 cells, the progression to tamoxifen resistance occurs over the course of a year.

1. Culture MCF-7 cells as described in **Subheading 3.1.1.**
2. After splitting cells to 1:10, allow cells to settle by incubating overnight in a 37°C incubator with 5% CO_2.
3. Once cells have attached to the plate, supplement the media with 1 μM of 4-OHT (*see* **Note 2**) by adding 10 μL of 1-mM 4-OHT. When adding 4-OHT, which is dissolved in ethanol, diligently add the drug directly to the media, because any direct contact of the ethanol to the cells will be lethal.
4. Cells with go through an initial growth arrest; continue to change the media and add drug every 2–3 d, but do not split cells until they are at least 70% confluent, which may take up to 1 mo.

5. Over the course of 6–12 mo, a population of cells will be selected that grow maximally, irrespective of the presence or absence of 4-OHT in the media. This is an in vitro model of drug resistance (*see* **Note 5**).

3.2. Development of In Vivo Models of Drug Resistance

3.2.1. Preparation of Cells for Injection

The following describes the harvesting of 4-OHT-resistant MCF-7 cells, ultimately, for inoculation into 30 athymic mice (described in **Subheading 3.2.2.**). Mice are bilaterally injected with 10×10^6 cells per side; therefore, we calculate the total number of cells based on the number of mice to be injected bilaterally.

1. To prepare cells for injection in 30 mice, 60×10^7 4-OHT-resistant MCF-7 cells, grown in the presence of 1 μM of 4-OHT, should be grown up to 80% confluence in T150 tissue culture flasks.
2. Cells should be rinsed once with 10 mL of sterile HBSS and released using 0.75 mL of 0.5% trypsin; then, gently disrupt cells before resuspending in 10 mL of RPMI for a single cell suspension. Place on ice until further use.
3. Cells should then be counted using a hemocytometer. Count number of cells in four large squares, and then use the following formula: no. cells ÷ 4 × 10^4 × dilution factor (if any) = total number of cells.
4. Pellet cells by spinning in a 4°C centrifuge and resupend pellet in sterile HBSS to a concentration 10×10^6 cells per 0.1 mL (*see* **Note 6**). Keep cells on ice and proceed directly to the next protocol.

3.2.2. Injection of Cells Into Athymic Mice

The use of animal models requires additional support from the animal care and use committee of each institution to provide approval for proposed protocols, maintenance, and veterinary care. The following protocol utilizes 30 mice to be separated into three treatment groups: no treatment, 1-cm estradiol capsule, and 1.5 mg of tamoxifen.

1. Once ovariectomized 4- to 5-wk-old old Balb/c nu/nu mice (Harlan Sprague Dawley) arrive and are set up; they should be allowed to 2–3 d to settle before any procedure is performed.
2. Divide mice into treatment groups by labeling cages. Generally, treatment groups consist of 10 mice each.
3. Spray surface of flow hood with disinfectant and cover work surface with sterile field. Set up surgical equipment and alcohol and Betadine swabs. Make up 0.8 mL of anesthetic in a 1-cc syringe with a 22-gage needle.
4. Before anesthesia, feed the 1.5-mg tamoxifen group by oral gavage. Specifically, using a 1-cc syringe, draw 1 cc of 0.5-mg/mL tamoxifen and attach gavage needle. Slightly bend gavage needle. Holding the mouse by the scruff and tail in one hand, with the other, work the gavage needle to the back of the throat and insert

needle into esophagus then to stomach; avoid significant resistance. For each mouse, inject 0.15 cc to deliver a dose of 1.5 mg tamoxifen (*see* **Note 7**).

5. Intraperitoneal anesthesia: to anesthetize a mouse, immobilize by grabbing scruff and tail with one hand, exposing the abdomen. With the other hand, tilt the mouse so the head is at the lowest point and inject into the lower left quadrant to avoid injecting colon or bladder. Swab with alcohol and inject 0.02 cc of anesthetic (*see* **Note 8**).

6. Prepare mouse for subcutaneous injection by swabbing area on the back, between the shoulders, first with Betadine, then with alcohol (*see* **Note 9**).

7. Using a 1-cc syringe, draw 0.4 mL of cell suspension (*see* **Note 10**), being careful to mix suspension to homogeneity, then attach 19-gage needle.

8. Cut a small hole in the intraclavicular area of the back and insert needle subcutaneously; carefully work syringe forward into axillary mammary fat pad and inject 0.1 mL of cell suspension, forming a pocket. Place a finger between pocket of cells and needle before pulling needle out to prevent dispersion of cells.

9. Implantation of estradiol capsule: irradiated estradiol capsule can be implanted subcutaneously by inserting the capsule, using forceps, through the same incision that was used to inject the cell.

10. Using forceps, pull the edges of the incision in the back together and staple.

11. Ensure mice recover from anesthetic before leaving them (*see* **Note 11**).

12. Tamoxifen is administered orally at 1.5 mg per mouse per day, 5 d/wk. Control and estradiol groups do not require any further treatment.

13. Tumor measurements should be performed weekly using vernier calipers. The cross-sectional tumor area is calculated using the formula: length $\times$ width $\div 4 \times \pi$ (*see* **Note 12**).

3.2.3 Retransplantation of Tumors

There are several benefits to retransplanting tumors compared to performing experiments by injecting cells. Retransplanting tumors allows the use of a single tumor for transplantation of up to 100 mice, resulting in a homogenous test population. In addition, retransplantation allows continued in vivo long-term treatment of tumor to acquire multiple drug resistant phenotypes.

1. Identify tumor for retransplantation (*see* **Note 13**) and label cages.

2. Before anesthesia, feed the 1.5-mg tamoxifen group by oral gavage as described in **Subheading 3.2.2.**, **step 4**.

3. One person should begin to anesthetize mice as described in **Subheading 3.2.2.**, **step 5**, concurrent with the harvesting of the tumor.

4. Place mouse bearing the tumor in an airtight chamber with dry ice until it dies. Remove the mouse promptly.

5. Using scissors and forceps, remove tumor, separating carefully tumor tissue from mouse tissue. Place tumor in sterile Petri dish.

6. Using a scalpel, promptly cut tumor into required number of 1-mm^3 pieces (implanting mice bilaterally, therefore, two pieces per mouse). When finished cutting, supplement with 2 mL of RPMI-1640 growth media.

7. Prepare anesthetized mouse with Betadine and alcohol as described in **Subheading 3.2.2., step 6**, and make a short, intraclavicular incision using scissors.
8. Load trocar with one tumor piece and insert trocar into incision and work to past axilla to mammary fat pad and then release tumor piece, place finger between tumor and trocar, and remove trocar.
9. Implant capsule in appropriate groups as described in **Subheading 3.2.2., step 9**.
10. Using forceps, pull the edges of the incision in the back together and staple.
11. Ensure mice recover from anesthetic before leaving them.
12. Tamoxifen is administered orally at 1.5 mg per mouse per day, 5 d/wk. Control and estradiol groups do not require any further treatment.
13. Tumor measurements should be performed weekly using vernier calipers. The cross-sectional tumor area is calculated using the formula: length $\times$ width $\div 4 \times \pi$.

4. Notes

1. A very important distinction must be made in the definition of drug resistance. Cases occur in which cells grow equally well being treated with or without an anti-estrogen present, as is the case of the in vitro model described here. However, certain in vivo models produce tumors that grow only in the presence of anti-estrogens; these tumors, too, are drug resistant, though they are anti-estrogen-stimulated. To this point, it has not been possible to derive an anti-estrogen-stimulated cell line in vitro. It is believed that certain host factors (i.e., stromal interactions) are necessary to support this type of growth.
2. Tamoxifen is a drug currently used for the treatment and prevention of breast cancer. When doing in vitro studies on tamoxifen, an important distinction must be made between the parent drug tamoxifen and the active metabolite 4-OHT. Tamoxifen cannot be metabolized in vitro; therefore, 4-OHT is used instead of tamoxifen for studies in vitro.
3. Tamoxifen at 0.5 mg orally per day resulted in serum levels of tamoxifen of 58 ± 7 ng/mL and at 1.5 mg 203 $\pm$ 100 ng/mL (mean $\pm$ standard deviation) *(20)*. Circulating levels of tamoxifen in patients are approx 160 ng/mL *(21)*.
4. The 0.3-cm estrogen capsules produced a mean 83.8 pg/mL of serum estrogen, whereas 1.0-cm estrogen capsules produced a mean 379.5 pg/mL of serum estrogen *(20)*. Each was designed to represent the low or high estrogen levels observed in post- or premenopausal women, respectively. Estrogen capsules must be replaced every 8–10 weeks.
5. Tamoxifen is tumoristatic, so cells will lie dormant for several weeks. Continue to change the media and supplement with 4-OHT. Cells will then begin to die, but do not split until cells have grown back to at least 25% confluence.
6. Anticipate that some cells will be lost in the harvesting and resuspending protocol, so start with more cells than the final amount needed. In addition, when resuspending cells for injection, make an additional 0.3 mL to insure adequate material for injection.
7. Volume of drug can be adjusted depending on the required dose of compound; however, the maximum allowable volume for gavage should not exceed 0.15 cc. Silastic E_2 capsules should be replaced every 8–10 wk.

8. It is important to inject only 0.02 cc of anesthetic, because mice vary in size, age, and sensitivity to the anesthetic and, therefore, may easily be overanesthetized, resulting in mortality. If mouse is inadequately anesthetized, an additional dose can always be given. In addition, after anesthesia is given, mice become hyperactive, so appropriate measures must be taken to secure mice from escaping (i.e., in cage with lid on).
9. Proceed in a timely manner to reduce decrease in cell viability.
10. Mix cell suspension (do not vortex) adequately before filling syringe to ensure consistent concentration of cells per injection site. In the beginning, start by filling the syringe with 0.2 mL (enough for bilateral injection of one mouse) until familiarity with the protocol occurs to prevent cells from settling in the syringe.
11. Once the procedure is finished, monitor the anesthetized mice until they wake up, and remove any dead mice.
12. Tumors can be snap frozen in liquid nitrogen for later use for protein, RNA, or DNA manipulations. It is important to remove tumors and freeze quickly to reduce RNA degradation.
13. To identify the best tumor for retransplantation, assess each tumor based on the following parameters: size (approx 1 cm^2), relatively round, and firm when gently squeezed. After harvesting tumor and removing any attached skin, ensure that the center of the tumor is not necrotic. Also, try to avoid using the fibrous center.

Acknowledgments

This work has been supported by the Department of Defense Breast Cancer Training grant DAMD 17-94-J-4466, DAMD 17-96-1-6169, P30 CA60553-09; National Research Service award T32 DK07169 (Dr. Schafer); NIH SPORE in Breast Cancer 1P50 CA89018-02 (Dr. Jordan); the Lynn Sage Breast Cancer Research Foundation of Northwestern Memorial Hospital; and the Avon Foundation.

References

1. Soule, H. D., Vazguez, J., Long, A., Albert, S., and Brennan, M. (1973) A human cell line from a pleural effusion derived from a breast carcinoma. *J. Natl. Cancer Inst.* **51,** 1409–1416.
2. Horwitz, K. B., Costlow, M. E., and McGuire, W. L. (1975) MCF-7; a human breast cancer cell line with estrogen, androgen, progesterone, and glucocorticoid receptors. *Steroids* **26,** 785–795.
3. Lippman, M., Bolan, G., and Huff, K. (1976) The effects of estrogens and antiestrogens on hormone-responsive human breast cancer in long-term tissue culture. *Cancer Res.* **36,** 4595–4601.
4. Brunner, N., Frandsen, T. L., Holst-Hansen, C., et al. (1993) MCF7/LCC2: a 4-hydroxytamoxifen resistant human breast cancer variant that retains sensitivity to the steroidal antiestrogen ICI 182,780. *Cancer Res.* **53,** 3229–3232.
5. Brunner, N., Boysen, B., Jirus, S., et al. (1997) MCF7/LCC9: an antiestrogen-resistant MCF-7 variant in which acquired resistance to the steroidal antiestrogen

ICI 182,780 confers an early cross-resistance to the nonsteroidal antiestrogen tamoxifen. *Cancer Res.* **57**, 3486–3493.

6. Levenson, A. S. and Jordan, V. C. (1997) MCF-7: the first hormone-responsive breast cancer cell line. *Cancer Res.* **57**, 3071–3078.

7. Early Breast Cancer Trialists' Collaborative Group (1998) Tamoxifen for early breast cancer: an overview of the randomised trials. *Lancet* **351**, 1451–1467.

8. Fisher, B., Costantino, J. P., Wickerham, D. L., et al. (1998) Tamoxifen for prevention of breast cancer: report of the National Surgical Adjuvant Breast and Bowel Project P-1 Study. *J. Natl. Cancer Inst.* **90**, 1371–1388.

9. Osborne, C. K., Hobbs, K., and Clark, G. M. (1985) Effect of estrogens and antiestrogens on growth of human breast cancer cells in athymic nude mice. *Cancer Res.* **45**, 584–590.

10. Osborne, C. K., Coronado, E. B., and Robinson, J. P. (1987) Human breast cancer in the athymic nude mouse: cytostatic effects of long-term antiestrogen therapy. *Eur. J. Cancer Clin. Oncol.* **23**, 1189–1196.

11. Gottardis, M. M. and Jordan, V. C. (1988) Development of tamoxifen-stimulated growth of MCF-7 tumors in athymic mice after long-term antiestrogen administration. *Cancer Res.* **48**, 5183–5187.

12. Gottardis, M. M., Wagner, R. J., Borden, E. C., and Jordan, V. C. (1989) Differential ability of antiestrogens to stimulate breast cancer cell (MCF-7) growth in vivo and in vitro. *Cancer Res.* **49**, 4765–4769.

13. Gottardis, M. M., Jiang, S. Y., Jeng, M. H., and Jordan, V. C. (1989) Inhibition of tamoxifen-stimulated growth of an MCF-7 tumor variant in athymic mice by novel steroidal antiestrogens. *Cancer Res.* **49**, 4090–4093.

14. Wolf, D. M., Langan-Fahey, S. M., Parker, C. J., McCague, R., and Jordan, V. C. (1993) Investigation of the mechanism of tamoxifen-stimulated breast tumor growth with nonisomerizable analogues of tamoxifen and metabolites. *J. Natl. Cancer Inst.* **85**, 806–812.

15. Smith, L. M., Wise, S. C., Hendricks, D. T., Sabichi, et al. (1999) c-*Jun* overexpression in MCF-7 breast cancer cells produces a tumorigenic, invasive and hormone resistant phenotype. *Oncogene* **18**, 6063–6070.

16. Schiff, R., Reddy, P., Ahotupa, M., et al. (2000) Oxidative stress and AP-1 activity in tamoxifen-resistant breast tumors in vivo. *J. Natl. Cancer Inst.* **92**, 1926–1934.

17. Song, R. X., Mor, G., Naftolin, F., et al. (2001) Effect of long-term estrogen deprivation on apoptotic responses of breast cancer cells to 17beta-estradiol. *J. Natl. Cancer Inst.* **93**, 1714–1723.

18. Gottardis, M. M., Robinson, S. P., and Jordan, V. C. (1988) Estradiol-stimulated growth of MCF-7 tumors implanted in athymic mice: a model to study the tumoristatic action of tamoxifen. *J. Steroid Biochem.* **30**, 311–314.

19. Yao, K., Lee, E., Bentrem, D. J., et al. (2000) Antitumor action of physiological estradiol on tamoxifen-stimulated breast tumors grown in athymic mice. *Clin. Cancer Res.* **6**, 2028–2036.

20. O'Regan, R. M., Cisneros, A., England, G. M., et al. (1998) Effects of the antiestrogens tamoxifen, toremifene, and ICI 182,780 on endometrial cancer growth. *J. Natl. Cancer Inst.* **90**, 1552–1558.

21. Langan-Fahey, S. M., Tormey, D. C., and Jordan, V. C. (1990) Tamoxifen metabolites in patients on long-term adjuvant therapy for breast cancer. *Eur. J. Cancer* **26,** 883–888.

32

Generation of Genetically Modified Embryonic Stem Cells for the Development of Knockout Mouse Animal Model Systems

Stephen D. Robinson, Stephen Wilson, and Kairbaan M. Hodivala-Dilke

Summary

The aim of our lab is to understand the contributions made by cell adhesion molecules in the processes of disease. Much of our recent work has focused on the role played by $\beta3$-integrin in mediating pathological angiogenesis. It is fair to state that without the ability to manipulate the mouse genome, and specifically to create knockout mice, the advances we have made in this field would not be nearly as significant as they are. The ability to generate knockout mice depends on the two technological breakthroughs of the ability to isolate and culture mouse embryonic stem (ES) cells and the methods employed for achieving targeted gene replacement in these cells by homologous recombination. Here, we present the methods we have found to be successful, and that we routinely employ to grow and manipulate ES cells, as well as those to screen and identify homologous recombinants.

Key Words: ES cells; knockout mice; gene-targeting; recombinase; homologous recombination.

1. Introduction

The ability to generate knockout mice has, unquestionably, revolutionized our understanding of multiple aspects of mammalian biology, from development to adult pathology, and the techniques involved have been applied across a broad spectrum of fields. Here, we provide the techniques used to generate homologously recombined embryonic stem (ES) cells carrying precise genetic alterations. The outcome of altering an endogenous gene to create a null, or "knockout," mutation comes with some inherent problems that can limit its use in many studies. These are worth considering when contemplating any knockout approach. The two most common problems encountered are embryonic lethality and developmental compensation by other genes. Both of these inhibit full analysis of a gene's function in the adult organism.

From: *Methods in Molecular Medicine, Vol. 120: Breast Cancer Research Protocols*
Edited by: S. A. Brooks and A. L. Harris © Humana Press Inc., Totowa, NJ

Recently, strategies have been designed that allow for site and/or time-specific DNA recombination in ES cells or living animals *(1–3)*. These strategies, in many instances, can circumvent an embryonic lethal phenotype, allowing for analysis in the adult. In addition, because not every cell in the organism carries the mutation, genetic compensation is frequently not an issue. The two most commonly used systems utilize either the cyclization recombination, or *cre*, gene of bacteriophage P1 *(4,5)* or the flippase, or *Flp*, site-specific recombinase from *Saccharomyces cerevisiae (6–9)*. *Cre* and *Flp* recombinases can efficiently excise DNA segments flanked by two *loxP* sites or two *Flp*-recombinase target sites, respectively. Spatially or temporally controlled recombination is accomplished by placing the appropriate recombinase under the control of a cell-specific or inducible promoter *(10–15)*. These systems are being improved and refined all the time, and it is becoming increasingly evident that combining cell-specificity with temporal regulation can be a very powerful tool *(16)*. In addition, by combining the two recombinase systems, additional subtleties may be introduced.

Because of space limitations, we will not discuss the methods involved in creating a targeting construct (however, *see* **Note 1**). In addition, the protocols we present stop at the production of genetically altered ES cells that are ready for blastocyst injection. The techniques involved in establishing chimeras from ES cells, and the breeding of these animals to produce mutant mice are discussed in **refs.** *17* and *18*.

2. Materials

1. 5% CO_2, 37°C tissue culture incubator.
2. Electroporation apparatus (we use a Bio-Rad [UK] Gene Pulser II, cat. no. 165-2105, with a capacitance extender).
3. Stratagene (UK) UV crosslinker.
3. Roller bottle hybridization oven.
4. Sealing film (cat. no. Z36,966-7; Sigma, UK).
5. Electroporation cuvets (cat. no. 165-2088, Bio-Rad).
6. Qiagen maxi plasmid purification kit (cat. no. 12263; Qiagen, UK).
7. Qiaquick nucleotide removal kit (cat. no. 28306, Qiagen).
8. Zeta Probe GT membrane (cat. no. 162-0197, Bio-Rad).
9. 0.25% Trypsin in ethylenediaminetetraacetic acid ([EDTA] cat. no. 25300-054, Invitrogen, UK).
10. Trypan blue solution (cat. no. T8154, Sigma).
11. Phenol/chloroform/isoamyl alcohol, 25:24:1 (cat. no. 77617, Sigma).
12. Chloroform/isoamyl alcohol, 24:1 ([v:v] cat. no. C0549, Sigma).
13. ES cell-qualified fetal bovine serum (FBS) (*see* **Note 2**).
14. High-glucose Dulbecco's modified Eagle's medium ([DMEM] cat. no. 11960, Invitrogen). Supplement with 1 m*M* sodium pyruvate, and 2 m*M* L-glutamine. Stock bottles can be prepared a couple of months in advance and stored at 4°C.

15. Murine embryonic fibroblast (MEF) growth medium DMEM, as above, supplemented with FBS (10%).
16. Freezing medium: 90% FBS and 10% dimethyl sulfoxide.
17. ES cell medium: DMEM, as above, supplemented with 15% FBS, 0.1 mM nonessential amino acids, 0.1 mM β-mercaptoethanol, 50 μg/mL gentamycin, and 1000 U/mL of leukemia inhibitory factor (Esgro®, available from Chemicon International [Temecula, CA], cat. no. ESG1107). After preparation, store at 4°C and use within 2 wk.
18. 96-Well plate freezing medium: 20% dimethyl sulfoxide and 80% ES cell medium.
19. 1% Roccal® solution. Roccal is a disinfectant that can be purchased as a 10X concentrate from any veterinary surgical supply company.
20. Sterile 0.1% gelatin (cat. no. G1890, Sigma). A 0.1% solution is prepared in distilled water and autoclaved to dissolve and sterilize. Store gelatin solution at 4°C and use within 2 mo.
21. DNA lysis buffer: 10 mM Tris-HCl (pH 7.5), 10 mM EDTA, 10 mM NaCl, 0.5% sarcosyl, and 2 mg/mL proteinase K. This can be prepared in advance and stored indefinitely at room temperature. However, proteinase K should be added just before use. Stock proteinase K is prepared at a concentration of 10 mg/mL in water. Aliquot the stock and store at –20°C. Do not refreeze the stock solution.
22. 10X loading buffer: one part 20X saline–sodium citrate (SSC) to one part glycerol, with addition of 0.3% bromophenol blue and 0.3% xylene cyanol. Can be stored indefinitely at room temperature.
23. 10 mg/mL of ethidium bromide solution. **Caution:** ethidium bromide is a potent carcinogen. Always wear gloves when handling and be extremely cautious if weighing out powder. In addition, ethidium bromide is light-sensitive and must be stored in the dark.
24. 0.5 M Phosphate buffer (PB): prepare 1 L of stock A as 0.5 M NaH$_2$PO$_4$ and 1 L of stock B as 0.5 M Na$_2$HPO$_4$. Mix 316 mL of stock A with 684 mL of stock B to make 1 L of 0.5 M PB, pH 7.2. Filter sterilize the PB. All three solutions can be stored at room temperature indefinitely.
25. Southern hybridization buffer: 0.25 M PB, 7% sodium dodecyl sulfate (SDS) and 1 mM of EDTA.
26. 10 mg/mL of random hexanucleotide primers (cat. no. 1034 731, Roche, UK). Dilute in water, aliquot, and store at –20°C indefinitely.
27. 1 N NaOH solution.
28. 1 M Tris-HCl, pH 7.5.
29. Random priming buffer (10X stock): 0.5 M Tris-HCl (pH 7.4), 50 mM MgCl$_2$, and 0.1 M β-mercaptoethanol. Aliquot and store at –20°C indefinitely.
30. Deoxynucleotide 5'-triphosphate mixture (cat. no. 1969 064, Roche). Prepare a mixture of 300 μM each of deoxyadenosine 5'-triphosphate, deoxyguanosine 5'-triphosphate, and deoxythymidine 5'-triphosphate. Aliquot and store at –20°C indefinitely.
31. ^{32}P-deoxycytidine 5'-triphosphate 3000 Ci/mmol (Redivue from Amersham [UK], cat. no. A0005). **Caution:** ensure handler is properly trained and licensed in the use of radioactive compounds.

32. Labeling grade Klenow enzyme (cat. no. 1008 412, Roche).
33. Southern rinse buffer: 20 m*M* PB, 1% SDS, and 1 m*M* of EDTA.
34. Salt extraction DNA buffer: 10 m*M* Tris-HCl (pH 7.4), 10 m*M* EDTA (pH 8.0), and 144 m*M* NaCl.
35. Sterile Tris-EDTA (TE): 10 m*M* Tris-HCl (pH 7.5), 1 m*M* EDTA (pH 8.0) solution, filter sterilized. This solution can be stored indefinitely at room temperature.
36. 13–14-d-postconception pregnant mice.
37. Low-passage ES cells.

3. Methods

3.1. Production of MEF Stocks (see Note 3)

1. Kill the 13–14-d-pregnant mouse and place in 1% Roccal solution for 5 min. Place mouse on paper towel and swab the abdomen with 70% ethanol. Dissect out the uterus aseptically into a sterile container.
2. Transfer the uterus into a 100-mm dish containing PBS, and dissect out each embryo, paying special attention to remove all membranes. Remove heads and all internal organs, and then place prepared embryo into a sterile glass universal containing DMEM. Repeat this until all embryos have been processed.
3. Wash embryos in DMEM at least three times to remove as much blood as possible. Remove the final wash and mince the carcasses, with scissors, into small pieces (approx 1 mm in diameter). Wash a further three times, allowing the tissue to settle between each wash.
4. Remove final wash and add prewarmed 0.25% trypsin/EDTA to a final volume of 20 mL. Add a sterile plastic stirring bar and incubate at 37°C on a stirring plate for 20–30 min. Occasionally, pipet suspension during this time to aid the digestion process.
5. Decant cell suspension into a 50-mL centrifuge tube containing 5 mL of FBS to neutralize the trypsin activity. Add DMEM to a final volume of 50 mL. Centrifuge at 200–300*g* for 10 min.
6. Aspirate supernatant and discard. Resuspend the pellet in 50 mL of MEF growth medium. Allow any undigested clumps of tissue to settle out and decant as necessary.
7. Perform a viable cell count using Trypan blue. Nonviable cells will stain blue. Count using a hemocytometer. **Note:** if this mixture stands for too long, viable cells will begin to stain with the Trypan blue as well.
8. Calculate cell concentration and plate between 5×10^6 and 10^7 viable cells per 100-mm tissue culture dish in 10 mL of MEF growth medium. Evenly disperse cells by rocking the dish gently, and then return it to the incubator and culture overnight.
9. Change the medium after 24 h to remove any cell debris.
10. Two to three days after plating the MEF, cells should have reached confluency. At this point, cells can be frozen, subcultured, or mitotically inactivated.

3.1.1. Freezing MEFs

If cells are to be frozen, between 5 and 10 dishes can be stored per freezing vial in 1 mL of freezing medium. Vials may be left at –70°C for short-term storage or placed in liquid nitrogen for long-term storage. When required, cells should be thawed rapidly at 37°C and plated onto twice the number of dishes from which they were frozen. Cells should reach confluency in 3–5 d.

3.1.2. Subculturing MEFs

If cells are to be subcultured, perform a 1:5 to 1:8 split. The cells should reach confluency after 3–4 d.

3.2. Mitotic Inactivation of MEFs

MEFs used to prepare feeder cells can either be thawed and subcultured or used from freshly prepared confluent MEFs. Under small-scale laboratory conditions, it is ideal to prepare stocks of frozen feeder cells. Each stock should be prepared from between 50 and 100 confluent 100-mm dishes of MEFs.

1. Remove the medium from the MEFs and wash twice with PBS.
2. Add 0.5 mL of 0.25% trypsin/EDTA to each 100-mm dish, then incubate at 37°C until cells have detached from the plate (approx 5 min). Plates may be tapped gently, if necessary, to assist in this process.
3. Neutralize the trypsin by adding 5 mL of MEF growth medium to each plate. Pool all the cell suspensions and break up any cell clumps by pipetting up and down.
4. Centrifuge cells at 200–300g for 5 min and resuspend pellet in 10 mL of DMEM. Repeat this rinse.
5. Expose the MEF cell suspension to 3000–10,000 rad of γ-irradiation.
6. Perform a viability count using Trypan blue.
7. Centrifuge cells at 200–300g for 5 min and resuspend pellet in MEF freezing medium. Cells should be frozen in 1 mL of freezing medium at a concentration of between 10^7 and 2×10^7 viable cells per milliliter. Store vials at –70°C for 1 d, and then transfer them to liquid nitrogen for long-term storage. A small volume of cells should be kept and plated in MEF growth medium. These plates should be left for 7–14 d and observed periodically for any contamination or unusual cell morphologies.
8. To make feeder plates, thaw a frozen vial of cells rapidly at 37°C. Resuspend the vial in 10 mL MEF growth medium. The cell density and viability should be checked with Trypan blue.
9. Mitotically inactivated MEF feeder cells should be plated at the correct density to allow a confluent uniform monolayer to be produced. As a guide: cells should be plated at a density of 7.5×10^4 and 7.5×10^5 cells/cm^2 (*see* **Note 4**).

3.3. Purification of Targeting Construct for Electroporation

1. Prepare a large-scale plasmid prep of targeting vector using the Qiagen plasmid maxi prep kit, following the supplied protocol.

2. Linearize the targeting vector with the appropriate restriction enzyme. Phenol/chloroform extract the DNA. This is accomplished by adding an equal volume of phenol/chloroform/isoamyl alcohol to the digested vector. Vortex vigorously and centrifuge at top speed in a microcentrifuge. Remove the aqueous (top) phase to a fresh tube and repeat the extraction with chloroform. Transfer the aqueous (top) phase to a fresh tube.

3. Precipitate the DNA by adding 0.1 volume of 5-M sodium acetate (pH 5.2) and 2 volumes of 100% ethanol. Leave at –70°C for 30 min then spin down at top speed in a microcentrifuge. Pour off supernatant and rinse twice with 70% ethanol. Air-dry the pellet.

4. Resuspend the pellet in sterile TE at a concentration of 1 mg/mL. Each electroporation requires 20–40 µg of linearized targeting vector. We recommend running an aliquot of the DNA on an agarose gel to ensure complete linearization.

3.4. Electroporation of ES Cells

1. ES cells used in this procedure should be morphologically normal, undifferentiated, and of a low passage (*see* **Note 5**). Cells should be passaged 24–48 h before being used and medium changed a few hours before harvesting. Approximately three to four 3.5-cm wells (from a 6-well plate) are required for each electroporation.

2. The day before commencing the experiment, prepare five 6-well plates of drug-resistant, mitotically inactivated fibroblast feeder cells for each electroporation.

3. Trypsinize ES cells with 0.25% trypsin/EDTA and resuspend as a single cell suspension in 10 mL of ES cell medium. Count the cells and adjust to between 5×10^6 and 5×10^7. If there are not enough cells, trypsinize further wells (or subculture the cells at a 1:2 dilution and carry out the electroporation when these cells have reached confluency).

4. Pellet the cells at 200–300g for 5 min.

5. Aspirate the supernatant and resuspend the cells in 10 mL of DMEM. Pellet at 200–300g for 5 min. Repeat the washing step.

6. Aspirate the supernatant and resuspend the cells in 0.9 mL of DMEM. Mix the cell suspension with 20–40 µg of linearized vector DNA and transfer into an electroporation cuvet. Leave for 5 min at room temperature.

7. Set the electroporation conditions to 240 V, 500 µF for the Bio-Rad Gene Pulser, using the capacitance extender.

8. Place the electroporation cuvette into the cuvet holder, observing the correct orientation. Deliver the electric pulse. A time constant of between 5 and 7 ms is expected. Remove the cuvet from the holder and leave for 5 min at room temperature.

9. Transfer the electroporated cell suspension to 15 mL of ES cell medium, mix, and then plate 0.5 mL of this solution to each of the 3.5 cm wells of the five 6-well plates. Disperse cells evenly by gently rocking the plate. Incubate at 37°C in a 5% CO_2 atmosphere.

10. 24 h after electroporation, change to ES cell medium containing the appropriate selective drug (*see* **Note 6**).

11. Change medium on cells daily with ES cell medium containing selection drug(s) for 7–10 d. At this point, individual drug-resistant colonies should be of a suitable size to pick.

3.5. Picking ES Cell Colonies (see Note 6)

1. The day before picking ES cell colonies, prepare an appropriate number of 96-well plates with feeders. Change the medium on these plates with 150 µL of ES cell medium before picking colonies.
2. Prepare a 96-well plate containing 25 µL of 0.25% trypsin/EDTA per well.
3. Wash the 6-well plate containing the electroporated ES cell colonies twice with PBS. Replace final wash with 1 mL of PBS. If necessary, after picking, the PBS can be replaced with ES cell medium and the plate returned to the incubator (if small colonies are visible and can be picked on subsequent days).
4. While viewing the colonies under a dissecting microscope, detach the colonies, using a yellow Gilson tip attached to a P20 Pipetman and transfer in a minimal volume (5–10 µL of PBS) to the 96-well plate containing trypsin/EDTA. Use a sterile pipet tip for each colony. Care should be taken that only a single colony is seeded per well to avoid the need for a further cloning step because of the presence of mixed cell colonies.
5. When 96 colonies have been picked, incubate the 96-well plate for 10 min at 37°C.
6. Neutralize the trypsin by adding 25 µL of ES cell medium to each of the 96-wells using a multichannel pipettor. Using fresh tips for each column, gently disrupt the cells by pipetting the cell suspension up and down, and then transfer to the prepared feeder plate, making sure to put the cells into the correct corresponding wells. Repeat this for each column of cells until all of the wells have been transferred.
7. Change the medium (using ES cell medium without selection drugs) the following day and then daily, until ES cells are confluent and ready to be subcultured to prepare duplicate plates for freezing and DNA isolation (usually 3–5 d).

3.6. Cryopreserving Drug-Resistant ES Cell Clones and Preparing a Duplicate Plate for Southern Blot Analysis

1. Once the cells have reached the desired stage of confluency (usually 3–5 d after picking, and when the medium has started to turn orange), they should be cryopreserved and a duplicate plate prepared for DNA analysis.
2. Prepare an appropriate number of gelatinized 96-well plates by preincubating wells with 0.1% gelatin approx 1 h before use. To coat wells, cover with gelatin solution and leave for at least 1 h. Remove the gelatin and replace with 170 µL of ES cell medium per well. Place in the incubator until required.
3. Aspirate the medium from each well of the 96-well plates containing the ES cell clones to be frozen.
4. Wash the cells twice with 150 µL of PBS.
5. Add 30 µL of prewarmed 0.25% trypsin/EDTA and incubate for 5–10 min at 37°C.
6. Observe cells using an inverted microscope, and once all the cells have detached from the plate, neutralize the trypsin by adding 50 µL of ES cell medium.

7. Gently disrupt cells by pipetting the solution up and down, and then using a multichannel pipettor, transfer 30 µL into the gelatinized 96-well duplicate plate containing 170 µL of ES medium per well. Repeat this for each column of cells, using fresh tips for each column. Return the duplicate plate to the incubator.
8. Add 50 µL of 96-well plate freezing medium to each of the wells (of the original plate) to be frozen.
9. Seal the edges of the plate with Parafilm, wrap with tissue, and transfer to a precooled polystyrene box in a –70°C freezer.
10. Change the medium on duplicate plates daily until ready for DNA extraction. Cells should be allowed to become over confluent, as it is ideal to obtain a maximum number of cells. For this reason, cell differentiation or poor morphology is not a concern on these plates.

3.7. DNA Extraction From Duplicate Plates of ES Cell Colonies

1. Once the cells have reached the desired stage of confluency (usually 3–5 d after plating and the media has started to turn yellow), DNA should be prepared.
2. Aspirate the medium from each well on the duplicate plate and wash twice with 200 µL of PBS.
3. Tap out any excess liquid onto a paper towel.
4. Add 50 µL of DNA lysis buffer to each well.
5. Cover the wells with sealing film, ensuring a good seal over wells containing cells. Incubate overnight at 56°C in a humidified atmosphere.
6. Allow to cool to room temperature (approx 30 min).
7. Tap the plate gently on the bench and then either place at 4°C or freeze at –20°C until required. Long-term storage at either temperature should be avoided and plates should be processed promptly.

3.8. Screening Picked Clones (see Note 7)

3.8.1. Restriction Digest of Isolated DNA

1. To precipitate DNA, add 50 µL of isopropanol to each well of the duplicate 96-well plate and allow the plate to stand at room temperature for 30 min.
2. Centrifuge the plate at 200–300g for 5 min at room temperature.
3. Empty the wells by slow and very careful inversion. Wash each well three times with 70% ethanol, inverting carefully after each rinse.
4. Allow the wells to air-dry for 20 min at room temperature.
5. Digest the DNA by adding 30 µL digest solution-appropriate restriction enzyme (10 U per digest), 1X digest buffer (appropriate for chosen enzyme), 0.2 mg/mL of bovine serum albumin, 1 mM spermidine, and 20 mg/mL of RNase A. Incubate overnight at 37°C in a humid atmosphere. Add a further 10 U of the restriction enzyme in a volume of 5 µL (using the same buffer components as above) and incubate for an additional 5 h at 37°C. Add 3.5 µL of 10X loading buffer and load the entire sample onto a 0.7% agarose gel prepared in 1X Tris-borate-EDTA and containing 1 µg/mL ethidium bromide.

3.8.2. Transfer of Electrophoresed Samples to Nylon

1. After running the gel, visualize on a short-wave ultraviolet transilluminator. Photograph with a ruler alongside for determining band sizes on the autoradiograph of the blot.
2. Acid depurinate the gel by soaking the gel in 0.25 M HCl for 15 min at room temperature.
3. Rinse the gel in distilled water and denature DNA by soaking in 0.5 N NaOH, 1.5 M NaCl for 30 min at room temperature.
4. Rinse the gel in distilled water and neutralize the NaOH by soaking the gel in 0.5 M Tris-HCl (pH 7.5) and 1.5 M NaCl for 30 min at room temperature.
5. Set up capillary transfer to ZetaProbe GT membrane in 10X SSC at room temperature. The membrane must be prewetted in distilled water and then soaked in SSC before setting up the transfer.
6. After transferring overnight, carefully remove the membrane from the gel and immediately crosslink using the Stratagene ultraviolet crosslinker/autocrosslink setting, ensuring that the side of the membrane that was closest to the gel is face up. The membrane can now be air-dried and stored at room temperature or immediately placed in hybridization buffer.

3.8.3. Southern Blot Analysis

1. Hybridize the nylon blot (in a roller bottle hybridization oven) for at least 4 h at 65°C in approx 20 mL of Southern hybridization buffer.
2. Meanwhile, prepare the random primed probe. Add 2 µL of random hexamer primers and 1 µL of 1-N NaOH to a tube containing 100 ng of probe template (in 6 µL of H_2O). Incubate at room temperature for 5 min.
3. Neutralize the reaction with 2 µL of 1 M Tris-HCl (pH 7.5) and add 2.5 µL of 10X random priming buffer, 1.5 µL of H_2O, 5 µL of deoxynucleotide 5'-triphosphate mixture, 5 µL of ^{32}P-deoxycytidine 5'-triphosphate, and 1 µL of Klenow. Incubate at room temperature for 2 h.
4. Purify the labeled probe using the Qiaquick nucleotide removal kit, following the supplied protocol. Denature the eluted radiolabeled probe at 100°C for 10 min and snap cool on ice for 5 min. Add directly to the blot in hybridization buffer and incubate overnight at 65°C.
5. The following day, pour off hybridization buffer and probe and rinse for 1 h at 65°C in Southern rinse buffer. Repeat this wash three times. We perform these rinses in the roller bottle using approx 100 mL per wash.
6. Wrap the membrane in plastic wrap and expose to X-ray film at –70°C, using an exposure cassette with intensifying screen.
7. Develop the autoradiograph and determine which clones demonstrate homologous recombination by giving a banding pattern indicative of the presence of both wild type and targeted alleles.

3.9. Expanding Positive Clones

Once the 96-well DNA plate has been screened, the positive clones should be recovered, expanded, frozen stocks generated, and a further DNA prep made for confirmation. **Note:** the frozen plate of cells can only be recovered once, so all positive clones must be recovered at the same time.

1. Prepare a sufficient number of 24-well plates containing a feeder layer the day before recovering the ES cell clones.
2. Remove the frozen plate of cells from the –70°C freezer and thaw rapidly either in a 37°C incubator or in a humidified box in a 37°C water bath (5–10 min).
3. Observe, and once all clones have thawed, add 100 µL of ES cell medium to each of the wells containing a targeted clone.
4. Using a yellow Gilson tip, pipet the cell suspension to mix thoroughly, and then transfer into two wells of a 24-well plate containing a feeder layer (100 µL/well).
5. Change the medium on the cells daily with ES cell medium until they become confluent. Once confluent, trypsinize and transfer one well into one well of a 6-well plate containing feeder cells. Change the medium on cells daily and once confluent, freeze three vials from each well of this plate (300 µL of freezing medium per vial). Transfer the remaining well into one well of a gelatin-coated 6-well plate containing no feeders. This is used for preparing DNA for confirmation.

3.10. Salt–Chloroform Extraction of DNA From ES Cells for Confirmation

1. Change the medium on the cells daily until ready for DNA extraction. Cells should be allowed to become overconfluent, as it is ideal to obtain a max. number of cells. For this reason, cell differentiation or poor morphology is not a concern on these plates.
2. Trypsinize cells with 0.25% trypsin/EDTA and pellet by centrifugation. Resuspend pellet in 500 µL of salt extraction DNA buffer and place into a microcentrifuge tube. Add 10 µL of 10% SDS and mix.
3. Add 10 µL of 10-mg/mL proteinase K solution and mix. Incubate at 55°C overnight.
4. Add 150 µL of 5-M NaCl and mix. Then, add 650 µL of chloroform/isoamyl alcohol and mix for 30 s.
5. Centrifuge at top speed for 10 min.
6. Transfer the aqueous (top) phase to a fresh tube and precipitate the DNA with an equal volume of 100% ethanol. Mix thoroughly and place into a –20°C freezer until required.
7. When ready to rescreen, centrifuge DNA at top speed in a microcentrifuge (10–20 min at room temperature). Rinse with 70% ethanol and air dry. Resuspend in 50–100 µL of TE. One well from a 6-well plate will provide approx 50–100 µg of DNA.

4. Notes

1. When designing a targeting construct, ensure that the vector backbone contains a unique restriction site on either side of the altered genomic sequence. This is used for linearization of the template before electroporation. Also, ensure that targeted and wild-type alleles can be easily distinguished from one another based on their restriction patterns using, preferably, single-enzyme restriction digests. Highest targeting efficiencies are achieved when the targeting construct is derived from DNA that is isogenic to the line of ES cells used.

2. FBS used for the culture of ES cells should be batch-tested by performing plating efficiency tests and selecting the most suitable batch for the particular ES cell line. If more than one ES cell line is going to be used, these should be included in the serum batch testing, as variations in growth rates and morphologies may be apparent and would contribute to the assessment of the suitability of a particular batch of serum to the conditions. Once a batch has been selected, we purchase a large quantity to suit our needs for a good amount of time, reducing the requirement for constant batch testing.

3. Most ES cell lines are maintained on a mitotically inactivated feeder layer of MEF cells. A healthy feeder layer will provide a suitable matrix for culturing ES cells, providing them with cellular factors to assist in maintaining an undifferentiated state. In addition, we supplement the medium with leukemia inhibitory factor to a concentration of 1000 U/mL of media. Feeders that are used during the drug selection step must themselves be resistant to the chosen selection drug—in most cases, this will be G418.

4. We recommend that feeder plates be recovered the day before they are required. Plates may be used for up to 10 d after they are seeded, but the integrity and condition of the monolayer should be assessed. Plates showing signs of poor morphology or signs of cell death should not be used, as they will not provide an appropriate environment for the ES cells. Medium should be replaced with ES cell culture medium before any ES cells are plated onto the feeder cells.

5. The quality, germline competence and pluripotency of ES cells used in these techniques are one of the key elements in the success of the experiment. For that reason, care should be taken when handling and culturing ES cells to provide them with a stable environment, otherwise, they may lose their pluripotent developmental state and consequently, lose the ability to colonize the germline when introduced into host embryos. Experience with aseptic cell culture techniques and obtaining quality reagents and equipment should not be overlooked. In our experience, many variables can contribute to the effective culture and use of ES cells. Low-passage ES cells should always be the starting point for any experiment. This can be achieved by in-house production of ES cell lines, or through collaboration with other researchers, thereby allowing the production of a frozen stock of low-passage ES cells. Commercially available ES cell lines are usually of a passage suitable for one or two experiments only, and not suitable for expanding and using as a stock.

6. The concentration of selection drug required will vary from batch to batch and for different ES cell lines. The level of selection should be determined by performing killing curves, and observing the lowest concentration of drug required to kill all unmanipulated ES cells within 7–10 d. Generally, between 150 and 200 µg/mL of G418 is sufficient for selection. If ganciclovir is to be used, add to a concentration of 2 mM and apply 48 h after electroporation. Transfection efficiency will vary from experiment to experiment, but generally, between two and six 96-well plates of clones are required to provide a suitable number of positive clones.

7. Of critical importance to the screening of drug-resistant clones for homologous recombination is the probe used for Southern blot analysis. For initial screening of clones, this probe needs to lie outside the region of the genome that is covered by the targeting construct, so that one can distinguish random integration from homologous recombination. It is vital to test a probe before screening—many probes can contain repetitive sequence that leads to high background on a Southern blot analysis; shorter seems to be better than longer in this respect.

Acknowledgments

The authors would like to thank the other members of their laboratories: Lorenza Wyder, Louise Reynolds, Andrew Reynolds, Francesco Conti, Garry Saunders, Colin Wren, Sue Watling, and the members of the Transgenic Services Laboratory for countless hours of help with writing and experiments.

References

1. Barinaga, M. (1994) Knockout mice: round two. *Science* **265,** 26–28.
2. Rossant, J. and Nagy, A. (1995) Genome engineering: the new mouse genetics. *Nat. Med.* **1,** 592–594.
3. Rajewsky, K., Gu, H., Kuhn, R., et al. (1996) Conditional gene targeting. *J. Clin. Invest.* **98,** 600–603.
4. Sternberg, N., Austin, S., Hamilton, D., and Yarmolinsky, M. (1978) Analysis of bacteriophage P1 immunity by using lambda-P1 recombinants constructed in vitro. *Proc. Natl. Acad. Sci. USA* **75,** 5594–5598.
5. Sternberg, N., Sauer, B., Hoess, R., and Abremski, K. (1986) Bacteriophage P1 *cre* gene and its regulatory region. Evidence for multiple promoters and for regulation by DNA methylation. *J. Mol. Biol.* **187,** 197–212.
6. Broach, J. R., Guarascio, V. R., and Jayaram, M. (1982) Recombination within the yeast plasmid 2mu circle is site-specific. *Cell* **29,** 227–234.
7. Andrews, B. J., Proteau, G. A., Beatty, L. G., and Sadowski, P. D. (1985) The FLP recombinase of the 2 micron circle DNA of yeast: interaction with its target sequences. *Cell* **40,** 795–803.
8. Senecoff, J. F., Bruckner, R. C., and Cox, M. M. (1985) The FLP recombinase of the yeast 2-micron plasmid: characterization of its recombination site. *Proc. Natl. Acad. Sci. USA 82,* 7270–7274.

9. Gates, C. A. and Cox, M. M. (1988) FLP recombinase is an enzyme. *Proc. Natl. Acad. Sci. USA.* **85,** 4628–4632.

10. Sauer, B. and Henderson. N. (1989) Cre-stimulated recombination at loxP-containing DNA sequences placed into the mammalian genome. *Nucleic Acids Res.* **17,** 147–161.

11. Gu, H., Marth, J. D., Orban, P. C., Mossmann, H., and Rajewsky, K. (1994) Deletion of a DNA polymerase beta gene segment in T cells using cell type-specific gene targeting. *Science* **265,** 103–106.

12. Kuhn, R., Schwenk, F., Aguet, M., and Rajewsky, K. (1995) Inducible gene targeting in mice. *Science* **269,** 1427–1429.

13. Tsien, J. Z., Chen, D. F., Gerber, D., et al. (1996) Subregion- and cell type-restricted gene knockout in mouse brain. *Cell* **87,** 1317–1326.

14. Akagi, K., Sandig,V., Vooijs, M., et al. (1997) Cre-mediated somatic site-specific recombination in mice. *Nucleic Acids Res.* **25,** 1766–1773.

15. Barlow, C., Schroeder, M., Lekstrom-Himes, J., et al. (1997) Targeted expression of Cre recombinase to adipose tissue of transgenic mice directs adipose-specific excision of loxP-flanked gene segments. *Nucleic Acids Res.* **25,** 2543–2545.

16. Metzger, D. and Chambon, P. (2001) Site- and time-specific gene targeting in the mouse. *Methods* **24,** 71–80.

17. Hogan, B., Beddington, R., Costantini, F., and Lacy, E. (1994) *Manipulating The Mouse Embryo, 2nd Edition.* Cold Spring Harbor Laboratory Press, Cold Spring Harbor, NY.

18. Joyner, A. L. (ed.) (1999) *Gene Targeting. A Practical Approach, 2nd Edition.* Oxford University Press, Oxford, UK.

33

In Vivo Xenograft Models of Breast Cancer Metastasis

Ursula Valentiner, Susan A. Brooks, and Udo Schumacher

Summary

If breast cancer patients are not cured, it is largely because of the fact that the cancer has spread beyond its primary site—the breast—to distant sites, such as, e.g., bone marrow, lung, brain, and/or liver. These secondary tumors are called *metastases*, and the underlying mechanisms leading to these secondary tumor deposits are complex and still ill understood. In this chapter, we report on how to develop clinically relevant human breast cancer cell line xenografts in severe combined immunodeficient mice. In severe combined immunodeficient mice, metastasizing human breast cancer cell lines were identified by their ability to bind the lectin *Helix pomatia* agglutinin, which was identified as a marker of metastasis in clinical studies. This model system was created to help to define the rate-limiting steps of the metastatic cascade.

Key Words: *Helix pomatia* agglutinin; HPA; metastasis; severe combined immunodeficient mouse; xenograft model.

1. Introduction

1.1. Background and Advantages of the Severe Combined Immunodeficient Mouse Model

In breast cancer, systemic spread of the disease is the cause of death for the majority of patients. Metastasis is a multistep phenomenon, and all steps have to be followed through successfully and consecutively until a clinically manifest metastasis occurs. Although all of these steps have been defined, and individual steps can be mimicked in vitro, the rate-limiting step of metastases formation is unknown. Hence, the significance of a particular in vitro test to the overall process of metastases formation is undefined. For example, a particular cell line may prove to have excellent capabilities to degrade the extracellular matrix, which would be one prerequisite to enter the circulation, but be highly vulnerable to proapoptotic factors within the circulation. Although

From: *Methods in Molecular Medicine, Vol. 120: Breast Cancer Research Protocols*
Edited by: S. A. Brooks and A. L. Harris © Humana Press Inc., Totowa, NJ

matrix degrading in vitro assays would indicate high metastatic potential, this cell line would be very unlikely to form metastasis in an in vivo (clinical) situation because of the subsequent cell death within the circulation. This is why whole-organism animal models, which cover the entire process of the formation of metastases, are still needed to put defined in vitro assays into a broader perspective.

Several animal models of metastasis have been proposed and evaluated over the past few decades. However, the main problem of these models is their relevance to the clinical situation. Murine breast cancer, for example, is caused by the mouse mammary tumor virus and is not hormone-dependent. In contrast, a considerable proportion of human breast cancer is estrogen-dependent, and no viral causes of human breast cancers have been shown. Therefore, murine breast cancer is of limited use as a model for human breast cancer *(1)*.

Not only do the different biological behaviors of animal cancers compared with human ones make it difficult to assess the clinical relevance of the animal models, but also, differences in antigen expression have to be taken into account, and they pose a problem. Most of the monoclonal antibodies that react with human epitopes do not crossreact with other species, making it impossible to evaluate the usefulness of a particular monoclonal antibody in cancer diagnosis and treatment using animal-derived tissues.

To overcome these problems, human cancers have been transplanted into immunodeficient animals, mainly mice. The first widespread model of an immunodeficient animal was the nude mouse *(2)*. Besides lacking hair, this mouse is characterized by the absence of a functional thymus; hence, mature and functionally active T lymphocytes are lacking. However, T-cell-independent B-cell response is still present in this mouse. The T-cell-independent B-cell immune response is active mainly against polysaccharides, such as those present in capsules of bacteria. Many thousands of studies in which human tumors were xenografted into nude mice have been published, but metastasis of human tumors is rarely observed; hence, the nude mouse is disappointing as a model for metastasis *(2)*. In recent years, a number of reports on the successful metastatic spread of human tumors transplanted orthotopically in the nude mouse model have been published *(3–6)*.

An alternative model in metastasis research is the severe combined immunodeficient (SCID) mouse. This mouse strain lacks the enzyme recombinase, which links the specific with the nonspecific parts of the immunoglobulins and the T-cell receptor, respectively. The original SCID mouse was derived from the Balb/c mouse and looks phenotypically normal, but lacks both immunoglobulins and functional T-cells, although macrophages and natural-killer cells are still present *(7)*. Because of this extended immunodeficiency, the SCID mouse has attracted our attention as a tool for metastasis research *(8)*.

1.2. Choice of Appropriate Cell Lines

A complete model of metastasis formation does not only require an appropriate animal (the "soil") but also requires the choice of the right cell line (the "seed"). A general assumption often made is that tumor cells derived from metastatic sites, e.g., from pleural effusions or from lymph node metastases, are metastatic, whereas those that are derived from apparently localized primary tumors are nonmetastatic. However, there is no experimental proof that this assumption is correct. Therefore, it is helpful to assess the metastatic potential of human tumor cell lines before they are transplanted into the animals in order to get a correlation with the clinical situation.

Such an analysis of metastatic capabilities for breast cancers has been performed by us and others using the lectin *Helix pomatia* agglutinin (HPA). The presence of HPA lectin-labeled primary tumor cells in clinical material correlatd with patients who had a poor prognosis and hence, suffered from a metastatic tumor *(9)*. It does not work as a prognostic marker in all types of tumors *(10)* but seems to be of particular value in adenocarcinomas (for review, *see* ref. *9*). However, especially in adenocarcinomas of the breast, some degree of controversy has existed over the prognostic significance of HPA lectin binding. One reason for this disagreement was the different methods of lectin histochemistry used by the different groups. It has been shown that methodology (including fixation and tissue processing) does indeed make a difference to the binding outcome *(11)*. In this connection, the indirect method using native, unconjugated HPA is superior to the direct method using conjugated HPA. According to the expected clinical behavior, human HPA-positive breast cancer cell lines metastasize in SCID mice, whereas HPA-negative ones generally do not *(8)*. The particular value of this system is the correlation between the behavior of the tumor cells in the clinical studies and the behavior of the human tumor cell lines grown in SCID mice. HPA-positive breast cancer cell lines were T47D, MCF-7, and DU4475. HPA-negative breast/breast cancer cell lines were BT20, HS578T, and HBL 100 *(9)*. Primary tumors of BT474 and HMT3522 cells showed areas of HPA-positive cells, although they did not metastasize in SCID mice (our unpublished results). However, these HPA-positive tumor areas were areas of squamous cells and for this cell type, HPA failed to predict outcome *(10)*. It should be kept in mind that antigen and glycotope expression can vary considerably between in vitro grown cells and tumor cells grown in vivo in SCID mice *(13)*. Thus, fixed and wax-embedded BT474 and HMT3522 cells grown in vitro showed no (HMT3533) and weak (BT474), respectively, HPA binding *(12)*. Therefore, the analysis of tumor cells from both sources is recommended. One breast cancer cell line, namely MDAMB435, did not fit well into the analysis with HPA. Although this cell line metastasized in our SCID mouse model, primary tumors, and wax-embedded cells showed only negligible HPA labeling.

Any other prognostic marker besides HPA can be applied to this kind of study. The only thing in common is the correlation between the expression of the marker of metastasis in clinical studies and in human tumor cells grown in the SCID mouse to give the model some clinical relevance.

Tumors other than adenocarcinomas (squamous cell carcinoma, small cell carcinoma of the lung) do not metastasize in SCID mice (our unpublished observations). The reason for this failure to metastasize is unclear. This may be owing to the selection of the cell lines or to the general nonsuitability of the SCID mouse as a host for these types of tumors. It may well be that adenocarcinomas in general, or at least of certain types, provide the appropriate seed and soil mechanisms for homing of metastasis, and that other tumor types use different recognition systems that are not represented in SCID mice, and hence, are unsuitable as a host to mimic metastatic spread.

1.3. The Scope of This Chapter

The handling of SCID mice, the treatment of the human tumor cell lines, and their processing will be described. The assessment of HPA-binding sites in tumor cells is described in Chapter 16.

2. Materials

2.1. Maintenance of the SCID Mouse Colony

The SCID mouse can be obtained from any of the large animal breeding farms (e.g., Jackson Laboratory, Bar Harbor, ME).

2.2. Treatment of the Cells for Injection Into SCID Mouse

1. 250-mL Flasks of human breast cancer cell lines, cultured according to standard laboratory protocols.
2. Standard cell culture medium appropriate for cell lines to be used (*see* **Note 1**).
3. Sterile phosphate-buffered saline (PBS), pH 7.1: Dissolve 8.5 g sodium chloride, 1.07 g disodium hydrogen phosphate (anhydride Na_2HPO_4), and 0.39 g of sodium dihydrogen phosphate ($NaH_2PO_4 \cdot 2\ H_2O$) in 850 mL of distilled water (*see* **Note 2**). Adjust to pH 7.1 with 0.1 M HCl or NaOH. Make up to 1 L in a measuring cylinder and filter under a sterile hood with 2 μm filter (*see* **Note 2**).
4. Trypsin/ethylenediaminetetraacetic acid (EDTA) solution is supplied by Invitrogen, Carlsbad, CA (GIBCO® cat. no. 45300-019).
5. Standard cell culture medium appropriate for the cell lines used, containing 10% (v/v) fetal calf serum.
6. Cell counting chamber, e.g., Neubauer.
7. 1-mL Sterile syringes fitted with small-gage needles (e.g., Becton Dickinson, Franklin Lakes, NJ; Microlance 2, 27 gage, 3/4 inch).
8. Saturated picric acid solution in distilled water.

2.3. Harvesting the Metastases for Microscopic Examination and Analysis

1. 70% (v/v) ethanol in distilled water.
2. Neutral buffered formalin, pH 7.1: 100 mL of formalin (40% formaldehyde in water) is added to 900 mL of PBS (*see* **Note 3**).
3. 4% (w/v) Difco Agar Noble.

3. Methods

3.1. Maintenance of SCID Mouse Colony

SCID mice are, despite their immunodeficiency, relatively easy to handle. Most pathogens that challenge the mice are bacteria, and because they are combated by granulocytes that are functional in SCID mice, these mice can resist infection. However, special care needs to be taken.

It is advisable to house SCID mice in a separate room within the animal house facility. Animal technicians should always take care of the SCID mouse colony first in the morning before they deal with other animal colonies in order to avoid cross-contamination. A barrier room to change clothes is advisable. Use disposable facemasks, hoods, and sterilized gowns, such as are used in operating theaters before entering the SCID mouse colony. Use fresh clothes every time the colony is entered. The cages have to be filter-top cages in order to minimize infection, and food, water, bedding, and cages have to be sterilized. The sterilization procedure can take place within the normal sterilizing procedure already in use for routine purposes in the animal facility. The cleaning of the cages and changing of bedding has to be done under sterile conditions in a laminar flow hood. Do this once a week. These conditions have allowed us to maintain the SCID mouse colony without special incubator facilities ("bubble"). The mice should weigh around 18–20 g when the experiments are started.

3.2. Treatment of the Cells for Injection Into SCID Mice

1. Grow the cell lines in their usual culture medium in culture flask I (250 cm^2). When confluent, remove the culture medium using a suction pipet. Rinse the cells with 15–20 mL of sterile PBS and aspirate them.
2. Add 5 mL of trypsin/EDTA solution to the flask. Incubate the flask for 5 min at 37°C. Tilt the flasks occasionally. The cells should come off by this time. The cells form white layers in the solution, which lift off from the bottom of the flask (*see* **Note 4**).
3. Add 5 mL of culture medium with 10% fetal calf serum added (*see* **Note 5**). Aspirate the solution using a 10-mL pipet several times to help to loosen the cells from each other. Empty this suspension into a sterile 15-mL centrifuge tube.
4. Rinse the bottom of the cell culture flask with additional 5 mL of medium and centrifuge this plus the initial solution at 1000*g* for 10 min.

5. Aspirate the supernatant, pool the cells, and resuspend in 5 mL of culture medium. Count the cell number using a cell-counting chamber (e.,g., Neubauer). Adjust the cell number to 10^6 cells in 200 µL of total volume. Use 1-mL syringes for injection and a small-gage needle (*see* **Note 6**).

6. Before injection of the cells, the mice should be weighed, individually labeled, and a record book should be initiated. Use saturated picric acid in water (itself a sterile solution) and apply the solution with cotton wool to the fur of the animal (*see* **Note 7**). Inject 200 µL of the cell solution between the scapulae of SCID mice (*see* **Note 8**).

7. Using estrogen receptor-positive breast cancer cell lines, tumor growth can be improved by supplementation with estrogen. One commonly used method is the implantation of slow release pellets of 17β-estradiol (Innovative Research of America, Sarasota, FL). A 90-d-release, 1.5-mg pellet will support the growth of the estrogen receptor-positive MCF-7 breast cancer cell line (from subcutaneous injection of 10^6 cells between the scapulae of the SCID mice).

3.3. Harvesting Metastases for Microscopic Examination and Analysis

1. The mice should be killed when the tumor reaches 20% of the body weight at the beginning of the experiments, or when the tumors start to ulcerate (*see* **Note 9**). Consult your local animal-care guidelines. Alternatively, perform survival surgery to remove the local tumor and allow established micrometastases to grow to a more readily detectable size.

2. The mice should be sacrificed by a Schedule 2 method (i.e., with rising concentrations of carbon dioxide). To harvest the primary tumors, wet the skin over the tumor with 70% ethanol solution to ease cutting and incise the skin over the tumor with a pair of scissors. Using forceps, hold one of the two sides of the skin flap open and dissect the tumors out of their bed (*see* **Note 10**). The tumors can be fixed in neutral buffered formalin for 2 d or can be frozen in liquid-nitrogen-cooled isopentane, embedded in optimum cutting temperature medium (Tissue-Tek, Miles, Naperville, IL) and stored in sealed containers in liquid nitrogen for histological or immunohistochemical examination. The specimens can be immediately frozen and stored in liquid nitrogen for molecular biological examination.

3. Turn the mouse around, wet the fur over the rib cage, and open it using a pair of scissors. Remove the lungs *en bloc* by cutting them out beginning at the trachea. Fix the lungs *en bloc* in neutral buffered formalin for 2 d or freeze in liquid-nitrogen-cooled isopentane and embed it in optimum cutting temperature medium (*see* **Note 11**).

4. Once the abdominal cavity is fully opened and the internal organs are removed, place them into neutral buffered formalin for 2 d (*see* **Note 12**). Alternatively, the organs can be stored in liquid nitrogen.

5. After 2 d, slice the lungs using a stereomicroscope. Cover graph paper with a glass plate and put this in the viewing field of the microscope. Section the lungs with a razor blade in 2-mm-thick slices. Place all the slices on a histological glass slide and cover the slices in 4% Agar Noble (*see* **Note 13**).

6. When the agar has solidified, trim the edges of the agar block (without any tissue slices) away and routinely process to paraffin wax in the same way as would be done with a piece of solid tissue (*see* **Note 14**). Cut 5-μm-thick sections using a microtome and prepare routine hematoxylin and eosin slides for microscopy. Use ×100 magnification to search for metastases (*see* **Notes 15** and **16**).

4. Notes

1. Different cell lines often require different cell culture media, and this makes the culture of a bank of cell lines expensive and difficult to maintain. By careful adjustment, many cell lines can be brought to grow in one of the better (and more expensive) media such as RPMI-1640. The ease of handling only one medium more than compensates for the extra costs of RPMI-1640.
2. Use fresh distilled water, which can vary considerably in pH. For cell culture purposes, it is advisable to use water supplied in 1-L bottles for clinical use. This is pyrogen-free and tested. Instead of filtering, this solution can be autoclaved, which is cheaper. If some of the water has evaporated after autoclaving, it has to be adjusted to 1 L again using sterile water.
3. During storage, formaldehyde decays to formic acid and hence, the pH drops. Therefore, buffering is necessary. For optimal results, it should be neutral or slightly alkaline. Check the pH of the solution before use. Prepare enough solution for optimal fixation results, 9 volumes of buffered formalin should be added to 1 volume of tissue.
4. Trypsin inhibitors in the serum block its activity.
5. If the cells do not come off, incubate them for 1 min longer in the trypsin/EDTA solution. Depending on the cell junctions, different cell lines need different incubation times, which have to be established for every cell line. If the cell line is embedded in agar to compare antigen expression of cells grown in vitro as compared to grown *in situ* in SCID mice, no trypsin should be used as this may digest the antigen under study. The use of agar-embedded cells will allow the processing of the cells according to the same protocol as blocks of tissue. Under those circumstances, cells should be harvested using a rubber policeman, fixed in buffered formalin, and embedded in agar for further processing.
6. Epithelia tend to self-aggregate. Take the cell suspension in a sterile centrifuge tube to the mouse colony. Shake the cells gently before injection, because some cell lines can aggregate while in the centrifuge tube or even in the syringe.
7. Devise a labeling scheme (e.g., mark on left foreleg = 1, right foreleg = 2, left hind leg = 3, right hind leg = 4, no label = 5, and so on). House up to five animals in a small cage or up to 10 animals in a large cage.
8. For normal subcutaneous injection, the mice do not need to be anesthetized. One person should hold the mouse while another injects the cells. The cells should be injected in a skin flap and should not be injected too deeply (subcutaneously).
9. The size and weight of the primary tumor may have a considerable influence on the number of metastases detected in the lungs. At least for the human colon cancer cell line HT29, it was shown that primary tumors weighing below 1 g

rarely show metastatic spread to the lungs, whereas primary tumors weighing more than 1.6 g lead to hundreds of metastases in both lungs (*see* **ref. 15**).

10. Primary tumors and lungs can be removed aseptically at this stage if further in vitro culture experiments are envisaged.

11. For most monoclonal antibodies, cryostat sections are necessary. Pretreatment of the sections using microwave treatment or digestion with trypsin will allow the use of paraffin sections. These give a superior morphology and are easier to handle for serial sections than frozen sections. If these pretreatment methods for antigen retrieval fail, one lung can be stored frozen and used for immunocytochemistry. The other lung should be embedded in paraffin wax, serially sectioned, and the number of metastases counted.

12. We generally only use liver, spleen, and sternum for histological examination. However, so far, only spontaneous metastases have been found in the lungs, so that not so much emphasis is placed on the examination of these organs; only sample sections are cut, no serial sections are prepared. It is, however, expected that metastases are absent from these sites. In the clinical situation, the primary tumor is often removed before gross anatomically visible metastases occur. To mimic this situation, the primary tumor should be removed at an earlier stage and the metastases should be allowed to grow independently (*see* **ref. 14**). Under these experimental conditions, the brain might additionally be investigated for the presence of metastases.

13. To prepare the agar solution, heat 100 mL of distilled water in a 200-mL beaker in a larger beaker used as a water bath on a hot plate stirrer. Adjust the magnetic stirrer to a slow-to-medium rotation. Add 4 g of agar. Stir until the agar is dissolved, has boiled, and turned into a yellowish solution. Use preheated glass pipets to add the liquid agar onto the lung slices. This will enable cutting the whole lung in one block that is only about 2 mm thick. This will largely reduce the workload for histological examination.

14. Process primary tumor, lungs, and internal organs, except for the sternum (which has to be decalcified) in parallel. If differences in the results of immuno- or lectin histochemistry between the primary tumor and its metastases are detected, different processing procedures as the reason for the results can be discounted.

15. For quantitative assessment of lung metastases, a simplified method can be used (*see* **ref. 15**). Keep every tenth section of the wax-embedded lung, and examine the ten sections from the middle of the block. Count all metastases found in the 10 middle sections and calculate the mean value of these (mean value$_{10}$). Multiply the mean value$_{10}$ −20% by the total number of serial sections in order to achieve an estimated value for the total number of lung metastases.

16. Human tumor cells are, in general, larger than the surrounding normal cells of the mouse lung. It is often helpful to compare the morphology of the tumor cells in the primary tumor with those in the lungs when in doubt. In particular, the structure of the often heterochromatin-rich large nucleus and the basophilic cytoplasm of the tumor cells are of help in assessing the presence of a metastatic cell. If in doubt, immunohistochemistry for human or tumor-specific antigens will help.

SCID mice do not have immunoglobulins, so that all mouse-derived monoclonal primary antibodies directed against human antigens can be used without background staining.

References

1. Van de Vijver, M. J. and Nusse, R. (1991) The molecular biology of breast cancer. *Biochim. Biophys. Acta* **1072**, 33–50.
2. Giovanella, B. C. and Fogh, J. (1985) The nude mouse in cancer research. *Adv. Cancer Res.* **44**, 69–120.
3. Fu, X., Guadagni, F., and Hoffman, R. M. (1992) A metastatic nude-mouse model of human pancreatic cancer constructed orthotopically with histologically intact patient specimens. *Proc. Natl. Acad. Sci. USA* **89**, 5645–5649.
4. Kubota, T. (1994) Metastatic models of human xenografted in the nude mouse: the importance of orthotopic transplantation. *J. Cell Biochem.* **56**, 4–8.
5. Furukawa, T., Kubota, T., Watanabe, M., Kitajima, M., and Hoffman, R. (1993) A novel "patient-like" treatment model of human pancreatic cancer constructed using orthotopic transplantation of histologically intact human tumor tissue in nude mice. *Cancer Res.* **53**, 3070–3072.
6. Furukawa, T., Kubota, T., Watanabe, M., Kitajima, M., and Hoffman, R. M. (1993) Orthotopic transplantation of histologically intact clinical specimens of stomach cancer to nude mice: correlation with metastatic sites in mouse and individual patient donors. *Int. J. Cancer* **53**, 608–612.
7. Bosma, C. G., Custer, R. P., and Bosma, M. J. (1983) A severe combined immunodeficiency in the mouse. *Nature* **301**, 527–530.
8. Schumacher, U. and Adam, E. (1997) Lectin histochemical HPA-binding pattern of human breast and colon cancers is associated with metastases formation in severe combined immunodeficient mice. *Histochem. J.* **29**, 677–684.
9. Mitchell, B. S. and Schumacher, U. (1999) The use of the lectin *Helix pomatia* agglutinin (HPA) as a prognostic indicator and as a tool in cancer research. *Histol. Histopathol.* **14**, 217–226.
10. Schumacher, D. U., Randall, C. J., Ramsay, A. D., and Schumacher, U. (1996) Is the binding of the lectin *Helix pomatia* agglutinin (HPA) of prognostic relevance in tumours of the upper aerodigestive tract? *Eur. J. Surg. Oncol.* **22**, 618–620.
11. Brooks, S.A., Lymboura, M., Schumacher, U., and Leathem, A. J. (1996) Histochemistry to detect *Helix pomatia* lectin binding in breast cancer: methodology makes a difference. *J. Histochem. Cytochem.* **44**, 519–524.
12. Brooks, S. A., Hall, D. M. S., and Buley, I. (2001) GalNAc glycoprotein expression by breast cell lines, primary breast cancer and normal breast epithelial membrane. *Br. J. Cancer* **85**, 1014–1022.
13. Schumacher, U., Mohamed, M., and Mitchell, B.S. (1996) Differential expression of carbohydrate residues in human breast and colon cancer cell lines grown in vitro and in vivo in SCID mice. *Cancer J.* **9**, 247–254.
14. Mitchell, B. S., Horny, H-P., and Schumacher, U. (1997) Immunophenotyping of human HT29 colon cancer cell primary tumours and their metastases in severe combined immunodeficient mice. *Histochem. J.* **29**, 393–399.

15. Jojovic, M. and Schumacher, U. (2000) Quantitative assessment of spontaneous lung metastases of human HT29 colon cancer cells transplanted into scid mice. *Cancer Lett.* **152,** 151–156.

34

Neoadjuvant Endocrine Therapy Models

Juliette Murray, William R. Miller, and J. Michael Dixon

Summary

Neoadjuvant therapy is therapy administered before surgical intervention and while the tumor remains in the breast. It may be given to treat large, locally advanced tumors, with the aim of shrinking them and thus making their surgical excision either simply possible or less radical. Most neoadjuvant therapy is chemotherapy, but adjuvant endocrine therapy is increasingly used in hormone-sensitive tumors; for example, those responsive to tamoxifen. Repeat biopsies aimed at assessing response to treatment—for example, by examining estrogen receptor status or markers of proliferation in tumor tissue—may be taken during the course of adjuvant therapy. In this chapter, the essential protocols associated with designing neoadjuvant trials are described, methods of assessing response to neoadjuvant therapy are detailed, and various approaches to collecting appropriate clinical samples and their assessment are presented.

Key Words: Neoadjuvant therapy; endocrine therapy; estrogen receptor; informed consent; trial ethics; tumor size; mammography; treatment response.

1. Introduction
1.1. Neoadjuvant Therapy

Neoadjuvant therapy can be defined as therapy that is given while the primary tumor is still *in situ* in the breast. **Figure 1** illustrates the concept of neoadjuvant therapy with the sequence of systemic therapy and surgery.

Neoadjuvant systemic therapy is now commonly used to treat large and locally advanced breast cancers (*see* **Fig. 1A**). It offers patients with large operable or locally advanced breast cancer the possibility of downstaging primary tumors *(1)*. This can allow inoperable tumors to become operable and tumors to be excised by wide local excision when mastectomy would have been required before treatment *(1)*. Most studies have focused on the use of chemotherapy, but endocrine therapy is increasingly being used in this setting for hormone-sensitive tumors. The majority of neoadjuvant endocrine studies

From: *Methods in Molecular Medicine, Vol. 120: Breast Cancer Research Protocols*
Edited by: S. A. Brooks and A. L. Harris © Humana Press Inc., Totowa, NJ

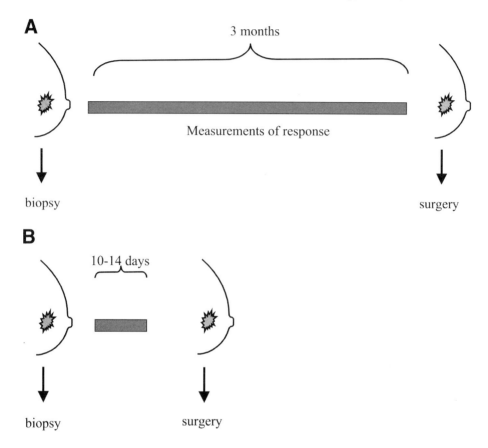

Fig. 1. The principle of two types of neoadjuvant therapy models. (**A**) neoadjuvant endocrine therapy is administered for 3–4 mo prior to surgery and sequential biopsies are taken during this period for pathological and/or biochemical analysis to monitor changes. Clinical response is also monitored by clinical examination and imaging. (**B**) alternatively, neoadjuvant therapy is administered for only 10–14 d between the time of diagnosis and surgical excision of the tumor. Tissue samples for pathological and biochemical analysis here are only taken at the time of diagnosis and again at surgery.

have involved tamoxifen *(2–5)*, but studies have also been performed with aminoglutethimide *(6)* and with the newer third-generation aromatase inhibitors letrozole, anastrozole, and exemestane *(7)*. Both tamoxifen and the aromatase inhibitors have been shown to be effective in the neoadjuvant setting *(6)*.

In vivo clinical studies offer the possibility of investigating the effects of neoadjuvant therapy at several time points in individual tumors. This allows early pathological changes to be correlated directly with clinical response and serial changes of factors, such as receptor status and proliferation, to be assessed at different stages of treatment. This allows a unique opportunity to relate changes in tumor biology to clinical response.

Studies have shown that 3 mo is the optimal time to give endocrine agents in the neoadjuvant setting in order to study tumor markers *(1,6,8–10)*. This is similar to the majority of neoadjuvant chemotherapy trials that have used three to four cycles.

1.2. Types of Study Models

There have been two main study models described to investigate the effects of endocrine agents on breast cancer in vivo.

The preoperative model involves giving patients preoperative endocrine therapy in the 14–21 d between diagnosis and surgery (*see* **Fig. 1B**). Tissue is taken at the time of diagnosis, and further tissue is obtained during definitive surgery from the same tumor. This allows for comparison of tumor tissue before and after exposure to endocrine therapy. A limitation of this model is that information on clinical response is not available to correlate with biological changes.

The other model system involves treating patients with neoadjuvant endocrine therapy for between 3 and 4 mo (*see* **Fig. 1A**). Tissue can be collected at several points during the study period. The clinical response is assessed by both clinical examination and imaging over the treatment period. This model has the advantage that clinical response can be correlated with pathological and biochemical changes in individual patients.

1.3. Future Directions

Neoadjuvant endocrine therapy models in vivo allow a unique opportunity to investigate the tumor response to treatment in a serial manner. In addition, it is possible to correlate pathological changes with clinical response to treatment.

The studies are relatively easy to set up and perform. It is important that tissue collection adheres to a strict protocol so that specimens can be analyzed accurately later. The scope for analysis of these samples is ever increasing.

2. Materials
2.1. Setting Up and Organizing In Vivo Studies

No specific materials are required for setting up and organizing in vivo studies, but the involvement of expert personnel to give advice on ethical considerations and study-appropriate statistics is necessary, as well as the involvement of a committed multidisciplinary clinical team.

2.2. Patient Selection

See **Subheading 2.1.**

2.3. Consent

See **Subheading 2.1.**

2.4. Methods of Assessing Tumor Response in Patients Having Neoadjuvant Therapy

Tumor response is measured in terms of change in size of the tumor, and this may be assessed by external measurement using calipers, mammography, and ultrasound or, if the tumor is excised, by pathological evaluation. For all of these approaches, trained specialist personnel and appropriate clinical facilities are required.

2.5. Collecting and Storing Blood and Urine Samples

Blood samples should be taken by appropriately trained personnel and standard equipment, including syringes, needles, and blood-receiving tubes are necessary. Urine samples may be collected by the patient themselves into appropriate screw-top containers. For storage, cryovials and −70 and −20°C freezer facilities are necessary.

2.6. Collecting and Storing Biopsy Samples

Surgical excision, core, or fine-needle biopsy samples should be taken in the clinic, using appropriate equipment and by specialist trained personnel. Standard materials for storing fresh biopsy material before analysis are given below.

1. 2-mL Round-bottomed cryogenic vials.
2. Cryogenic marker pen.
3. Liquid nitrogen.
4. RNA Later solution.
5. Distilled water.

2.7. Snap-Freezing Biopsies

1. 2.5 L of isopentane.
2. Dewar flask to contain liquid nitrogen (1 L capacity).
3. Cryomatrix.
4. Cork mounting disks.
5. Freezing pots.
6. 2 × 50-mL Pyrex™ beakers.
7. String (approx 45 cm).
8. Forceps with long, slender points.

9. Masking tape.
10. Scissors/scalpel.
11. Large spatula.
12. Cryogenic marker pen.

2.8. Formalin-Fixed Tissue Samples

Biopsy material will normally be fixed and processed to paraffin wax as part of routine in any hospital-based pathology department; thus, appropriate facilities and trained specialist personnel are necessary.

2.9. Analysis of Tissue Samples

Materials required for analysis of tissue samples depend on the analyses chosen, which are not given in detail in this chapter.

3. Methods

3.1. Setting Up and Organizing In Vivo Studies

A detailed protocol outlining the background and reason for the study, as well as its aims and objectives, should be prepared. Statistical advice on the number of patients who need to be treated to obtain clinically meaningful results is also required. The protocol together with a patient information sheet, consent form, and general practitioner information sheet should then be submitted to a local ethics committee to obtain permission to recruit patients for any trial or study (*see* **Note 1**).

Suitable patients for a study are best identified at the time of initial diagnosis. This also has the advantage that when core biopsies are taken for diagnosis, additional cores can be taken and stored for research purposes at the same time. This reduces the need to perform repeat core biopsies to obtain tissue specimens for research studies (*see* **Note 2**).

As an illustrative example, in the Edinburgh Breast Unit, a standard consent form is used at the time of taking the initial diagnostic core biopsy to allow extra samples to be taken and stored for research purposes (*see* **Appendix 1**). This consent form has been approved by the local ethics committee before being used. Core biopsy is performed in the outpatient clinic under local anesthesia and is well tolerated. These core biopsies can be routinely assessed for estrogen receptor (ER) status, as described in Chapter 12, which is used to select patients suitable for any neoadjuvant endocrine trials. Patients with a tumor that is ER-positive potentially benefit from endocrine therapy, but tumors with an ER category score of 6, 7, or 8 (within a range of 0–8) are most likely to respond. When a patient returns to the clinic to obtain results of the core biopsy and to make a definitive treatment plan, neoadjuvant protocols are discussed as part of that plan. It is important that all aspects of the patient's management, including any potential trial involvement, be discussed at a multidisciplinary meeting to ensure appropriate patients are selected, and that there is unanimous agreement that the patient is suitable for the proposed treatment. It is also important to record a copy of the multidisciplinary meeting decision in the patient's case notes.

3.2. Patient Selection

In terms of preoperative endocrine therapy, theoretically, any patient having surgery as primary treatment can be enrolled, regardless of clinical stage providing the tumor is ER-positive. In practice, this means that patients with distant metastatic disease are excluded, because surgery is not usually part of their primary treatment. Patients with severe renal or hepatic impairment are usually excluded, as are patients who may risk transmitting HIV or hepatitis B or C. Anyone unable to give informed consent is automatically excluded. Individual trials will have additional entry and exclusion criteria, for example, whether patients need to be pre- or postmenopausal. It is important to have these clearly established before the trial is ready to start recruiting (*see* **Note 3**).

The patient group considered eligible for the neoadjuvant study model is quite different. In general, patients must have an inoperable or advanced tumor or a large operable cancer to derive a potential benefit from tumor shrinkage, following successful primary endocrine therapy. In Edinburgh, patients enrolled into these studies are predominantly elderly patients with a tumor greater than 3 cm clinically (2 cm on imaging), which has been proven to be ER-positive on core biopsy. The majority of these patients go on to have surgery at the end of the treatment period, but some who are considered unfit or decline surgery may continue on primary endocrine therapy if their tumor shows evidence of clinical response. Younger patients who have large primary tumors are enrolled into neoadjuvant studies as they may derive benefit from having their proposed surgery downscaled from mastectomy pretreatment to breast conserving surgery following treatment (*see* **Note 4**).

3.3. Consent

It is imperative to obtain informed consent for any trial. Often, patients who are suitable for treatment with neoadjuvant endocrine therapy are elderly and may be confused or suffer from dementia. They may still be suitable for neoadjuvant therapy, but treatment without a clinical trial is necessary if they are unable to give informed consent.

In addition to the diagnostic biopsy consent form that allows patients to give permission for extra tissue to be taken for research purposes, patients need to sign separate consent forms for the particular trials being entered. Before doing this, they need to discuss all aspects of the trial with one of the study personnel. It is also important to give patients and their general practitioners written information about the trial. Contact details for trial personnel should be included at the end of the information sheets, so that further questions can easily be asked and any problems discussed.

3.4. Methods of Assessing Tumor Response in Patients Having Neoadjuvant Therapy

Trial patients have their tumor response assessed by multiple modalities; first, by clinical examination, using bidimentional caliper measurement. Size of the primary tumor may be determined by measuring two different diameters at 90° intervals using calipers. Tumor size is determined by multiplication of the longest diameter by the greatest perpendicular diameter (bidimentional measurements). Response can also be assessed on the basis of tumor volume changes, calculated with the formula for the volume of an ellipsoid *(11)* using the two different diameters measured at 90° intervals and the thickness of the primary breast lesion (tridimentional measurements).

This allows the tumor volume to be calculated using the formula *(31)*: $V = D^3 \times \pi$, where V is the volume, and D is the mean diameter.

Second, ultrasound scan performed in two different planes allows accurate volume assessment using the formula: $V = D^2 \times d \times \pi$, where V is the volume, D is the mean diameter, and d is the mean thickness.

Clinical examination and ultrasound scan are performed at diagnosis, half-way through the treatment period (6–8 wk) and at the end (3 or 4 mo).

Two-view mammography (oblique and craniocaudal views) is performed at the start and end of the study period. Bidimensional assessment and percentage change in volume is used to assess response to therapy. Finally, in those patients who go on to have surgery, pathological response is assessed. Ultrasound examination has been shown to correlate most closely with pathological size and response *(12)*.

Modified World Health Organization criteria are used to evaluate tumor response as follows:

1. Complete response: no measurable tumor.
2. Partial response: reduction in tumor size 50% or greater from pretreatment size.
3. Minor response: reduction in tumor size 25% or greater and less than 50% from pretreatment size.
4. No change: less than 25% decrease or less than 25% increase in tumor size from pretreatment size.
5. Progressive disease: 25% or more increase in tumor size from pretreatment size.

3.5. Collecting and Storing Blood and Urine Biological Samples

Blood samples, which might be taken as part of neoadjuvant studies to assess the side effects of endocrine agents, ideally should be taken in the morning when the patient is fasting. Blood samples that will be used for serum analysis of markers of bone and lipid metabolism and clotting factors need to be centrifuged at 5°C for 15 min and then stored in a freezer at –70°C (*see* **Note 5**). This allows delayed analysis of the whole group together at the end of the study when serial samples from the same patient can be processed as part of the same run.

Urine samples should be the second voided urine of the day and should ideally be taken after fasting as well. The markers of bone metabolism are robust, and the urine samples can simply be frozen at –20°C and analyzed at the end of the study. It is important when measuring other markers in either blood or serum to know exactly how samples should be taken and stored in order to facilitate accurate measurement of the desired markers.

3.6. Collecting and Storing Biopsy Samples

Collection and storage of frozen biopsies is the subject of Chapter 2 and is therefore not detailed here. Tissue may be obtained by fine-needle aspirate, core biopsy, or wedge biopsy. Fine-needle aspirate samples need to be frozen in a suitable storage medium, and do not give as much information as biopsies that show tissue architecture. The core-biopsy gun used in Edinburgh is a Bard Max Core Disposable Biopsy Instrument with a 14-gage needle. Ideally, four cores are taken for diagnostic purposes, and four are taken to be fresh frozen in liquid nitrogen for research use. The availability of mammotome biopsies allows large samples of tissue to be taken under ultrasound guidance. It is important that fresh samples be frozen in liquid nitrogen as quickly as possible (within a few minutes of being taken). In practice, this requires a container of liquid nitrogen to be available in the adjacent clinic to where the samples are taken.

In preoperative studies, repeat tissue samples are taken at the time of surgery, and both fresh-frozen and formalin-fixed tissue can be obtained. Chapters 1–3 detail appropriate methods and approaches. In order to be able to do this, either a pathologist should be available to take a piece of fresh tissue from the excision specimen, or a surgeon or trained technician can take core biopsies from the sample or excise part of the tumor as soon as possible after the specimen has been removed. The sample can then be fixed in formalin, and paraffin wax-embedded sections can be obtained after processing.

In the neoadjuvant studies, patients may have an optional repeat core biopsy performed a few days to weeks after starting endocrine therapy (currently, 10–14 d in the Edinburgh Breast Unit). Again, both fresh frozen and formalin-fixed tissue are taken from the tumor. A final tissue sample is taken at the time of surgery. If the patient is not fit enough for surgery at 3 mo, at this point another core biopsy can be taken to evaluate histological response.

Fresh-frozen samples are stored in 2-mL round-bottomed cryogenic vials, with identification details marked clearly with a suitable cryogenic pen. The details of the patient are coded to prevent identification and are clearly recorded together with the date the biopsy was performed and in which study the patient is enrolled. After being taken, they are immediately put into liquid nitrogen before being transferred to the tissue bank. If samples from wide local excision or mastectomy specimens cannot be stored immediately, they should be placed on ice while awaiting storage.

If the practicalities of tissue collection are such that fresh tissue samples cannot go straight into liquid nitrogen, it is possible to store specimens for short periods in RNA Later. Cores stored in RNA Later need to be less than 0.5 cm thick. They should be put in the standard cryogenic vial and fully immersed in 1.5 mL of RNA Later solution. The vials should be stored on ice if they cannot be frozen immediately, and can then be stored at 4°C overnight or at –20°C for up to 1 mo. Before transferring the samples into liquid nitrogen in the tissue bank, the RNA Later solution should be drained from the tubes and the samples washed in distilled water for 5 min before being put into liquid nitrogen. There are concerns that using RNA Later can destroy the tissue morphology, limiting the use of the fresh-frozen tissue in future. It is considered preferable to store the samples directly in liquid nitrogen wherever possible.

3.7. Snap-Freezing Biopsies

To improve tissue architecture when assessing morphology it is also possible to use isopentane to freeze the samples before storing them in liquid nitrogen. To do this the following protocol may be used:

1. Wear lab coat, gloves, and safety glasses at all times during procedure. All work should be done in a fume cupboard (although it does not need to be a class 2 cabinet).
2. Fill the Dewar flask with liquid nitrogen until it is almost full.
3. Prelabel all freezing pots and cork mounting disks using a cryogenic pen. Then, prechill the freezing pots (but not their lids) in the liquid nitrogen.
4. Tie string around each beaker with enough remaining to suspend it in the liquid nitrogen container.
5. Cut the cork mounting disks using scissors or a scalpel to make it easy for them to fit into the freezing pots.
6. Fill the two beakers with 30 mL isopentane. Dip both beakers into the liquid nitrogen and secure in place (*see* **Note 6**). Leave for at least 15 min to allow the isopentane to freeze (it becomes a white solid).
5. Remove one of the beakers from the liquid nitrogen and leave it to defrost for 30 s (on an insulated surface).
6. Deposit approx 5-mm diameter Cryomatrix™ (Shandon, Pittsburgh, PA) onto a cork-mounting disk. Position the sample into the Cryomatrix, laying it longitudinally and parallel to the cork-mounting disk.

7. Stab the corkboard with the fine-nose forceps and submerge both the sample and the corkboard into the partially defrosted isopentane for 30 s.
8. Using the large spatula, remove the freezing pot from the liquid nitrogen and immediately transfer the frozen tumor and cork mounting board into the freezing pot. Put the lid on the pot and store the sample in liquid nitrogen or dry ice for transportation to the tissue bank.

If there is still 1 cm of frozen isopentane in the bottom of the beaker, it can be used for the next sample. If not, it needs to be refrozen and the other beaker used for the next sample. After the procedure is finished, the isopentane can be left to evaporate off in a fume cupboard.

3.8. Formalin-Fixed Tissue Samples

Formalin-fixed tissue samples are placed directly into formalin as soon as possible in clinic or theater and then transported to the pathology department for processing and paraffin wax-embedding within 24 h.

3.9. Analysis of Tissue Samples

Formalin-fixed, paraffin wax-embedded tissue blocks can be used for a wide range of analyses. Serial blocks from the same patient can have immunohistochemical staining performed at the same time, during the same run to exclude experimental error. (Immunohistochemistry is the subject of Chapter 15.) In Edinburgh, the preliminary staining that has been performed on these neoadjuvant tissues samples includes ER, progesterone receptor, and markers of proliferation, such as Ki67, but a wide variety of end points may be assessed if antibodies are available that can detect antigenic determinants in fixed paraffin-embedded material. Immunohistochemistry for ER determination is the subject of Chapter 12, and its application for detection of other markers of interest in breast cancer include altered glycosylation (the subject of Chapter 16), angiogenesis (the subject of Chapter 14), and gene expression (the subject of Chapter 23).

However, fresh tissue is required if end points involve enzyme activity or the analysis of genetic material by reverse transcriptase-polymerase chain reaction or microarrays (the latter described in Chapters 27 and 28). It is wise to examine the morphology of core biopsies on frozen section before submitting material to analysis. In this way, it can be ensured that sufficient malignant tissue is present within the biopsy for analysis. This is where mammotome biopsies become useful, as more tissue is available for analysis. Frozen sections can be performed to ensure that there is adequate tumor in the cores before it undergo costly investigation. The tissue morphology is often slightly damaged by being stored in liquid nitrogen or especially RNA Later. In some samples, it is necessary to microdissect specimens (described in Chapter 8) to enrich the sample for malignant tissue.

4. Notes

1. The process of submitting forms to get ethical permission to perform studies can be very time-consuming. It is important to be aware of local procedures and to follow them closely. It may be necessary to obtain separate permission from the hospitals where patients will be recruited, as well as from an ethics committee. It is advisable to submit forms several months before recruiting patients—ideally, as soon as the protocol is written. If protocol changes are then made, an amendment can usually be granted by the committee much faster than granting permission for the original application.

2. Practically, this is best achieved by having a dedicated research team. The team can simply consist of a research fellow (e.g., surgical trainee who can perform core biopsies) and a research nurse. They are then able to screen patients and identify those who are potentially suitable to be enrolled in trials. They can then organize and perform the diagnostic core biopsy and arrange the immediate storage of fresh tissue in liquid nitrogen. By having dedicated staff, research is always being considered and the team can be well integrated into the work of the unit.

3. It is useful to display laminated colored-card copies of trial entrance criteria in clinical areas, so that staff are reminded of the trials that are currently running; thus, they can consider if their patients may be suitable.

4. It is important that all the clinicians in a unit are aware of which trials patients may be suitable for, so that they may be discussed. Often the doctor who has been involved in making the diagnosis will discuss potential options for treatment with the patient and introduce the possibility of taking part in a trial to them. This doctor can then go on to discuss it fully and recruit the patient, or they can pass the patient onto a dedicated member of research staff with whom the patient can discuss the trial more fully.

5. When the blood sample has been spun, the serum can be pipetted off into small cryogenic storage vessels. Red tops can be used for serum and yellow tops for urine to allow easier specimen identification later. It is important to label the tubes using a cryogenic pen in a manner that allows easy identification later but preserves anonymity.

6. When placing isopentane into liquid nitrogen, it is important to ensure that no isopentane gets into the liquid nitrogen and that no liquid nitrogen gets into the isopentane. To secure the beakers in the liquid nitrogen, tie the string around the Dewar flask handles, as well as taping it in place. It does not matter if the isopentane is in the liquid nitrogen for longer than 15 min before the procedure starts.

Appendix
Edinburgh Breast Unit
Surgical and Associated Services Division
Western General Hospital, Crewe Road, Edinburgh, EH4 2XU

Consultants:	Miss EDC Anderson, Mr U Chetty, Mr JM Dixon, Mr GT Neades, Mr RJ Salem
Unit Co-ordinator:	Mrs S Watchman
General Office:	0131 537 1611 Ward 6: 0131 537 1631 Fax No: 0131 537 1004

Patient Information

Studies on Breast Disease

You are about to have a core biopsy performed to determine the cause of your breast lump. Following injection of local anaesthetic, thin slivers of tissue obtained by a biopsy needle will be taken and sent to the pathology department to diagnose the cause of your breast lump.

The Edinburgh Breast Unit is involved in a number of research projects looking at the effect of drugs on breast lumps. We write to invite you to allow us to take extra slivers of tissue from your lump which might be used in future research should you receive any drug treatment.

If a definite diagnosis is not obtained from the specimens we send to the pathology department, then the stored samples will be made available to the pathology department to help diagnose the cause of your breast lump.

Page 1 of 2   Generic Consent Form120302

Edinburgh Breast Unit
Surgical and Associated Services Division
Western General Hospital, Crewe Road, Edinburgh, EH4 2XU

Consultants:	Miss EDC Anderson, Mr U Chetty, Mr JM Dixon, Mr GT Neades, Mr RJ Salem
Unit Co-ordinator:	Mrs S Watchman
General Office:	0131 537 1611 Ward 6: 0131 537 1631 Fax No: 0131 537 1004

Patient Information

Studies on Breast Disease

Please Initial Boxes

I have read the attached information sheet.

I agree to undergo the procedure of core biopsy. I understand that the purpose of the core biopsy is to determine the cause of my breast lump.

I agree to allow extra samples of my breast lump to be taken. I understand how the sample will be collected and that giving this sample is voluntary and that I am free to withdraw my approval for use of the sample at any time without giving a reason and without my medical treatment or legal rights being affected.

I understand that the research performed on the extra sample may include research to improve our understanding of how drugs influence breast disease.

I understand that if these extra samples are used for research, ethical approval will be obtained for the research project and that I will be asked to sign a separate consent form giving permission so these extra samples can be used.

I have read and understood the consent form.
I consent to having a core needle biopsy.

Signature of Patient ....

Name of Patient ....

Date ....

Consent Witnessed by ....

References

1. Anderson, T., Hawkins, R. A., et al. (1999) Neoadjuvant endocrine treatment: the Edinburgh experience, in *ESO Scientific Updates, Volume 4. Primary Medical Therapy for Breast Cancer* (Howell, A., Dowsett, M., eds.). Elsevier, Amsterdam, The Netherlands, pp. 1–11.
2. Mustacchi, G., Milani, S., Pluchinotta, A., et al. (1994)Tamoxifen or surgery plus tamoxifen as primary treatment for elderly patients with operable breast cancer. The GRETA trial. *Anticancer Res.* **14**, 2197–2200.
3. Gazet, J. C., Ford, H. T., Coombes, R. C., et al. (1994) Prospective randomized trial of tamoxifen vs surgery in elderly patients with breast cancer. *Eur. J. Surg. Oncol.* **20**, 207–214.

4. Van Dalsen, A. D. and De Vries, J. (1995) Treatment of breast cancer in elderly patients. *J. Surg. Oncol.* **60,** 80–82.

5. Bates, T., Riley, D. L., Houghton, J., et al. (1991) Breast cancer in elderly women: a Cancer Research Campaign trial comparing treatment with tamoxifen and optimal surgery with tamoxifen alone. *Br. J. Surg.* **78,** 591–594.

6. Anderson, E. D. C., Forrest, A. P. M., Levack, P. A. et al. (1989) Response to endocrine manipulation and oestrogen receptor concentration in large operable primary breast cancer. *Br. J. Cancer* **60,** 223–226.

7. Dixon, J. M. (2001) Neoadjuvant endocrine therapy, in *Aromatase Inhibition and Breast Cancer* (Miller, W. R., Santen, R. J., eds.) Marcel Dekker, Basel, Switzerland.

8. Keen, J. C., Dixon, J. M., Miller, E. P., et al. (1997) The expression of Ki-S1 and BCL-2 and the response to primary tamoxifen therapy in elderly patients with breast cancer. *Breast Cancer Res. Treat.* **44,** 123–133.

9. Dixon, J. M., Love, C. D. B., Tucker, S., et al. (1997) Letrozole as primary medical therapy for locally advanced and large operable breast cancer. *Breast Cancer Res. Treat.* **46(Suppl),** 54.

10. Kenny, F. S., Robertson, J. F. R., Ellis, I. O., et al. (1999) Primary tamoxifen versus mastectomy and adjuvant tamoxifen in fit elderly patients with operable breast cancer of high ER content. *Breast* **8,** 216.

11. Forouhi P., Walsh, J. S., Anderson, T. J., and Chetty, U. (1994) Ultrasound as a method of measuring breast tumour size and monitoring response to primary systemic therapy. *Br. J. Surgery* **81,** 223–225.

12. Dixon, J. M., Renshaw, L., Bellany, C., et al. (1999) Efficacy of anastrozole as neoadjuvant therapy in postmenopausal women with large operable breast cancers: reductions in tumor volume. *Breast* **8,** 215.

35

Primary Mouse Endothelial Cell Culture for Assays of Angiogenesis

Louise E. Reynolds and Kairbaan M. Hodivala-Dilke

Summary

The growth of new blood vessels, known as angiogenesis, is a dynamic but highly regulated process involving many different regulatory pathways. Endothelial cell migration and proliferation is also essential for this process to occur. Studying the behavior of endothelial cells and how they repond to the factors involved in angiogenesis is important in understanding how the process is controlled. The ability to generatic primary endothelial cells allows for such detailed studies. In this chapter, we present the method for endothelial cell isolation that we have found to be successful and that we routinely employ to isolate and culture primary endothelial cells.

Key Words: Angiogenesis; endothelial cells; macrophages; cell sorting; cell culture.

1. Introduction

Angiogenesis (neovascularization) is the formation of new blood vessels from preexisting vasculature and involves coordinated migration, proliferation, and differentiation of vascular endothelial cells, resulting in tubule formation *(1)*. It is important in both physiological conditions (including during embryonic development, ovulation, menstruation) and wound healing *(2)* and is also a hallmark of certain pathological conditions including tumor growth and ocular diseases, such as retinopathy of prematurity and age-related macular degeneration *(3)*. In both these pathological and physiological conditions, neovascularization is stimulated by the local production of proangiogenic factors, such as basic fibroblast growth factor and vascular endothelial growth factor. During tumor angiogenesis, newly formed microvessels supply oxygen and nutrients to developing tumors, without which they would not grow beyond a few cubic millimeters. Therefore, the study of endothelial cells and their response to angiogenic factors is an important aspect of several angiogenic

From: *Methods in Molecular Medicine, Vol. 120: Breast Cancer Research Protocols*
Edited by: S. A. Brooks and A. L. Harris © Humana Press Inc., Totowa, NJ

conditions. Quantitative assays of angiogenesis in breast cancer is the subject of Chapter 14.

Angiogenesis can be studied both in vivo in whole animals and in vitro using endothelial cells *(4)*. Each in vitro assay described below reflects a particular step involved in the development of endothelial cell into new vessels, and their response to angiogenic stimuli. During the earliest stages of angiogenesis, endothelial cells become activated by vascular endothelial growth factor and basic fibroblast growth factor, which in turn activates molecules (matrix metalloproteinases) that allow the endothelial cells to invade the surrounding matrix. After invasion, endothelial cells migrate and permeate the matrix. These two biological processes can be investigated in vitro using migration assays and proliferation assays, allowing the study of the effects of proangiogenic factors on endothelial cells. The final stage of angiogenesis involves endothelial cell differentiation to form new lumen-containing vessels. Analysis of the specific steps involved in capillary tube formation can be studied in a variety of in vitro endothelial cell assays. These assays include the tube formation assay, where endothelial cells are embedded in a substrate, such as collagen, fibrin, or Matrigel® that has been impregnated with angiogenic growth factors. The endothelial cells reorganize into capillary networks *(5)*, which can subsequently be used for analysis. An assay involves coating latex beads with endothelial cells, also embedded in Matrigel, which sprout and proliferate to produce microvessels.

This chapter describes the isolation of mouse lung endothelial cells. Briefly, mouse lungs are excised, collagenase-digested, and further disaggregated to produce a single cell suspension. Because the cells that are initially isolated are a mixed population of endothelial cells, macrophages, and fibroblasts, they are subjected to a series of negative and positive sorts that result in a greater than 90% pure population of endothelial cells. The endothelial cell monolayers produced by this method can be used for almost all cell and molecular biological techniques from immunohistochemistry (the subject of Chapter 15) to retroviral infection *(6)*.

2. Materials

Prepare all solutions under sterile conditions.

2.1. Flask-Coating Medium: Stock Solutions

1. 0.1% Gelatin: dissolve 0.4 g of gelatin in 400 mL of distilled H_2O and autoclave at 65°C for 30 min. Store at 4°C. This flask-coating medium is stable up to 2 mo.
2. Bovine plasma fibronectin (Sigma, UK): add 5 mL sterile phosphate-buffered saline (PBS) to 5 mg of fibronectin and allow the fibronectin to dissolve at room temperature for 5 min. Aliquot and store at –20°C. Before use, thaw an aliquot of fibronectin for 5 min at 37°C. Store at 4°C for up to 3 wk.

3. Concentrated stock (3 mg/mL) Vitrogen (Vitrogen Cohesion, Palo Alto, CA). Use directly from stock. Store at 4°C (*see* **Notes 1** and **2**).

2.2. Cell-Sorting Reagents

1. Rat antimouse FCγRII/III antibody (Pharmingen), UK: aliquot and store at 4°C.
2. Rat antimouse intercellular adhesion molecule (ICAM)-2 antibody (Pharmingen). Aliquot and store at 4°C.
3. Magnetic beads coated with sheep antirat antibody (Dynal Biotech, UK). Store at 4°C. Before use, resuspend thoroughly to create a single-bead suspension.

2.3. Collagenase Preparation

1. 0.1% Type I collagenase (Gibco®, Invitrogen, UK): dissolve 0.2 g of collagenase in 50 mL of PBS. Incubate at 37°C for 1 h. Add a further 50 mL of PBS, then filter sterilize using a 0.2-μm filter and store at 4°C for up to1 mo.

2.4. Mouse Lung Endothelial Cell Medium

Stock solutions:

1. Low-glucose Dulbecco's modified Eagle's medium ([DMEM], Biowhittaker, Walkersville, MD). Store at 4°C.
2. Hams F-12 medium. Store at 4°C.
3. Fetal calf serum. Thaw at room temperature and heat inactivate at 55°C for 30 min. Store at 4°C for up to 2 mo.
4. Heparin (Sigma). Store as purchased in powder form at 4°C.
5. Endothelial mitogen (Biogenesis, UK). Store as purchased in powder form at 4°C.
6. 100 U/mL Penicillin and 100 μg/mL of streptomycin. Store the stock at –20°C.
7. 2 mM Glutamine. Store the stock at –20°C.
8. To prepare 400 mL of mouse lung endothelial cell medium (MLEC) medium:
   a. Mix 200 mL of DMEM with 200 mL of Hams F-12 in a single sterile bottle.
   b. Dissolve 50 mg of heparin in 5 mL of Hams F-12 medium immediately before medium preparation and add to the DMEM/Hams F-12 medium.
   c. Add 5 mL of 100X penicillin/streptomycin stock and 10 mL of 200 mM of glutamine stock to the medium and filter sterilize using a 0.2-μm disposable filter (Nalgene, Rochester, NY).
   d. Finally, add 25 mg of endothelial mitogen and 100 mL of fetal calf serum (do not filter sterilize the two components). Store the medium at 4°C.

3. Methods

3.1. Preparation of Coated Flasks

1. Prepare fresh flask-coating medium by combining 100 μL of Vitrogen stock, 100 μL of fibronectin stock, and 10 mL of 0.1% gelatin. Apply 10 mL/75 cm^2 of tissue culture plastic.
2. Incubate flasks for 2 h to overnight at 37°C.
3. Aspirate medium from the flask before adding cell suspension (*see* **Note 2**).

3.2. Collagenase Treatment of Lungs

All procedures must be carried out under sterile conditions in a tissue culture hood.

1. Kill the mouse by cervical dislocation and spray down the fur using 70% ethanol. Transfer it into the tissue culture hood, spray again, and begin dissecting. Using a pair of forceps and scissors, make an anterior–posterior incision down the midline of the mouse, peel back the skin, and pin it down to reveal the ribcage. Using a fresh pair of forceps and scissors, cut open the chest cavity and dissect out the lungs (*see* **Notes 3–5**).
2. Place the lungs in a sterile 50-mL tube containing fresh Hams F-12, supplemented with penicillin/streptomycin and place on ice until beginning the cell isolation procedure (*see* **Note 6**).
3. To clean and dissect the lungs, prepare three 10-cm diameter Petri dishes. Into the first Petri dish, pour the lungs and Hams F12. In the second dish, pour 7 mL of 70% ethanol, and into the third, pour 7 mL of MLEC medium.
4. With the lungs floating in Hams-F12, use sterile forceps to remove any fat, blood clots, and connective tissue from the lungs.
5. Using forceps, gently transfer the lungs into 70% ethanol and wash briefly (no more than 10 s), followed by a longer wash in MLEC medium.
6. Place lungs on an inverted lid of a sterile 10-cm diameter Petri dish. Using sharp scissors, mince the lungs for 5 min to produce a pâté-like consistency (*see* **Note 7**).
7. With a sterile metal spatula, transfer the minced lungs to a sterile 50-mL tube containing 10 mL of collagenase and incubate in a water bath for 1 h at 37°C, swirling the tube occasionally (*see* **Note 8**).
8. Transfer the collagenase-digested lungs into the tissue culture hood and add 10 mL of MLEC medium to the solution.
9. Pour the solution into a Petri dish, and with a 20-mL syringe, extract the digested lungs. Place a 19.5-gage needle on the syringe and force the solution though the needle into the Petri dish. Repeat four times (*see* **Note 9**).
10. Pass the solution though a 70-μm cell strainer into a 50-mL tube containing 20 mL of MLEC medium and centrifuge for 5 min at 3000g.
11. Remove the supernatant, leaving approx 5 mL of liquid and the cell pellet in the bottom of the 50-mL tube (*see* **Note 10**).
12. Carefully resuspend the pellet in the remaining liquid by gentle pipetting.
13. Plate the cell suspension into a coated 75-cm^2 tissue culture flask containing 10 mL of MLEC medium.
14. Culture cells at 37°C, 10% CO_2, for 24 h.

3.3. Removal of Macrophages From a Mixed Cell Culture

The cell suspension will contain many cell types that need to be removed from the culture to produce a greater than 90%-pure population of endothelial cells. The most abundant contaminating cell type present at this stage of the culture process is the macrophage. These cells are removed by a "negative sort."

Preparation of antibody solution and beads for negative sort:

1. Prepare anti-FcγRII/III antibody: mix 3 mL of sterile PBS with 10 μL of antibody for each 75-cm² flask. Store at 4°C until required (approx 20 min).
2. Prepare a fresh suspension of magnetic Dynabeads (Dynal Biotech): mix 50 μL and resuspended beads with 3 mL of MLEC. Store at 4°C until required (approx 1 h).

3.4. Negative Sort

1. Remove MLEC medium from flasks and replace with 5 mL of fresh MLEC medium. Incubate at 4°C for 20 min (*see* **Note 11**).
2. Replace the MLEC medium with 3 mL of antibody solution, ensuring the solution coats the bottom of the flask and incubate for 30 min at 4°C. Swirl the solution around the flask occasionally to ensure even coating.
3. Remove antibody solution and wash the adhered cells gently once with PBS (*see* **Note 12**). Add 3 mL of bead solution and incubate for 30 min at 4°C. Swirl the solution around the flask occasionally to ensure even coating.
4. Remove the bead solution and wash the adhered cells gently three times with PBS. Using an inverted microscope, check that the beads have bound to the macrophages. The macrophages will appear as very small, round cells.
5. Trypsinize cells with 2.5 mL of 0.25% trypsin stock for approx 2 min or until all the cells have detached.
6. Add 9.5 mL of MLEC to the flask and resuspend cells by gentle resuspension, using a 10-mL pipet.
7. Place a 15-mL tube into a magnetic holder and pipet the cell suspension gently into it (*see* **Note 13**).
8. Allow the beads to attach to the side of the tube for 5 min. Because the beads are attached to the macrophages, and these are not wanted, pipet off the medium carefully and transfer it into a fresh precoated tissue culture flask (see **Note 13**).
9. Feed flasks every 2 d. Once colonies of approx 20 cells are apparent, a positive sort can be carried out (*see* **Note 14**).

3.5. Positive Sort for Endothelial Cells

This step separates endothelial cells from the remaining mixed cell population, using an antibody against an endothelial cell marker, ICAM-2.

1. Prepare an antibody solution using anti-ICAM-2 antibody: mix 3 mL of sterile PBS with 10 μL of anti-ICAM-2 antibody for each flask (approx 20 min).
2. Prepare a suspension of magnetic beads using Dynabeads: mix 50 μL of resuspended beads with 3 mL of MLEC (*see* **Note 15**). Store at 4°C until required (approx 1 h).
3. Remove medium from the flasks and replace with 5 mL of fresh MLEC medium. Incubate at 4°C for 20 min (see **Note 11**).
4. Replace MLEC medium with 3 mL of antibody solution, ensuring the solution coats the bottom of the flask and incubate for 30 min at 4°C. Swirl the solution around the flask occasionally to ensure even coating.

5. Remove antibody solution and wash the cells once with PBS (*see* **Note 12**). Add 3 mL of bead solution and incubate for 30 min at 4°C. Swirl the solution around the flask occasionally to ensure even coating.
6. Remove the bead solution and wash the adhered cells gently three times with PBS. Check that the beads are bound to endothelial cells. Endothelial cells have a cobblestone-like appearance.
7. Trypsinize cells with 2.5 mL of 0.25% stock trypsin until all the cells are detached from the flask.
8. Add 9.5 mL of MLEC to the flask and resuspend cells by gentle pipetting.
9. Place a 15-mL tube into a magnetic holder. Pipet the cell suspension gently into the tube.
10. Allow the beads to attach to the tube for 5 min. Pipet off the medium carefully and discard. Resuspend the beads in 10 mL of MLEC medium and transfer to fresh, precoated tissue culture flasks.
11. Feed flasks every 2 d. Once the cells are 50% confluent, repeat the positive sort to enhance the endothelial cell culture. This step is normally carried out approx 5 d after the initial positive sort.
12. Cells will reach confluency approx 7 d after final sort.

4. Notes

1. Vitrogen should be kept at 4°C at all times. Do not freeze the stock solution and do not allow it to warm while preparing the flask-coating medium.
2. Vitrogen solution is very acidic, and it is important to aspirate the dish after the coating incubation, because any residual acidity may kill the cells.
3. When sacrificing mice for endothelial preparation, they must *not* be sacrificed by CO_2 inhalation, but by cervical dislocation. CO_2 inhalation will damage the endothelial cells in the lungs and compromise the endothelial cell culture.
4. Lungs from three mice are required for each endothelial cell preparation for 75-cm^2 tissue culture flasks. Only two lungs are needed for 25-cm^2 flasks. Use a clean set of instruments for each different genotype of mouse.
5. When dissecting the lungs from the mouse, use separate pairs of instruments for cutting the skin and the lungs. This prevents contamination from bacteria on the skin entering the body cavity.
6. It is possible to store the lungs for up to 6 h on ice before beginning the cell-isolation procedure. Longer storage may result in a lower yield and reduced viability of cells.
7. Cut the lungs into the smallest pieces as possible, as this will increase the final cell yield.
8. When collagenase digesting the lungs, incubate for exactly 1 h, because longer or shorter incubations will compromise the final cell yield.
9. Do not oversyringe the digested lungs. Oversyringing can cause whitish strands of DNA to precipitate out of the cells. This is potentially toxic to the other cells and will compromise the culture.

10. At this stage, avoid creating bubbles in the tube, as these can dislodge beads that are attached to the magnet.
11. If there are too few endothelial cells in a colony, then a poor endothelial cell culture will be achieved at a later stage of the preparation.
12. Do not pipet the PBS directly onto the cells, as they will detach from the flask. Pipet the PBS onto the opposite surface, and gently swirl the PBS over the cell layer.
13. Depending on the cell density, the volume of magnetic beads can be reduced or increased (to a max. of 50 µL per 3 mL of MLEC medium).
14. After centrifugation, the pellet at the bottom of the tube is extremely fragile and is easily dislodged. Therefore, gently remove the supernatant using a 25-mL glass pipet.
15. Prechilling reduces phagocytosis of the magnetic beads.

References

1. Folkman, J. and Shing, Y. (1992) Angiogenesis. *J. Biol. Chem.* **267,** 10,931–10,934.
2. Folkman, J. (1974) Tumor angiogenesis. *Adv. Cancer Res.* **19,** 331–358.
3. Cockerill, G. W., Gamble, J. R., and Vadas, M. A. (1995) Angiogenesis: models and modulators. *Int. Rev. Cytol.* **159,** 113–160.
4. Bischoff, J. (1995) Approaches to studying cell adhesion molecules in angiogenesis. *Trends Cell Biol.* **5,** 69–74.
5. Bach, T. L., Barsigian, C., Chalupowicz, D. G., et al. (1998) VE-Cadherin mediates endothelial cell capillary tube formation in fibrin and collagen gels. *Exp. Cell Res.* **238,** 324–334.
6. Reynolds, L. E., Wyder, L., Lively, J., et al. (2002) Enhanced pathological angiogenesis in β3 and β3/β5 double knockout mice. *Nat. Med.* **8,** 27–34.

Index

A

Affinity purification, 445
Agarose gel electrophoresis, 149, 398
Albumin, removal from samples, 223
Aneuploidy determination, 299
Angiogenesis, 30, 161–187, 390, 498
  in vitro assay, 503–509
  quantitation using immunohistochemistry, 161–187
Animal models
  athymic mouse xenograft, 30, 453–464
  knockout mouse, 465–477
  nude mouse, 480
  SCID mouse xenograft, 479–488
Annexin-VI, 370
Antibodies, phospho-specific, *see* phospho-specific antibodies
Antigen retrieval, 130, 131, 192, 198, 299, 300
Apoptosis, 29, 35, 36, 37, 147–160, 390, 455
  DNA ladder assay, 154, 155
  ELISA for histone/DNA fragment, 155, 156
  PARP assay, 156, 157
  TUNEL assay, 158
Archive, clinical, 3–24
Aromatase inhibitors, 364
Arrays, *see* microarrays
Athymic mouse, 454
Autoradiography, 337
Automatic tissue processors, 12, 131, 136, 137

Avidin–biotin immunohistochemical method, 193, 204, 205, 210, 211
Axillary lymph node dissection, 91–94

B

Basic fibroblast growth factor, 503, 504
Bax, 37, 148
Bcl-2, 37, 148
Biomarkers, treatment-induced changes, 29
Biopsies, serial, *see* BRCA1 assessment, serial biopsies
Biopsy sample storage, 496, 497
Blood sample storage, 495, 496
BRCA1 assessment, 441–452
  antibody preparation, 447, 448
  immunohistochemistry, 450
  polyacrylamide gel electrophoresis and Western blotting, 448–450
  sample preparation, 448

C

Carcinoma *in situ*, 87, 88, 96, 170, 172
Caspases, 147, 148
Cathepsin D, 366, 371, 372, 374, 375, 379
Cationic amino acid transporter E16, 374
CD9, 370
CD31, 165; *see also* angiogenesis quantitation
CD34, 161–187; *see also* angiogenesis quantitation
CD59, 370

CD63, 370
Cell culture models of drug resistance,
    453–464
c-erb-2, see HER-2
Chalkley counting, 169
c-jun, 454
c-myc, 270, 297–307
Colony hybridization, 366
Comparative genomic hybridization
    (CGH), 269–295
Confocal microscopy, 38, 299
Coomassie brilliant blue stain,
    225–226, 239
Cryostat sectioning, *see* frozen
    (cryostat) sectioning
Cyclin D1, 30, 374–376
Cytochrome p450-II b, 374, 377
Cytokeratins, 95, 172

D

DEME-2, -12, -31, -40, and -47, 366
Desmoplakin, 370
DET-2, 372
Differential display, 369, 370, 375
Differential hybridization, 367, 375
DNA
    template, 324
    plasmid, 324, 326
    extraction, 61–63, 72, 272, 273
    ladder assay, 154, 155
Downstaging, 31, 489, 490

E

E$_2$-induced genes, 371
EIT-6, 372
Electrophoresis, *see* agarose gel
        electrophoresis,
        polyacrylamide gel
        electrophoresis, and
        two-dimensional gel
        electrophoresis
ELF-1 BS69, 378

ELISA, *see* enzyme-linked
    immunosorbant assay
Endocrine responsiveness models,
    453–464
Endocrine therapy, 133–135,
    363, 364; *see also*
    neoadjuvant endocrine
    therapy trials
Endothelial cell isolation and culture,
    503–509
Endothelial cell markers, 172
Enzyme-linked immunosorbant assay
    (ELISA), 149, 155, 156, 191,
    245–265
Epidermal growth factor, 454
Epidermal growth factor receptor, 37
ER-ICA, *see* estrogen receptor
    immunohistochemistry
Estrogen receptor, 36, 37, 39, 85, 86,
    127–146, 363, 365, 374–376,
    453, 498
    immunohistochemistry 127–146
Ethical issues in tissue banking,
    19–21
Expression profiling using cDNA
    microarrays, 403–414,
    415–424
    amplification of mRNA,
        407, 408
    cDNA labeling, 408, 409,
        419, 420
    hybridization and posthybridization
        washing, 409, 410, 420
    production of filter cDNA arrays,
        418–419
    RNA extraction, 405–407
    scanning and analysis, 410–412,
        421, 422

F

Fatty acid synthetase, 366
Filter cDNA microarrays, *see*
        expression profiling using
        cDNA microarrays

Fine-needle aspirates/biopsies, 29–41
Flavin-containing mono-oxygenase-5, 370
Fluorescence *in situ* hybridization (FISH), 45, 297–307, 269–295, 309–322; *see also* comparative genomic hybridization
deparaffinization, 303
DNA extraction, 282–285
FISH hybridization, 305, 314
posthybridization wash, 289, 305, 314, 315
probe preparation, 285–287, 305
quantification, scoring, and analysis, 290, 291, 305, 306, 315
slide pretreatment, 304, 312–314
slide/sample preparation, 279–281, 303
FOXA1, *see* hepatocyte nuclear factor 3α
Freezing protocol for biopsies, 497, 498
Frozen (cryostat) sectioning, 14, 15, 70, 118
Frozen tissue sample collection and storage, 3–24, 25–28

G

Gap junction protein, 374
GATA-3, 374, 376–378, 381
Gene amplification, detection, 297–307, 309–322
Gene copy number determination, 68
Gene regulated by estrogen in breast cancer *GREB1* and *GREB2*, 368
Glycosylation, 201–216, 498
G protein-coupled receptor GPR30, 370

H

hDlg5, 370
Heat shock proteins
1-β, 371
E2IG1, 371
Hsp27, 365, 366, 374–376, 378, 379
Helix pomatia agglutinin (HPA), 202, 203, 481–482
Hematoxylin and eosin stain, 5, 9, 12, 13, 45, 105, 115, 119, 120, 304
Hepatocyte nuclear factor 3α, 376–378, 381
HER-2, 37,39, 300, 270, 309–322
Herceptin, 310
High-mobility group 1 protein, 371
Hormone-regulated genes, *see* steroid hormone-regulated genes
Hormone resistance models, 453–464
Hypoxia inducible factors (HIFs), 166

I

Icere-1, 370
Image analysis, 136, 175, 176, 232, 274
Immunohistochemistry
before microdissection, 66, 71
for BRCA1 analysis, 450
for CD34/angiogenesis, 165, 167, 168
for cytokeratins, 95, 105, 115, 120, 121
for estrogen and progesterone receptor, 374, 127–146
for lectin binding/glycosylation, 201–216
or micrometastasis detection, 83, 84
for *TP53* determination, 390
general methodology, 191–200

in adjuvant therapy trials,
498–499
on serial biopsies, 36
on tissue microarrays, 44
section preparation for, 15–16
with *in situ* hybridization,
323–346
In situ hybridization, *see also*
fluorescence *in situ*
hybridization (FISH), 271,
297–307, 309–322, 323–346
Insulin-like growth factor, 365, 376
Insulin-like growth factor binding
protein, 4, 374, 375, 376
Integrins, 165, 427
Interphase nuclei, 272, 298
Isoelectric focusing, 235–237
Isotopic *in situ* hybridization, *see*
in situ hybridization

K

Ki67, 29, 30, 35, 36, 498
Knockout mouse model, 465–477

L

Ladder, *see* DNA ladder assay
Laser-assisted microdissection, *see*
microdissection
Lectins, 201–216
LIV1, 374, 375, 376, 377, 378, 380
Lymphatic invasion, 84

M

6-Maleimedo-caprolyl
N-hydroxysuccinamide
(MCS) coupling, 443
Mass spectrometry, 232, 240
Matrix metalloproteinases (MMPs),
504
Metaphase chromosomes, 272, 298
Metastasis, 479–480
Microarrays, *see also* expression
profiling using cDNA
microarrays

cDNA, 36, 38, 366, 372–378, 375,
403–414, 415–424
comparative genomic hybridization,
271
gene, 347 370–372
mRNA, 372–374, 375
tissue, 38, 43–50, 270–271, 324
Microdissection, 16–17, 65–75
Micrometastases, 83–84
Migration assay, 504
Mitogen activated protein (MAP)
kinase family, 429
Mouse mammary tumor virus, 480
MUC1, 378
Multicolor FISH, 270
MYB, 378

N

Na$^+$/H$^+$ exchanger regulatory factor, 369
Na$^+$/K$^+$ ATPase α-1, 370
Necrosis, 85
Neoadjuvant endocrine therapy trials,
489–502
analysis of samples, 498–499
collection and storage of samples,
495–498
consent, 494–495
methods of assessing response, 495
organization, 493–494
patient selection, 494
role of serial biopsies, 31
Neu, *see HER–2*
Neuropeptide Y and Y1, 368
N-myc, 300
Northern blotting, 347, 368
Nude mouse, 480

P

p53, *see TP53*
p27^{kip1}, 30
Paraffin wax-embedded samples
fluorescence *in situ* hybridization,
297–307
immunohistochemistry, 35–36,
191–200, 498–499

in situ hybridization, 35–36
in situ hybridization with
    immunohistochemistry,
    323–346
    preparation and storage, 3–24,
      129–130, 197, 209, 498
    sectioning, 14–16, 119, 120
PARP, *see* poly-ADP-ribose
    polymerase
PBX1, 378
PCR, *see* reverse transcriptase
    polymerase chain reaction
PDZK1, 368, 374, 375
Pescodillo 1, 371
6-Phosphofructo-2-kinase/fructose-2,
    6 biphosphatase, 370
Phospho-specific antibodies, 441–452
Plasmid DNA, 324
Polymerase chain reaction (PCR), 5,
    299, 367, 369
    cDNA microarrays, 416
    TP53 determination, 395–398
Ponceau red S stain, 226–227
Polyacrylamide gel electrophoresis
    for analysis of uPA system, 337
    for BRCA1 DNA damage,
      442–443, 448–450
    for differential display, 369
    for identification of steroid
      hormone regulated genes,
      365–366, 375
    for ribonuclease protection assay,
      347–362
    general methodology, 217–229
    in two dimensional gel
      electrophoresis (proteomics),
      237–238
Poly-ADP-ribose polymerase (PARP),
    148–150, 156–157
Probes, gene, 298–299
Progesterone receptor, 36, 37, 39,
    85–86, 127, 365, 374,

375, 376, 453, 498
Prognostic markers, 79–89
    angiogenesis, 163, 165, 175
    estrogen receptor, 127–146
    grade, 84
    Helix pomatia agglutinin (HPA)
      binding, 202–203, 481–482
    Her2/neu, 301
    histological types, 85
    historical and traditional, 79–80
    Hsp 27, 378–379
    nodal status, 83–84, 91–111
    ras-related and estrogen-regulated
      growth inhibitor (RERG), 380
    stage, 80–82, 92
    steroid hormone-regulated genes, 363
    urokinase-type plasminogen
      activator (uPA) system, 166,
      246, 261, 428
Proliferating cell nuclear antigen
    (PCNA), 442
Proliferation assay, 504
Proliferation markers, *see also* Ki67,
    29, 30, 36–37, 498
Protein quantification, 235
Protein precipitation using chloroform/
    methanol, 223–224
Proteomics, 38, 231–243, 366

R

Radionucleotide-labeled probes for
    in situ hybridization, 298,
    323–346
ras-related and estrogen-regulated
    growth inhibitor (RERG),
    374, 380–381
Reverse transcriptase polymerase
    chain reaction (PCR), 14,
    38, 68, 347, 498
Ribonuclease protection assay,
    347–362
Riboprobes, 310, 324–325
RNA
    extraction, 51–53, 55–59, 72

quantitation by ribonuclease
protection assay, 347–362

S

SAGE, *see* serial analysis of gene
expression
SCID mouse, *see* severe combined
immunodeficient (SCID)
mouse xenograft model
SDS-PAGE, *see* polyacrylamide gel
electrophoresis
Sentinel lymph node, 83–84, 91–111,
113–125
operative technique, 96–104
evaluation, 95–96, 113–115,
118–121
accuracy of assessment, 96–104
surgeon experience, 105–106
clinical implications, 106–107
Serial analysis of gene expression
(SAGE), 370–372, 374, 375,
380
Serial biopsies, 29–41
Severe combined immunodeficient
(SCID) mouse xenograft
model, 479–488
Silane treatment of slides, 196–197,
208
Silver nitrate stain, 239–240
Snap freezing, *see* freezing protocol
for biopsies
Spectral karyotyping (SKY), 270
Staging, *see* TNM staging system
Stanniocalcin 2, 371, 374–378, 380
Stem cells, 465–477
Steroid hormone-regulated genes,
363–388
Subtraction hybridization, 366–369,
375
Surgical margins, 86–87

T

Tamoxifen, 29, 37, 346, 454
Terminal deoxynucleotidyl
transferase-mediated
dUTP-biotin nick-end
labeling, *see* TUNEL
Thrombospondin, 368
Tissue banking, 3–24, 26–28
Tissue microarrays, 324
TIT-5, 372
TNM staging system, 80–82, 96
Touch print preparations
fluorescence *in situ* hybridization,
297–307
sentinel lymph node preparations,
118
Transcription activator protein-1,
454
Transforming growth factor-1, 368
Trefoil factor family (TFF), 366, 368,
371, 374–380
Trials, *see* neoadjuvant endocrine
therapy trials
3-(Triethoxysilyl)propylamine
treatment of slides, *see* silane
treatment of slides
Tube formation assay for angiogenesis,
504
Two-dimensional gel electrophoresis,
see proteomics
TUNEL, 35, 37, 147–160

U

UDP-glucose dehydrogenase, 370
uPA, *see* urokinase-plasminogen
activator (uPA) system
Urine sample storage, 495–496
Urokinase-plasminogen activator (uPA)
system, 166, 427–440

V

Vascular endothelial cell growth
    factor, 164, 166, 503, 504
Vectabond treatment of slides, *see*
    silane treatment of slides

W

Western blotting
    apoptosis analysis, 150,
    BRCA1 analysis, 442, 443, 445,
        448–450

general methodology, 217–229
uPA system analysis, 437–438
Wnt-1 inducible signaling pathway
    protein 2 (WISP2), 371

X

X-box binding protein-1 (XPB-1),
    376–378, 382
Xenografts in athymic mouse model,
    30, 453–464